Counseling Skills for Speech-Language Pathologists and Audiologists

SECOND EDITION

Lydia V. Flasher, Ph.D.
Director, Psychology Training Programs
Licensed Psychologist
Children's Health Council
Palo Alto, California

Paul T. Fogle, Ph.D., CCC-SLP
Private Practice
Sacramento/Elk Grove, California

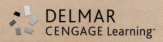

DELMAR
CENGAGE Learning™

Australia • Brazil • Japan • Korea • Mexico • Singapore • Spain • United Kingdom • United States

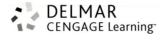

DELMAR
CENGAGE Learning·

Counseling Skills for Speech-Language Pathologists and Audiologists, Second Edition
Lydia V. Flasher, Ph.D. and Paul T. Fogle, Ph.D., CCC-SLP

Vice President, Editorial: Dave Garza

Director of Learning Solutions: Matthew Kane

Senior Acquisitions Editor: Sherry Dickinson

Associate Acquisitions Editor: Tom Stover

Managing Editor: Marah Bellegarde

Product Manager: Laura J. Wood

Editorial Assistant: Anthony Souza

Vice President, Marketing: Jennifer Ann Baker

Marketing Director: Wendy E. Mapstone

Associate Marketing Manager: Jonathan Sheehan

Production Manager: Andrew Crouth

Senior Art Director: David Arsenault

Content Project Management: PreMediaGlobal

Cover Image: Open door © Elsar/ Shutterstock. Used with permission.

Library of Congress Control Number: 2011923633

ISBN-13: 978-1-4354-9936-2

ISBN-10: 1-4354-9936-0

Delmar
5 Maxwell Drive
Clifton Park, NY 12065-2919
USA

Cengage Learning is a leading provider of customized learning solutions with office locations around the globe, including Singapore, the United Kingdom, Australia, Mexico, Brazil, and Japan. Locate your local office at: **international.cengage.com/region**

Cengage Learning products are represented in Canada by Nelson Education, Ltd.

To learn more about Delmar, visit **www.cengage.com/delmar**

Purchase any of our products at your local college store or at our preferred online store **www.cengagebrain.com**.

Printed in the United States of America
2 3 4 5 6 7 17 16 15 14 13

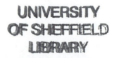

DEDICATION

*This book is dedicated to
my mentor Dr. Hans H. Strupp
and my husband Dr. Dawson S. Schultz.*

L. V. F.

*This book is dedicated to
the students and professionals who will be using
what they learn to help their clients, patients,
and families. I also wish to dedicate this book to
my lifelong friend Ed Little, to my wife,
V. Carol Fogle, R. N., and to my daughters,
Heather B. Morrison and Heather Lea Fogle.*

P. T. F.

TABLE OF CONTENTS

PART I   FOUNDATIONS OF COUNSELING SKILLS

Chapter 1   THE BASICS

Chapter 2   THEORIES OF COUNSELING: APPLICATION TO SPEECH-LANGUAGE PATHOLOGY AND AUDIOLOGY

Chapter 3 THE THERAPEUTIC RELATIONSHIP AND THERAPEUTIC COMMUNICATION

Chapter 4 INTERVIEWING AND THERAPY MICROSKILLS

Chapter 5   COUNSELING IN A MULTICULTURAL SOCIETY: IMPLICATIONS
FOR THE FIELD OF COMMUNICATION DISORDERS

Marlene B. Salas-Provance, Ph.D., F-CCC-SLP
Associate Professor, New Mexico State University
Las Cruces, NM

Chapter 6   WORKING WITH FAMILIES

PART II   **COUNSELING SKILLS FOR WORKING
WITH SPECIFIC DISORDERS**

Chapter 7   COUNSELING SKILLS FOR WORKING WITH SPEECH, LANGUAGE, FLUENCY,
VOICE, AND CLEFT LIP AND PALATE DISORDERS

Chapter 8 COUNSELING SKILLS FOR ADULT NEUROLOGICAL DISORDERS AND DYSPHAGIA

Chapter 9 COUNSELING FOR ADULTS AND CHILDREN WHO HAVE HEARING LOSS

Nancy Tye Murray, Ph.D., CCC-A
Professor, Washington University School of Medicine
Department of Otolaryngology
St. Louis, MO

PART III THE THERAPEUTIC PROCESS WITH CHALLENGING SITUATIONS AND BEHAVIORS

Chapter 10 DEFENSE MECHANISMS RELEVANT TO SPEECH-LANGUAGE PATHOLOGISTS AND AUDIOLOGISTS

PREFACE

We are pleased to have the opportunity to update, expand, and improve upon *Counseling Skills for Speech-Language Pathologists and Audiologists*. This expanded edition includes five new chapters: Counseling in a Multicultural Society, Working with Families, two new chapters on Counseling with Specific Disorders, and a chapter on Counseling with Adults and Children Who Have Hearing Loss. The primary goal of this text is to provide students as well as beginning and experienced clinicians with the best and most thorough information on counseling skills that will help them better serve their clients, patients, and family members. While some counseling skills may be intuitive for many clinicians, all clinicians can benefit from enhanced training in the foundations of counseling skills as well as learning more advanced skills, particularly for working with challenging emotions and situations that sometimes vex clinicians.

This text combines the knowledge and nearly six decades of experience of both a speech-language pathologist and a clinical psychologist. Because it is the only text on counseling in the fields of speech-language pathology and audiology that has a clinical psychologist as a co-author, this text can cover important topics in both the breadth and depth that are needed by our professions. Dr. Flasher's extensive knowledge of the psychology literature (including clinical psychology, counseling psychology, and family therapy) and her many years of clinical work with children, adults, and families provide additional understanding of clients and their families, insights into the many subtle and challenging situations in which speech-language pathologists and audiologists may find themselves, and therapeutic techniques to better manage these situations. Finally, her current work in a multidisciplinary clinic for children, adolescents, and families underscores the way in which non–mental health professionals frequently need to draw upon psychological and counseling skills in order to enhance their practice.

One focus of this text is on building counseling skills by placing the theories and techniques into real-life contexts. Speech-language pathologists (SLPs) and audiologists (Auds) working in various school settings, medical and rehabilitation centers, clinics, home health agencies, and private practices have suggested many of the counseling situations and sensitive issues that are described and addressed in this text. Similarly, numerous examples of counseling issues and situations are provided that come directly from the clinical work of the speech-language pathologist (Paul Fogle), with additional case examples provided from the perspective of the clinical psychologist who currently works in a multidisciplinary clinic and frequently collaborates with SLPs (Lydia Flasher).

With the goal of providing relevant and usable skills to individuals in the sciences of communication and hearing disorders, the authors present therapy skills, techniques, and strategies in user-friendly language without the burden of unnecessary psychological terminology. At the same time, the text shows how clinicians can gain a better understanding of client, patient, and family attitudes, emotions, and behaviors by employing concepts from a variety of psychological and theoretical perspectives. SLPs and Auds, like other educational and health care professionals, need to be aware and have the knowledge and skills to understand and appropriately and professionally manage challenging emotions, behaviors, and situations. All of the situations discussed in this text have been experienced by many clinicians, particularly those working in medical settings. Additionally, individuals developing and refining their counseling skills can reflect on their own clinical experiences and how they might manage challenging emotions, attitudes, situations, and behaviors in a more therapeutic manner using the techniques presented in this text.

Although substantial new material is presented in this text, the authors have been selective in what they have chosen to include. Other topics and literature that SLPs and Auds may find useful are provided in the extensive reference list at the end of this text.

ORGANIZATION AND FEATURES OF THE SECOND EDITION

Part I of the text is designed to help students and professionals understand the foundations of counseling skills and includes Chapter 1, The Basics, and Chapter 2, Theories of Counseling: Application to Speech-Language Pathology and Audiology. Other chapters discuss aspects of the therapeutic relationship and therapeutic communication (Chapter 3) and the specifics of interviewing and therapy microskills (Chapter 4) during interactions with clients and their families. There is a new chapter (Chapter 5) on multicultural competencies, written by Marlene B. Salas-Provance, Ph.D., F-CCC-SLP, an internationally recognized expert in this important area of our professions. We also include a new chapter on working with families (Chapter 6), which focuses on the rationale and skills for understanding the client's family system and working with family members.

Part II, Counseling Skills for Working with Specific Disorders, illuminates the psychological, emotional, and social effects of communication disorders on children and adults, as well as how these disorders affect family members. Chapter 7 focuses on counseling skills for working with speech, language, fluency, voice, and cleft lip and palate disorders in children and adults, and Chapter 8 focuses on counseling skills for working with adult neurological disorders and dysphagia. Chapter 9 is a new chapter on counseling for adults and children who have hearing loss, written by Nancy Tye-Murray, Ph.D., CCC-A, an internationally recognized expert in the area of aural rehabilitation.

Part III, The Therapeutic Process with Challenging Situations and Behaviors, goes beyond providing essential information about counseling skills for speech-language pathologists and audiologists and emphasizes the challenging situations and behaviors that our clients and their families sometimes present, such as resistance and defenses, catastrophic reactions, crises, and threat of suicide or self-harm. Individual chapters present information on defense mechanisms relevant to speech-language pathologists and audiologists (Chapter 10), working with challenging and difficult emotions (Chapter 11), communicating bad news and working with challenging situations (Chapter 12), working with resistance and anger (Chapter 13), and working with crisis situations (Chapter 14). In Chapter 14, new information is presented on working with active duty military and combat veterans that is not available in any other text in our professions. The material is written by Paul Fogle, who is a veteran of war (combat medic, Vietnam, 1969). The final chapter of this text provides updated information on clinician strategies for self-care and prevention of burnout: Taking Care of Ourselves (Chapter 15).

Each chapter begins with a *Chapter Outline* listing major headings and an *Introduction* that places the material in context, and ends with *Concluding Comments* that recap and synthesize the information presented. A variety of special features bring counseling skills to life. Numerous *Personal Experience* boxes give readers access to Dr. Fogle's four decades of experience providing therapy and counseling individuals with communication disorders. These personal experiences offer glimpses into what it can be like working with a wide range of clients and patients with a variety of disorders in various work settings and the sometimes challenging situations they present. The *Case Study* feature provides real-life therapy and counseling situations but does not present the authors' approach to the situation. Each case study asks the student to try to determine reasonable approaches to manage the challenging situation. Additionally, *Counseling Skills in Action* boxes demonstrate issues, experiences, and techniques that provide a broader foundation for the application of counseling skills. (Note: All of the Personal Experience, Case Study, and Counseling Skills in Action features are provided by Dr. Paul Fogle unless it is specifically indicated that they are provided by Dr. Lydia Flasher.) *Key terms* appear in boldface on their first occurrence in the text. A corresponding *Glossary* at the end of the text includes all boldface key terms for quick identification and understanding. Each chapter concludes with thought-provoking *Discussion Questions* that are intended to spark introspection and debate about the topics presented. These questions encourage the sharing of experiences, application of theories and therapy techniques to specific scenarios, and critical thought about how clinicians might become more effective therapists and rehabilitation counselors.

An important addition to this second edition is the *Role Play* section at the end of each chapter (except for Chapter 1) that instructors and students can use to practice scenarios in class in order to increase skills that are discussed throughout the text. Instructors can use these exercises to expand discussions regarding the application of skills discussed in each chapter. In this section, it can be assumed that "client" always refers to a student who is role playing a client, rather than a real client. The skills may be practiced in dyads or in small groups to enhance counseling skills that may later be used with actual clients and their family members. An *Appendix* provides numerous Internet resources that provide general and specific websites that are applicable to this text and are intended to be helpful to clinicians, clients, and families. The *References* section has been substantially expanded and enhanced and now includes over 750 references, providing readers with a wealth of resources for further reading and research. The *Index* is detailed for easy location of specific topics and concepts. All of the carefully thought-out organization and features of *Counseling Skills for Speech-Language Pathologists and Audiologists* are designed to enhance the learning and enjoyment of the material presented in this second edition.

HIGHLIGHTS OF WHAT'S NEW TO THE SECOND EDITION

- A new chapter (Chapter 5), Counseling in a Multicultural Society: Implications for the Field of Communication Disorders, written by Marlene B. Salas-Provance, Ph.D., F-CCC-SLP, a well-known expert in this area of study.

- A new chapter, Working with Families (Chapter 6), focuses on the rationale and skills for understanding the client's family system and working with family members.

- Two new chapters focus on counseling clients and patients with specific disorders: Counseling Skills for Working with Speech, Language, Fluency, Voice, and Cleft Lip and Palate Disorders (Chapter 7) and Counseling Skills for Adult Neurological Disorders and Dysphagia (Chapter 8).

- A new chapter, Counseling for Adults and Children Who Have Hearing Loss (Chapter 9), written by Nancy Tye-Murray, Ph.D., CCC-A, an expert in the area of aural rehabilitation.

- Chapter 14 presents new information on working with active duty military and combat veterans that is not available in any other text in the CSD professions.

- Updated information on clinician strategies for self-care and prevention of burnout is provided in Chapter 15.

- Role play activities presented at the end of each chapter (with the exception of Chapter 1) offer prompts for in-class group activities. Instructors can use these exercises to expand discussions regarding the application of skills discussed in each chapter.

Thank you for your interest in studying counseling skills—some of the most important skills that any clinician can develop. The authors hope that this text will serve you well throughout your education and professional career and that you will continue to further your professional development in this vital area.

ACKNOWLEDGEMENTS

FOR DR. LYDIA FLASHER

I would like to acknowledge Dr. Hans H. Strupp and Dr. Ira Turkat for their outstanding teaching, support, and inspiration during my graduate school experience at Vanderbilt University. I would also like to acknowledge my colleagues in the Department of Psychology at the Montreal Children's Hospital, especially Carol Schopflocher and Dr. Phil Zelazo, who enriched my early stages of professional growth. In addition, I am indebted to Dr. Joan Baran, Clinic Director, as well as my colleagues at Children's Health Council (CHC) in Palo Alto, California for their flexibility and support while I finished the second edition of this manuscript. Special appreciation goes to my psychologically astute speech-language colleagues at CHC who helped me to reflect upon relevant and common counseling issues that were instrumental in creating a plan for the new chapter on working with families. I am extraordinarily grateful to all the graduate students, interns, postdoctoral fellows, and clients and families who have compelled me to refine my conceptual thinking and clinical skills. Special thanks go to my dear and loyal friend Margaret Lovett, who has brightened my life for almost 30 years. Finally, I want to thank my husband Dr. Dawson S. Schultz, for his unconditional love, support, and companionship as well as his insightful conceptual and editing comments.

FOR DR. PAUL FOGLE

I would like to acknowledge the people who made this text "real"—the clients, patients, and their families with whom I have worked for over 40 years. They are my best teachers. All of the "Personal Experiences," "Case Studies," and "Counseling Skills in Action" actually occurred as described.

I also would like to acknowledge Dr. Joseph and Vivian Sheehan for their years of friendship and for training me at the University of California, Los Angeles to work with adults who stutter. They will be forever missed. Dr. Dean Williams, an internationally recognized expert in stuttering, was my professor and mentor at the University of Iowa. Dr. Williams used to tell his students, "I hope all of you find someone who helps you become more than you ever thought you could be." Dr. Williams was that person for me, and he also will be forever missed.

Thanks go to the various organizations and universities for providing me the opportunity to present seminars on the topic of counseling skills throughout the United States, as well as in Australia, New Zealand, and Singapore, to speech-language pathologists, audiologists, physical therapists, occupational therapists, and nurses.

Special thanks go to my lifelong friend Ed Little for his insights, counsel, and support. Most importantly, I want to thank my wife, Carol Fogle, R. N., for her love, support, and encouragement for this and all of my other writing projects.

JOINT ACKNOWLEDGEMENTS

This second edition would not have been possible without the support of two important people at Delmar Cengage Learning: Sherry L. Dickinson, senior acquisitions editor for health care, and Laura J. Wood, product manager, for her expert managing of the numerous steps in the production of this text. We are extremely grateful to them for recognizing the value of this text and the potential for its expansion.

Reviewers

Lisa R. La Salle, Ph.D., CCC-SLP
Board Recognized Specialist—Fluency Disorders
Professor, Communication Sciences & Disorders
University of Wisconsin-Eau Claire
Eau Claire, WI

Adrienne McElroy-Bratcher, SLP.D., CCC-SLP
Assistant Professor, Graduate Coordinator/
Program Director
Eastern New Mexico University
Portales, NM

Jean Sawyer, Ph.D., CCC-SLP
Assistant Professor
Illinois State University
Normal, Illinois

Debra Schober-Peterson, Ph.D., CCC-SLP
Clinical Associate Professor
Georgia State University
Atlanta, GA

Laura Teague, M.A., CCC-SLP
Clinical Instructor
LSHA, ASHA, Louisiana State University
Baton Rouge, LA

ABOUT THE AUTHORS

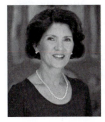

Lydia V. Flasher, Ph.D., earned her baccalaureate summa cum laude and Phi Beta Kappa from Duke University, and her masters and doctorate in clinical psychology from Vanderbilt University. Her mentor at Vanderbilt was Hans H. Strupp, a pioneer in psychotherapy research and short-term dynamic psychotherapy. She completed her internship at the Montreal Children's Hospital, a McGill University teaching hospital, and then worked there as a staff psychologist specializing in personality assessment, family therapy, and pediatric psychology. Dr. Flasher was previously a professor at Colorado State University and the University of the Pacific and has many years of experience teaching graduate students in clinical and counseling psychology. She has been director of a university training clinic for doctoral students in counseling psychology and has over 20 years of experience supervising psychology graduate students, interns, and postdoctoral fellows. Currently, she is Director of the Psychology Training Programs and a clinical psychologist at Children's Health Council in Palo Alto, California. In her administrative role, she is co-director for an APA-approved predoctoral psychology internship consortium between Stanford University's Packard Children's Hospital and Children's Health Council. She also directs a clinical psychology postdoctoral fellowship program. In her direct clinical work, she specializes in multidisciplinary assessments, anxiety disorders, and family therapy. She has published professional literature and presented at professional conferences on varied topics including supervision competencies, multiculturalism, interpersonal psychotherapy for children, medical narrative, and pediatric palliative care. Dr. Flasher lives in the Santa Cruz Mountains above Los Gatos and enjoys hiking and running in the redwood forest. You can learn more about this author by accessing www.chconline.org and going to the Staff Bio section. Her e-mail address is lflasher@chconline.org.

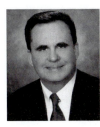

Paul T. Fogle, Ph.D., CCC-SLP, (Fogle is pronounced with a long *o*, as in FO-GULL) has been studying, training, and working in speech-language pathology for over 40 years. Although he earned all of his degrees in speech-language pathology, he minored in psychology throughout each degree. He earned his Bachelor of Arts in 1970 and his Masters of Arts in 1971, both at California State University, Long Beach. After receiving his M.A., he worked for two years as an aphasia classroom teacher for the Los Angeles County Office of Education and started the first high school aphasia class in California, teaching and working with adolescents who had sustained traumatic brain injuries, strokes, and other neurological impairments. Between 1970 and 1973, Dr. Fogle worked as a therapist at the University of California, Los Angeles (UCLA) Psychology Adult Stuttering Clinic, training under Dr. Joseph Sheehan and Mrs. Vivian Sheehan. Concurrently, he trained on human brain autopsy procedures at Rancho Los Amigos Medical Center.

Dr. Fogle earned his doctorate in 1976 from the University of Iowa. He specialized in neurological disorders in adults and children and in stuttering. His dissertation was directed by Dr. Dean Williams and he was awarded membership in Sigma Xi, the Scientific Research Society of North America, for his research. Since receiving his Ph.D. he has taught undergraduate courses on Introduction to Speech-Language Pathology and Audiology, Anatomy and Physiology of Speech, Speech Science, and Organic Disorders. At the graduate level he has taught Neurological Disorders in Adults, Motor Speech Disorders, Dysphagia/Swallowing Disorders, Gerontology, Voice Disorders, Cleft Palate and Oral-Facial Anomalies, and Counseling Skills for Speech-Language Pathologists. Since the early 1990s, he has been training in counseling psychology and family therapy. Most recently he has been receiving education and training in neuropsychology.

Dr. Fogle has worked extensively in hospitals, including Veterans Administration hospitals, university hospitals, and acute, subacute, and convalescent hospitals. He has maintained a year-round private practice for over 30 years. He has presented numerous seminars, workshops, and short courses on a variety of topics at state, ASHA, international (IALP), and Asia-Pacific Society for the Study of Speech-Language Pathology and Audiology conferences and conventions. Dr. Fogle has presented all-day workshops in cities around the United States and in countries around the world on counseling skills for speech-language pathologists and audiologists. He has been involved with forensic speech-language pathology (testifying in court as an expert witness) for over 25 years and has published and presented on this topic. Most recently he has been the speech-language pathologist on Rotaplast (Rotary) International Cleft Palate teams in Venezuela and Egypt.

Dr. Fogle's primary publishing has been textbooks and clinical materials. He is the author of *Foundations of Communication Sciences and Disorders* (Delmar Cengage Learning, 2008), *Essentials of Communication Sciences and Disorders* (Delmar Cengage Learning, 2012), and coauthor of the *Ross Information Processing Assessment-Geriatric* (2nd ed.) (Pro-Ed, 2011), *The Source for Safety: Cognitive Retraining for Independent Living* (LinguiSystems, 2008), and the *Classic Aphasia Therapy Stimuli* (CATS) (Plural Publishing, 2006). His forthcoming publications include *Court Testifying as an Expert Witness: A Survivor's Guide* (2012), *The Complete Dictionary for Speech-Language Pathologists and Audiologists* (Delmar Cengage Learning, 2013), and *Neuroscience for Speech-Language Pathologists and Audiologists* (Delmar Cengage Learning, 2015). His website is www.PaulFoglePhD.com and his e-mail address is paulfoglephd@gmail.com.

PART

I

Foundations of Counseling Skills

Part I of this text provides a framework for considering the essential ingredients involved in counseling skills for speech-language pathologists (SLPs) and audiologists (Auds). Defining the scope of practice and professional parameters is important for new professionals getting their bearings and for practicing clinicians who want to hone their counseling skills. This text also discusses the ethics of counseling and some factors that must be kept in mind during any interaction with people we are trying to help. This section provides an outline of various theoretical frameworks that can help the clinician to better understand and respond to clinical situations. These psychological theories help organize the wealth of information that comes from our interactions with clients. In addition to having good instincts and positive personal characteristics, we need to have a systematic rationale for our behavior with clients, patients, and their family members.

While psychological theories may help to orient the clinician to understand and organize certain client phenomena (e.g., existential struggles, family dynamics, and cultural behaviors), the clinician also needs to have a repertoire of basic counseling skills that transcend theoretical boundaries. Chapters 3 and 4 provide detailed information about therapeutic communication and the specific skills that provide the foundation of any good therapeutic approach. These skills are practiced unknowingly by many, but we believe that all clinicians can benefit by making a self-conscious assessment and evaluation of the skills they use. Speech-language pathologists and audiologists can continually learn by taking stock of themselves and the ways that they interact with clients. It is through this ongoing process of self-reflection and evaluation that we continue to become better clinicians.

The Basics

CHAPTER OUTLINE

- Introduction
- Definition of Counseling for SLPs and Auds
- Using Counseling Skills Versus Being a Counselor
- Counseling: Science *and* Art
- Overlap in the Work of SLPs, Auds, and Psychologists
- Personal Qualities of Effective Helpers
- Purposes of Counseling for SLPs and Auds
- Counseling Boundaries and Scope of Practice
- Ethical and Legal Aspects of Counseling for Our Professions
- Bioethical Considerations
- Concluding Comments
- Discussion Questions

INTRODUCTION

Welcome! You are beginning the study of what is considered by many speech-language pathologists and audiologists to be one of the most crucial aspects of a student's education and training: counseling. Clinicians in the field consistently report that counseling is something they do with every person with whom they work, whether it is a child, adolescent, adult, or elderly person. Often the clinician is involved in counseling family members as well, including parents, grandparents, spouses, siblings, children, and even grandchildren. Any interaction with a client, patient, or family member involves using counseling skills, even though you may not be doing counseling per se.

Corey (2008) states that counseling is a process of engagement between two people, both of whom are bound to change through the therapeutic venture. Studying counseling and counseling skills will help you develop a deeper understanding of people, their problems, and how they cope. You also will develop a deeper understanding of yourself, your interpersonal style, and how you cope. You will learn skills that will help you better manage challenging interactions with family, friends, and co-workers, and you will learn how to help other people cope with life's vicissitudes and challenges.

This text is not a course in psychology or psychopathology, but it is about helping ordinary people (our clients, patients, and their families) deal with disorders of hearing, communication, and swallowing. It will help you learn the essentials of counseling as well as the essentials of how to deal with the inevitable challenging situations and behaviors that arise in therapy. This text is about both you and the people you are trying to help.

DEFINITION OF COUNSELING FOR SLPS AND AUDS

Counseling began to take form in the early research and writings in psychology by Carl Wundt and Sigmund Freud in the late 1800s (Baron, Kalsher, & Henry, 2008). Within the broad field of psychology is the specialty of counseling psychology, with its goal of assisting individuals in dealing with personal challenging life situations that do not involve psychological disorders. Even more recent than the development of counseling psychology is the development of marriage–family–child counseling (now more commonly called marriage and family therapy or family therapy). In this text we will draw heavily from counseling psychology literature as well as family therapy literature.

The American Speech-Language-Hearing Association's (ASHA) 2007 Scope of Practice statement under Clinical Services specifically states that counseling is an appropriate function of SLPs and Auds; for example, counseling individuals, families, co-workers, educators, and other persons in the community regarding acceptance, adaptation, and decision making about hearing, communication, and swallowing. Standards for certification, minimal competencies for the provision of audiologic rehabilitation and speech-language pathology services, and best practice patterns all emphasize the importance of counseling in our professional roles.

The counseling we do in speech-language pathology and audiology is educational and rehabilitation counseling. The terms *counseling* and *interviewing* are often used interchangeably by some professionals. Though the overlap is considerable, interviewing may be considered an interactive process for information gathering in which the professional uses listening, rapport-building, and empathic skills to understand the unique person. **Counseling** may be used more broadly to refer to the interactive process used to understand the unique characteristics and circumstances of individuals and to facilitate positive change in situations where individuals are suffering emotional distress and/or coping with challenging life situations (Ivey, Ivey, & Zalaquett, 2009). In our professions we do interviewing, therapy, and counseling, often without a clear distinction. The skills used in interviewing and counseling overlap and are used throughout the various stages of the therapy process.

Counseling for the professions of speech-language pathology and audiology may be defined as an applied social science and a helping, interpersonal relationship in which the clinician's intentions are to assist a person or family member to understand a hearing, communication, or swallowing disorder and its impact on the person's life, as well as ways of preventing, managing, adjusting to, or coping with these disorders. As an applied social science, counseling has a considerable body of literature to support its effectiveness. Counseling is a helping, interpersonal relationship, which means that it involves at least two people and that a relationship, no matter how transient or superficial, always develops. Both the helper and helpee have some kind of interaction that leads to opinions and feelings about one another.

Ideally, every counseling statement, gesture, or silence may be regarded as purposeful (Feltham & Dryden, 2005). Although sometimes our best intentions may not always result in the positive effects that we anticipated, we must always have the client's best interests as our primary goal. Further, we should be *reflective practitioners* (Schon, 1983, 1987) who carefully select the communication techniques and strategies we use and calibrate or modify those that have not been helpful with a particular individual.

Conducting the initial telephone contact or first meeting with a client or parent with warmth, genuineness, and professionalism can set the tone for future interactions. However, if the clinician is perceived as cold or indifferent and just "going through the motions" during this first contact, the client might easily have negative expectations. A client's initial impressions of a clinician and a clinician's initial impressions of a client are often difficult to overcome, even when further interactions appear contrary to the first.

In counseling we attempt to help children, clients, patients, and families understand ways of preventing disorders. For example, we help children and adults understand how they can prevent further hearing loss and preserve the hearing they have. We help parents learn to be better listeners to their young children who are beginning to be unusually disfluent and to try to give their children more opportunities to produce fluent speech. We also help individuals manage their communication disorders by understanding what motivates them to improve and what factors, both personal and environmental, may interfere with maximizing their therapy gains.

Sometimes counseling involves helping individuals and their families adjust to and cope with long-lasting or even permanent communication disorders (Friehe, Bloedow, & Hesse, 2003). A child's severe hearing loss may be lifelong; a child's hypernasal speech caused by a cleft palate may affect speech intelligibility throughout life; a young adult with a traumatic brain injury (TBI) may always have difficulty with communicating and problem-solving for activities of daily living (ADLs); and an elderly person developing dementia will likely see abilities to communicate and function independently slowly erode over time.

One of the challenges of counseling individuals with communication disorders is the possibility that their communication disorder may interfere with their ability to understand some of the more subtle (or even the most direct) messages and information that we present. Likewise, their communication disorder can interfere with their ability to explain to us what they are thinking and feeling. Moreover, when working with family members of some clients and patients, there is the possibility that they may have some of their own auditory processing, language (both receptive and expressive), and cognitive problems that prevent them from fully understanding what we are trying to communicate or clearly expressing their thoughts and feelings. Sometimes at the end of counseling with clients, patients, or family members, clinicians wonder what was really accomplished and what clients and their family members will take away from the interaction.

USING COUNSELING SKILLS VERSUS BEING A COUNSELOR

Although speech-language pathologists and audiologists do counseling and use counseling skills when working with clients, patients, and families, it is not appropriate to identify ourselves as counselors. There are several areas in which we have education and training, yet it is not ethical or legal to identify ourselves with those professional titles. For and how to use counseling skills and the interpersonal sensitivity to use the best timing possible. The scientific aspect is unique to professional helpers and differentiates them from nonprofessional helpers. The scientific aspect emphasizes objective observations, testing hypotheses, and employing empirically validated assessment and treatment strategies.

We cannot make a clear distinction between the science of counseling and the personality and behavior of the person doing the counseling. In the psychotherapy literature, these are referred to as specific (i.e., technical) and nonspecific (i.e., interpersonal) factors (Strupp, 1992; Strupp & Hadley, 1979). Although counselors can learn attitudes and skills and acquire knowledge about personality dynamics and the therapeutic process, a considerable part of effective counseling is developing the art. The artistic aspects of counseling suggest that it is a flexible, creative process. Timing of the counselor is often a crucial part of the art, not only saying the right thing but also saying it at the right time. At any given moment when working with an individual, we may need to empathize, teach, model, support, question, restructure, interpret, or remain silent. The therapeutic value of these interventions can depend upon the timing used by the therapist.

The artistic aspect also includes the concept of giving of ourselves, such as our concern, support, and empathy. This giving of ourselves is a delicate, balanced process that is learned over time: when to give, how much to give, in what way to give. This concept is derived from humanistic psychology and emphasizes the importance of being authentic and human in the counseling approach (Nystul, 2005). SLPs and Auds can give support as they empathize with their clients. Sometimes just listening carefully to clients may be the best gift clinicians can give at the time, bearing witness to their suffering (Frank, 2002) and helping them overcome feelings of aloneness and isolation.

Luterman (2008) says that counseling can be demystified so clinicians understand it is something we do, even when we are not aware we are doing it. Counseling skills are used in every encounter, whether intentionally or spontaneously (Crowe, 1997; Fogle, 2008). Strict stimulus-response therapy may not be counseling, but our facial expressions, body language, and tone of voice give strong messages about our acceptance and feelings about the person we are working with. Our feelings about people inevitably color our interactions with them.

Counseling is not reserved for a particular group of professionals who call themselves counselors or psychologists. The following are brief definitions of various professionals who are commonly seen by individuals seeking what most people typically think of as counseling (Feldman, 2005). This list is provided to help clarify each professional's education and role.

Clinical psychologist

Possesses a Ph.D. or Psy.D. and specializes in assessment and treatment of psychological disorders and their symptoms.

Counseling psychologist

Possesses a Ph.D. or Psy.D. and usually treats day-to-day adjustment problems in a counseling setting, such as a university or mental-health clinic.

Marriage and family therapist

Usually a professional with an M.A. who attempts to change the structure and interaction processes of the client's family.

Licensed case social worker

Usually a professional with an M.A. who works with individuals and families and mobilizes community support systems.

Psychiatrist

Physician (M.D.) with postgraduate training in abnormal behavior, psychotherapy, and psychopharmacology who can prescribe medications as part of treatment for mental disorders.

Psychiatric social worker

Professional with an M.A. and specialized training in treating people in home and community settings.

Psychoanalyst

Either a physician or a psychologist who specializes in psychoanalysis, the treatment approach first developed by Sigmund Freud.

School psychologist/counselor

Usually possesses an M.A. in school psychology or educational psychology who works in school settings with children and parents.

Essentially all professionals working with people use some counseling skills as part of their interaction with clients, patients, and families. While counseling comes more naturally to some, counseling skills can be learned. Burnard (2005) says counseling is never simply a matter of learning a generic list of skills that we then apply in a range of settings. Instead, counseling involves working with particular clients, listening carefully, and using counseling skills to help address the issues at hand. The application of these skills requires our understanding and selection of which skills to apply, with whom, and at what time.

A client with a delay, disorder, or disability almost always exists within a family context. The communication disorder usually affects more than a single individual. For clinicians to be most effective we must deal with the client and at least some of the important people (family and sometimes close friends) in the client's life, as well as other professionals on the treatment team. The focus, however, must always be on the communication problems and how they are affecting the client and family's coping abilities.

Although Luterman (2008) says that counseling needs to be at the forefront of students' clinical education and our professional research, the professions of speech-language pathology and audiology typically do not have a history of extensive training in the area of counseling. This deficit in education and training is not unique to our professions. In informal surveys conducted by the author (P. F.) of over 3,500 SLPs, Auds, occupational therapists (OTs), and physical therapists (PTs) throughout the United States and foreign countries who have attended my seminars on counseling, 100 percent of them acknowledge that they use counseling skills in every interaction with clients, patients, and family members, although fewer than 20 percent of clinicians surveyed say they had a specific course in their education dealing with counseling. It is interesting to note that most clinicians who attend these seminars have between 5 and 20 years of professional experience, with some having 25 to 30 or more years of experience. Even after decades of working with clients, patients, and families, most rehabilitation clinicians still feel uncomfortable with counseling skills that they consider an essential and ongoing part of their evaluations and therapy.

When working with clients, patients, and families we cannot easily interrupt a person who is discussing sensitive issues surrounding a communication disorder and say we cannot discuss the issue and would like to refer the person to a psychologist. We definitely have our boundaries and scope of practice (to be discussed later), but must work with many issues and emotions as they arise. These issues and emotions may become critical in our understanding of the client and our selection of appropriate interventions. Being unresponsive or interrupting the person would be nontherapeutic, and an immediate referral to a psychologist to continue the discussion is seldom practical and can negatively affect our rapport with a client. Co-treatment with a psychologist present is also an unlikely occurrence.

In a study by Culpepper, Mendell, and McCarthy (1994) in which training programs accredited by ASHA were surveyed, it was found that approximately 40 percent of the programs offered a course on counseling within the department that emphasized relating counseling theories and skills to the profession. Approximately 35 percent required students to take a counseling course outside of their department, and approximately 25 percent of programs did not offer or require speech-language pathology or audiology students to have any course work in counseling. This lack of classroom and clinical training in communication disorders programs continues to be a problem (Kaderavek, Laux, & Mills, 2004). The lack of counseling courses being offered may reflect a lack of education and training of individuals qualified to teach such courses. Some programs try to infuse counseling into their various course offerings; however, in that model it is difficult for students to get a holistic understanding of counseling as well as specific approaches and counseling strategies that will be helpful with a wide variety of speech, language, cognitive, swallowing, and hearing disorders. The infusion approach follows a top-down model where students try to learn some specific counseling principles or techniques in a course (e.g., aural rehabilitation) and then, along with counseling techniques infused in other courses, attempt to develop a unified approach that fits their world view and ways of working with clients.

When students have a counseling course offered in their major they learn that counseling principles and skills are applicable to all disorders. When clinicians begin to understand counseling approaches and techniques, they begin generalizing them to a variety of disorders and situations. This follows the bottom-up model, in which a particular approach or technique may apply to a variety of situations. The bottom-up model allows students to build a foundation of knowledge in the area of counseling and see how that knowledge is applicable to all of their clinical work.

Beyond education and training in counseling psychology or family therapy, it is helpful for the individual who teaches a counseling course to be actively involved in the challenges of direct client or patient care. In this way, the professor can put into practice and refine what is being taught. Fogle (2001), in an article on "Professors in Private Practice," noted several benefits for professors working with clients and their families on a regular basis. These benefits translate into improved teaching and student training:

- The continual stimulation of working with challenging clients and families
- The direct hands-on experience that cannot be appreciated when observing student clinicians through a two-way mirror
- The satisfaction of working with clients from the initial interview to termination of therapy and knowing that we have been an important part of the person's improvement
- New therapy stories for students to help relate theoretical information to clinical practice
- A more realistic empathy with students struggling with therapeutic dilemmas
- The opportunity to collect data for research studies or develop new assessment or therapy materials

OVERLAP IN THE WORK OF SLPS, AUDS, AND PSYCHOLOGISTS

Counseling and psychotherapy have similarities and differences (Rollin, 2000). At no time, however, should the SLP or Aud say she is doing psychotherapy. Some disorders, though, lend themselves to more of a psychotherapeutic or counseling approach. Sheehan (1970) said that stuttering therapy is a modified form of psychotherapy because the clinician is helping the client change attitudes about stuttering as well as the stuttering behaviors themselves. Adults with voice disorders often have interpersonal conflicts and/or anxieties that contribute to laryngeal tension as well as generalized tension. SLPs who address the whole person in a holistic approach are concerned with more than just communicative behaviors; they are concerned with the person's emotions, mind, body, and spirit.

SLPs and Auds occasionally see individuals with emotional or mental disorders who have diagnoses specified in the *Diagnostic and Statistical Manual of Mental Disorders Fourth Edition, Text Revision* (*DSM-IV-TR*) (American Psychiatric Association, 2000). We work with individuals who have substance and alcohol abuse problems, adjustment disorders, mood disorders such as depression, conduct disorders, and anxiety disorders. However, we do not focus on or address those emotional or mental disorders per se; we work with the speech, language, and cognitive problems that may be a part of those disorders. We try to work around or through those disorders but do not try to do the counseling and psychotherapy to manage those disorders.

There are several *DSM-IV-TR* (2000) disorders that we as professionals frequently encounter. SLPs are qualified to make some of these diagnoses, but we are not qualified to make the vast majority of them. In some cases we may be the main professional treating a client who has been diagnosed by a psychologist. For example, the *DSM-IV-TR* discusses in considerable detail "amnestic (amnesia) disorders" (294.0) that are characterized by memory impairment that affects the person's ability to learn new information or to recall previously learned information or past events. These memory disturbances must cause marked impairment in social or occupational functioning and must represent a decline from a previous level of functioning. This *DSM-IV-TR* diagnosis reflects the memory impairments SLPs work with when patients have had strokes, TBIs, tumors, or other neurological damage. The *DSM-IV-TR* also has a considerable discussion of various types of dementia, such as Vascular (multi-infarct) Dementia (290.4x) and Alzheimer's Disease (290.0). SLPs working in convalescent hospitals (skilled nursing facilities or SNFs) see many residents with dementia.

Attention Deficit/Hyperactivity Disorders, Predominantly Hyperactive-Impulsive Type (ADHD) (314.01), Attention Deficit/Hyperactivity Disorder, Predominantly Inattentive Type (314.00), and Attention Deficit/Hyperactivity Disorder Not Otherwise Specified (314.9) are *DSM-IV-TR* diagnoses. We see many children in our public school case loads who have ADHD with comorbid language disorders, including problems with pragmatics. The *DSM-IV-TR* has specific sections on Expressive Language Disorders (315.31), Mixed Receptive-Expressive Language Disorders (315.32), Phonological Disorders (315.39), and Stuttering (307.0). There are *DSM-IV-TR* classifications for Learning Disorders, including Reading Disorders (315.00), Disorders of Written Expression (315.2), and Mental Retardation with severity levels ranging from Mild (317) to Profound (318.2). Autistic Disorder (299.00) and Pervasive Developmental Disorder (299.80) are *DSM-IV-TR* classifications. It is clear that there are a variety of disorders that psychologists, psychotherapists, and psychiatrists are able to diagnose, but the SLP may be a critical member of the treatment team involved in the habilitation or rehabilitation of these disorders.

PERSONAL QUALITIES OF EFFECTIVE HELPERS

Before we begin discussing personal qualities of effective helpers (counselors), we should first explain what is meant by "helper." The term *helper* tends to show up in the counseling and psychotherapy literature and refers to several professionals who are trained in and use counseling as their way of helping people. As clinicians we know that we are helpers, but it is a term we do not typically apply to ourselves. Ultimately, our goal for helping a client is for that person to not need our help any longer, to become independent of us, to become a self-helper (Brammer & McDonald, 2002; Nystul, 2005). Like most helpers, our job is to work ourselves out of a job.

The term *helper* is useful to us in our understanding of counseling. Rogers (1957) identified three core conditions as "necessary and sufficient conditions" to help individuals with personal growth (these will be discussed further in the section on Humanistic Therapy in Chapter 2). These conditions must first be characteristics of a counselor before they can be conditions the counselor brings into the client–clinician relationship.

■ Congruence: The clinician is genuine in terms of what she experiences and communicates. Congruence implies that the clinician is in touch with her thoughts and feelings, she voices them when it is perceived to be helpful, and her body language and tone of voice mirror her words and statements.

■ Empathic understanding: The clinician attempts to understand the client from the client's point of view (i.e., tries to understand what the person is thinking, feeling, and experiencing and communicates this understanding back to the client).

■ Unconditional positive regard: The clinician needs to communicate a sense of acceptance and respect to the client. The clinician is consistently nonjudgmental, which allows the client to relax, trust, and be open with the clinician. It means being accepting of the client, but not necessarily all of the client's behaviors; we can "separate the deed from the doer" (Martin, 2000; Nystul, 2005).

The challenge with these characteristics is that they are difficult to teach. SLPs and Auds typically possess these characteristics before their training begins, which may be one of the reasons they have gravitated to these professions. Their training helps to further develop their natural tendencies.

Clinicians, like other people, often have difficulty being congruent, although we always need to be striving to become more congruent in our own lives (Luterman, 2008; Rogers, 1980). It is sometimes difficult to know just what we are thinking or feeling, and we are often taught to be polite rather than to be congruent or authentic in social situations. Perhaps due to our social training, it is sometimes difficult to know the difference between a thought and a feeling. Feltham and Dryden (2005) define *thought* as cognition or mental activity, using words such as thinking, remembering, reasoning, concentrating, questioning, figuring, calculating, projecting, and pondering. *Feeling* is defined as affect or emotion, using words such as happy, joyful, delighted, sad, depressed, lonely, eager, apathetic, surprised, curious, indecisive, fatigued, courageous, protective, powerful, satisfied, overwhelmed, loved, hopeful, angry, and fearful. Like primary colors, there are primary emotions of joy, anger, and sadness. Many of our emotions are variations or degrees of these primary emotions.

Clinicians sometimes struggle with understanding their own thoughts and feelings and how they interact and influence each other. Baron, Kalsher, and Henry (2008) and Stirling and Elliott (2008) discuss how affect influences cognition and how cognition influences affect. For example, our affect (feelings) and affective states (moods) influence our perceptions of ambiguous stimuli or experiences. In general, we perceive and evaluate these stimuli and experiences more favorably when we are in a good mood than when we are in a negative mood. Positive and negative feelings exert a strong influence on memory. In general, when we are feeling positive we tend to retrieve positive memories, and vice versa. We need to be aware or mindful (i.e., possess a calm consciousness or awareness of our own thoughts and feelings) of how our feelings and affective states may be influencing our thoughts and interactions with a client.

At the same time, clinicians try to have their body language, facial expressions, and tone of voice congruent (match or be in agreement) so that listeners do not get mixed messages (Burgoon, Buller, & Woodall, 2002; Fogle, 2009a). Clients and patients (particularly those with neurological disorders) are often confused enough without us confusing them more by saying one thing with our words and something else with our body language, facial expressions, and tone of voice.

Empathic understanding, that is the attitude and skill of following, grasping, and understanding as fully as possible the client's subjective experiences (Feltham & Dryden,

Emotionally Stable

Most SLPs and Auds are at least fairly well-adjusted people who are coping with life's challenges adequately to maintain their mental health. We, like every other person, have stresses in our lives and have days where we feel less "together," focused, and energetic. We may even feel sometimes that our problems are worse than those of the people we are trying to help, although we never want to suggest or imply that to them.

Sometimes the problems we are working on with clients may be similar to those that we are working on in our own lives. For example, an SLP may have a child with ADHD, a spouse with a stroke or head injury, or an elderly parent with dementia. We may identify with the struggles the client, patient, or family members are trying to manage, and sometimes have to work hard not to allow our personal emotions to come forward. We may have to try to distance ourselves just enough to maintain our professional stance in order to be helpful to the people who have come to us for therapy. When we feel we cannot be sufficiently objective and professional because of issues in our own lives, we need to consult with a supervisor, co-worker, or mental health professional to try to help us better manage ourselves so we can meet the needs of our clients. If we find we cannot be effective clinicians because of temporary personal or professional interferences, we need (if at all possible) to make appropriate referrals to other clinicians. We later may be able to effectively help such clients, but for a time we may be too fragile or self-absorbed to do our job professionally.

As professionals, we need to actively practice those things we find helpful to maintain our own good mental health. Many clinicians think in terms of staying "centered," meaning knowing: "I'm OK. I usually do things right. I'm an honest person. I'm a good person. I complete tasks. I'm a good clinician. People usually like me. I'm basically a happy person. My family loves me. People are basically good. My faith will sustain me. Tomorrow is a new day." Clinicians attending counseling seminars have suggested a variety of ways they find helpful to care for themselves, for example, going outside for a few minutes to look at the grass and trees, going for a brief walk, exercising, deep breathing, praying, meditating, or talking to a friend. Baker (2003) and Weiss (2004) offer additional suggestions for learning to manage ourselves and environmental stresses. For example, Weiss discusses the importance of learning to set limits and listening to our body's signals in order to recognize and avoid burnout. We always need to be in the process of learning how to take better care of ourselves so we can take better care of others.

Self-Aware

Self-awareness appears to be related to other concepts of self, such as self-acceptance, self-esteem, and self-realization. Having a positive sense of self and being comfortable "in our own skin" is important for us to maintain our emotional stability. Self-awareness also helps us appreciate our strengths and limitations as clinicians. We have awareness that we can do good therapy with certain kinds of clients and a realization that we may do merely adequate therapy with others. We are aware of the areas in which we need to seek further training and continuing education. We also are aware of areas in which we can be helpful to other clinicians in their attempts to continue their training and education. There is a general sequence in our professional lives that is passed on from generation to generation. The sequence is: "I need help" (education, training, experience); "I can do it alone" (I'm able to be independent now); and "I can help you" (I'm ready to help educate, train, and provide experiences for you).

Positive Self-Esteem

A positive self-esteem, tempered with humility, can help clinicians cope with the trials and tribulations of therapy. Also, when clinicians feel positive about themselves they tend to see the positive attributes of their clients. When clinicians feel negatively about themselves they are more likely to become defensive when suggestions are made by supervisors about how to improve their work.

Patience

One of the hallmark characteristics of SLPs and Auds is patience. It is the ability and willingness to persevere during the often long, slow road of speech and language development or rehabilitation of our clients and patients. We need to practice patience. The challenge for many people we work with is their impatience to improve, to be able to communicate without difficulty. Our ability and willingness to be patient gives them a model and someone to help temper their **anxiety** and frustration about their pace of improvement.

Tolerance for Ambiguity

There are few absolutes in our professions, although there are three that should be emphasized to students: (1) you are going to make mistakes; (2) you are going to get tired; and (3) you are never going to know everything. Ambiguity is a part of our incomplete knowledge and understanding of every area of our professions. The data are never all in. At the end of almost every research article is the standard statement, "Further research is needed." Speech-language pathology and audiology, like medicine and psychology, are inexact sciences. An ability to tolerate ambiguity reflects our flexibility and ability to work at the fringes of our knowledge and competencies. As David Luterman said in a seminar on counseling at the 1999 ASHA Convention, "In our professional lives we need to always be working on the fringes of our competencies. If we wait to be 'certified' in everything we do we have probably missed helping a lot of people." The only way we become competent is by doing what we are not yet competent to do, and by seeking education and consultation during this process.

Spirituality

Although this may seem like an inappropriate personal quality to discuss, spirituality is an emerging concern in the counseling and psychotherapy literature. The value of addressing and utilizing spiritual-religious dimensions in the helping process is being recognized (Aten & Leach, 2009; Plante, 2009). For the professional, appropriate ways of honoring and respecting spirituality include being sensitive to and accepting of the religious and spiritual values and beliefs of our clients, patients, and their families as well as ourselves.

The majority of people in this country profess some belief in God, as they understand God. For many of our clients and patients, their spiritual beliefs provide comfort and support beyond what any person can provide. In many cases, our own beliefs may be similar to theirs, and it can be comforting to the people we are working with if they have the sense that we are on the "same wavelength." No matter what the spiritual or religious beliefs are of the people that we are working with, we need to honor and respect them, not just tolerate them.

Amazing Grace

One day after finishing work at a convalescent hospital I was about to leave the facility when the Director of Nursing (DON) came running up to me and grabbed my hand. She had me in tow when she grabbed another SLP's hand. As we were rushing down the hall she said, "We are going to sing 'Amazing Grace' to Mr. Williams." I thought to myself, my singing is *not* going to be therapeutic. One of the resident's last requests was to hear his favorite hymn (even if it was poorly sung). The DON, the other SLP, and I stood at the end of the resident's bed, his wife and son behind us. We gave our best rendition of the hymn and it seemed important to everyone present. We honored his request and spirituality. Not long after that he rested in peace.

This story illustrates that sometimes the smallest things we do may have the most important impact on a person's life, even at the end of life. Had I not been very familiar with the words to "Amazing Grace," I would have done the best I could anyway to meet the resident's needs.

CLINICAL QUESTIONS

1. If you do not have a faith in God, how would you have handled that sensitive moment?

2. What benefits do you think the family received from hearing the hospital employees singing "Amazing Grace"?

Riley (2002) and Gladding (2009) define several other personal qualities of an effective counselor, including:

■ Curiosity and inquisitiveness: a natural interest in people

■ Ability to listen: finding listening stimulating

■ Emotional insightfulness: comfort dealing with a wide range of feelings, from anger to joy

- Introspection (self-awareness): the ability to be self-reflective and accurately analyze oneself
- Capacity for self-denial: the ability to set aside personal needs to listen and take care of others' needs first
- Ability to laugh: the capability of seeing the bittersweet quality of life events and the humor in them

SLPs and Auds may choose their professions partly because they naturally have many of the personal qualities that are important in being good counselors. Much of their clinical training with children and adults either directly or indirectly helps enhance or strengthen those qualities, and the training continues throughout their professional careers.

PURPOSES OF COUNSELING FOR SLPS AND AUDS

Holland (2007) states that one of the goals of counseling clients and their families is to support decisions and behaviors that optimize their quality of life. In addition, Riley (2002) points out that the goal of counseling is to facilitate individuals to find their own answers, experience an internal sense of control, and leave with new perspectives and the confidence that they can continue to care for themselves. Riley lists several outcomes expected from counseling with an SLP:

1. The client will be more self-aware and able to observe herself with some objectivity.
2. The client will exhibit reduced limitations that inhibit choices.
3. The client will experience increased internal (vs. external) control.
4. The client will be able to recognize and accept responsibility for her feelings.
5. The client will demonstrate an increased use of "I" statements rather than "you" statements.
6. The client will be able to deal with uncertainty with less anxiety.
7. The client will have a more positive view of self and others.
8. The client will have made a commitment to continue to grow.

Crowe (1997) and Parkinson and Rae (1996) identify numerous purposes of counseling for our professions:

1. Listen actively and empathically to clients and families.
2. Gather and convey information (e.g., interviewing and presenting diagnostic information).
3. Prevent disorders from developing or from becoming more severe and involved (e.g., teaching parents how to listen to their child who is at risk for stuttering).
4. Explore the feelings, thoughts, and behaviors so that individuals may come to terms with their problems.

5. Help clients adjust emotionally to their disorders and resist developing counterproductive behaviors in reaction to them (e.g., helping a child with a repaired bilateral complete cleft lip accept her appearance and recognize other kinds of beauty in herself).

6. Help be supportive of families and significant others in coping with a client's disorder or disability (e.g., helping the parents of a child with traumatic brain injury deal with the new and difficult behaviors of their once loving child).

7. Help clients improve their overall function and independence by learning decision-making and problem-solving skills and maintain high motivation levels for therapy (e.g., helping patients with strokes recognize their abilities and appreciate the small gains they are making).

8. Assist clients to exercise autonomy so they can take responsibility for making changes in their lives.

9. Provide an environment for clients that is optimal for change and improvement (e.g., helping a family realize the negative impact of their chiding and criticism of the client as an ineffective way of encouraging her to work harder.)

10. Help clients develop the self-reinforcement behaviors and coping strategies that are critical to successful carryover and generalization of therapy results (e.g., helping clients see their progression of improvement and ways they can continue to help themselves once they are discharged from therapy).

Overall, every aspect of our work as diagnosticians and clinicians includes counseling as an integral part of interactions with clients, patients, and their families. The people we try to help may not remember our therapy techniques that helped them improve their abilities to communicate as much as they remember how we listened to them and talked with them about the sensitive issues surrounding their hearing, speech, language, cognitive, or swallowing problems.

COUNSELING BOUNDARIES AND SCOPE OF PRACTICE

In order for SLPs and Auds to do our work professionally and ethically, we need to understand our scope of practice. As mentioned earlier, ASHA (2007) includes counseling our clients, patients, and their family members as within our scope of practice *as the counseling relates to the communication problem.*

Within Boundaries and Out of Boundaries

Stone and Olswang (1989), Stone, Shapiro, and Pasino (1990), and English (2002a) say that in order to better understand our scope of practice we can divide boundaries into "within our boundaries," "out of our boundaries," and "challenges to our boundaries." The ideal stance is to have a firm understanding of the within-boundaries and out-of-boundaries areas for our professions, and to recognize the situations that present challenges to our boundaries and require our thoughtful discernment about how to best manage those challenges.

Within Boundaries

Within-boundaries areas are the legitimate areas within the scope of practice of SLPs and Auds, including but not limited to:

- Interviewing the client, patient, or family
- Presenting the diagnosis of delays or disorders
- Providing information about the delays or disorders
- Discussing interventions for the delays or disorders
- Dealing with the client or patient and family's reactions to the diagnosis
- Planning for educational or health care needs beyond our therapy
- Supporting the strengths of the person and her efforts to regain function and to be independent
- Supporting the strengths of the family to help them interact optimally with the client or patient
- Creating supportive empowerment for the client or patient and family to develop the ability to manage their own problems and be independent of the clinician

The within-boundaries areas are broad, and most young clinicians learn to develop some level of comfort with these during their clinical training. New clinicians, however, sometimes do not realize that all their clinical work in some way involves counseling skills and that their counseling must relate to the communication problems of their clients.

Beyond Boundaries

Beyond-boundaries areas for SLPs and Auds are areas or issues that are clearly out of our scope of practice to work on directly, although we know they may have contributed to the cause or continuation of the communication problems with which we are working. Several of these issues need immediate referral to other professionals. Examples of issues beyond our scope of practice include (in alphabetical order):

- Chemical dependence
- Child or elder abuse
- Chronic depression
- Legal conflicts
- Marital problems
- Personality or character disorders
- Sexual abuse and sexual problems
- Suicidal ideation

A recent study by Atkins (2007) on graduate SLP and Aud clinicians' self-awareness of professional boundaries found that while clinicians demonstrated 91 percent accuracy in the identification of topics within professional boundaries, they demonstrated only 55.6 percent accuracy regarding topics that are not within their professional boundaries. Clearly, there is a need to better educate clinicians in this area.

Challenges to Boundaries

Challenges to our boundaries can occur in our first interactions with any client. We cannot avoid possible encounters with situations that challenge our boundaries, so we need to recognize them and have the tools to respond to them appropriately. We sometimes start therapy working within our boundaries but find that there are issues affecting our therapy that are beyond our boundaries. In these cases, we may find ourselves on a slippery slope. For example, a mother may appear angry or displeased with the clinician about the way he is working with her child. After the clinician discusses with the mother his concerns, the mother begins to disclose marital difficulties that are increasing her irritability. The clinician can communicate an empathic response but needs to be alert not to slide into a discussion of her marital issues, even though they may be affecting the mother's perception of the clinician's work.

Another type of challenge to our professional boundaries occurs when we must make a decision about whether we are equipped to accept a particular client or venture into a particular discussion with a client or family member. In these cases, we may not have preset boundaries, but must assess our resources in the moment and decide whether or not to work with that client or venture into a discussion of a very challenging issue. We must ask ourselves what resources (e.g., professional knowledge, experience, understanding of the problem, or support from other professionals) we have to address these problems.

Other challenges to our boundaries occur when parents want us to help them with behavior problems of siblings of the child with whom we are working, or when individuals request a diagnosis of a problem over the telephone. Many of these challenges to our boundaries involve ethical issues, which are discussed in more detail in Lubinski, Golper, and Frattali (2007), and Shipley and Roseberry-McKibbon (2006). Stone, Shapiro, and Pasino (1990) give the following rule of thumb: if a clinician is feeling tense, anxious, uncomfortable, or develops headaches while working with a particular client, patient, or family, it may be a "red flag" that the clinician is in a beyond-boundaries area for our profession or the clinician's level of training and expertise.

Stone and colleagues (1990) use the metaphor of smooth concentric circles to represent the boundaries for counseling within our professions. They suggest that we think of the circles as an ocean and that as professionals we are willing to go into the water. The boundaries are the depth of water. The inner circle is within our boundaries; the middle circle challenges our boundaries; and the outer circle is out of our boundaries.

A modification of the model may help better visualize the concept. Rather than smooth concentric circles, the challenges to our boundaries may be represented as a serrated middle concentric circle. The serrated edges represent areas where we may tread carefully, for instance, deciding whether to pursue a topic a client has brought up (see Figure 1-1).

Stone and colleagues (1990) present the following metaphor. When we are students or newly graduated we tend to stay very close to the shore. As we gain more experience we venture out farther but we must first know how to swim. The water can get choppy and even have big waves. It can get deep very rapidly and we can quickly be in over our heads. It is more comfortable for us if we always know where the shoreline is (within boundaries). If we get too deep in the water (e.g., discussing marital relations) we start to thrash around and may even drown, but if we keep our heads clear and start to swim back to shore we will be safe. If we are working with complex family dynamics, we are in very strong weather

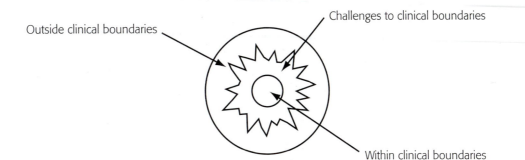

Outside clinical boundaries

Challenges to clinical boundaries

Within clinical boundaries

Figure 1–1 Concentric circles with uneven edges representing clinical boundaries for counseling (adapted from Stone et al., 1990).

and need to stay close to shore. There also may be sharks (challenging issues) in the water or a strong undertow, which means we should not be swimming alone (we need another professional we can consult with about challenging issues). We may need a lifeguard (a supervisor who can help us better manage a situation). The better and more experienced swimmer we are, the farther out we can go. If we are going to swim we are going to get wet, and jumping in the water can be very uncomfortable. However, to become a stronger swimmer we need to get wet often, practice our various strokes, and build our strength.

If both the clinician and client bring considerable strengths (professional knowledge, experience, understanding, insight, patience, etc.) to the relationship, more issues may be addressed. We need to ask ourselves, "What 'baggage' (personal biases or things that bother or limit us) may potentially affect our therapy with clients?" (See the discussion of transference and countertransference in Chapter 3.) Some days we can work with certain emotional issues more easily than others, but we still must do our professional job no matter how we are feeling and maintain stable, predictable boundaries and therapeutic environments. Sometimes the client or family's emotional pain will be similar to pain we have felt or are currently experiencing. During these occasions we need to stay focused on our client's experience and not our own.

Stone and colleagues (1990) present three levels of a therapeutic relationship as they apply to SLPs and Auds.

LEVEL I: "I CAN WORK WITH YOU"

When considering boundary issues we need to not only consider our expertise in an area but also safety issues of the clinician. The clinician must create conditions in order to feel physically safe. A realistic assessment of safety includes knowing whether you are in a safe part of town (but not being complacent about alertness even in a safe area), whether there is sufficient lighting, what distance needs to be walked, and the possibility of severe weather. Inside a building (e.g., a hospital) the therapist needs to be alert to patients who have a history of acting out or violence. (The code 5150 is often used to denote a patient who has potential for self-harm or harming staff. In some hospitals Code Green is used to alert personnel that a patient is being unusually uncooperative and that people in nearby areas should come to assist the health care provider with a silent show of force rather than physical intervention or combativeness.) In home health care, the wise clinician is very alert to any signs that reflect potential danger. Beyond our systematic assessment of the environment, we may use our gut-level feeling to alert us to potential dangers (De Becker, 1997, discusses the importance of listening to our fear). Clinician physical safety is always the first consideration. SLPs and Auds need to go about their business and provide their services with an awareness of safety issues but not be paralyzed with fear.

CASE STUDY

A Client in a Bad Area of Town

An insurance company asked me to evaluate a young man in his home (apartment) who had sustained a TBI from being attacked with a baseball bat. When I scheduled the appointment I learned that the 19-year-old young man was from Southeast Asia and his native language was Hmong. He had become fairly fluent in English during the years he lived here, but spoke little English since the trauma. His girlfriend agreed to translate during the evaluation.

I knew the area where he lived was not the safest part of town, but I was willing to do the evaluation. The young man lived with his family in a small, second-floor apartment. When I was invited into the living room I noticed that all the furniture was against the walls (this may have been a cultural arrangement, but it was somewhat disconcerting to me). The father brought me a folding chair and set it in the middle of the room and invited me to sit down to wait for the client (I felt like I was sitting in the "hot chair" with everyone staring at me). The young man and his girlfriend later came out of a back room and she showed me to what had been a laundry room where a small table had been set up for us to work. A second visit was needed to complete the evaluation. The young man definitely needed therapy, but it was potentially unsafe for a therapist to make frequent visits to the residence.

CLINICAL QUESTIONS

1. What factors or variables would you consider in determining the safety of a particular home environment?
2. What would you do if you worked for a home health care agency that sent you to a part of town where you did not feel safe to see a client?

We structure our environment to create a formal or casual atmosphere. An informal or casual structure invites more testing of the boundaries while increased structure increases the clearness of the boundaries. The clinician must be the one to structure the session and environment. We can do this by staying focused on the communication disorder (behaviors) but still deal with the emotions and other issues that arise. Our general demeanor, the way we dress (professionally or inappropriately casual), and body language (posture, gestures, facial expressions) are important in structuring the therapy environment and maintaining a professional stance.

Private practice and home health care may be settings that most challenge our structuring of therapy because of their typically inherent casual atmospheres compared to clinics, offices, hospitals, and so forth. It is wise for clinicians working in private practice and home health care to be particularly cautious of their own and the client's behavior and to maintain appropriate structure and boundaries.

Seeing Clients in Their Homes or Offices

I find that working in private practice is ideal for working with clients in their homes. I typically work with a child in his room with toys on the floor. I get to know the child's brothers and sisters, pets, and sometimes friends. I also get to work with the parents at their kitchen or dining room table where they are comfortable and perhaps more their real selves. (I have had fathers offer me a drink or beer while we are talking. I *always* decline the offer.)

With adults and children who stutter or have voice disorders I get to see and better understand some of the family dynamics that I would not be able to observe in a more sterile clinic environment. With clients who have had a CVA or TBI, I often work at the kitchen table and have their own household items available to incorporate into therapy.

By seeing a client with vocal nodules in her home I was able to observe the floor plan and acoustics of the home. I observed that the floors were hardwood with no carpeting or rugs, and that the walls were sparsely decorated, causing excessive reverberation of sound. I noted that I automatically raised my voice volume, as did the client, when in her home as a natural effort to talk over the reverberation and ambient noise. I suggested that constant loud voice use in her home, along with other factors, may have contributed to her vocal nodules. She discussed this with her family and they decided to make some changes by adding some throw rugs and sound-absorbing wall hangings.

Another voice client was a high-powered attorney with an otolaryngology diagnosis of muscular tension dysphonia. I saw her for several sessions in her home and then she asked me to have a therapy session at her law office. The client had a very large, imposing (distancing) desk. With the client on one side of the desk and me on the other, I noted how automatically we both raised our voice levels to be more easily heard. I then noticed that there was a heater/air conditioner vent almost directly over her desk that was very noisy. I suggested that it would be easier to talk with her, as well as easier on her voice, if she sat closer to me on her side of the desk. I also noticed a small conference room adjacent to her office and asked if we could try working there. With both of us at the small round conference table we were away from the noisy heater/air conditioner vent and we automatically lowered our voice loudness levels. She stated that she was willing to begin working with her clients in the smaller room to help conserve her voice.

Continues on next page

Continued from previous page

CLINICAL QUESTIONS

1. What advantages can you imagine when working in a client's home?

2. What disadvantages or risks can you imagine when working in a client's home?

3. What can you do as a clinician to minimize the risks of working in a client's home?

LEVEL II: "I CAN CONTINUE WORKING WITH YOU, BUT . . ."

Once again, we may not choose to say these words aloud, but we may need to consciously consider what we need to do to restructure the therapy environment. Whenever we restructure the environment our tone of voice and body language are essential components of our messages. The clinician needs to restructure or refocus the therapy session to work on the problems and issues on which she is comfortable. The clinician might say, "Let me stop you there and ask you about . . ." or "I would like to stay focused on . . ." The client usually will follow the clinician's lead, but if not the clinician may need to redirect or refocus the client again. In some instances a more direct approach may be needed, such as stating that the conversation is going into areas that are outside the clinician's scope of practice or that the area of conversation is not really appropriate in the therapy setting. (See Chapter 4 for more detailed discussions of skills and strategies that may be helpful in this situation.)

In medical settings clinicians always need to be alert to patients who potentially may be harmful to caregivers. For example, patients with TBIs at Level 4 (confused, agitated) on the revised Rancho Levels of Cognitive Functioning (Hagen, 1998) may be verbally abusive or strike out in anger as a result of their neurological impairment (see Chapter 13 for strategies to manage patient anger). Although aggressive behavior can be understandable as a result of the neurological damage, therapists can be injured. We should consider that the patient is, even with the worst behaviors, doing the best he can to manage himself. When the patient cannot manage his behaviors appropriately we need to structure the environment and our responses and to minimize inappropriate or potentially injurious behaviors.

Kriege (1993) emphasizes that we can best help patients by accepting them exactly where they are (cognitively, emotionally, and physically), treating them with respect, and giving sufficient personal space. If we are seeing a patient at bedside we need to approach the patient confidently, but cautiously, and in a nonthreatening manner. We need to try to understand what triggers the patient's behaviors and what the risks are for harm to himself or us. We need to know our own reactions when our emotional buttons are pushed. The threat may be more psychological than physical, with our professional qualifications or self-worth being attacked. We need to know our limits, be in complete control of ourselves, and remain calm.

It is very helpful to speak to the patient in a soothing, calm, and reassuring tone of voice. Speaking slowly and using short, simple sentences (Rule of Fives: five-letter words, five-word sentences) help decrease the amount of information the patient has to process and, therefore, the amount of frustration. We need to try to decrease noise and confusion in the patient's room. Dimming the lights can be soothing to the patient. Gently touching the patient can help him adjust to our presence. We need to share with the other rehabilitation team members and health care providers what we find helpful when working with a particular patient. We need to encourage other staff to interact with the patient who has difficult or challenging behaviors. A patient who feels avoided or isolated may begin to behave in an irritable or aggressive manner. As always, it takes a team approach to appropriately manage challenging patients.

CASE STUDY

Confabulation of a 17-Year-Old

I was asked to evaluate and then provide private therapy for a 17-year-old female high school student who had sustained a severe TBI when hit by a car as she was crossing the street after getting off her school bus. I learned during the interview with the parents that the girl had made accusations about sexual abuse by a family member, but that the accusations were unfounded and the likely result of confabulation secondary to the head injury. I told the parents that I would be willing to evaluate and provide therapy for their daughter under certain strict conditions that would allow me some level of comfort and feeling of professional safety, namely, that an adult observer would be in the room at all times.

CLINICAL QUESTIONS

1. What types of clients may alert you to the need for special precautions?
2. What are some conditions you might request to reduce the risk of a patient making false claims against you?
3. If a client makes any false claims of inappropriate behavior by a therapist, what might be the consequences?

LEVEL III: "I CAN'T CONTINUE WORKING WITH YOU"

When a client continues to try to take us beyond our boundaries and we have repeatedly tried to stay focused on the communication problems the person presents, we need to make explicit statements and give clear messages that we cannot help the person in general or specific ways. In most cases a gentle voice is sufficient, but in others a firmer voice is needed. For example,

> Gentle voice: "I have really enjoyed working with you and I care about you, but what we are dealing with is beyond what I can work with (my scope of practice)."

Firmer voice: "I know that this is important to you, but I cannot be a resource for you in this area. It is beyond my scope of practice. We need to find someone else who can help you with these issues."

In such cases where we feel that the client's needs are beyond our scope of practice, we have a few options. The first, of course, is to refer the client to another professional such as a family therapist, counselor, or psychologist. The client may need to work with that professional before we can continue our therapy, or we may continue working with the client concurrently while the client is seeing the other professional. Another option is to encourage the client not to bring up issues that are clearly outside of our scope of practice or realm of expertise.

In summary, the within-boundaries areas are legitimate professional areas for SLPs and Auds to communicate with clients and families. The beyond-boundaries areas are issues that are clearly out of our scope of practice. Challenges to our boundaries are not always clearly delineated and may arise at any time in our work. We need to be very careful not to go beyond our education, training, and skill levels.

Setting Boundaries in the Therapeutic Relationship

Pipes and Davenport (1998) emphasize that "boundary" does not mean "wall" (with all the pejorative connotations accompanying such a term). Rather, from a counseling perspective, it refers to the characteristics of the relationship along the dimensions of (a) role behavior and (b) identification with the person with whom we are working. The concerns often are whether we are "getting too close" to the client and not maintaining our professional role, or whether we are identifying too closely with the issues the client is working on and losing our objectivity.

Counselors and psychotherapists use the term **therapeutic alliance** (Gelso & Samstag, 2008; Greenson, 1967) to mean the helping relationship and the relationship factors that maximize therapeutic effectiveness. It is frequently thought of as the bond or rapport between the client or family and the therapist (Feltham & Dryden, 2005), but also includes mutual respect, honesty, trust, and the agreed upon goals of therapy. The therapeutic alliance can be threatened or damaged, rather than enhanced, if the therapist tries too hard to establish rapport (e.g., too vigorous of a handshake, too warm of a greeting), or the therapist goes beyond professional boundaries in her discussions and interactions with a client.

The therapeutic alliance involves the establishment of the appropriate therapeutic distance (Gabbard & Wilkinson, 1994). **Therapeutic distance** refers to the interpersonal distance that we establish with clients. This distance can be too close, too far away, or optimal. **Therapeutic errors** occur when clinicians fail to adequately distinguish between the client's problems and their own problems, or when clinicians inadvertently violate boundaries in the therapy setting. If we are emotionally too involved with our clients, we are probably too close to be able to assess their situation with reasonable objectivity. For example, if a mother is discussing family conflicts that have been occurring because of her child's ADHD and the clinician starts recalling and focusing on the emotional difficulties in her own family with a younger sibling who has similar problems, the clinician may not be able to continue listening to the mother with sufficient therapeutic distance or focus. On the other hand, if we are too distant and detached from our clients we are unable to appreciate their problems with the necessary sensitivity. For example, if the client's lifestyle is very different from yours and impedes your ability to respond empathically you may run the risk of treating the client in a detached, distant manner.

Maintaining an optimal therapeutic distance places a priority on the client's needs rather than our own and always respects the professional nature of the relationship. Optimal therapeutic distance allows clinicians to view their clients holistically. Gladding (2009) explains that if a person is to be evaluated completely we need to understand the person's physical (e.g., general health, pain, or discomfort), intellectual (general intelligence and educational level), social (friendships and support systems), emotional (anxieties, fears), and environmental (home life and work) processes. The ideal is to understand the person as a whole, including beliefs, perceptions, and goals, and to realize that the mind and body are interacting systems, not separate entities (Nystul, 2005).

Another way of talking about excessive therapeutic distance is to identify the person's actions and behaviors that create this condition. Therapeutic distance is not just an attitude or frame of mind. Some professionals use distancing techniques (being aloof, cold, detached, monotone, having little facial expression, or showing lack of interest or concern about the person's thoughts and feelings) to prevent or decrease emotional involvement. Some professionals may avoid another person's pain in order to protect themselves emotionally, that is, so they do not need to confront their own feelings. Thus, excessive therapeutic distance involves the clinician's refusal of vulnerability, which likely has a deleterious effect on the client–therapist relationship (Adams, 1993).

Adams (1993, p. 35) also says that "Bedside manner has nothing to do with information about the patient. Bedside manner is the unabashed projection of love [of all people], humor, empathy, tenderness, and compassion for the patient. Scientific brilliance is an important tool, but it is not the magic inherent in healing." Many clients and patients are motivated to work in therapy and to practice their exercises not just to see their own improvement, but to please the clinician who has established a healthy and mutually rewarding therapeutic relationship.

CLIENTS AND FAMILIES SOMETIMES QUESTION THE CLINICIAN'S LIFE EXPERIENCES

Occasionally our professional credibility will be questioned on the basis of inadequate life experiences. This concern may be voiced in the form of questioning the clinician's apparent youth, status as an unmarried person, lack of experience in raising children, and so forth. Whatever the concern, the clinician needs to keep in mind the value of not reacting defensively. What clients are usually most concerned about when asking these kinds of questions is, "Are you competent to work with me with my kinds of problems?" The inquiry is likely one for information about the clinician and not necessarily an expression of resistance. (Note: Young psychologists, counselors, and psychiatrists have similar experiences.) A possible response to this challenging situation may sound like this: "That is a reasonable question (observation), and I believe you and I will get along fine. You are right in saying I'm younger than you (have not raised children, etc.), but I believe I can help you. My education and training have provided me knowledge and skills designed to help you, and I have been helpful to other people with similar problems. However, if you feel I am not able to do that, I will help you find someone you feel will be more helpful to you."

and tolerance of her speech. This feedback can then be shared with the parents as a *recommendation* rather than as a *criticism* of a particular family member's behavior.

Gladding (2009) suggests that counselors establish guidelines with parents and the minor about the nature of information that can be released to parents at the outset of the therapy. The American Counseling Association (ACA, 2005) provides an ethical code that can help structure guidelines for SLPs and Auds: "When counseling minors or persons unable to give voluntary informed consent, counselors act in clients' best interest" (Section A:3). The counselor can therefore release confidential information to parents when the counselor believes it is in the child's best interest. Examples of situations in which the therapist *must* communicate information to parents and/or to other authorities are situations where child abuse or neglect is suspected or the minor reveals a plan to harm himself. These situations are examined more fully in Chapter 14.

COUNSELING SKILLS IN ACTION

Concurrent Therapy with a Mental Health Professional

Some private clients I have worked with have voluntarily informed me that they are also concurrently working with a counselor, psychologist, or psychiatrist. I have, quite appropriately, not received reports from these other professionals working with my clients. A brief 10–15 minute telephone call to the psychologist can sometimes add or clarify relevant information about a client that can help me with my therapy. A client's work with a mental health professional is confidential and a client may choose what, if anything, to share with me. My evaluation and treatment progress reports are provided to clients, who have the option then of sharing them with other professionals in any way that they choose.

CLINICAL QUESTIONS

1. What kinds of information could a psychologist provide that could be helpful to a speech-language pathologist or audiologist?

2. How would you handle the confidentiality issue if you made a referral to a psychologist after your client told you details of her verbal arguments with her husband?

For the protection of both the client and clinician, it is wise to state the terms of confidentiality within the work setting, including who will see any information and why. If a court (judge) requests our documentation we *must* submit all documents (Fogle, 2003). If an attorney subpoenas our records we do not have to submit them until there is a court order. However, it is important to contact the client to inform him that his records have been subpoenaed and ask if he would like the records released. In any case, we must respond to a subpoena; we cannot ignore it (Nagy, 2005). The clinician must be the interpreter of his own reports; that is, the attorney or court will likely call upon the clinician to interpret the findings and specific statements in any subpoenaed reports (Fogle, 2000).

Team Approach

SLPs and Auds always work as team members with clients, families, and other professionals. The most important person on the team is the child, client, or patient, and without that person no other team members are necessary (Fogle, 2008). Therefore, at a minimum the team includes the child, client, or patient and the clinician. Additional team members may be parents, grandparents, spouses or partners, teachers, other school personnel, psychologists, administrators, nurses, physicians, PTs, OTs, respiratory therapists, social service and discharge planners, counselors, or psychiatrists. Professionally, we do not work in a vacuum. What we communicate and how we communicate to the other team members about our clients and patients can have significant impact on the other team members' interactions with the people we are trying to help. Much of what we communicate is data and observation-based information; for example, what is included in an evaluation of a child's speech, language, and hearing report or a medical note. However, as objective as we may try to sound or appear, our feelings about the child, client, or patient may emerge. If we have very positive feelings about the person we are trying to help, our choice of words, tone of voice, facial expressions, and body language will likely reflect our feelings. The same is true if we have negative feelings.

As team members, we need to be aware of the primary and secondary messages we are communicating. For example, we may be discussing our evaluation results about a client (primary message) and at the same time unknowingly revealing our negative feelings about the person (secondary message). Listeners (observers) note our words as well as our affect. If we are trying to sound positive about a client but our tone of voice, facial expressions, or body language belie our words, the other team members will receive mixed messages and may believe our nonverbal communications more than our verbal ones. The unintended messages that have "leaked out" may influence or alter their perceptions of the client or patient, and therefore possibly their interactions with the person. It is appropriate for us to alert other team members about concerns we have about a client or patient's behavior, affect, and cognition; although we need to be particularly careful to not unduly bias other team members.

Making Referrals

Shipley and Roseberry-McKibbon (2006) state that the referrals SLPs or Auds make to other professionals indicate the clinician's attempts to serve the client's best interests. We may make referrals to educational specialists such as reading specialists or to medical specialists such as otolaryngologists. We may refer a client to a psychologist or counselor when we feel the client's problems are beyond our scope of practice. We also may refer clients to other SLPs or Auds who have greater expertise in a particular area than we might have.

When we make referrals to other professionals we need to give clear, straightforward, but tactful reasons for our recommendations. Some clients may be reluctant to see another specialist, particularly a psychologist, psychiatrist, or other mental health professional. Clients may be concerned about the cost of other therapy, whether insurance will cover it, or the imagined stigma of seeing such a professional. We may avoid this stigma by suggesting that the client consult with or talk with another specialist, avoiding words such as *evaluate* or *psychotherapy*. *Talk with* is less threatening and likely to be more easily accepted by the client. The word *counselor* is often less threatening than psychologist, psychotherapist, or psychiatrist. Another method is to use descriptive phrases such as "see a specialist who can help with problems like you are experiencing." You also may emphasize the importance of the client's experiences, thus validating them rather than simply giving the impression that you want someone else to deal with the client's less desirable qualities, which may be what the client fears. Referrals, particularly to mental health professionals, should be done judiciously, carefully, and with tact. A client is most likely to follow through with seeking a referral when the clinician and client have developed a trusting relationship and the clinician feels the client will be receptive to the referral.

Referring a client or patient to another professional indicates that the clinician has provided the best service she can to that individual. It does not mean that she is inadequate or that her professional scope of practice is too narrow. It means that she recognizes her professional limitations (we all have them) and that she is working within her profession's scope of practice. When we receive referrals from another professional such as an otolaryngologist, psychologist, or education specialist it means that the person also recognizes his professional limitations and scope of practice, and that our education and training in speech-language pathology or audiology is the expertise needed to help the client or patient.

COUNSELING SKILLS IN ACTION

Another Therapist Was a Better Match

Over the years I have referred a few private clients to other SLPs whom I felt would be better suited (a better match) for a particular client. For example, I began working with a young adolescent girl with a voice problem and by the second session had the feeling that she could be better helped by a female SLP. I discussed this with the client and her mother, and then found an SLP to whom I felt confident referring the client.

In another case, I began working with a five-year-old boy with language problems, particularly word finding. I saw the young boy in his home. He was cooperative and willing to work with me, and I liked him. However, after several sessions I felt that I was not the best therapist for him and could not pinpoint just what was lacking in our working relationship. I discussed the issue with the parents and the child and, although they wanted me to continue, agreed that if I did not feel I was the best therapist to serve his needs, they would be willing to have another SLP take over. The SLP I chose to replace me developed an excellent working relationship with the child and family, was his therapist for quite a long time, and accomplished the goals that were needed.

CLINICAL QUESTIONS

1. What types of experiences or feedback would lead you to make a referral to another SLP or Aud?

2. How would you explain this decision to the client or family?

BIOETHICAL CONSIDERATIONS

To assist clinicians and allied health professionals in making ethically troublesome choices, several ethical principles have been identified that are important in health care. **Bioethical** concerns and problems may be evaluated with the following principles in mind (Aiken, 2008; Beauchamp & Childress, 2008).

Autonomy

The first ethical consideration involves the principle of respect for patient **autonomy**. This principle suggests that patients, rather than clinicians, are in the best position to evaluate and decide which interventions are in their own best interest. Not only is this principle bioethically important, it has important legal standing as well. The law upholds the right of patients to make their own decisions about their health care, including refusal of treatment, even if that treatment is necessary to maintain or save the patient's life. Furthermore, the principle of respect for patient autonomy leads to another important bioethical concept, namely informed consent.

Informed consent means that patients have a right to know the risks and benefits of treatment so that they can make their own care decisions in a fully informed manner. This right is matched by the clinician's corresponding duty to disclose the risks and benefits of the treatment in question. Both the principle of respect for patient autonomy and the duty of informed consent suggest that clinicians need to be direct and straightforward in their communications and recommendations for patient care. Clinicians must keep in mind that clients and their family members do not have to follow or accept our professional recommendations.

Beneficence and Nonmaleficence

A second bioethical consideration involves the principle of **beneficence**. According to this principle, health professionals have the duty to help patients while preventing harm to them. In general terms, the above ideas are often understood as the duty to help promote the patient's best interest and to contribute to their welfare. The desire to help is often a motive for deciding to become a health professional. It is important to keep in mind that the clinician's desire to help must at all times be carefully weighed against the patient's right to make his own health care decisions—a delicate balance that sometimes can play out in ways that lead to bioethical concerns and dilemmas.

The principle of beneficence is related to another bioethical consideration which involves the ancient Hippocratic mandate "Do No Harm!" This consideration is normally referred to as the principle of **nonmaleficence**. What this principle means in practical terms is that clinicians are ethically prohibited or prevented from inflicting injury or harm on their patients, although these notions do not necessarily always mean the same thing. While the idea of *injury* pertains mainly to interventions that can cause damage to the patient's physical body, *harm* is usually understood to refer to the infliction of damage to the patient's person (as distinct from her physical body) as such. Hence, it is possible for a clinician to harm a patient simply by failing to respect the patient's preferences or wishes for care, that is, by failing to respect her right to make her own health care decisions without interference from the clinician. In this light, it is easy to see that harm can apply to situations that involve no physical injury whatsoever to the patient.

In general, ethical considerations involving respect for the principle of patient autonomy as well as the duty to help and not to harm the patient apply to all aspects of our counseling. These principles require that professionals need to become well educated and trained in this essential area of our interactions with clients and their families so that what we say and do will be helpful to them and will reflect recognition of our scope of practice and the limits of our expertise.

CONCLUDING COMMENTS

This chapter provides a definition of counseling for speech-language pathologists and audiologists and explains the counseling processes that are inevitably intertwined with our everyday clinical work. Counseling is both a science and art, and we begin our study of this topic by distinguishing between the technical or scientific aspects of this process and the interpersonal aspects of creating a caring, professional relationship. You are likely to already have many, if not most, of the personal qualities of effective helpers fairly well developed. Knowledge of relevant psychological concepts and counseling skills can facilitate the process of more intentionally and thoughtfully selecting strategies to use when counseling clients. Throughout our discussion of counseling skills we must keep in mind the scope of our professional competencies and the limits of our practice so that we can recognize and refer clients when needed to a mental health professional.

Discussion Questions

1. What counseling skills do you view as most critical to your professional work?

2. Discuss the differences between using counseling skills and being a counselor.

3. Discuss the importance of having a counseling course in your education that relates specifically to speech-language pathology and audiology.

4. Of the numerous personal qualities of effective helpers discussed in this chapter, which ones do you feel are some of your strongest? Some of your weakest? How might you strengthen your weakest personal qualities?

5. How would you rate your tolerance for ambiguity on a 1–10 scale (1 = low tolerance, 10 = high tolerance)? What improvements can you make in this area and how would you go about improving this aspect of your clinical performance?

6. What are some challenges to boundaries you have been confronted with in your clinical work thus far? How did you respond and what was the result of that response? How would you respond now?

7. When you have difficulty achieving an optimal therapeutic distance from clients, do you tend to be too distant or too close? What do you need to do differently?

8. How do you structure your therapy environment to maintain comfortable boundaries?

9. What life experiences do you have or lack that you feel may affect your credibility with the parents of a child? An adolescent who stutters? A married woman with a voice disorder? An elderly man with aphasia?

10. What might you say to:
    a. A parent who asks you how you could know anything about raising a child with problems when you are not even a parent? Or do not have a child with a problem (or the same problem)?
    b. An adolescent who stutters who asks you how you know anything about what it feels like to stutter when you have never had the problem?
    c. A married woman whose voice disorder appears to be partly the result of family stress when she asks you how you could know anything about the stresses of married life and being a parent when you are not married or do not have children?
    d. An elderly man with aphasia who communicates that you do not understand what it is like to be old and not be able to understand or talk to other people?

11. Discuss a counseling experience you had or can imagine in which you were uncertain about breaking confidentiality by sharing information with a parent.

Theories of Counseling: Application to Speech-Language Pathology and Audiology

CHAPTER OUTLINE

- Introduction
- Humanistic Approaches to Counseling
- Interpersonal Approaches to Counseling
- Behavioral Approaches to Counseling
- Cognitive Approaches to Counseling
- Family Systems Approaches to Counseling
- Existential Approaches to Counseling
- Multicultural Approaches to Counseling
- Theoretical Integration
- Concluding Comments
- Discussion Questions
- Role Plays

INTRODUCTION

Many exceptional practitioners have learned to integrate a number of theories of psychotherapy with their personal therapy experiences and over time have developed an individual style of therapy (Corsini & Wedding, 2008; Gladding, 2009; Truscott, 2010). Meanwhile, most beginning therapists are working to master a particular theory and its applications. However, no one theory or therapy approach fits all situations, and a clinician may actually apply multiple therapy approaches with any one client, patient, or family. The theoretical and therapy approaches that an individual clinician selects and uses often depends on the clinician's personal orientation (e.g., humanistic, behavioral, or multicultural), what the clinician has learned in her training, and what has worked for the clinician in the past. There is no one "right" theoretical or therapeutic framework, although empirical research during the last couple of decades has provided more validation for some therapeutic approaches than for others (e.g., American Psychological Association, 2005; Hibbs & Jensen, 2005; Messer, 2004). As it is impossible to learn and use the over 400 counseling and psychotherapy approaches that are currently in the literature (Prochaska & Norcross, 2009), speech-language pathologists and audiologists can be most effective by learning about a few of the major theories that offer relevant concepts that can be applied to our professions. The theories presented in this chapter are among those that are considered to form the conceptual and clinical bedrock of the fields of clinical psychology and counseling (Corsini & Wedding, 2008; Wachtel & Messer, 1997).

There is much value in a clinician having multiple theoretical and therapeutic frameworks from which to draw. If a clinician only has one or two to select from, she is limited in ability to understand and help clients, patients, and families. ("If a person only has a hammer, then everything looks like a nail.") Theoretical purity (i.e., following a singular approach) is seldom helpful with the vast variety of people and problems we work with. Lazarus and Beutler (1993) found that 60 to 70 percent of professional counselors identify themselves as *eclectic* in the use of theory and techniques. However, beyond a piecemeal eclectic approach we can use an *integrative* approach in which we tie together concepts and approaches that have commonalties or are complementary to each other. For further reading in the area of psychotherapy and counseling theories, the student or clinician may wish to refer to one of many excellent textbooks in the area, for example, Capuzzi and Gross (2003); Corey (2008); Corsini and Wedding (2008); George and Cristiani (1995); Gurman and Messer (2003); Prochaska and Norcross (2009). A personal favorite of the author (L.V. F.) is the Prochaska and Norcross text, which inspired the format for this chapter and the presentation of a case example seen through the lenses of various theoretical perspectives.

This chapter begins with two therapy approaches that emphasize the clinician–client relationship: understanding how to use the relationship to promote therapeutic change. It then moves into therapies that emphasize helping people change their ways of thinking about particular issues and their problematic behaviors as they relate to our professions. Additional therapy approaches are discussed that help expand our way of seeing the client or patient's world as well as our own.

HUMANISTIC APPROACHES TO COUNSELING

Carl Rogers (1951, 1957, 1961, 1980) developed in the 1940s and 1950s what is known today as humanistic therapy and client-centered (person-centered) therapy. Rogers emphasizes that people are rational and inclined toward positive growth or **self-actualization** (realizing one's potential). This viewpoint is considered the central assumption of humanistic therapy. Healthy personality development occurs if the person receives sufficient **unconditional positive regard**, that is, love and acceptance from parents or significant others for her unique, individual self. Often times the best example of unconditional positive regard is the love and acceptance a parent has for her child. For example, the parents of a child with hearing impairments who show consistent love and acceptance help the child to grow and develop feelings of self-worth. The child learns **congruence**, that is, to be in touch with her own thoughts and feelings, and to communicate with facial expressions and body language that mirrors (i.e., is consistent with) verbal or sign language.

Unhealthy personality development occurs when an individual experiences conditions of worth, repeatedly receiving messages from parents that she will be loved and accepted only if certain conditions are met; for example, the child must never cry or show anger and, instead, must be compliant, studious, and easy to get along with. As a result of these experiences, the child learns to conceal her real self and present a façade that is incongruent (discrepant with what the child thinks, feels, and expresses verbally or nonverbally) with her genuine feelings. In presenting a façade, the child sacrifices natural tendencies toward positive growth in order to receive conditional love and approval. For example, a child with a hearing loss may not feel accepted by parents when she observes that they give more attention and love ("regard") to siblings. The child with a hearing impairment may try to conceal from parents that she could not hear or understand them in order to appear more like her siblings.

SLPs or Auds using humanistic or person-centered techniques attempt to promote the client's natural positive striving and growth. The clinician's role is **nondirective** (not trying to influence; being primarily reflective) and supportive. The clinician avoids engaging in confrontation or direct attempts to change the person's behavior.

Conditions Necessary and Sufficient for Therapeutic Change

Rogers (1957) discussed therapeutic conditions that he regards as necessary and sufficient for therapeutic change, which are outlined in the following sections.

GENUINENESS

The genuine clinician presents herself in an open manner and is not showing a façade. The clinician behaves in a way that is congruent (consistent and genuine) with her real feelings. For example, if a client comments to the clinician, "You look tired today," the clinician may say, "Yes, you're right, I am a little tired today." In this response, the clinician validates the client's (correct) perceptions.

Presenting a congruent response is challenging when how we feel toward a client is not congruent with how we think we *should* feel toward the client. For example, we may feel irritated with a client who has not followed through with exercises or comes late to sessions. Yet we are striving to respond respectfully and therapeutically. If we are not careful, what the client may experience is a mixed message based upon our real feelings "leaking out." Our behavior may be polite on the surface but contain undertones of anger or resentment. Another example of incongruence may occur when the clinician is not aware of how angry or annoyed he actually is with the client.

In either case above, the clinician focuses on presenting a positive and warm response to the client. However, the client may perceive both levels of the clinician's response: the polite surface behaviors and the angry, irritated undertones. The incongruence between the two levels of communication will likely cause discomfort in the client, and the client may respond negatively. The clinician, unaware of the client's perceptions, may view the client as uncooperative, unappreciative, or difficult. In order to work with this challenging situation, the clinician first needs to become aware of any tendency toward an incongruent response, and work through the negative feelings toward the client rather than just trying to conceal them. The clinician also may choose to express feelings to the client in a non-threatening manner using "I-messages" (e.g., "When you do . . . , I feel . . .") As we have seen in the above example, trying to conceal negative feelings often does not work and can impair the clinician's working relationship with a client.

Working through negative feelings towards a client involves trying to better understand the client's viewpoint (empathy). The clinician may want to ask herself some questions, such as, "What stops the client from coming on time?" or "What is the client afraid of?" Usually if the clinician can better understand the client's fears, behaviors, and life circumstances, she will feel more empathic and less annoyed with the client. The point is that the clinician needs to reflect on her own behavior toward the client and not simply blame the client. By taking these steps the clinician will be better able to develop or return to a stance of unconditional positive regard toward the client. It is important to note that Rogers' (1957) concept of clinicians' genuineness has sometimes been misunderstood as a license for clinicians to talk about themselves or engage in excessive self-disclosure. This was not Rogers' intention; he was primarily concerned with the idea that clinicians should not feign interest or caring, as this façade is likely to be detected by clients and damage the therapeutic relationship.

EMPATHY

Empathy involves "being with" the person and his experiences on a moment-to-moment basis. It involves a personal encounter, not simply an objective appraisal of the person's problems. In order for the clinician to experience and show empathy, she must understand not only the communication disorder (e.g., stuttering), but how the communication disorder is affecting the person's self-image and life. Although we can never truly feel what the client is experiencing, we can try to get a sense of what the person must cope with almost every time he tries to talk.

In striving to be empathic, clinicians should take care not to go overboard. Sometimes excessive efforts to appear friendly, caring, and empathic, especially in the early stages of the working relationship, can appear phony and disingenuous to the client. This is a different kind of incongruence than discussed above. In this case the clinician is trying to appear warmer and more empathic than she is truly feeling. The clinician may have good intentions, for instance, to help the client feel understood and valued, but a saccharine (i.e., too sweet and overly caring) presentation may be viewed negatively by clients.

UNCONDITIONAL POSITIVE REGARD

When SLPs and Auds communicate genuine respect and caring in a consistent manner to clients they are demonstrating unconditional positive regard. This allows clients to experience a nonjudgmental environment in therapy, which may encourage them to be more honest with the clinician, such as when they cannot (or will not) perform therapy tasks with maximum involvement or effort.

In humanistic therapy there is an emphasis on providing a positive relationship rather than on therapeutic techniques. As the person expresses himself, however, the clinician is alert for statements pertaining to the self (for example, "I haven't felt like doing my exercises lately" or "I don't understand how these exercises will help"). The clinician also attends to the person's nonverbal communications that are incongruent with verbal communications (e.g., smiling while discussing a negative feeling or personal loss).

In order to help both the client and clinician understand the client's feelings, the clinician may provide reflections that paraphrase the statements or, when needed, point out discrepancies in the communications (these skills, rooted in Rogers' theory, are expanded in Chapter 4). To provide a simple reflection the clinician should let the person know she has been heard and that the clinician is interested in hearing more. The clinician's reflections should, however, not simply mimic or parrot the client's last words. For example, a patient may mention symptoms that suggest penetration of food or liquid into the larynx (e.g., episodes of coughing or choking), and then deny that they are a problem. The clinician may reflect on both of these statements and then ask about the person's feelings. The patient may be feeling embarrassment or have fear around meal times. For example, the clinician might say, "You say you are doing some coughing and choking while eating, but that it's not really a problem for you. Are you sometimes a little embarrassed about coughing and choking, or are you a little afraid that you won't be able to continue eating regular food?" While it is important not to force a particular interpretation on a client or to assume what he is feeling, the clinician can ask questions such as these which express empathy for the client's probable experiences. Providing an environment where all of the client's feelings and experiences are respected and validated is central to humanistic therapy and can maximize disclosure in therapy sessions.

COUNSELING SKILLS IN ACTION

Reflecting Empathy to a Child Who Stutters

A 13-year-old boy was brought to therapy by his parents because of the child's stuttering problem.

Clinician: "Tell me what it's like to talk in different situations."

Child: "I don't talk much at school. It makes me nervous."

Clinician: "You don't talk much because it makes you nervous."

Child: "Yeah, and I get *really* nervous about speaking out in front of the class."

Clinician: "Speaking out in front of the class. Is that one of the hardest things for you to do?"

Child: "Uh huh, especially if the teacher wants me to read from the science book."

Clinician: "You don't like to read out loud from the science book." (The clinician is staying very close to what the child says, but not sounding like a mechanical parrot.)

Child: "Yeah, the words are tough and I get stuck on them and I make a fool of myself."

Clinician: "So you are afraid of stuttering or making a mistake and being embarrassed about that."

Child: "The guys will laugh at me."

CLINICAL QUESTIONS

1. How might you encourage a child to continue to provide helpful information without the child feeling judged or criticized?

2. How might you respond if the child tells you that one of his classmates has teased him, calling him "retarded" and "dumb"?

CASE STUDY

Michael and a Humanistic Counseling Approach

Throughout this chapter Michael and his family will be used to illustrate how various therapy approaches and strategies can be applied to working with a fairly complex case.

Michael is a 12-year-old seventh-grade boy who sustained a closed head injury from a motor vehicle versus bicycle accident. He was not wearing a helmet at the time of the accident. He is in an acute-care hospital in his small hometown. Prior to the accident, Michael, according to his parents and teacher, was well adjusted, well liked by his peers, and a good student with no learning disabilities. He was athletic and enjoyed soccer and baseball.

Michael's father, John, is a computer programmer, and his mother, Margaret, is a third-grade elementary schoolteacher at the school Michael attends. Michael has a 14-year-old brother, Steven, and an eight-year-old sister, Lisa. Steven has reportedly always had difficulty in school and has been a behavioral challenge at home. Lisa is doing well in school and has no significant behavioral problems. Michael's maternal grandparents (Joe and Martha) live near the family and are very involved in the lives of all three grandchildren.

Michael's neurological injuries include frontal lobe damage, contrecoup damage, and damage to both left and right temporal lobes. He has been diagnosed with moderate receptive and expressive aphasia, moderate cognitive impairments affecting his attention, immediate and recent memories, and sequencing and organizational abilities. His judgment, reasoning, and problem solving also are moderately impaired. His speech is characterized by mild to moderate dysarthria with respiration and phonation within normal limits, but mild hypernasality and moderate weakness of the mandible, lips, and tongue. He is approximately 90 percent intelligible at the single-word level, 80 percent at the phrase and short sentence level, and 70 percent at the conversational level. He does not have dysphagia.

Michael is currently at a Rancho Level 6, Confused-Appropriate, with some emerging Level 7, Automatic-Appropriate, behavior as evaluated from the Revised Rancho Levels of Cognitive Functioning (Hagen, 1998). Michael shows the following signs and symptoms from the Rancho Scales: inconsistent orientation to person and place; able to attend to highly familiar tasks in non-distracting environments for 30 minutes with moderate redirection; remote memory with more depth and detail than recent memory; vague recognition of some staff; emerging awareness of appropriate responses to himself, family, and basic needs; emerging goal-directed behavior related to meeting basic personal needs; lack of awareness of impairments, disabilities, and safety risks with unrealistic planning for the future (Fogle, Reece, & White, 2008); following simple commands; and verbal expressions appropriate in highly familiar and structured situations.

The parents are experiencing guilt related to not requiring Michael to wear a helmet when riding his bicycle. His older brother is concerned that Michael may now be "retarded" and an embarrassment to the family. His sister is confused about why Michael does not understand what she says, why he sounds so different and acts so funny. Michael's grandmother, Martha, has been concerned for some time about the freedom his mother has given him, which has been a source of tension between the parents and grandparents. The grandfather just wants his favorite grandson to get better.

Patients with TBI commonly have behaviors that are disagreeable to both the family and the rehabilitation staff. Michael's father, who is known for his impatience and somewhat intolerant attitudes, is having difficulty accepting the "new" Michael. John is demonstrating cold and distancing behaviors (aloofness, detachment, monotone voice, little warmth in facial expressions, and stiff, noncomforting touch) toward Michael. The SLP notices the father's behaviors and knows that it is important for Michael to receive as much warmth and acceptance as possible from everyone in contact with him. The SLP also knows that the father is an important communication partner for Michael, and the father's withdrawal may interfere with Michael's improvement in rehabilitation. The SLP shows genuine empathy for the father and his difficulty accepting his son as he is now. The SLP does not distance herself from the father, but rather presents unconditional positive regard so the father does not feel judged. The therapist realizes that her relationship with the father is very important for the total team approach; interventions with Michael's family members as well as with Michael directly are essential to Michael's rehabilitation.

Some clinicians may feel distressed by the father's withdrawal and lack of involvement with his son. They may even feel irritated with the father for not providing more unconditional love and support. In experiencing these responses to Michael's father, the SLP may find it challenging to maintain a congruent relationship. The SLP may feel a need to suppress the urge to criticize the father for his failure to provide more support in Michael's time of need. The clinician will need to empathize with the father's fears and anxieties in order to feel less judgmental toward him. Once the clinician can do that, she has a better chance to approach the father with a genuine and caring manner, even if she does not approve of all his responses toward his son.

The father's behaviors also may contain incongruencies. He may indicate that he is having difficulty spending time with Michael and seeing him as the same son he was before. John may try to smile while saying this to the SLP. The clinician may

CASE STUDY

Michael and a Behavioral Counseling Approach

Michael has a variety of excesses, deficits, and inappropriate behaviors. Michael tends to have perseverative behaviors, responding to different verbal stimuli with the same answers. He has deficits in his immediate and recent memory, making it difficult for new learning to occur. He has inappropriate behaviors such as swearing and occasional striking out at caregivers.

In patient care conferences and rehabilitation team meetings, the SLP will want to describe specific behaviors Michael is demonstrating that can then be care-planned so that all the team members respond to Michael's behaviors in consistent, nonpunitive ways. The family and other visitors should be informed how the rehabilitation team members are managing various behaviors and how the family can respond to Michael in ways that are consistent and reinforce the work of the therapists.

COGNITIVE APPROACHES TO COUNSELING

Behavioral therapists now include the role of cognitions (thoughts) in determining behavior (Beck, 1995; Mahoney, 1974, 2004; Meichenbaum, 1999; Wilson & Franks, 1982). However, cognitive therapists have always recognized that thoughts influence behaviors. People do not just respond to events but to their interpretations and beliefs about events. For example, when a student clinician arrives late to a therapy session one supervisor may feel the student has a legitimate reason for being late and, therefore, treats the student in an accepting manner. Another supervisor, however, may interpret the student's lateness as a sign of the student's irresponsibility and lack of professionalism, and therefore respond to the student in an aloof, cold manner.

Cognitive therapists recognize that there are countless perspectives or interpretations of any given event. Furthermore, the way in which people think about events (their perceptions) determines how they feel about themselves, others, and the future (Beck, 1995; Corey, 2008; George & Cristiani, 1995; Gladding, 2009; Prochaska & Norcross, 2009). For example, a patient who is discharged from therapy before feeling he has reached maximum potential may interpret the discharge to mean that he is not worth the clinician's time, the clinician is uncaring, and the patient will never get better now. It is clear that this sequence of thoughts can affect a patient's mood and behavior.

Cognitive theorists believe that certain core beliefs affect our behavior with others (Beck, 1995; Mahoney, 2004). These core beliefs are often learned early in life and become part of the assumptions we make about people. For example, "People are basically good" and "I can trust medical professionals to take good care of me" may represent some individuals' core beliefs. These thoughts and beliefs are automatic and we are not likely to evaluate them, so they persist in an unscrutinized form. In many situations a person's core beliefs work to the clinician's advantage. The person may have had an earlier positive experience with an SLP (e.g., the person's child benefited from speech therapy), and now the person has sustained a traumatic brain injury and maintains the automatic belief that an SLP will help her too. Any previous experience with a clinician, whether positive or negative, may influence the client's thoughts and behaviors toward a clinician.

Cognitive therapy has been applied to understanding and treating depression as well as many other mood, behavior, and anxiety disorders (Beck, 1967, 1995; Christner, Stewart-Allen, & Freeman, 2007; Clark & Beck, 2009; Persons, Davidson, & Tompkins, 2001). Depressed individuals are regarded as having pessimistic assumptions about themselves, other people, and the future in general. For example, a depressed individual might think, "I can't win," "People don't like me," and "I can't control what happens to me." Further, they might be inclined to selectively attend to negative experiences that confirm their beliefs and to ignore experiences that are inconsistent with their beliefs. For example, a child with an auditory processing disorder (APD) and attention deficit disorder who has had numerous failures in school and poor peer relationships may have negative expectations for the new school year that has just started. He may tend not to notice positive events such as a teacher's praise or a classmate's attempts to get him involved in play activities. What the child tends to notice (or misinterpret) are the behaviors that confirm his negative beliefs about himself.

The essential purpose of cognitive therapy is to help the individual recognize and examine tightly held but problematic beliefs and replace them with more adaptive and flexible ways of thinking. The goal in therapy is to examine the evidence that these beliefs are true, to refute them if erroneous, and then to construct rational, behavioral steps for coping with the erroneous thinking (Beck, 1995; Craighead et al., 1994; Ellis & Grieger, 1986; Mahoney, 2004; Persons, Davidson, & Tompkins, 2001; Prochaska & Norcross, 2009).

Many times SLPs and Auds work with a person's faulty beliefs surrounding the communication problem. This is frequently seen in children and adults who stutter (Conture & Curlee, 2007; Guitar, 2006; Zebrowski, 2002; Zebrowski & Kelly, 2002). For example, children and adults may have negative beliefs that affect their expectations of their ability to improve. The child or adult who has been stuttering for years will likely have low expectations of her potential to become more fluent. The person may lack experience with interactions with someone else who stutters and, therefore, may believe that her stuttering problems are unique. The clinician may want to help the person recognize that she is not alone, and that there are many people who stutter, even though the person has not encountered them. In this way the clinician is helping the person to recognize and modify her faulty beliefs.

Cognitive Distortions

Common types of erroneous thinking or **cognitive distortions** (Beck, Rush, Shaw, & Emery, 1979; Craighead et al., 1994; Prochaska & Norcross, 2009) include:

■ **Catastrophizing**   The person frequently believes the worst will happen, or, if something bad can happen, it will happen to him. For example, "If I don't get my voice back by next week, I may lose my job." A cognitive therapy intervention may include helping the person see the actual probabilities of the worst happening and focusing on evidence that the worst will not likely happen.

■ **"I Should" Statements**   These typically reflect perfectionistic tendencies and an intolerance of personal flaws. For example, a patient with dysphagia may say, "I should be able to eat my meals without any help." Or a patient with speech apraxia declares, "I should be able to say it, but I can't." A cognitive therapy intervention may include helping the person "free" herself from her "I should" self-statements and understand that what she has been able to do easily before her swallowing or communication problem cannot be done safely or easily now.

■ **Dichotomous Thinking**   The person views events and experiences as one extreme or the other (i.e., all good or all bad). For example, the client talks very negatively about his abilities or about another clinician. A cognitive therapy intervention may include helping the person view his abilities and other people and experiences on a continuum, where he (the client) is not the worst at some skill but can see himself as having some nascent skills. The clinician may no longer be viewed as "all bad" but as a competent professional who made an error at one point.

■ **Overgeneralizations**   The person believes that if something is true in one case, it applies to any case that is similar. Disfluent children, for example, overgeneralize fears of speaking situations such as speaking up in class to speaking in front of small groups of children. Many discouraged patients make incorrect inferences based upon one or two isolated events. After a new patient with a laryngectomy fails to easily learn esophageal speech, the patient may think, "I'll never be able to do this." After one hospital staff member treats a patient rudely or sternly, she concludes, "Everyone here is a jerk. No one here cares about me." A cognitive therapy intervention may include helping the person understand that her logic (thinking) may not be accurate and to help the person recognize exceptions to her rule.

SLPs using cognitive therapy techniques vary in how confrontational they choose to be with individuals who are demonstrating various forms of faulty thinking. However, the common theme is that they do not take a person's beliefs at face value; they question them and help the person develop more positive and realistic interpretations of experiences. While recognizing that people may have developed their negative beliefs early in their lives, the clinician using cognitive therapy techniques focuses on challenging and changing the current beliefs that interfere with a logical and rational approach to the communication problem.

COUNSELING SKILLS IN ACTION

Using Cognitive Therapy Techniques with a 13-Year-Old Girl

Lisa, a 13-year-old girl with a repaired cleft lip and palate who continues to have some hypernasality, is anticipating a future surgical revision of her lip. She says, "If I don't get my lip repaired perfectly, I'll never be pretty and no one will like me. I won't get invited to a prom, no one will ever marry me, I'll never have children, and I'll die alone." The SLP may begin to gently challenge the girl's beliefs in the following way:

SLP: "It sounds like you are really feeling discouraged now. I'm wondering, though, how much of what you are saying is actually true. For instance, when you say no one will like you, I'm wondering if you have some friends now, despite the scar on your lip and your speech problem."

Lisa: "Yes, I do have a couple of friends."

SLP: "And have they seen the scar on your lip and heard you talk?"

Lisa: "Well, of course. Who could miss it or not hear me sound like I talk through my nose?"

SLP: "So they haven't refused to be your friend because of your lip and speech."

Lisa: "Well, I guess not."

SLP: "Even though your lip and speech bother you, they don't prevent your friends from liking you. What do you think they like about you?"

Lisa: "Well I like to do a lot of things, so we play volleyball and go shopping together."

SLP: "So if these girls like you, what are the chances that you will find other friends in the future, even boyfriends?"

Lisa: "Well, maybe you have a point. Maybe I was getting a little carried away."

CLINICAL QUESTIONS

1. What are examples of Lisa's catastrophizing? Dichotomous thinking? Overgeneralization?
2. What might be some other ways you could help Lisa with her cognitive distortions?

CASE STUDY

Michael and a Cognitive Counseling Approach

As you recall, Michael is a 12-year-old seventh-grade boy who sustained a closed head injury from a motor vehicle versus bicycle accident. He has been in rehabilitation receiving speech therapy, physical therapy, and occupational therapy for the past four weeks, making steady but slow progress. However, for the past two weeks Michael has refused to actively participate in his speech therapy as well as physical and occupational therapy. Michael is showing depressed affect and expressing a sense of hopelessness about his future, getting back to school, and playing soccer and baseball again.

Michael is making statements such as, "If my speech doesn't get better, I'll fail school and lose all of my friends" (a catastrophizing statement), "I should be able to talk right by now" (an "I should" statement), and "You're not helping me" (an overgeneralization). The SLP may begin by gently challenging Michael's perceptions that he is not making progress in therapy. The clinician may ask Michael if his speech and memory are better now than they were a few weeks ago. The clinician may also show Michael a graph with his improvement in various areas of his speech therapy. The clinician may ask how often he now has to repeat what he says in order to be understood by others. Michael may then realize that he has to repeat himself much less frequently than he did a few weeks ago. Through these various methods of providing evidence of Michael's progress, the clinician challenges the patient's pessimistic beliefs and helps him to develop more positive and realistic beliefs about his therapy.

FAMILY SYSTEMS APPROACHES TO COUNSELING

A variety of schools of family therapy emerged in the 1950s to 1960s, which presented a radical alternative to mainstream approaches to clinical psychology and the study of mental illness in individuals (Bateson, Jackson, Haley, & Weakland, 1956; Bowen, 1978; Haley & Hoffman, 1968; Minuchin, 1974, 1978; Satir, 1976, 1983). Pioneers of these theories emphasized that a person's emotional problems must be viewed in the context of the family's roles, communications, and interactions. Individuals do not have emotional or behavioral symptoms in a vacuum, but rather develop and maintain their symptoms in a dysfunctional family context where there are faulty communication and interaction patterns and/or faulty family structure. Because these theories focus on family relationships and systems rather than individuals, they are often referred to as systems theories (Becvar & Becvar, 2009; Doherty & McDaniel, 2010; Hoffman, 2002).

A basic premise of the family therapy model is that each person (family member) in the family system affects all other members and the system is *inter*dependent. Within the family system are subsystems, for example, mother–father, mother–son, father–daughter, grandparent–grandchild, and so forth. Another basic premise is that separate elements (e.g., an individual's behavior) cannot be understood apart from the whole system (the family). Thus, a person's behavior that appears problematic or puzzling may be better understood by examining it in the family context.

While there are at least a half-dozen separate schools of family therapy, some concepts are universally accepted (Gladding, 2009; Goldenberg & Goldenberg, 2007; Prochaska & Norcross, 2009). Many of these were developed by two institutes in Palo Alto, California, which shared the assumption that communication is the key to understanding human behavior. Some of the well-known pioneers of this communications approach to family therapy include Bateson et al. (1956), Satir (1976, 1983), Watzlawick (1978), and Weakland (1976). These individuals studied the complex patterns of communication occurring in families, looking at verbal and nonverbal dimensions and overt versus covert messages. They believed that emotional and behavioral symptoms might develop in children and adults because of repeatedly receiving mixed messages from family members. Typically, these mixed messages are ones in which the verbal and the nonverbal (covert) messages are contradictory. The covert message may be conveyed through voice inflection, body language, and facial expression.

Jack and His Parents

A six-year-old boy with moderate to severe disfluency was referred to me by the Stuttering Foundation of America. When I work with a child who stutters much of my focus is on the parents, helping them identify attitudes and behaviors they may have that may be contributing to disfluencies of their child and how they can change those attitudes and behaviors (Fogle, 1978; Ramig & Dodge, 2010; Zebrowski & Kelly, 2002). Parents are often unaware of many of the overt and covert attitudes and behaviors they present to their children. Therefore, when working with the parents I use the *Modified Children's Report of Parental Behavior Inventory* (MCRPBI) (Fogle, 1978; Schaefer, 1965; Yairi, 1970; Yairi & Williams, 1971) to identify many of these attitudes and behaviors. The MCRPBI is a 192-item questionnaire which is divided into 19 scales that assesses various areas of attitudes and behaviors parents may have toward their child, for example, acceptance, rejection, positive involvement, hostile control, withdrawal of relations, positive attitudes toward speech, and negative attitudes toward speech. Assessing parental attitudes and behaviors can help to identify areas for needed change.

Jack's parents told me that their son's stuttering sometimes annoyed, upset, or embarrassed them, but that they did not think he noticed their feelings. When Jack tried to talk to his parents they would tell him how much they enjoyed hearing his stories about school, but their tense body language and facial expressions and loss of eye contact telegraphed a different message to the child. The overt message was an invitation for the child to tell the parents about his school day, while the covert message was the parents' communication of disapproval, anxiety, and embarrassment about his stuttering.

The child's natural response to the perceived covert messages was to withdraw. Such mixed messages placed the child in a quandary where he might be punished (e.g., reprimanded for not talking about his school day) for correct interpretation of covert messages. After several weeks of therapy with the parents, they became aware of and were able to modify many of their attitudes and behaviors that were contributing to Jack's disfluency, and the child's stuttering diminished significantly. This left fewer changes for the child to make in his stuttering and allowed for a more permanent improvement of his speech problem. Had the therapy focused solely on the child, the family dynamics would likely have changed little, creating a more difficult environment for the child to make and maintain improvements in his fluency.

CLINICAL QUESTIONS

1. What might you say to parents if you are concerned that their parenting behavior may be hindering their child's speech production and fluency?

2. How might you respond if the parents protest your interpretation and declare, "You are wrong. We really do want Jack to speak more!"

Continues on next page

> *Continued from previous page*
>
> **3.** Without an instrument such as the *Modified Children's Report of Parental Behavior Inventory*, how might you identify overt and covert attitudes and behaviors parents may have toward their child?

Hospitalized patients also may receive mixed messages that make it difficult to know what to do. Elderly people and stroke survivors, in particular, may receive contradictory messages that cause them to wonder just what their family truly wants. For example, many elderly individuals stoically accept the situation when their adult children offer for the elderly parent to come to live with them but then do nothing to help the parent make the transition. The real message is unstated but clear. When stroke survivors or elderly people are able to return home, they are often excluded from normal family activities, sometimes because they are unable to participate in physical or communication activities, and at other times because no one makes sufficient effort to include the person. When a person is unnecessarily excluded from family activities, the communication disorder becomes a true handicap (Tanner, 2008).

Individuals like the patient in the following case study may become especially sensitive to covert messages that are expressed repeatedly and, as a result, develop behavioral symptoms such as food refusal or incontinence. The key ideas here are that mixed messages (e.g., "I really want you to come home, but . . .") put the recipient in a bind in which no course of action seems acceptable. Meanwhile, the person who gives the complex communication is typically unaware of the double-sided nature of the message. However, the complex message may reflect internal conflicts and feelings that are viewed as unacceptable such as, "I really don't want to take care of my mother after she leaves the hospital," or "My child's stuttering embarrasses me." Rather than directly expressing feelings that may go against a person's principles, they "leak out" in the form of mixed messages. A clinician who understands this communication process can help the family to identify the incongruent messages being conveyed and to work towards therapeutic decision making without negatively labeling any of the family members.

CASE STUDY

Mom and Her Son

An elderly person who is convalescing after a stroke may hear her grown son's invitation, "Mom, we want you to come live with us now so that you have someone to help take care of you." At the same time, however, the elderly patient hears her son's heavy sighing and worries about space in the home and financial matters. The patient may experience this as a lose-lose situation. Neither response (i.e., to accept her son's offer or to decline it) solves the dilemma. If she accepts her son's offer, she may feel (correctly) that he will be burdened by her presence and needs. If she declines his offer and tries to live alone, she may contribute to his further worry and rumination about her safety. The patient in this situation may act strangely, refuse medication, or behave in other ways that postpone medical recommendation for hospital discharge. In effect, her behavior serves to stall decision making in a no-win situation. The SLP who is aware of the patient's situation is likely to be empathic and better understand her occasional difficult behaviors.

CLINICAL QUESTIONS

1. How might you communicate your understanding of the patient's predicament to help increase her compliance and cooperation in therapy?

2. What might you say to the adult son about his mixed feelings?

SLPs and Auds have used family systems therapy concepts for decades with a variety of disorders (Boles & Lewis, 2003; Guitar, 2006; Holland, 2007; Luterman, 2008; Tye-Murray, 2009; Shames, 2006). Watts Pappas and McLeod (2009), Andrews (1986) and Andrews and Andrews (1990) emphasize family system therapy concepts with language-impaired children. Mary Andrews, a trained family therapist, and James Andrews, an SLP, describe techniques for helping children with language disorders within a family-based approach. The blueprint for family-centered early intervention is the Individualized Family Service Plan (IFSP) which includes (1) making a contract with the family, (2) planning for and conducting an assessment of the child, (3) identifying family strengths and needs, (4) developing outcome statements, (5) implementing the plan of treatment, and (6) evaluating the plan. This process is discussed in detail by McGonigal, Kaufman, and Johnson (1991). Andrews and Andrews emphasize the value of encouraging all family members to participate in the evaluation and treatment of a child with a hearing or communication impairment. Family members are likely to accept an invitation to participate when it is made clear that they can be helpful to their child by being involved from the initial evaluation and throughout therapy.

Family systems concepts also can be used by paying attention to the labels that family members give to one another (e.g., my "bright" child, my "problem" child, my "handicapped" child) and the way those labels affect the therapist's perceptions of the client. Negative comments or innuendoes from family members may bias the clinician in subtle ways about the client. Novice clinicians may have a tendency to be compliant with family members who present themselves as the authority in the family, affecting the therapist's perceptions of the client and their treatment efforts.

Family therapy emphasizes concern about the negative labels family members use to describe the client or patient that may bias the clinician (Minuchin, 1978; Hoffman 1981, 2002). Often clinicians interview family members to obtain information about the client, their concerns, and goals for treatment. Potential problems arise when the family members' comments and labels regarding the client bias the clinician's perceptions. In addition, the family member's statements may diminish the client's credibility in describing her own strengths and weaknesses, and, therefore, reduce the clinician's perceived need to have an extended dialogue with the client. For example, a clinician may respond differently to a young client depending upon whether the parent describes his child as motivated and co-operative versus whether the parent describes his child as unmotivated and difficult. The parent who describes the child in positive terms is likely to be having better experiences with the child and will be supportive of the child's best interests in therapy. However, the parent who uses negative terms and descriptions may present more challenging attitudes and behaviors for the clinician.

We also need to be aware how labels may be used to control a family member's behavior (e.g., my "hard-working" child, my "lazy" child, my "demented" father). Typically, assigning a label gives one family member power over another. If a family member informs a clinician that the client is lazy, unmotivated, uncooperative, or demented, it gives that family member the appearance of a legitimate basis for claiming power over the labeled person and taking authority and control over the person's treatment. The actions, opinions, or preferences of the client or patient then may be disqualified or disregarded. Clinicians who accept at face value the family labels of a person (e.g., *lazy, demented*) may not be as open and willing to take into consideration the client or patient's perceptions and requests.

Another broadly accepted concept in family therapy concerns recurrent behavioral patterns that keep the family system functioning within tolerable limits. Each family has a predictable pattern of behavior that serves to maintain its balance or **homeostasis** (Bateson et al, 1956). Serious illness or injury inevitably disrupts the family's current homeostatic equilibrium. Even in crisis, healthy families are able to maintain homeostasis, but still be flexible enough to adapt to change. For example, a family of four may function well until the father sustains a TBI. In response to this event, the wife and two adolescent children may shift roles and responsibilities in order to take care of mortgage payments and daily household chores. In contrast to this family, other families may exhibit less flexible and more rigid patterns of behavior, for example, a father with a TBI in which the family members deny the severity of his impairment, maintain unreasonable expectations for his recovery, and refuse to take on new household responsibilities.

Family therapists such as Ackerman (2002) and Bowen (1978) examined family patterns that were repeated in one generation after another. The concept of multigenerational transmission of symptoms suggests that symptoms are caused by the family's failure to separate themselves from the immediate family and the problems of prior generations. The family's ability to cope with a current illness or crisis may be strongly and negatively affected by their previous experiences with illness and crises that may have occurred in previous generations (usually grandparents). SLPs and Auds need to be aware of this possible family dynamic that limits the family's current coping and make a referral to a family therapist.

Concepts originally defined by Minuchin (1974) in his description of **structural family therapy** also are widely accepted by family therapists. Minuchin was primarily interested in the structure of family systems and the belief that unhealthy family structures support emotional symptoms. He believed that a healthy family has a **hierarchy** wherein the parents are in charge and in control of the children. The parents also form a subsystem in which they are close to each other and communicate clearly with each other about the family's functions. Siblings generally get along harmoniously, have a special bond with one another, and thus form another subsystem within the family.

A family with healthy organization also has clearly marked **boundaries** (Goldenberg & Goldenberg, 2007; Minuchin, 1974; Minuchin, Nichols, & Lee, 2007). Boundaries are invisible lines of demarcation between two or more family members that help to demarcate and maintain healthy family member roles. When healthy boundaries are present, family members are allowed to experience appropriate levels of autonomy. In contrast, when healthy boundaries are absent, family members may be too close and unable to experience healthy levels of autonomy. Family members may function as one instead of as two individuals. Problematic or insufficient boundaries may be present when one family member assumes too much responsibility for another or one family member relies excessively on another. Unhealthy boundaries may be present in the following examples: (a) a father who needs comforting after learning of a serious medical diagnosis goes to his daughter rather than to his wife for solace, or (b) a mother who is upset by her husband's hospitalization goes to her ex-husband for support. Boundaries in a family may be assessed by observing who takes responsibility for whom and who spends time with whom, especially in times of emotional distress. Disruption of a healthy family hierarchy and boundaries can contribute to increased emotional and behavioral symptoms in family members.

Frequently seen in educational and medical settings are cases where well-meaning but overly protective parents "speak for" and exert excessive control over the behavior of their children. **Enmeshed** families occur when boundaries between members are blurred and members are overly concerned or overly involved in each other's lives (Goldenberg & Goldenberg, 2007; Minuchin, 1974). When parents are overly involved in their child's life the child may not be allowed to make independent decisions. An enmeshed parent–child relationship may serve to lower parental anxiety regarding the child. This may, for example, inhibit the child from using the problem-solving skills that the SLP has been working on in therapy that also are designed to help the child develop self-confidence in his own abilities.

At the other end of the family dynamics spectrum, some families experience excessive **disengagement** where family members have overly rigid boundaries and members feel isolated or disconnected from each other (Goldenberg & Goldenberg, 2007; Minuchin, 1974). Each member may function separately, autonomously, and with minimal involvement in the day-to-day activities of the family. There is little sense of family loyalty, and interpersonal distance is significant, with little ability to ask for or receive much-needed emotional support. Communication among family members is often strained and guarded. In some cases this can lead to a child's behavioral difficulties and inappropriate age roles in a family. This may occur when there is a severely medically ill or chronically depressed and withdrawn parent who is relatively unavailable to the child, either physically or emotionally. The child may become "parentified"; that is, she takes on adult-like roles and responsibilities. The SLP may want to encourage the parents to assume some of the adult activities and responsibilities so that the parentified child can resume a more age-appropriate child role. In a disengaged family, parents may be encouraged to become more involved in their child's school and play activities.

Triangulation refers to the process in which two family members recruit a third family member into an unhealthy alliance, often in order to avoid conflict with one another (Bowen, 1978; Doherty & McDaniel, 2010; Goldenberg & Goldenberg, 2007; Minuchin, 1978; Minuchin et al., 2007). There are at least two common versions of triangulation. In the first, the parents avoid conflict with one another by banding together and focusing

but not successfully. The SLP confers with social service staff and the hospital psychologist to ask if there is a way the parents can be encouraged to take a day off and just take care of one another rather than taking care of Michael.

The SLP hears Michael's parents tell him that he is "still our bright boy," and wonders how often that is said to Steven, who has difficulties in school and presents behavioral challenges at home. Does Steven feel equally validated and appreciated by his parents? The SLP may take care to present praise to the child who appears to get less parental attention. This simple SLP intervention may remind the parents to pay attention to the healthy children as well. The SLP can discuss with the parents the need to praise their other children and model desired behaviors, such as acknowledging the accomplishments of the healthy children as well as the gains Michael is making in therapy.

The clinician hypothesizes that some degree of enmeshment appears to be present. The parents, particularly the mother, are overly involved with Michael and are doing things for him that he is capable of doing himself, such as speaking for him and helping him dress when he can generally manage these tasks, but with considerable difficulty. The SLP recognizes, however, that in times of crisis families often pull together so tightly that they appear enmeshed. This enmeshment is usually temporary and will decrease as the child improves. However, the SLP knows that she needs to encourage both parents to allow Michael do to all that he can for himself even though he struggles.

The SLP recognizes that while she is involved with Michael's rehabilitation she is not a neutral outsider. The mother is competing for the clinician's attention, trying to get the SLP to address comments about Michael to her rather than to the father. The clinician takes care to join with all family members. For example, the SLP tries to look at both parents when conferencing with them, and not just the parent who asks most of the questions. She makes certain that she asks each parent individually what questions the parent might have. She also speaks to Michael's brother and sister and his grandparents, sharing information with them so that they do not feel left out of Michael's rehabilitation. The SLP tells and shows each family member how to best communicate with Michael, how to use the "Rule of Fives" (five-letter words, five-word sentences), and how to be alert to possible agitation when he is feeling overwhelmed. She explains her goals to the family and provides hope that Michael will make maximum improvement because of the excellent medical care and strong rehabilitation team working with him as well as his premorbid status.

EXISTENTIAL APPROACHES TO COUNSELING

Existential therapists are interested in the ultimate conditions of life and how people deal with the tragedies of existence (Corey, 2008; Gladding, 2009; Prochaska & Norcross, 2009). Yalom (2004) describes existential psychotherapy as a dynamic approach to therapy that focuses on concerns that are rooted in the individual's existence. People face conditions of existence that are awesome and profound. We grow up, we grow old, we become ill, we die. Yet knowing these conditions, we still strive to be good children, good adults, good workers, and good to our neighbors. Somehow we strive to find meaning to pursue our goals and to be responsible despite the inevitability of our own demise. Understanding and finding meaning in our existence, despite its sometimes bleak conditions, was the focus of early existential writers (Bugenthal, 1965; Frankl, 1959; May, 1953, 1961, 1994).

SLPs and Auds inevitably encounter existential issues in their work, for example, when a clinician counsels parents of a child whose seizure disorder is contributing to his impaired speech, language, and cognition, and the impairments are altering the parents' expectations of their child's future; when the clinician is working with an adult patient who is struggling with his cognitive losses and the meaning of life after a stroke; and when the clinician grows fatigued because she has encountered so many cases in which human loss and suffering takes an increasing toll on her abilities to cope with and manage anxiety about dealing with more loss. However, for many SLPs and Auds existential principles may become more relevant as they encounter increasing losses in their own professional or personal lives.

Existential therapy is concerned with each person's unique experience of being-in-the-world (Boss, 1963; May, 1994), how people perceive themselves and their surroundings, and how they manage to create meaning in their lives. In this context, people are understood to be in a constant state of flux, and this is reflected in how they deal with their lives. This includes how we treat and take care of ourselves and others, as well as our relationship to the existential conditions of life such as the uncertainty of our own health, the meaninglessness of tragedies, and the isolation associated with losing loved ones (George & Cristiani, 1995; Prochaska & Norcross, 2009; Yalom, 2004). The following describes some of the specific concepts considered by existential therapists that are relevant to clinicians.

Existential Uncertainty

Existential uncertainty involves the fact that as much as we attempt to control events in our lives, we discover that many events are outside our control (Fromm, 1941). We may lead a healthy lifestyle, practice good nutrition, exercise regularly, and wear seat belts when driving. Yet we may develop a brain tumor or a chronic illness or be struck by a drunk driver. In an attempt to protect loved ones who are disabled we may provide protective devices in the home. However, we still cannot eliminate all uncertainty regarding when or how they may fall. We cannot eliminate uncertainty even though we can try to decrease the risk of harm or danger to our loved ones and ourselves. Our beliefs that we should be able to eliminate uncertainty can leave us with feelings of guilt when we are unable to control tragic events, especially for those whom we love. For example, a grandparent has a serious fall in the shower resulting in a TBI, even though the adult children had just installed safety bars. Or a mother briefly loses sight of her two-year-old who falls into the swimming pool and has a near-drowning that results in severe anoxia.

Existential Meaninglessness

Once a tragic event occurs, questions and doubts around meaninglessness emerge. **Existential meaninglessness** refers to our anxieties about the meanings we have created for ourselves that may be obliterated by a single event. If a child is born with a severe neurological impairment, or an adolescent has a TBI from a motor vehicle accident, or an elderly adult has a severe stroke, previous meanings may be challenged or destroyed and we may be left with a sense of meaninglessness. Such tragedies may lead to the terrifying thought that there is no meaning, no significance in existence. The challenge we all face is to find meaning in our lives despite the adversities in order to endure life on a daily basis. Frankl (1959) emphasized that the primary force in life is our own search for meaning. Each person must create a unique and specific meaning that gives life coherence and significance. While some people look to religious beliefs to give their lives meaning, others develop secular meanings that provide them with direction and dignity in an indifferent world. Many health care professionals find meaning in their efforts to help others.

Many existential issues came to the forefront in the tragedy described in the story of Major Janet Deltuva and in the responses of the individuals involved. Tragedies of this kind challenge our usual, day-to-day beliefs and leave us face-to-face with these universal concepts of meaning, uncertainty, isolation, and death. Some individuals are able to modify their beliefs in healthy ways, so that they accept what they cannot control but still feel a sense of effectiveness and meaning in their lives.

COUNSELING SKILLS IN ACTION

Air Force Major Janet Deltuva

On September 11, 2001, Air Force Major Janet Deltuva, a speech-language pathologist and hospital administrator assigned to the Pentagon in Washington D.C., was in her office directly across the courtyard from the point of impact of the jetliner that flew into the Pentagon that morning. Major Deltuva had been trained in medical readiness and her role was to assist senior medical officers, who immediately set up a triage area in the center courtyard.

Major Deltuva performed a variety of extraordinary tasks that day that went beyond her speech-language pathology training and hospital administrator duties. She comforted injured victims, handed out surgical gloves, distributed glucose saline and other supplies, and did whatever was asked. Major Deltuva sought out victims who were alone and assisted them in any way she could, helping them make cell-phone calls to family and giving reassurance to the injured. Later that day she was asked to find volunteers to separate the living from the dead, and then was sent to count body bags.

In spite of tragedies, including terrorist attacks, Major Deltuva stated, "We have to establish a new 'norm' in our lives. If you choose to live in fear, the enemy has achieved their objective. And unlike many things in our lives, we do have control over how we deal with fear" (Moore, 2001, p. 6).

CLINICAL QUESTIONS

1. In the face of a tragedy, what are the positive personal characteristics that you can bring to bear on the situation?

2. What helps you to have strength in the face of existential conditions of life?

Existential Isolation

A third existential concern is isolation or our ultimate aloneness in the world (Fromm, 1956; Yalom, 2004). Yalom explains that **existential isolation** refers to an unbridgeable gulf between any other person and ourselves. We can have close family or friends who share important events in our lives with us, but ultimately, no one knows what it is like to be us, to undergo the pain and loss caused by our illness or our process of dying. For many people, it is not death itself that is so frightening, but the sense that it highlights our ultimate aloneness. No matter how close we become to another person, each of us must depart our existence alone. No one can go with us on that journey (Yalom, 2004).

Elderly people in convalescent hospitals may represent a readily apparent example of feelings of isolation and aloneness. They often have lost most of their family and close friends, and may have few if any visitors. The only interactions they may have with people are the brief nursing care and meals that are delivered throughout the day. Beyond this physical isolation and aloneness, elderly people are likely to feel existential anxiety and isolation about confronting their own demise—alone. However, SLPs and Auds need to be aware that nonhospitalized people are not immune from these existential anxieties and may experience a profound sense of isolation in the midst of their illness and suffering, even when surrounded by loving family and friends.

Another example of existential isolation concerns a child with a hearing impairment whose parents choose not to learn sign language, the child's preferred mode of communication. The child's only extensive conversations may be with other children who are hearing impaired and sign, or perhaps with a classroom teacher. However, the child with a hearing impairment who is fortunate to have parents and siblings who have learned sign language may still be isolated during some family time, such as visiting family or friends who do not sign, or watching television when there is no closed captioning. The child may be left out of important conversations, the humor of programs, or important news messages.

Both of these children inevitably experience isolation, even though the second family has tried to minimize the child's psychological isolation. The sense of isolation felt by these children stems from feeling different from other children and feeling that their families, no matter how loving, can never fully understand what it is like to be hearing impaired. No matter how well meaning an SLP or Aud is, she can never completely close the gap of existential isolation. Even if the clinician has a similar experience, for example, a hearing loss, the clinician can still never know what that experience is like for the client.

Maurer and Martin (2001) state that no communication environment is a positive one for people with hearing impairments. Environments where older people reside or spend much of their time, such as private homes, high-rise apartments, nursing homes, extended-care facilities, and senior centers, often are located in high-traffic areas where average outside noise levels exceed that of normal conversation. Interior noises of buildings negatively affect a person's hearing as well. In turn, older adults often feel isolated because of their hearing loss, which is compounded by the unmanageable environmental noise levels. Adults with hearing impairments often find themselves isolated from family and friends because people communicate less with them, and what is communicated may not be heard accurately or completely.

False reassurance that the SLP or Aud understands or knows what it is like to have a particular impairment is not helpful. In fact, false reassurance (such as, "I know what you are going through") can make the person feel even more isolated. We can never fully understand all of a person's emotional pain and suffering. Also, clumsy attempts at empathy in which the clinician says, "I understand" may sound arrogant to the person who knows that the clinician does not truly understand. Therapeutically, it is better for the clinician to say, "I'm trying to better understand how you are feeling and what you have to deal with." In the face of these existential conditions of life, as well as others, emotionally healthy people try to find meanings that make their lives worthwhile. They also try to find a balance between facing the dread brought on by these conditions versus a healthy denial and compartmentalization of these existential facts of life.

It is not necessarily the professional responsibility of the SLP or Aud to have extended conversations with clients or patients and their families about their struggles with uncertainty, sense of meaninglessness, or isolation. However, the clinician, particularly in acute-care settings or other crisis environments, may be confronted with patients and families who are dealing with such issues. Statements that signal such struggles may be, "Why is my family suffering so many tragedies all of the time?" "How can I ever forgive myself for letting this happen to my child?" "What did I miss that could have made me aware that my husband was having little strokes?"

In response to the client's struggles to find meaning, the SLP or Aud may want to make empathic responses acknowledging the person's anxiety and distress by saying, "It's understandable that it is difficult to make sense of this experience." This statement helps the person feel understood. If the person continues to ruminate along these lines, the clinician may wish to go a step further by helping the person regain a sense of meaning by asking, "What has helped you in the past make sense of difficult situations?" The clinician should not feel compelled to impose her own meanings on events, such as "I'm sure your family will become stronger and closer by dealing with this together" or, "I'm sure God has a plan for you."

Existential Nonbeing (Death)

Yalom (2004) discusses **existential nonbeing** and death anxiety in his classic text *Existential Psychotherapy*. Although death arguably is the single most important issue of life, it is a topic that most people avoid. In fact, most people spend considerable energy avoiding the terror of death, losing ourself, and becoming nothing. The experience of the inevitability of our end, of our death, is referred to as the realm of *nonbeing*. This experience or death anxiety motivates many people to turn to diversions in life, a lust for lasting fame, and reckless activity that seems to defy the possibility of death (e.g., race-car driving, sky diving, and extreme sports).

Although the physicality of death destroys a person, the idea of death and the closeness of death saves him. The awareness of death encourages a mindfulness of being, that is, attempting to live authentically and living life to the fullest. Near-death experiences (resulting from automobile accidents, heart attacks, etc.) often lead to a strong sense of the shortness of life and how precious it is; a greater sense of zest for life; a heightening of perceptions and emotional responsiveness; an ability to live in the moment and to savor each moment as it passes; a greater awareness of life and living things; and the urge to enjoy life now before it is too late (May, 1975, 1994; Yalom, 2004).

Anxiety and fear of death may occur on many levels, for example, the act of dying, fear of pain during dying, causing grief for family and friends, loss of caring for other people, regretting unfinished business (personal and professional), mourning the end of personal experiences, and being forgotten (Jeffreys, 2004). Death anxiety and difficulty discussing death may contribute to the limited discussion of death of clients and patients in the speech-language pathology literature on counseling. Luterman (2008) and Scheuerle (1992) have brief discussions of the topic. Other writers on counseling in speech-language pathology and audiology do not include discussions of death.

The reality is that clients, patients, and their families likely think about death much more than might be imagined. Patients, given the slightest encouragement, will often discuss their concerns about death. They may discuss the death of family members, friends, or themselves. Because clinicians may have had limited experience with death or are uncomfortable with the subject, they may avoid any conversations or reference to death. Denial-based strategies (e.g., suppression, repression, displacement, and belief in personal omnipotence) are ubiquitous and powerful defenses that play a central role in selective inattention to potential conversations about death. This denial is present in many of the helping professions (Yalom, 2004).

Facing Death with a Client

I have been willing to openly discuss death with many of my patients in hospitals, particularly those in convalescent hospitals where death becomes a way of life. Also, the topic of death has seemed relevant and/or imminent for some private clients. Other professionals and family members have appeared too busy or unwilling to talk with patients about their thoughts and feelings on this important part of life.

I worked with a private client, a woman in her mid-60s with Parkinson's Disease and dysarthria that affected all of her speech systems, for several months in her home at her kitchen table. Over the months her physical strength and ability to ambulate and communicate deteriorated. While she still was able to verbally communicate she occasionally, with no other family members present, would begin to talk about her imminent death and that she did not fear it. She said that she welcomed it. My willingness to listen and openly talk about death helped create richness in the therapy relationship. A few months after I ended my therapy with her, she died and I was asked by her family to do the eulogy at her funeral. It was a tremendous honor and responsibility to prepare the eulogy for this prominent figure in the community.

CLINICAL QUESTIONS

1. What counseling skills might you use if a client begins to discuss issues about loss and death with you?

2. Under what circumstances would you feel the need to consult with another professional?

Children often have a pervasive concern about death that exerts far-reaching influence on their experiential worlds (Jeffreys, 2004; Sourkes, 1982, 1995). Death is a great enigma to them, and one of their major developmental tasks is to deal with fears of helplessness and obliteration. "All gone" is one of the first phrases in many children's languages, and "all gone" is a common theme in childhood fears. Young children often fear being devoured, flushed away, or sucked through the bathtub drain. Perhaps the true facts of life for children involve the realization of death. However, adults confuse children about death with their idioms, for example: "My car died on the way to work." "I was just dead at the office today." "I'm feeling dead. I'm going to take a little nap." Many children are confused about the permanence of death.

Children with chronic illnesses (e.g., asthma) or life-threatening medical conditions (e.g., cancer, leukemia, severe burns) are often more knowledgeable and even precocious in their understanding of death than the adults around them believe (Brown & Sourkes, 2010; Sourkes, 1982). SLPs working in school settings may have children on their case loads who have asthma attacks or seizures during therapy. Children may bring up discussions about death at unexpected times, and it is important for the clinician to be willing to engage in these discussions. Children often feel isolated about their concerns of death, and clinicians should inform the parents about discussions they have had with children about this matter. If a child brings up the topic of death more than occasionally, or if the child appears troubled by thoughts of death, the SLP can encourage the parents to seek a consultation with a psychologist or family therapist. In medical settings, particularly acute-care hospitals and children's hospitals, ongoing death concerns and fears may be prominent in children's thoughts and conversations. It is important to listen to children and speak openly with them but to rely on each child's existing knowledge about death. Adding to their knowledge of death may be counter-therapeutic as it may create new fears or exacerbate existing fears.

Death of a Child

I received a referral from a physician to work with a two-year-old girl who had severe, spastic quadriplegic cerebral palsy, and I continued working with her for 18 months. She had been born without neurodevelopmental impairments but had a heart defect that required open-heart surgery when she was six months old. All went well with the surgery; however, she had severe complications afterwards and "died," but was resuscitated after many minutes without oxygen, which resulted in the cerebral palsy.

Neurodevelopmental Therapy (NDT) was appropriate for this child with primitive reflexes and no functional form of communication. I worked with the child twice a week in her home on the living room floor with her mother present. We had bonded well and she worked very hard in therapy, often smiling. One week she developed a bladder infection and died suddenly. On a Thursday afternoon at one o'clock when I would normally be doing therapy with her I attended her funeral.

Continues on next page

Continued from previous page

CLINICAL QUESTIONS

1. In speaking with a client's family, what therapeutic skills might you use in responding to news of a client's death?

2. Are there circumstances when you might feel too uncomfortable to attend a client's memorial service or funeral? Explain.

Yalom (2004) expresses a fundamental principle in this beautiful and profound passage:

> Count your blessings! How rarely do we benefit from that simple homily? Ordinarily what we *do* have and what we *can* do slip out of awareness, diverted by thoughts of what we lack or what we cannot do, or dwarfed by petty concerns and threats to our prestige or our pride systems. By keeping death in mind, one passes into a state of gratitude, of appreciation for the countless givens of existence. This is what the Stoics meant when they said, "Contemplate death if you would learn to live." The imperative is not, then, a call to a morbid death preoccupation but instead an urging to keep both figure and ground in focus so that being becomes conscious and life richer (p. 163).

CASE STUDY

Michael and an Existential Counseling Approach

Michael and his family are experiencing a classic existential crisis: uncertainty, meaninglessness, isolation, and death anxiety. Michael is likely feeling some existential isolation: feeling alone, not understanding what other people are saying to him, and not being able to communicate his wants, needs, thoughts, and feelings easily or clearly. He is likely experiencing a sense of meaninglessness about the accident that has left him with so many impairments; he may be asking himself why this has happened to him or what he has done to deserve this. He is probably feeling uncertainty about his future, whether he will be able to do well in school again, be as athletic as he was before the accident, and still be liked by his friends—or whether they will abandon him because he is not the same "old" Michael. He may be thinking about how close he came to dying. The SLP needs to be willing to listen to Michael's confused and sometimes disorganized conversations about himself that are occasionally punctuated with existential concerns. It is important to listen empathically, although the clinician may not be able to help him fully process his concerns. The SLP may want to discuss openly with the parents Michael's concerns as well as make a referral to the hospital psychologist for ongoing sessions to give Michael the opportunity to process his concerns.

Each of Michael's family members will likely be going through their own existential crises, including uncertainty as to how Michael's impairments will not only affect him, but the entire family; whether Michael will be accepted by his peers or be socially isolated; and how meaningless this tragedy is—how could it serve any good purpose? They are thankful that he survived the accident, but are very aware of how close they were to losing their son. The parents may have a heightened sense of gratitude for Michael's life and their relationship with him.

The SLP needs to be willing to listen to each of the family member's existential concerns and make appropriate referrals to the hospital psychologist. It is very important for the SLP to not trivialize any of the family's concerns by making what could be construed as condescending, naive statements. See Figure 2-1 for examples of therapeutic and nontherapeutic statements.

It is important for clinicians to acknowledge the family's existential concerns rather than deny them. Overly optimistic responses to the family may quell the clinician's anxiety, but may feel invalidating to the family.

Nontherapeutic Statements	Therapeutic Statements
"I understand what you must be going through."	"I understand that you are going through a lot of difficult adjustments right now." (This response makes fewer assumptions that the clinician knows exactly what the child's family is feeling.)
"I'm certain that some good will come out of all this."	"It sounds like you are considering how all this is going to affect Michael and the whole family." (In this statement the therapist is encouraging the family to find their own meaning for this experience rather than the clinician imposing his or her own meaning.)
"I'm sure that Michael's friends will welcome him back and he will be just as popular as he ever was."	"You're concerned about Michael's relationships with peers and hoping he won't be isolated, teased, or rejected." (The clinician acknowledges the possibility of changes to Michael's social relationships rather than denying this inevitable change.)
"Michael is a survivor. He is going to come out of this better than any of us might expect."	"Michael has made it through the acute phase. The medical and rehabilitation teams will work with Michael to help him make the best recovery possible. (The clinician acknowledges the collaborative efforts and uncertainty present in the therapeutic processes.)

Figure 2-1 Nontherapeutic and therapeutic statements

MULTICULTURAL APPROACHES TO COUNSELING

The development of multicultural theory since the 1960s has coincided with the increase of cultural diversity in the United States, particularly in the increase of African American, Hispanic, Asian, and Middle Eastern populations (Prochaska & Norcross, 2009). These groups have challenged the traditional male European perspective that has dominated North American thinking in areas as diverse as science, social policy, ethics, and family values. These diverse cultural groups have not always experienced the European/

North American perspective as fair or applicable to them, and therefore have called for a reevaluation of traditional attitudes and beliefs, a striving for equality for all people, and an appreciation of diverse beliefs and lifestyles (Fouad & Arredondo, 2007; Pedersen, Crethar, & Carlson, 2008; Saba, Karrer, & Hardy, 1995).

The role played by culture has increasingly come to be recognized in all aspects of counseling, from assessment to intervention. The cultures of both the clients and their families as well as the cultures of the clinicians influence the counseling process both pervasively and profoundly. Salas-Provance, Erickson, and Reed (2002), for example, confirmed the general concept that culture plays an important role in folk and medical belief systems regarding health and illness within a multigenerational Hispanic family. Their study also pointed out that the experiences and beliefs professionals hold may be in stark contrast to those held by clients. Overall, it is recognized that all counseling occurs in a multicultural context, and the cultures are crucial components of the counseling experience. Multicultural theory and principles are applicable to all counseling approaches used by clinicians, whether behavioral, humanistic, interpersonal, family, existential, or others (Gladding, 2009; Kuo & Hu, 2002; Pedersen, Draguns, Lonner, & Trimble, 2002).

Much of the recent speech-language pathology literature on multicultural populations focuses on children and the demands for services in the public schools (e.g., Battle, 2002; Langdon, 2002; Roseberry-McKibbin, 2008); however, we need to keep in mind that many adult clients, patients, and their families have diverse cultural backgrounds as well. It is often advantageous for clinicians to be bicultural or bilingual to be able to communicate with clients from different backgrounds.

The terms *race* and *ethnicity* are often used interchangeably, although they have different meanings. Race is defined as a classification that distinguishes groups of people from one another based on physical characteristics such as skin color, facial features, and hair texture. Two people can be the same race but differ widely in cultural identity. Ethnicity (ethnography) is a term that is sometimes confused with race, but is the social definition of groups of people based on various cultural similarities and includes race as well as factors such as customs, nationality, language, and heritage. Understanding of ethnicity implies a developed sense of the complexity of perceptions, symbols, meanings, and behaviors of a culture (Battle, 2002; Roseberry-McKibbin, 2008).

Culture may be defined in several ways, including ethnographic variables such as ethnicity, nationality, religion, and language; demographic variables of age, gender, place of residence, and so forth; status variables such as social, economic, and educational background and a wide range of formal or informal memberships and affiliations (clubs, churches, organizations, etc.). A broad definition of **culture** is any group of people who identify or associate with one another on the basis of some common purpose, need, or similarity of background (Gladding, 2009). Culture refers to shared beliefs, traditions, and values of a group of people. Culture is a term that implies explicit behaviors such as clothing and ways of dressing, food preferences, customs, lifestyle, and language. Implicit cultural variables include such factors as age and gender roles within families, child-rearing practices, religious and spiritual beliefs, educational values, and attitudes. Speech, language, and communication are embedded in culture (including the Deaf culture). The social rules of discourse and narratives are culturally determined (e.g., who speaks to whom, when, where, the physical distance between communicators, eye contact, who initiates the conversation, who selects the topic, and who ends the conversation). Communication and language are reciprocal: culture and communication influence each other. Culture is the lens through which people perceive and interpret their worlds (Canino & Spurlock, 2000).

Multicultural societies contain a diversity of cultures with varieties of religions, languages, customs, traditions, and values, and in which there are numerous racial and ethnic backgrounds living and working together (Battle, 2002; Roseberry-McKibbin, 2008). Multicultural counseling involves two or more people with different ways of being socialized and perceiving their social environment being brought together in a helping relationship (Nystul, 2005).

Acculturation refers to the learning, incorporating, and adopting of some of the values, customs, and beliefs of the dominant culture in order to fit in and get along with the society in which a person is living. It does not mean people must give up their cultural or religious heritage. People who retain their original cultural identity but simultaneously become acculturated to the American way of life have achieved **bicultural adjustment**. Distress often occurs in the family context when certain family members (usually the younger ones) are more acculturated to the dominant culture than are the elder members. This may lead to conflicts in decision making when, for example, the parents' wishes reflect their culture's traditional beliefs but their children's preferences reflect their more acculturated status. Here, the clinician should listen to, respect, and strive to understand the different world views that are expressed so that a culturally sensitive decision can be made.

Multicultural theory emphasizes the importance of taking into account culturally diverse world views. **World view** pertains to an individual's assumptions and perceptions about the world (i.e., existence, history, society) from a moral, social, ethical, and philosophical perspective. It is the source of a person's values, beliefs, and assumptions. These are derived from cultural, social, religious, ethnic, and/or racial perspectives (Pedersen et al., 2002). Multicultural theory rests on the assumption of cultural relativism, that there are few universal standards for evaluating right or wrong, healthy or unhealthy human behavior. What people believe and how they behave is significantly influenced by the culture in which they are raised. Thus, clinicians have a responsibility to understand the cultural variables that affect their clients' beliefs, rather than simply passing judgment on a client's beliefs that differ from their own.

CASE STUDY

A Japanese American Boy Who Stuttered

I received a rather desperate telephone call from an American man who was born and raised in Stockton, California, but was now living in Japan teaching English in the schools. He had been in Japan for 10 years and married a Japanese woman, and they had a five-year-old son who had begun to stutter. The father contacted the Stuttering Foundation of America to receive the name of an SLP in the Stockton area who had experience working with individuals who stutter. My name was provided to him. The family planned to return to Stockton for the summer and was hoping their son could receive therapy while here. I explained to the father that much of the therapy would include working with the parents and not just the child. Appointments were scheduled, and in their second week in Stockton I began working with the child and parents on a regular basis.

In this case I was working with three cultures in the same family: the father, Caucasian American; the mother, Japanese; and child, Japanese American. I had a little understanding of Japanese culture from spending some time in Japan many years ago and having five Japanese foreign exchange students live with my family over parts of various summers. I understood how a child with a handicap or disability might be perceived by some Japanese parents as a reflection on their parenting or on their family. Extra sensitivity was needed when talking with both parents, but particularly the mother, about their child's speech problems and things they could do when interacting with the child that could help improve his self-esteem and speech fluency.

CLINICAL QUESTIONS

1. How might you adjust your clinical approach to working with a Japanese family? A Hispanic family?
2. What signs might let you know that your therapeutic approach was not being positively received?

Lack of knowledge or inability to communicate fluently in the host society's language may contribute to members of other ethnic groups experiencing a disadvantaged status. In a medical setting, a language barrier may inhibit a patient's attempts to communicate with the medical team and his silence mistakenly may convey consent, or the patient's medical questions may go unanswered. If at all possible, it is helpful to have a translator present in these cases to facilitate communication and understanding of medical information.

Multicultural Work Environments

In many of the hospitals I have worked, there have been professionals from numerous cultures involved with a single patient. I recall a female Vietnamese patient who had a male Indian physician, several female and male Filipino nurses, female and male African American and Hispanic CNAs, and me, a Caucasian male SLP from California. This example illustrates that clients and patients may receive medical care and treatment from professionals representing a variety of cultures with varying languages, dialects, accents, and world views. It also highlights that as SLPs and Auds we not only work with clients and patients from different cultures, but that we also work with other professionals from diverse cultures.

Continues on next page

Continued from previous page

CLINICAL QUESTIONS

1. With professionals from such diverse cultural backgrounds, who do you think this patient trusted most easily? Why?

2. Since we work with professionals and colleagues from multiple cultures, why is it important to get to know them as individuals when possible?

A primary issue of concern for multicultural counseling is the dominance of theories and perspectives based on European/North American cultural values. Some of the predominant beliefs of European/North Americans include an emphasis on individual rights, an action-oriented approach to solving problems, a strong work ethic, the scientific method, and an adherence to strict time schedules (Gladding, 2009). Other cultures may not place the same value on these characteristics (Fouad & Arredondo, 2007; Pedersen, Crethar, & Carlson, 2008).

Stereotyping and overgeneralization are inherent dangers when considering culture, race, and ethnicity. Stereotyping may be defined as rigid preconceptions individuals hold about other people who are members of a particular group. Stereotyping fails to take into consideration logic or experience and distorts all new information to fit preconceived ideas (Nystul, 2005). To avoid stereotyping and overgeneralizing it is important for clinicians to treat clients as unique individuals first and as people from a particular culture second. Part of being a culturally competent professional is the ability to recognize that there is tremendous diversity that exists within each culture and that each person in any cultural group must be viewed first and foremost as an individual (Battle, 2002; Kuo & Hu, 2002; Pedersen et al., 2002; Roseberry-McKibbin, 2008).

As clinicians we need to be aware of our own cultural, racial, and ethnic backgrounds and how they influence us. Even individuals who deny any form of racial or ethnic prejudice often implicitly value certain types of people and devalue others. We are also a part of a variety of subcultures that may influence our beliefs, values, and assumptions. Some subcultures may include the part of the country and the state we live in; whether we were raised in or work in an urban or rural area; our family's educational and economic backgrounds; the type of university or employment setting we are in; and many others. We need to be very aware of the influences of our larger cultural and ethnic backgrounds and the subcultures we are a part of and how they affect our interaction with clients, patients, and their families as well as other professionals.

Shipley and Roseberry-McKibbin (2006) discuss numerous assumptions and values of Americans with mainstream backgrounds that may differ significantly from other cultures. For example:

■ "Punctuality is important and is an intrinsic part of a professional relationship based on mutual respect."

■ "In professional situations such as meetings, it is important to 'get down to business' as quickly and efficiently as possible."

- "Informality and social equality are the ultimate goals in all interactions between professionals and clients."

- "Frankness, openness, and honest discussion of situations and feelings are important."

- "The gender of the clinician and the client is not important; the clinician's competence is the most important variable."

- "The age of a clinician, relative to the client, is unimportant as long as the clinician is competent."

- "Written documentation is a necessary and intrinsic part of professionals' interactions with clients and families."

- "Speech and language therapy are usually necessary even if the client does not have an overt physical handicap."

- "Rehabilitation is usually necessary because the goal for all individuals, including those with speech and language impairments, is to be as independent as possible."

- "When clients display speech-language disabilities, Western forms of intervention are the most effective and appropriate."

- "When a particular client is receiving rehabilitative services or therapy, the family must be as active as possible in collaboration with the clinician."

- "Individuals have control over their own destinies."

- "Families who speak other languages at home need to speak English to their children so that the children will learn English."

- "Counseling individuals in isolation can be quite effective."

These assumptions are often such a basic part of the way we think about the world and interact with people that it may not occur to us that other people may make different assumptions. We also tend to elevate these values and consider them ideals, and may judge negatively people who have different or opposing values. For example, a person who does not value punctuality and is late for appointments may be judged negatively.

There is no one multicultural theoretical perspective or approach that is appropriate for working with all cultures. Realistically, it is impossible for any SLP or Aud to be well educated and understand the numerous cultures and subcultures within her community, much less the countless variations and nuances within any recognized cultural group. However, Battle (2002) presents several helpful "dos" and "don'ts" when considering a person's cultural background:

- Consider your own personal cultural beliefs, attitudes, and values and how they may be contributing to the clinical encounter.

- Learn the name of the person's cultural or geographic group that is commonly used by that group. For example, use *Japanese* for someone from Japan, not *Asian*. Use *Guatemalan* for someone from Guatemala, not *Hispanic* or *Latino*. (It may be helpful to inquire about the client's preferences, for example, how the client would like to be addressed.)

- Avoid using terms with questionable or negative connotations such as *culturally deprived, culturally disadvantaged,* or *minority*.

- Do not overgeneralize or stereotype individuals or groups of individuals.
- Be aware of the nonverbal sources of miscommunication between people from different cultural groups, such as styles of greeting behavior, the role of touch during conversation, and appropriate topics of conversation.

Culturally sensitive clinicians clearly have multiple responsibilities. One is to learn about cultural diversity (Kuo & Hu, 2002; Pedersen et al., 2008). Clinicians cannot possibly learn all the values and customs of all societies of the world. They can, however, learn about common beliefs and values held by people belonging to the major ethnic groups in their communities. This provides a foundation for learning about other cultural groups and respecting diverse systems of thought. Clinicians also can strive to develop empathic relationships with individuals of all cultures and express curiosity about understanding others' beliefs and customs (Pedersen et al, 2008).

Shipley and Roseberry-McKibbin (2006) make several suggestions for effectively communicating when interviewing and counseling clients who are experiencing difficulties communicating in English.

1. Loudness: Do not increase the volume of your voice. Unnecessary loudness may make clients feel they are being treated like children.

2. Rate of speech: Decrease your rate of speech and pause often. The slower rate makes it easier for individuals to understand, and the pauses between sentences allow them time to process the information.

3. Articulation in connected speech: Articulate each word clearly, but do not exaggerate mouth movements. Avoid using contractions such as "don't," "wouldn't," and so forth.

4. Sentence length and complexity: Avoid multisyllabic words. (Using the "Rule of Fives," i.e., five-letter words, five-word sentences, may be helpful.) Avoid slang and idioms, technical jargon, and abstract terms.

5. Repeat key information: Clients typically need to hear key words and concepts several times, especially clients for whom English is not their primary language.

6. Nonverbal cues and body language: Proxemics (the use of physical distance) and kinesics (the use of gestures and facial expressions, including eye contact) differ among cultures.

7. Size of interaction groups: During interviews clients may be more comfortable and bolstered by having other family members or close friends present.

8. Allow extra time for meetings and be patient: Avoid appearing hurried.

9. Use translators when needed: Be cautious to choose translators who have good communication skills and act in a professional manner, including maintaining confidentiality.

Fortunately, many departments of communicative disorders in universities and colleges around the country are providing education and training in the area of multicultural populations to assist SLPs and Auds to begin to develop multicultural competencies. There is a need for clinicians in all work settings to have extensive and ongoing education in this important area to better help our clients, patients, and their families. Awareness and understanding of multicultural issues also can help us with our interaction and sensitivity with colleagues and co-workers.

CASE STUDY

Michael and a Multicultural Counseling Approach

In order not to stereotype Michael and his family's racial, ethnic, and cultural backgrounds, and to avoid stereotyping the SLP's racial, ethnic, and cultural backgrounds, the authors have chosen not to continue this case study in relationship to multicultural theory. The reader is encouraged to consider her own race, ethnic, and cultural background and to imagine how these factors may influence interactions with Michael and his family by varying their backgrounds, for example as an African American family, a Hispanic family, an Asian family, and so forth. That is, what adjustments and modifications might you need to make to your counseling approach and what challenges to effective therapy implementation might you encounter?

CLINICAL QUESTIONS

1. Given your family's background and culture, what clinician style or values would likely be the best fit or match?

2. Given your family's background and culture, what clinician behaviors might be perceived as unappealing or incompatible with your family's values?

THEORETICAL INTEGRATION

A number of prominent theorists have attempted to integrate or combine elements from various theories (Moursund & Erskine, 2003; Safran & Segal, 1990; Stricker & Gold, 2006; Wachtel, 1977, 2007), or have traced this movement (Goldfried, 1982; Prochaska & Norcross, 2009). There is also a journal entitled *Journal of Psychotherapy Integration*.

During interactions with a client or family, an SLP or Aud may apply various theoretical concepts discussed in this chapter (humanistic, interpersonal, behavioral, cognitive, family systems, existential, and multicultural). The clinician may integrate theoretical principles and use what is believed to be the most therapeutic intervention at the moment. Integrative counseling is the process of selecting concepts and methods from a variety of therapeutic approaches (Corey, 2008). Surveys of clinical and counseling psychologists report that 30 to 50 percent of the respondents consider themselves to be integrative or eclectic in their therapeutic practice (Norcross & Newman, 2005; Norcross & Prochaska, 1988; Prochaska & Norcross, 2009). As SLPs and Auds working with a wide variety of hearing, speech, language, cognitive, and swallowing disorders of individuals of all ages, we need to be able to draw upon concepts, strategies, and techniques from a variety of counseling frameworks to communicate effectively with our clients, patients, and their families. The integrative approach is characterized by openness to various ways of combining diverse theories and techniques. An integrative approach to counseling attempts to look beyond and across the confines of single-theory approaches to see what can be learned from—and how clients can benefit from—other perspectives (Corey, 2008).

There are three primary methods for achieving integration: technical eclecticism, theoretical integration, and common factors (Arkowitz, 1997; Corey, 2008). **Technical eclecticism** is a collection of techniques chosen from a variety of different approaches. The clinician chooses at any moment during an interaction with a person the technique that will be most helpful without necessarily subscribing to the theoretical position from which the technique is drawn. **Theoretical integration** refers to development of a conceptual or theoretical framework that synthesizes the best of two or more theoretical approaches with the assumption that the synthesis will be richer than the individual theories alone. The **common factors approach** attempts to distill, from different theoretical systems, nonspecific elements (Frank, 1982) that are common among the theories. Nonspecific elements include such factors as positive expectations, a warm, trusting relationship, and faith in the clinician. This perspective on integration is based on the premise that these common factors are at least as important in accounting for therapy outcomes as the unique factors that differentiate one theory from another (Corey, 2008). Patterson (1986) cites seven commonalities among counseling approaches:

1. The counseling approaches agree that humans can change or be changed.
2. The approaches agree that some behaviors are undesirable, inadequate, or harmful, or result in dissatisfaction, unhappiness, or limitations that warrant change.
3. Counselors expect people to change as a result of their particular techniques and interventions.
4. Individuals who seek counseling experience a need for help.
5. Clients generally believe change can and will occur.
6. Counselors expect clients to be active participants.
7. Intervention characteristically includes encouragement, support, and instruction.

Overall, because no one theory, strategy or technique is always effective when working with a wide range of ages, delays and disorders, and personality types, it is wise to not limit ourselves to a single theory (Corey, 2008; Kelly, 1991; Lazarus, 1996). Corey states,

> Practitioners who are open to an integrative perspective will find that several theories play a crucial role in their personal counseling approach. Each theory has its unique contributions and its own domain of expertise. By accepting that each theory has strengths and weaknesses and is, by definition, "different" from the others, practitioners have some basis to begin developing a theory that fits for them. Developing an integrative perspective is a lifelong endeavor that is refined with experience (p. 459).

CONCLUDING COMMENTS

Several theories and therapy approaches of counseling have been presented to help clinicians develop a framework from which they can work effectively with clients, patients, and their families. Clinicians need to remember that no one counseling theory or therapy approach fits all situations and that clinicians will likely draw upon several therapy approaches with a particular client or family member.

The foundation of counseling is the clinician–client relationship; therefore emphasis is first placed on "connecting" with the client and family (including appreciating cultural differences), and second on cognitive and behavioral changes. Existential concepts may seem unusual for SLPs and Auds to consider when working with clients and their families, but many of the life problems we are trying to address often involve uncertainty, meaninglessness, isolation, and sometimes even death. Most of the other theories and therapy approaches discussed involve analysis of culturally influenced behavior, family functioning, and values development, while these existential concepts tend to address more universal life experiences. Finally, it is important to remember the theories and therapy approaches presented here are just a few of the hundreds in the counseling and psychotherapy literature, and that there are other theories and approaches that contain relevant concepts as well.

Discussion Questions

1. Discuss why no one theory or counseling approach fits all situations.

2. Discuss a few of the counseling approaches that you would likely use with any counseling interaction.

3. What does "unconditional positive regard" mean to you? How do you demonstrate this quality to your clients?

4. What types of erroneous thinking or cognitive distortions do you occasionally use?

5. Discuss a client with whom you had to work closely with other family members. What were the subsystems that were involved? Was there any triangulation involved?

6. How do you respond to existential uncertainties in your life?

7. Discuss the death of someone with whom you were close. How did that affect the way you see life and relationships?

8. Discuss the primary cultures and subcultures you are a part of. How do those cultures affect the way you interact with people from other cultures? Discuss whether you think that being an SLP or Aud places you in another subculture.

Role Plays

1. Have two students in the class play the roles of parents seeking a consultation for their seven-year-old daughter who has speech and language delays. The identified client (the daughter) is described by her parents as timid and shy and tends to avoid situations where she anticipates failure. She has an older brother who is more extraverted and outgoing. Have a third student (or a pair of students) play the role of the SLP conducting an initial interview and asking questions about the family functioning that is relevant to understanding the speech and language problems. After 5–10 minutes, have the class discuss behavioral, interpersonal, and family systems concepts that arose during the interview.

2. Have two students in the class play the roles of a 60-year-old man who recently had a stroke and his wife of 35 years. The man expresses a strong sense of pessimism regarding his ability to recover his former speech, language, and cognitive capabilities. He also expresses resentment about the roles his wife must now assume in caring for him. Have two additional students play the roles of SLPs who are conducting an initial interview. After 5–10 minutes, have the class discuss humanistic, cognitive, family, and existential concepts and issues that arose during the interview.

3. Add to role play exercises 1 or 2 the element that the family has recently moved here from Mexico. What are the additional considerations in these cases? Discuss concepts from multicultural theory and how this may impact the clinician's approach to this family.

The Therapeutic Relationship and Therapeutic Communication

CHAPTER OUTLINE

INTRODUCTION

Technical expertise is necessary but not sufficient to be a competent speech-language pathologist or audiologist. It is not only the clinician's knowledge of our profession and therapeutic techniques that define what we do, but the ability to enter into the person's world and to develop a therapeutic working relationship. The child or adult's subjective experiences of communication problems are inevitably affected by the quality of the relationship with the clinician (Brammer & MacDonald, 2002; Guitar, 2006; Holland, 2007; Luterman, 2008; Rollin, 2000; Shames, 2006; Shipley & Roseberry-McKibbon, 2006). Similarly, it has long been known in the area of psychotherapy and counseling that the therapeutic alliance, or the quality of the relationship between the therapist and the client, is a key element that impacts therapeutic outcome (e.g., as reviewed in Crits-Christoph, Gibbons, & Hearon, 2006; Lambert, 2004; Norcross, 2002). The quality of the relationship, once it begins, has its own dynamic quality that inevitably is affected by what the clinician and client bring to it. The client and the clinician continue to influence each other as their relationship evolves. How clients behave toward us is inevitably linked to how we think, feel, and behave toward them. Thus, the evolution of the therapeutic relationship during the counseling process involves a reciprocal feedback loop in which each person's actions continually influence the other's. This chapter describes some of the essential relationship factors and communication strategies that can be used to enhance the cooperative, working alliance between client and clinician.

VARIABLES CONTRIBUTING TO THE THERAPEUTIC RELATIONSHIP

The variables contributing to the therapeutic relationship are illustrated in Figure 3-1. The client–clinician relationship is dynamic, meaning that it is constantly changing. The relationship emphasizes the *affective* mode because, like any relationship, there is an emotional quality to the interaction. Ideally, a positive working relationship begins upon the initial contact between a client and clinician. However, for new and inexperienced clinicians, there is often a feeling of anxiety when meeting a new client, working with a disorder for the first time, or working with an adult for the first time. This is normal. Clinician anxiety, however, can interfere with how we are perceived by clients and their willingness to trust and work with us.

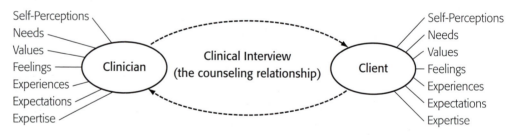

Figure 3-1 The counseling relationship in the clinical interview (adapted from Brammer & McDonald, 1999).

Inexperienced and experienced clinicians alike enter into evaluations and therapy with clients with self-perceptions of their education and knowledge, training, and competence. Clinicians have the desire to feel good about their clinical work and to feel that their clients respect them. Clinicians have values about what is important to them, and they may sometimes impose those values onto the client. However, novice clinicians may have feelings of uncertainty, anxiety, and even fear about how the evaluation and therapy sessions will go, including considerable anxiety about their supervisor's reactions and appraisals. Clinicians have experiences with other children and adults that they draw upon to help them feel comfortable with clients. Clinicians have expectations of themselves, sometimes hoping to do a "perfect" evaluation or therapy session, and soon find that perfection is elusive even to the most well-educated and experienced clinicians (Kottler, 2010; Kottler &

Blau, 1989). Clinicians often have expertise in areas other than speech-language pathology or audiology that help give them confidence that with enough education, training, experience, and time, they also can develop expertise in their profession.

It is important to keep in mind that the client also is likely to have some level of anxiety upon meeting a clinician. It may be the client's first experience with an SLP or Aud, and there may be considerable uncertainty about the diagnosis and how much benefit he will receive in therapy. Clients who come to us for help may have negative self-perceptions and may not be optimistic about receiving help. Children sometimes have had years of frustration because they cannot be understood easily or have difficulty communicating with peers, teachers, and even their family. Adults who have functioned well all their lives but now have a significant loss of hearing, speaking, understanding, communicating, or swallowing may have negative self-perceptions because they compare themselves to how they used to be and may not appreciate their potential for rehabilitation. For some clients whose potential for rehabilitation is poor even with the best of care, their negative self-perceptions of their communication or swallowing problems may be fairly accurate.

Some clients, however, have overly optimistic and unrealistic expectations for improvement, the rate of improvement, and the clinician's ability to facilitate those improvements. While clients' positive expectations can initially contribute to a positive client–clinician relationship, the client eventually may experience disillusionment with the clinician and the therapy if the clinician does not discuss during the interview, evaluation, or therapy the amount, rate, and effort needed for improvement. By discussing these factors, the clinician can prepare the client for a realistic view of the work that needs to be done in order to achieve improvement.

Clients need to feel they are getting the best of care and that they have potential for improvement. Clients have values about what is important to them in therapy and, ideally, experience therapy as a collaborative problem-solving activity with the clinician. This sense of a shared understanding and an agreement upon the therapy goals and tasks constitutes an important element of the therapeutic alliance (Bordin, 1979; Norcross, 2002; Safran & Muran, 2000). Clients have feelings of uncertainty, anxiety, and even fear about how they will perform during the evaluation and in therapy with the clinician. They may have considerable anxiety about the qualifications and skills of the clinician. The dimension of trust–mistrust has important implications for the development of the therapeutic relationship (Brammer & MacDonald, 2002). Will the clinician be able to help? Clients, like most people, hope that the other person will like them. The clinician's skills at showing empathy and respect for the client and accurate understanding of her problems are some of the ways that clinicians may begin to earn the client's trust.

Despite the clinician's behaviors, however, clients have interpersonal schemas (i.e., expectations based upon previous experiences with other adults and professionals) that inevitably influence them as they get to know a new clinician. Thus, two different clients may interpret the same clinician behaviors in very different ways. For example, a client who has a more trusting schema may interpret a clinician's lateness to an initial appointment to mean that the clinician has a busy, successful practice. Meanwhile, a client who has a less trusting schema may interpret the same clinician behavior to mean that the clinician does not care about him. This concept of interpersonal schemas is closely related to the concept of transference, which is discussed later in this chapter. Suffice it to say here that psychotherapy research has shown that it is important to be attuned to client perceptions of the therapist and be ready to provide information that will help to correct and repair initial misunderstandings or ruptures in the therapy process (Muran, Safran, Gorman, Samstag, Eubanks-Carter, & Winston, 2009). Ruptures in the therapeutic relationship can occur because the client feels disrespected, misunderstood, judged, intimidated, or lectured.

Clients have expectations of themselves, sometimes expecting that they will be "cured" quickly of their hearing, speech, language, cognitive, or swallowing problems. Adult clients often have expertise in a variety of areas in their personal and professional lives, e.g., raising a family, being a valued employee for many years, and being a contributor to society. Clients can usually draw upon successes in other areas of their lives to experience self-confidence and motivation to address the challenges in therapy.

Both clinicians and clients enter the therapeutic relationship with these historical experiences, but approach the therapy from different perspectives (Lambert, 2004). While the client is seeking symptom reduction, improvement in functioning, and wellness, it is important for the clinician to be clear about serving the client's best interests rather than her own. Clinicians need to become aware of their needs and resolve them beforehand so that they can better attend to their client's concerns and anxieties. Otherwise, clinicians run the risk of using other people (clients) to help themselves (Brammer & MacDonald, 2002). When clinicians understand their clients' self-perceptions, needs, values, feelings, experiences, expectations, and areas of expertise, they can begin to tailor their behaviors, communication, and treatment strategies so that the potential for success is optimal.

In addition to the variables discussed above, clinicians have general styles and ways of approaching clients that can affect their relationship. As supervisors, we have found that how clinicians talk about and think about their clients can set the stage for how a particular clinician–client relationship develops. Some ways of talking about clients objectify them (i.e., treat them as though they are objects rather that people). ASHA has a "person first" policy, for example, referring to the "person with a hearing impairment" rather than the "hearing-impaired person," or the "person who stutters" rather than the "stutterer," or the "patient who had a TBI" rather than the "TBI patient." In medical settings, patients are particularly vulnerable to feeling decreased worthiness. While we know that most SLPs and Auds are empathic, they may inadvertently objectify patients by using objectifying language (e.g., "The new stroke is in room 302"). Sometimes patients hear this language when clinicians and medical personnel are discussing them and may perceive it as dehumanizing. Patients' emotional suffering is increased when clinicians treat them as objectified anatomic parts and, conversely, suffering can be alleviated when clinicians acknowledge and respect their personhood (Fogle, 2008; Frank, 2002).

"Oh, You're a New TBI."

In 2003 I was invited by the Director of Speech-Language Pathology and Audiology at Walter Reed Army Medical Center (WRAMC) in Washington, D.C. to provide

Continues on next page

Continued from previous page

an in-service to her team of SLPs on "Counseling Combat Casualties and Their Families" from the Iraq and Afghanistan wars. The specific topic I chose to discuss was "Giving Bad News." When I entered WRAMC I needed help finding the director's office and I was about to ask a receptionist when a young soldier struggled to tell her his name and tried to ask a question. Without any apparent appreciation of the effect her words might have, she briefly looked up at him and said, "Oh, you're a new TBI." I immediately saw his eyes and head turn downward with an expression of "That's all I am now." I began my in-service presentation with that brief story.

CLINICAL QUESTIONS

1. How would you attempt to rectify this error if you heard another professional or staff say this to your patient?

2. Can you recall a situation where you or a family member were labeled by your illness or disability? How did you feel about being labeled in this way?

One remedy to the overemphasis on medical technology and the increasing neglect of the human side of illness and treatment is a renewed appreciation and attention to the therapeutic relationship. This focus is consistent with the writings of medical ethicists (Schultz & Carnevale, 1996; Zaner, 1993, 2004), psychologists (Burnard, 2005; Kottler, 2010), nurses (Bishop & Scudder, 1990; Keltner, Schwecke, & Bostrom, 2007; Tschudin, 2003), and physicians (Cassell, 1996) who have urged health care professionals to put the "care" back into medical care. Caring for patients may not cure illness but it can contribute to the lessening of patient suffering and provide the foundation for a trusting and cooperative patient–clinician relationship. For these reasons, clinicians should be guided by an ethic of health care.

For SLPs and Auds, the question is not whether they have time to develop a relationship with a client. The client–clinician relationship is an inevitability and, therefore, the question is how therapeutic that relationship will become. Therapeutic relationships can either enhance or diminish treatment gains (Duncan, 2010; Martin, Garske, & Davis, 2000).

Personal qualities of effective helpers have been discussed. There also are guidelines to follow to develop better therapeutic relationships with our clients and patients. It is helpful to analyze some of the skills that can contribute to a positive working relationship. Increased awareness of these skills can help clinicians be more mindful and intentional in our interactions with people, especially with those individuals who are challenging. Although the elements of a therapeutic relationship are intertwined in our daily work, they are discussed in sequence here to better understand them.

TRANSFERENCE AND COUNTERTRANSFERENCE

We have all developed a pattern of feelings, expectations, perceptions, and attitudes that shape our new experiences with others. Some laypersons refer to this phenomenon loosely as the emotional "baggage" they are carrying. These personal templates or schemas typically operate automatically and can have a powerful impact on the process and outcome of a new relationship (Henry, Schacht, & Strupp, 1990; Henry, 1997; Kiesler, 1996). The client's feelings, expectations, perceptions, and attitudes toward the clinician are referred to as transference, while the clinician's feelings, expectations, perceptions, and attitudes toward the client are referred to as countertransference. Both are inevitable experiences (Butler, Flasher, & Strupp, 1993; Gabbard, 2005; Kahn, 1999), and clinicians are wise to understand that these forces can exert a powerful influence over the therapeutic climate. Depending upon the type of transference or countertransference responses, these can either facilitate or interfere with the therapeutic process (Levenson, 1995, 2010).

Transference

In addition to the conscious needs, values, and expectations that each person brings to the therapeutic relationship, the client also brings a set of unconscious wishes, perceptions, and fears. These unconscious forces that shape the client's perceptions of the therapist are referred to as **transference** (Freud, 1912; Gill, 1982; Gabbard, 2005). While this concept was originally used by psychoanalytic theorists, it has in more recent years been understood in broader terms by psychologists from many theoretical camps (Kahn, 1999; Safran & Segal, 1990; Stricker & Gold, 2006). While this concept has many ramifications for the therapy process that are beyond the scope of this text, a basic understanding of transference phenomena can provide SLPs and Auds with important tools for understanding and nondefensively addressing certain aspects of the therapeutic relationship.

The basic idea is that people view others through the lenses of their past experiences. The transference, then, simply refers to the lenses through which we perceive new situations and people. We all are influenced by our past relationships and, for example, have grown to trust easily or remain skeptical of others based upon our past experiences. Every time we meet a new person, we encounter a multitude of incomplete or ambiguous stimuli that we must organize in some way. Our transference can be thought of as an organizing principle (Stolorow, Brandcraft, & Atwood, 1987; Kahn, 1999) that helps us to filter, organize, and attend to certain characteristics or behaviors in other people. Becoming sensitive to transference phenomena can help clinicians make sense of situations and avoid defensive countermoves when clients behave in puzzling or irritating ways (Strupp, 1996).

In some therapeutic situations, the transference may be "invisible" or unnoticed by the clinician and not require any special skills or interventions (Gabbard, 2005). These are often situations in which a relatively well-adjusted client approaches the therapist with a trusting and positive therapeutic relationship. In a specific case, a child may have a positive impression of the SLP or Aud who reminds her of a gentle and loving mother or aunt, or an elderly patient may respond to the younger clinician as if he were a loyal son. In these cases, the client takes in a certain amount of information about the new clinician and then fills in the "blanks" with old experiences. The fact that transference is occurring does not mean that the client is blind to the actual characteristics of the clinician. To some degree, there is a *hook* or *peg* on which the transference is "hung" (Wachtel, 1993, p. 58).

With some clients, however, the transference interferes with the development of the therapeutic relationship and accomplishing therapeutic tasks and goals (Henry et al., 1990). These cases are often ones in which a negative transference develops. Here, the client's perceptions of the clinician are colored or clouded by past negative experiences. For example, a child may respond in a guarded and tense fashion to a new speech therapist as if the SLP is her critical mother or teacher, or an adolescent may respond argumentatively to his clinician as if she is an authoritarian parent. Bearing in mind Wachtel's (1993) point about needing a peg on which to hang the transference, the clinician should always reflect on her behavior to examine what she may have done that was interpreted as authoritarian or critical.

Clinicians may learn to use special caution with some clients so that their behavior is less likely to be misinterpreted. What is important to remember is that we all establish transference relationships in our everyday lives (Wachtel, 2007). Therefore, clients should not be criticized or told that they are wrong for how they perceive us. It is not appropriate, for example, to declare "I am not your critical (or authoritarian, punitive, etc.) parent!" If you sense that your client perceives you in a negative way, you might ask (in a nondefensive tone) what you have done or what makes it seem that way to him. For example, "I'm wondering what I may have done or said that sounded critical." In this way, you gather information about your client's perceptual style and sensitivities and your impact on the client. In some cases, talking about their perceptions resolves the tension. In other cases, you may need to calibrate your future behavior, for example, by making certain to discuss recommendations in a collaborative tone so that you are not perceived as authoritarian.

COUNSELING SKILLS IN ACTION

A Client's Romantic Transference

A female client asked her male SLP in private practice to schedule an appointment at her home. The SLP did not know her husband would be at work. Once they were seated at her dining room table, the client began to compliment the SLP's kind, gentle manner and sensitivity to her feelings and to lament her husband's shortcomings in these areas. The client had apparently begun to develop a romantic transference onto the therapist. It was likely the SLP's kind and sensitive manner stimulated her fantasy. In cases like these, it is extremely important to maintain professional boundaries and to recognize and avoid responding to the client's projections, for example, that the clinician will be the knight in shining armor who rescues the client from a less than satisfactory marital relationship.

CLINICAL QUESTIONS

1. How might you respond to a client who flirts with you so that you maintain appropriate professional boundaries while maintaining your working alliance with the client?

2. How might you phrase your response to a client who has very low self-esteem?

Countertransference

The counterpart to the transference concept is **countertransference**. Since its introduction (Freud, 1910), this concept has undergone many changes in meaning and has become increasingly important to an understanding of the therapeutic relationship (Butler, Flasher, & Strupp, 1993; Gabbard, 2005). The countertransference concept originally referred to the clinician's personal psychological "baggage" that interfered with the therapy. For example, a clinician who avoids giving a clear and detailed explanation of a child's communication disorder to the parent may have her own issues with loss and giving bad news. She may have experienced personal losses that make it difficult to face losses in her professional work. In such cases, countertransference is viewed as an impediment to therapy because it prevents the clinician from adequately performing aspects of clinical work. Historically, the clinician's personal psychotherapy was viewed as the appropriate forum in which to work through and eliminate these interfering emotions and behaviors.

More recently, the countertransference concept has been expanded to include all of the clinician's emotional responses to the client (Anchin & Kiesler, 1982; Butler et al., 1993; Kernberg, 1965; Kiesler, 1996). Many of these responses do not reflect the clinician's psychological problems and shortcomings, but are understandable responses to certain kinds of client behavior. For example, friendly and agreeable clients typically elicit a friendly response from the clinician. An SLP or Aud may do extra favors for a well-behaved child who reminds her of a younger sibling, or a clinician may consider providing extra help to a client, thinking of him as if he were a kind, elderly grandparent. These examples demonstrate that some countertransference responses involve positive emotional reactions to clients. Typically, these therapist responses are benign. Clinicians need to be alert, however, for positive countertransference responses that can create threats to appropriate professional boundaries with clients.

Other countertransference responses involve negative emotional reactions to clients. A clinician who dislikes a particular sullen and depressed client may "forget" to reschedule the client's missed appointment. A client who speaks in a harsh, critical manner to the clinician may elicit a more terse and less friendly greeting than the clinician offers other clients. In these cases, the clinician's countertransference responses represent deviations from the clinician's usual friendly, conscientious, and professional style.

An important concept articulated by interpersonal theorists (e.g., Anchin & Kiesler, 1982; Kiesler, 1996) is that countertransference responses should not simply be concealed or eliminated. They can be used as a tool to understand clients better. The clinician's countertransference response may provide important clues about what the client is feeling or thinking about the clinician. For example, a clinician who is bored with a particular client may realize that the client appears apathetic and unmotivated to put forth effort in therapy. The clinician who gets angry with a particular client may reflect (privately) on what that client has done and what he may be trying to communicate. Is the client resisting the clinician's recommendations because he feels efforts will be futile? Is the client feeling rejected by the clinician who appears hurried or preoccupied? What can we learn about the client based upon our countertransference responses? Clients are often responding to how we have treated them or what they perceive we have communicated to them (Henry, Schacht & Strupp, 1986).

The goal here is to become comfortable and nondefensive about our own emotional responses so that we can reflect on what factors have triggered them. As clinicians, our reactions to clients are seldom neutral even though we are trained to maintain a professional stance. This does not mean that we should feel free to express all of our emotions to clients, but rather that we should admit them to ourselves. Once we do this, we may develop insight into the factors that are impeding a particular therapy or therapeutic relationship. For example, if a clinician finds herself feeling angry with a client, she may reflect on this emotional response and realize that it is a reaction to the client's chronic lateness for therapy appointments. The outcome may be that the clinician discusses this (lateness) issue with the client or asks the client how he is feeling about the therapy. It is vital that the clinician explore these issues with the client using a nonjudgmental tone so that the client feels comfortable to discuss whatever is getting in the way. In countless situations, the clinician's countertransference can be used as a tool to analyze what is happening in the therapeutic relationship (Betan, Heim, Conklin, & Westen, 2005; Butler, Flasher, & Strupp, 1993; Levenson, 1995, 2010).

ATTENDING AND LISTENING

A foundational and prerequisite element of a therapeutic relationship is attending to the client through both auditory and visual channels. The purpose of clinical observation is to take in as much information as possible about the client and to obtain a sample of the client's behavior. Riley (2002) provides several suggestions about what the clinician should observe when the client enters the room. For example, does the client smile or is she serious? Does she start talking or wait for the clinician to ask a question? Is the client open in her comments or cautious? Does her body language appear tense or relaxed? Is there appropriate eye contact or avoidance? Are the arms crossed or in a relaxed position? Is the voice tense or natural? If the voice becomes tense, what is being discussed? When asked what the client observed about herself since the last session, how does she respond? Does the client appear interested in observing herself in an objective manner?

First impressions during an interview or the beginning of a therapy session provide clues as to how the initial portion of the meeting may be focused. Riley says that through observations the clinician looks for signs of fear, anger, sadness, interest, excitement, reticence, eagerness, and so on. When a clinician reflects back to the client something that he perceives but that the client is not aware of, there is the experience of being heard. For example, if the clinician observes tension in the client's voice and body when the discussion is about work being difficult, the client is often pleased and surprised, wondering how the clinician knew. Schow and Nerbonne (2006) say that rehabilitative audiologists need to begin their work by listening to their clients' attitudes toward hearing loss and their goals in seeking help. By listening to the person with a hearing impairment, the audiologist begins to build a bridge between the client's life experiences with a hearing loss and the audiologist's understanding of the results of the formal audiologic assessment.

Barkley (2005) explains that attending (attention) includes arousal (being alert), selective attention (choosing what to attend to), sustained attention (staying focused), and how much information can be attended to or processed at one time. Clinicians must first attend to their clients before they can listen to them. Most clinicians have had the experience of clients speaking to them while the clinician is attending to something else. There are a variety of obstacles to attending and listening to clients, a few of which are:

- The clinician's stress and anxiety
- Negative value judgments of the client
- The clinician being so eager to respond that she listens only partially to what the client is saying
- Rehearsals of what the clinician is planning to say
- Problems the client is presenting that are very similar to problems the clinician is personally trying to manage, resulting in splitting the clinician's attention between the client's problems and her own problems
- The client's experiences which are very different from the clinician's and the clinician having difficulty relating to the client
- The clinician not feeling well or being preoccupied by her own physiological needs such as hunger or fatigue.

Listening to a person may sound deceptively simple, but it may be partially or completely omitted when clinicians feel pressured by a busy schedule and demanding environment. Under these circumstances, clinicians may be too fatigued or distracted, or simply forget to genuinely listen to their clients, patients, and their families. Instead, they may operate on automatic pilot, explaining to clients about their communication problems and the intended therapy procedures rather than listening to their clients for information about how they are feeling and thinking about their problems. To listen to a client or patient, the clinician should take note of the person's responses to stimulation (e.g., the therapeutic exercises). Is the person physically and psychologically ready to engage in therapeutic tasks? Is the person motivated to take part in therapy? Does the client understand the purpose of the therapy or exercises?

Joseph Wepman's conceptual model for the therapeutic processes involved in recovery from aphasia considers the following questions (Brookshire, 2007; Chapey, 2008; Wepman, 1951). Wepman discusses *stimulation* as the auditory, visual, or tactile stimuli the clinician presents to the patient. *Facilitation* refers to the patient's physical and psychological readiness to benefit from the stimuli (therapy) presented. *Motivation* is the patient's interest and even enthusiasm to attend and work for improvement both in the therapy session and outside it. Wepman's overall conclusion is that when stimulation, facilitation, and motivation are operating optimally, therapy has its best opportunity for success.

Listening to our clients and patients will probably take more time in the short run than simply going about our preplanned therapy; however, time may be saved in the long run. Listening to our clients' thoughts, feelings, and experiences requires patience, compassion, and investment of time and energy on our part. When we listen to people, we open ourselves to the experiences of human tragedy, loss, and suffering. Hearing our clients' and patients' stories "touches" us and reminds us that we are vulnerable to life's vicissitudes as well. To listen to people involves being attuned to their messages and needs, no matter how bluntly or subtly expressed. It means listening to a person's clear statements about physical discomfort as well as listening for nonverbal messages such as a cough that signals reluctance to comply with the clinician's request or a raised finger that signals that the person wants to say something. Our attunement to people involves paying attention to multiple channels of communication (verbal, nonverbal, and tactile) they use and learning to recognize their needs so that we are less likely to miss important signals (Fogle, 2009a).

On a pragmatic level, careful listening can lead to a modification of our therapy plans to better meet the client's needs and preferences. For example, a client may hint at a desire to focus on a particular area in therapy that is important to her, such as remembering grandchildren's names, that helps the clinician better understand the client's priorities. On an interpersonal level, our listening helps clients feel understood, appreciated, respected, and cared for. Simple listening can go a long way toward building the person's trust in the clinician and therapy. At the same time, it is sometimes necessary to put limits on listening to a person's concerns. Because of time constraints, as well as professional scope of practice, a client or patient's concerns (complaints) may need to be directed to another health care or mental health specialist, for example, a nurse, psychologist, or pastoral staff. Careful and therapeutic listening involves making decisions about what is relevant to our area of practice and what information warrants another professional's evaluation.

TONE OF VOICE

In professional as well as personal relationships, tone of voice communicates an immense amount of information and can be even more powerful than the content of the message. Throughout a person's life, the voice often mirrors the person's emotional state (Boone, McFarlane, & Von Berg, 2009; Colton, Casper, & Leonard, 2006). How we feel may be heard in the sound of our voices as well as in changes in our prosodic rhythm patterns. Our emotional status plays a primary role in the control of respiration; for example, nervousness can be heard in our shortness of breath.

From the client's perspective, the clinician's tone of voice may be recalled long after instructions or therapy is forgotten. A warm and friendly, yet confident and authoritative, voice helps clients both like and respect clinicians without fully knowing how competent they may be. A tone of voice that sounds blaming, belittling, or critical may discourage clients from following recommendations, no matter how good they are. A gentle and accepting voice tone may make it easier for clients to accept the clinician's words, even when difficult news or information has to be shared. However, the clinician should avoid sounding saccharine or excessively sweet. This may be perceived by clients and other professionals as being disingenuous and in some settings (particularly medical) can quickly diminish professional credibility. On the other hand, a tone of voice that reflects false confidence or bravado can sound equally insensitive or arrogant and can diminish a client's respect for a clinician.

EMPATHY

Empathy is central to the development of a therapeutic relationship. It is the principal route to understanding clients and their families and helping them to feel understood. Adler (1956) characterized empathy as the ability to "see with the eyes of another, hear with the ears of another, and feel with the heart of another" (p. 135). Empathy involves careful listening, understanding, and *communicating* that understanding to the client (Kahn, 1999). Important skills for empathic understanding include attending, listening, paraphrasing, reflection of feeling, and summarizing (these skills will be discussed further in Chapter 4). The clinician strives to accurately paraphrase the client's main thoughts or feelings, often using the important words of the client and distilling and condensing the principal thoughts and feelings (Nystul, 2005). The clinician tries to communicate to the client that she not only has technical expertise and understands the communication problems, but is trying to understand what it is like to walk in that person's shoes. The clinician, while maintaining a professional posture, is allowing herself to feel something of the person's distress or emotional suffering and what it might be like to go through that experience (Brammer & MacDonald, 2002; Ivey et al., 2009).

A distinction needs to be made between empathy and sympathy (Schultz & Carnevale, 1996). Sympathy does not require as much interpersonal connection with someone as does empathy. We may genuinely feel sorry for someone's loss (sympathy), but we may not engage in the dialogue that is required to achieve true empathy. To have sympathy, a person feels sorry for another's situation or loss, yet remains relatively detached (e.g., we send sympathy cards, not empathy cards). With sympathy, friends or families may cry with one another, but there is not necessarily a personal responsibility to become involved and an ongoing responsibility to help. Sympathy often includes sharing mutual or similar experiences in commiseration. Sympathy is not a professional stance with clients, patients, and families, and in counseling it may be nontherapeutic. For example, if, while listening to a particularly tragic case history, a clinician begins to cry in front of a client, the client may view the clinician's response as somewhat unprofessional. The client may change the topic or edit the information he is presenting to avoid further upsetting the clinician.

Therapeutically, empathy is the better response to clients' and families' difficulties and tragedies. Although you may genuinely feel sympathy toward a person, empathy allows you to feel, as best you can, what the person is experiencing, while functioning at an interpersonal level that is sufficient to maintain your professional composure. Your composure assures people who are suffering that you can maintain the professional perspective necessary to support them and help them find their internal and external resources to cope with life's challenges (Brammer & Mac Donald, 2002).

An important skill in determining an appropriate empathic response is reading the client's nonverbal behavior (Brammer & MacDonald, 2002; Fogle, 2009a). Body communication of feelings and needs often is more revealing than words. By carefully attending to clients' and family members' verbal and nonverbal messages we can answer important questions about what the person is feeling that will help guide our responses to the person. For example, What is the person feeling right now? How does the person view this problem? How does the person view her world right now? Other important questions include, Why is the person so upset? What is causing this strong emotional reaction from the person? Through nonjudgmental understanding of the client's experiences and feelings, clinicians can better construct treatment plans that are meaningful to their clients and help meet the emotional needs that are within our scope of practice.

Ivey and colleagues (2009) discuss different levels of clinician empathy, from subtractive levels to basic empathy to additive levels. Subtractive responses are less-than-desirable responses and subtract something from the client's experience. They do not adequately capture the client's story and usually indicate poor listening skills on the part of the clinician. Basic empathy indicates that the clinician's responses are compatible with the client's experience; the clinician is using good attending skills with paraphrasing, reflection of feeling, and summarization. In additive empathy the clinician adds congruent ideas and feelings and furthers the depth of understanding in order to facilitate client exploration of additional or alternative thoughts. By deepening the client's understanding, the additive level of empathy also opens up some degree of hope. The following are examples of five levels of empathy to a client:

> Client: "I don't know what to do with my son since he was in the car accident. He doesn't seem to want to be part of the family anymore and he just stays in his room all of the time. I've tried everything I can think of and everything anybody else can think of!"

> Clinician (Level 1, *subtractive response*): "You seem to have a rather negative view of your son. I think you ought to consider the fact that he has had some neurological damage."

> Clinician (Level 2, *slightly subtractive response*): "It sounds like you are very frustrated and maybe feeling like giving up on your son."

> Clinician (Level-3, *basic empathy*): "You're discouraged and confused about how to help your son become more involved with the family. The things you have tried so far haven't worked, and you're not sure what to try next."

> Clinician (Level 4, *slightly additive*): "You have tried every way you can think of to get your son back involved with the family, but nothing is working. You've tried hard and are getting tired and a little frustrated with the situation. What does all this effort that you've made for your son tell you about your feelings for him?"

> Clinician (Level 5, *additive*): "I sense your confusion and frustration right now, and your feeling that maybe you should give up. Based on what you have told me, your thoughts and feelings make a lot of sense. It is also understandable that you keep trying to bring your son back into family activities together (i.e., the clinician expresses hope for the future, and suggests that the parent's efforts are not futile). You have told me how loving and happy he was before the accident and how different he is now. It sounds like the adjustment to these changes has been very difficult for you. I imagine it takes a while to adjust your expectations, especially because you care so much for him."

This last response, at the level 5 additive level, takes a risk of adding the clinician's perceptions. It is always important to observe how the client responds to empathic statements so that you can return to safer level 3 responses if needed.

Overall, empathic responses involve the use of nonblaming language so that the client or family member can feel that whatever they have done, or whatever they are thinking or feeling, is normal. SLPs' and Auds' training help them learn to avoid subtractive responses (levels 1 and 2); use effectively basic empathic responses (level 3); and occasionally employ slightly additive empathic responses (level 4). Psychologists and counselors may have the training and the skills to more appropriately use additive (level 5) responses.

Providing empathic responses follows a 1–2–3 pattern (Ivey et al., 2009) and requires that we listen to the client's responses to determine whether our statements should be recalibrated.

1.   The clinician attends to, listens to, and observes the client's verbal and nonverbal behaviors. The clinician selects a key thought or feeling the client has communicated, and paraphrases, reflects, or summarizes the thought or feeling to the client.

2.   The client responds to the clinician's reflective or summary statements with verbal and nonverbal behaviors. The client's response may indicate general agreement or disagreement with the clinician's empathic remark.

3.   The clinician again attends to, listens to, and observes the client's verbal and nonverbal behaviors and responds to the client's behaviors. For example, "That observation seemed to have resonated with you in some way," or, if the clinician's response was not sufficiently empathic she might say, "The observation I just made got a reaction from you. Can you tell me what you are thinking?" This question provides an opportunity to continue the dialogue with the client and to repair the empathic error if necessary.

Empathic responses are often important to communicate as the clinician is sharing a diagnosis with a parent or client. Many times children with hidden problems such as auditory processing disorders are brought to the clinic for an evaluation. The parents initially may have no idea what is wrong with their child, why he is not listening, learning, or obeying them. Parents have usually given much thought to their child's difficulties and have tried to figure out the problems. They may have taken the child to various specialists including a pediatrician, reading specialist, or psychologist. However, often it is not until the child is seen by an SLP or Aud that a determination is made that the child may have an auditory processing disorder (Bellis, 2003; Musiek & Chermak, 2007; Kelly, 2001; Roeser & Downs, 2004).

After the child has been evaluated and the clinician and parent(s) are in the exit interview, the clinician may want to reinforce the parents for all they have done to try to determine the nature of the child's problems. It may be helpful for parents who are experiencing guilt for not getting an earlier evaluation or therapy to say, "Don't be hard on yourself. You have been searching for a long time to better understand your child's difficulties. It has been perplexing, but I think we are beginning to understand some of the foundational issues that are impeding his language development. There are strategies that can improve your child's ability to understand you and to communicate."

It is not necessary that clinicians have gone through situations and experiences identical to their clients and patients in order to empathize with them, although clinicians who have faced loss and suffering in their own lives may be somewhat more capable of feeling and expressing empathy for others. Along these lines, a clinician may respond to a client with, "I know that this slow process of recovery is really hard on you." This example highlights the point that empathy needs to be communicated, not just privately felt by the clinician. Empathy is not a static quality or a personality trait of the clinician; it occurs in an interpersonal context. Clients are not likely to know that their clinicians are feeling empathy unless it is communicated (Brodley, 2001; Ridley & Lingle, 1996).

Two types of cautions regarding clinicians' expressions of empathy need to be described. The first caution involves failures in empathy that occur when a well-meaning SLP or Aud unwittingly projects her own reactions to a situation onto a client. For example, an SLP may think it would be terrible not to be able to read newspapers, magazines, or books. Yet this client, who did little reading anyway, is not particularly concerned about decreased reading ability. In this case, it would not sound empathic for the clinician to tell the client, "Not being able to read must be very hard on you." This may not accurately reflect the client's appraisal of the situation. The clinician needs to gain an accurate understanding of the client's experience before she can make an accurate empathic statement or reflection (Brammer & MacDonald, 2002).

The second caution involves expressions of empathy that side with the client's pessimism instead of fostering hopefulness. While it is important to communicate to people an understanding of their experiences, a clinician's communications should avoid excessive indulgence in their pessimism or self-pity. The clinician should try to balance empathy for how the person feels at the moment with expressions of hopefulness that are realistic and appropriate to that person's situation. A clinician may reflect something along the lines, "It sounds as though you are feeling frustrated with the slow pace of your progress, but you should make significant improvements if you keep up your current speech exercises." It is critical for the clinician to convey hope rather than dwelling on despair. Hope gives the person some sense that the future may bring some relief from suffering (Brammer & MacDonald, 2002).

Expressing Empathy

Jason, a 14-year-old boy, sustained a severe traumatic brain injury when hit by a drunk driver as he and his family were walking along a country road while on vacation. He was taken to a large children's hospital in Northern California where he remained in a coma for several months. When he was capable of receiving rehabilitation, physical therapy, occupational therapy, and speech therapy, professionals began working with him. After a few months of rehabilitation, Jason was discharged home, and the hospital referred him to me so that he could continue speech, language, and cognitive therapy.

During my initial interview with the parents in the family home, I learned that Jason was a very bright high school freshman who was very well liked and athletic. Although both parents appeared to have gone through the grieving process, bringing Jason home from the hospital with his numerous severe physical, speech, language, and cognitive limitations made the reality of his impairments and disabilities even more tragic. Both parents were understandably mourning the loss of the child they knew (just as Jason was lamenting the loss of the self he previously knew). The parents appeared to have considerable pessimism and fear about their son's future improvements, his eventual independence, and his quality of life. The father was particularly concerned that his son could not continue being the athlete he

Continues on next page

Continued from previous page

was before the TBI and play football as he (the father) had done in high school and college. Jason understandably also had considerable pessimism about his future in school, athletics, and social life.

I felt it was important when talking with both the child and parents to be both empathic ("It's understandable how frightening it must be not knowing how much recovery can be made"), realistic, and hopeful. Over the two years that I worked with Jason, I sometimes conveyed to Jason and his parents that he was likely going to continue having problems with his speech, language, and cognition, but with supportive parents, hard work, and continued therapy he would maximize his potential. With strong support from his family and long-term speech, language, and cognitive therapy, Jason eventually graduated from high school and community college and is now living semi-independently.

CLINICAL QUESTIONS

1. As the clinician in this case, how might you balance providing realistic feedback and support to this family?

2. What feedback from the client would you expect if your empathic efforts "missed the mark"?

RESPECT FOR THE PERSON

Another crucial building block for the therapeutic relationship is the clinician's respect for the person. Clinicians' questions, suggestions, and interventions should always convey respect for individuals and should affirm that they are doing the best they can under difficult circumstances. The delicate balance is always between acceptance of individuals for who they are (and how they feel at the moment) and encouragement to change (Dimeff, Koerner, & Linehan 2007; Linehan & Kehrer, 1993; Linehan, 1993; Siegel, 2007). For example, an SLP can convey empathy and respect to a client who is disfluent, but simultaneously present therapy that instills hope and encourages the person to develop healthier attitudes toward his disfluency and ways of improving his speech. We can hope that, over time, the client will internalize our messages and become both more self-accepting and more encouraging of self-change.

Respect for the person is most often communicated through daily interaction rather than through direct statements. In other words, the clinician's behaviors convey an implicit respect for the person's dignity, privacy, autonomy, and vulnerability. In medical settings in particular, patients may feel that their dignity and privacy are invaded because of needing assistance with dressing and toileting. They may feel that they have lost autonomy because doctors, nurses, and rehabilitation staff make decisions for them. SLPs, for example, may decide what food textures and liquid consistencies are safe for the patient, thereby taking charge of areas the patient has controlled most of his life. The patient may feel vulnerable to the "whims" of the medical staff caring for him, and even the rehabilitation staff who are attempting to help the patient return to his home and community. The patient may feel that the SLP is being arbitrary in her decision about the patient's limits in problem solving and reasoning through safety issues in the home. Clinicians need to act in ways that protect and support patients' basic human rights by giving them adequate information, respecting their physical modesty, and providing them with an environment in which they are encouraged to develop their potential (Fogle, 2004; Fogle, Reece, & White, 2008).

One way that SLPs and Auds protect their clients' and patients' rights is by maintaining professional boundaries. The clinicians' actions should serve the clients' needs rather than their own. Although clinicians should relate to clients as people who are sensitive to life's trials, relationships with clients are generally nonreciprocal. Therefore, clinicians should not slip into a social posture of reciprocal sharing of feelings and problems. Occasional clinician self-disclosures may enhance the therapeutic relationship and the clinician's credibility (Kahn, 1999). Self-disclosure can best be used sparingly and on occasions when the client expresses doubt in the direction of treatment. On these occasions, the clinician might provide a relevant or parallel example in which obstacles were overcome. Empathic self-disclosures may be meaningful to the client if they accurately reflect the client's current feelings and simultaneously instill hope. Clinician self-disclosures are not likely to promote the therapeutic relationship when they are used to help the clinician increase her self-confidence, credibility, or need for a social connection with the client.

Occasionally a clinician may work with a client who has a similar disorder or problem as a clinician's family member, such as a parent or grandparent. For example, the clinician may be working with a young girl who has an attention deficit disorder and significant language problems, and the clinician may have a child with similar problems. It would not be therapeutic to commiserate with the parents of the client about the mutual challenges they experience with their children. However, it may be helpful to mention briefly that the clinician has a child with similar problems and how important it has been to get a thorough diagnosis and ongoing therapy. Similarly, if the clinician has a parent or grandparent who sustained a CVA, it may be therapeutic to mention to the patient or family member the experience and how important it has been to have the help of an SLP, but not to present details of how the clinician has coped with the challenges. These very brief self-disclosures may support the importance of therapy but should not be overused or used in a self-indulgent way by the clinician.

THERAPEUTIC COMMUNICATION

Communicating in a therapeutic manner with clients can help support, develop, and maintain a therapeutic relationship. Therapeutic communication refers to the actions, utterances, and behaviors that contribute to the therapeutic relationship. While the therapeutic relationship describes the context in which therapy occurs, dimensions of therapeutic communication provide therapists with the "how to" skills or the methods for conveying respect, empathy, understanding, and warmth to our clients.

Therapeutic communication encompasses our verbal and nonverbal communication; it includes our physical presentation, body language, tone of voice, and wording of responses or interventions. The moment we meet a client we begin to communicate both nonverbally and verbally. Even when a person has no voice or ability to speak, he is "shouting" nonverbally to anyone and everyone (Tanner, 2008). The old adage is true: we *cannot not* communicate. In other words, even our silence is not neutral (Anchin & Kiesler, 1982; Kiesler, 1996); it can convey respect and patience or indifference and disrespect. The following discussion addresses different aspects of therapeutic communication.

Nonverbal Communication

Our nonverbal communication can convey our professional role and authority in a friendly, non-intimidating manner (Burgoon, Buller, & Woodall, 2002; Ciccia, Step, & Turkstra, 2003; Fogle, 2009a). Our nonverbal communication can also convey respect and acceptance for people. Nonverbal channels of communication include our physical appearance and dress, our postures and movements, and how we position ourselves in relation to our clients. Clients are not the only ones who may develop a guarded posture in the therapeutic setting. Sometimes clinicians present themselves in a guarded fashion, either because they lack confidence with certain types of clients or because they are uncomfortable with a client's interpersonal style (e.g., angry, hostile, or sullen). Optimally, our nonverbal communication should convey our professional confidence and poise, and it should be consistent with our verbal messages.

PHYSICAL APPEARANCE

Obviously, there are aspects of our physical appearance that we cannot change, for example, our height and general body type. However, we can choose to dress professionally to enhance our credibility, particularly when working on sensitive issues with clients, patients, and family members. Some hairstyles and colors, excessive piercings, or tattoos may look unprofessional or even threatening to some people. The task here is to balance personal preferences with the demands of our professional roles. In our professions of speech-language pathology and audiology being well groomed is an asset; however, we do not want to appear to be prima donnas to our clients or co-workers. Deciding upon our physical presentation (e.g., hair and dress) may also depend upon the particular setting, client population, ethnicity, and regional standards. Wearing a white lab coat, for example, may enhance professional credibility in some settings (i.e., medical) but unnecessarily intimidate or distance clients (e.g., children) in other settings. Dressing very casually may convey comfort and poise with clients in some settings, but disrespect in others.

Children often wear clothing and styles to project particular images, and adults often do the same. However, hospitalized patients usually have that form of expression curtailed when they are required to wear unattractive and often uncomfortable and poorly-fitting gowns. Patients can reestablish some of their self-image when they are allowed and encouraged to wear clothing that reflects their personal style.

COUNSELING SKILLS IN ACTION

Helping Clients Feel Good

In convalescent hospitals some residents choose to wear clothes that may appear unnecessary for the environment. Some women like to dress in their finest attire before going into public areas, and some men wear a tie throughout the day, much like they may have worn through much of their professional careers. When I see a resident well groomed and dressed I like to compliment him or her and make a little fuss over how nice the person looks, but not in a patronizing manner. Residents seem to always appreciate people who notice when they are dressed up. They may have precious few opportunities to express their pride and dignity and to garner positive comments from others.

CLINICAL QUESTIONS

1. In what ways can your communication with an inpatient be used to express respect and support for positive self-esteem?

2. What kinds of compliments may be "too much" or run the risk of being misconstrued?

BODY LANGUAGE

There are other aspects of our physical presentation that affect clients, and these generally are referred to as body language. We convey to people how we feel about them through an assortment of macrogestures (e.g., body postures, arm and hand positions, and gestures), and microgestures (e.g., eye contact, eye blinks, and intentional and unintentional facial expressions). Clients are keen observers of clinicians' movements and gestures that convey comfort or tension in their presence. Clinicians who feel comfortable with their clients typically have an open body language, for example, their arms and legs are uncrossed. Clinicians who are tense or unsure of themselves may communicate these feelings with more of a closed body language, for example, crossing their arms over their chest or holding their note pad as if it is a shield between them and their clients. Clinicians need to monitor the degree of confidence, comfort, and engagement that is conveyed by their body language with clients. Clients can be very sensitive to the emotional barriers clinicians create with their arms, note pads, table and chair arrangements, or other objects. In general, clients feel you are interested in them if you face them squarely and lean forward slightly, have an expressive face, and use encouraging gestures (Burgoon et al., 2002; Fogle, 2009a; Ivey et al., 2009).

Clinicians also can monitor how they pace themselves (e.g., walking or arm gestures) with different kinds of clients; for example, adjusting our pace to be consistent with an elderly client's slower pace can communicate patience and empathy. On the other hand, maintaining a pace that is much faster than a client's may communicate impatience, insensitivity, or intolerance. Slowing our pace or adjusting it to be more similar to a client's may pose a challenge to clinicians who are very energetic and achievement or activity (versus relationship) focused.

PROXEMICS

One of the first signals we give people about how we feel about them is where we stand or position ourselves in relation to them. Burgoon and colleagues (2002), Ciccia, Step, and Turkstra (2003), and Fogle (2009a) discuss personal space and interpersonal or conversational distance (proxemics). Personal space refers to the minimum amount of spatial distance a person needs to feel comfortable, which can vary considerably depending on the relationship, interaction, or activity with another person, as well as cultural backgrounds.

COUNSELING SKILLS IN ACTION

A Stranger at the Door

I received a request from a home health agency to evaluate and treat an elderly woman who had sustained a CVA. The woman lived in an older part of town and it was not generally safe when strangers came to the door. I had scheduled the appointment through a lady friend of the client who was planning to be present during my visits. I followed my typical procedures, which include, immediately after ringing the door bell, stepping back two paces so that when the door is opened I do not present a physical threat by having invaded the person's comfort zone. I am also out of arms' reach. (This practice was learned during my ambulance driving and EMT years; the driver and attendant never knew what to expect when a door opened.) I handed the client's friend my business card and she looked it over carefully. She then asked to see my driver's license (a very wise request) and I took it out of my wallet and handed it to her. She told me to wait a moment while she showed my identification to my new client. The door was closed, but after a couple of minutes the woman returned and invited me into the home. I was very aware that both elderly women were initially uncomfortable with a strange man in the home, and that the utmost decorum was needed in their presence.

CLINICAL QUESTIONS

1. What strategies can you use to help clients become comfortable with your presence?

2. What attitudes are important for you to convey?

3. What feedback can you be alert for in order to determine whether you are being perceived as too intrusive?

Appropriate distance can convey respect, but standing too far from a person can convey (accurately or inaccurately) discomfort or dislike of the person. According to Hall (1966) and Burgoon et al. (2002), public distance is about 10 feet or more apart; however, this is not considered a distance for effective therapeutic interaction or communication. Social-consultive distance (4 to 10 feet) is used for both social conversations and business transactions. However, social conversations frequently occur in the close range (4 to 6 feet) and business transactions in the far range (6 to 10 feet). Both people are out of touching range. Stewart and Cash (2003) recommend that for interviewing and counseling a distance of 2 to 4 feet is generally appropriate. SLPs and Auds frequently use the personal-casual distance (1 1/2 to 4 feet) when working with clients and patients, for example, when doing table work; however, the intimate distance (0 to 18 inches) is often needed during evaluations and hands-on therapy.

When entering a patient's intimate zone, observe his nonverbal messages. Note the patient's facial expressions and body language for signs of how he is tolerating your close presence and physical contact. It helps to verbally express appreciation of the patient's willingness to let you come near and touch the person's face or neck. Although counseling is not done in the close range, counseling skills are used, including eye contact, appropriate facial expressions, choice of words, and tone of voice. We need to keep in mind that the various proxemic distances and the comfort levels of both the patient and clinician are culturally based and often gender based, and what may be comfortable to the clinician may be very uncomfortable to the patient.

COUNSELING SKILLS IN ACTION

Evaluating Mr. T.

An attorney contacted me and requested that I evaluate a man's language and cognitive functioning because he had a history of various closed head injuries. The man I was to evaluate was in jail. I had to pass through various levels of security and entered into a small visitor's room. My client was brought into a small holding room. Cameras recorded everything being said and done. We both sat on hard, round stools separated by a low wall and a heavy wire mesh. I had to lay all the testing materials on the metal counter on my side of the wire mesh. No physical contact with the materials was possible for the examinee other than during a writing task where I slipped a piece of paper and pen through a narrow slot. Although we were within the personal-casual distance, there was nothing personal or casual about the interaction. The environment was highly structured and not particularly well suited for developing rapport.

CLINICAL QUESTIONS

1. In highly formal situations such as the one described above, what strategies can you use to develop rapport with the client?

2. What typical alliance-building strategies might be contraindicated?

Hospitalized individuals, particularly those in skilled nursing facilities, often stake out their territory in the hallway near the nursing station or the activities room. Many residents have their place to eat in the dining room area, and they become upset if someone inadvertently sits in that place and, because of inability to communicate well, may give strong nonverbal messages to indicate their displeasure. A sense of personal territory helps patients feel that they have some control over their environment and that they possess something. Asking patients if you may join them, for example, during meal time shows respect and consideration for their territorial needs (Tanner, 2008; Fogle, 2009a).

COUNSELING SKILLS IN ACTION

The Holocaust Survivor

I received an order to evaluate a patient's swallowing in a skilled nursing facility. I was advised by nursing staff that the patient was an elderly woman who had survived the Holocaust and that she was still very fearful of men, particularly men wearing any kind of uniform. I chose to take off my white lab coat before entering the room. I knocked on the door frame and softly said her name to get her attention before entering the room. Her bed was next to the door and I made certain she was watching me as I approached so that I would not startle her. I bent down slightly as I walked toward her so my eyes would be nearer her eye level and to try to make myself appear less threatening. I pulled up a chair and sat beside her bed so that I was not standing over her, and I did not touch her. This approach apparently worked well, along with noninvasive gestures, a soft tone of voice, and quiet conversation. I did not attempt to evaluate her swallow during this time, but only gain her trust. I came back later and was able to successfully do a bedside swallow evaluation.

CLINICAL QUESTIONS

1. What other kinds of clients might require an especially sensitive initial approach?

2. How might you adapt your usual professional manner in these cases?

SEATING ARRANGEMENTS

Seating arrangements and postures can have an influence on our clients' level of trust and comfort. Frequently, clinicians and clients sit across from one another in therapy with a table between them. Various assessment or therapy materials may be scattered over the table. However, during both therapy and counseling with clients it is often better not to have a table (a physical barrier) between you and the person. Sitting at right angles facing one another with just the corner of the table to one side and an open area on the other can facilitate a sense of openness in the communication. Sitting on the same side of the table facing one another is also helpful for a feeling of openness. If a table must be between you and the person to whom you are talking, try to have the evaluation or therapy materials moved to the side so they are not distracting or adding to the physical barrier.

When discussing sensitive issues or presenting bad news, it is helpful to have cups or glasses of water on the table for each person present, including yourself. Sometimes when we are uncomfortable about what we are sharing with someone our mouths may become dry and a sip of water can give us some moisture as well as help soothe our nerves. During extended counseling, clients and families also may need a little water to drink to relieve a dry mouth or to sip during anxious moments. Having water available to clients and families is a small gesture that reflects thoughtfulness and sensitivity.

EYE CONTACT

Even though clients sometimes have poor eye contact, it is important for clinicians to position themselves so that they can make direct eye contact to demonstrate respect, interest, and sensitivity to clients. Standing up while the client is sitting down interferes with comfortable eye contact and may appear intimidating, especially to children. (Children often are more comfortable if a clinician drops down on one knee to be more eye to eye.) Clients may interpret how well clinicians like them based upon the clinicians' amount of eye contact. Clinicians also can stay alert for signs that certain clients are uncomfortable with eye contact, which may reflect their cultural or ethnic backgrounds and social customs.

By maintaining good eye contact with the people to whom we are talking we can more easily note their responses to our comments. Good eye contact allows clinicians to observe facial expressions and helps us interpret what clients understand or how they may be feeling in response to our statements. Clients often look away when discussing topics that particularly distress them, and we also may find ourselves avoiding eye contact when we are uncomfortable with a topic or uncertain of our information (Fogle, 2009a; Ivey et al., 2009).

When talking to clients or family members, as well as professionals such as teachers, administrators, nurses, and physicians, it is often helpful to establish eye contact for one to two seconds before speaking. This can help listeners recognize that we are serious about what we are going to communicate and also can help us appear more confident than we may actually be feeling. A clinician who has poor eye contact when communicating may be perceived as less confident or trustworthy than a clinician who establishes and maintains good eye contact (Burgoon et al., 2002; Sheehan, 1970).

TOUCH

Patients in medical settings often feel that physicians and rehabilitation therapists disregard their need for personal space and privacy (Frank, 2002; Malkin, 2002). As SLPs and Auds we typically must touch clients and patients in our work with them, for example, during oral-peripheral and swallowing examinations, oral-motor exercises, and audiological testing and hearing aid fitting. It is respectful to clients of all ages to ask them if you may touch them, particularly around the head, face, or throat areas, which are the most sensitive areas for many individuals. A surprise touch from a clinician can be startling and offensive to many clients. Advising the client and asking permission to touch the client shows respect for personal space and communicates a desire to avoid being overly intrusive; for example, "Mrs. Cohen, I would like to place my fingertips on your throat while you are chewing and swallowing to see how you are doing with your swallowing today. Is that okay?" Some clinicians typically have warm hands, which may feel comforting to clients and patients. Other clinicians may tend to have cold hands that are at first uncomfortable to the person they are touching. Clinicians who tend to have cold hands can tell the client that they are going to warm them up by rubbing them together for a moment. This sometimes amuses clients, but they also appreciate the clinician's thoughtfulness. Although it is difficult to generalize about individuals' sensitivity to touch, we need to appreciate that even though we are accustomed to touching both children and adults on and around their faces and even inside their mouths, such touching may be very uncomfortable to the client or patient because of their cultural, medical, or family backgrounds. A client's personal (and possibly traumatic) experiences (Linehan, 1993; Masterson & Lieberman, 2004), sensory integration disorder (Kranowitz, 2005), or Asperger's Disorder (Emmons & Anderson, 2005) can also be associated with being over- or under-sensitive to touch. In addition, some patients with CVAs or TBIs may have either hypersensitivity or hyposensitivity to touch, and therapists need to be aware of this possibility. Those with hypersensitivity may not appreciate or easily tolerate touch around the face and neck. Those with hyposensitivity may not perceive the tactile cues that are presented.

COUNSELING SKILLS IN ACTION

Hypersensitivity to Touch

After a particularly emotional psychotherapy session in which the client exposed significant emotional pain, the client, a mother of four children, stood up and began walking towards the office door. The psychologist (L. V. F.) followed behind her and gently reached out to momentarily put her hand on the client's shoulder in a gesture of compassion and support. The sobbing woman whirled around and glared at the psychologist and ordered her to "Never do that again!" A review of the client's history revealed that she had been raped years earlier by a trusted authority figure and had subsequently developed a hypersensitivity to touch, especially unexpected touch, by other adults. In this case, the client's trauma history had created a sensitivity to touch and even misperceptions regarding the supportive intentions of people in her current life.

CLINICAL QUESTIONS

1. How might you try to repair this therapeutic error if you were the clinician in this situation?

2. What other factors may alert you that a particular client finds touch to be aversive or frightening?

CONSISTENCY OF COMMUNICATION

Consistency of communication is extremely important in creating a therapeutic climate. There are two types of consistency: (1) communication consistency in the moment and (2) communication consistency over time (Ivey et al., 2009). The first, communication consistency in the moment, refers to the clinician's ability to send a consistent message through both verbal and nonverbal channels of communication (e.g., Benjamin, 1996; Henry, 1997; Kiesler, 1996). If a client perceives inconsistent messages from the clinician, the efforts at therapeutic communication may be negated. For example, if a clinician is careful to use friendly, nonblaming language but has her arms folded and a tense jaw, she may betray a negative attitude toward the client. Any positive efforts may go unnoticed by the client, and the client may feel mistrustful of the clinician.

Initially, this may sound like too much for a clinician to keep track of; however, consistently positive communication skills will probably come automatically to the reflective and well-trained clinician in most circumstances. When a clinician notices inconsistencies in his communication with a client, it may signal ambivalence or suppressed feelings (e.g., frustration) toward a client. It is time, then, to reflect on our feelings and reactions toward the client so that consistent communication can be resumed.

Consistent communication over time is also very important to the maintenance of the therapeutic relationship. This involves clinician stability of attitude and behavior toward clients. We should treat clients the same way next week as we did this week. Clients should be able to predict how we will treat them rather than wonder what mood we will be in, how kind or understanding we will be. Clients are inevitably experiencing uncertainty in their lives because of their hearing, communication, or swallowing problems, and our relationship with them should contrast with that uncertainty. The professional relationship should offer a safe haven from all the other unpredictable events in their lives.

NONBLAMING LANGUAGE

When clients do not follow through or complete assigned therapy tasks (or when the nature of their symptoms or complaints is unclear), the clinician's manner of inquiry can either encourage the client to examine her behavior or increase the client's resistance or defensiveness (Kahn, 1999; Teyber, 2005; Wachtel, 1993, 2007). The clinician's language can encourage the client to open up, or it can create an adversarial climate. Even if the clinician feels frustrated by the client's low motivation or lack of commitment to the therapy, clinicians should resist the urge to sound disapproving or blaming toward clients. Such messages are not likely to encourage clients to work harder in therapy. On the contrary, clients who feel blamed are more likely to feel ashamed or embarrassed and more likely to hide their true feelings from the clinician.

It is important to maintain focus on the tasks of therapy without blaming the client for noncompliance or behaviors that interfere with therapy. Blaming clients (even when done unintentionally) can cause them to feel even worse about themselves and therefore less likely to follow through with future tasks (Levenson, 1995, 2010). Instead, the clinician can try to reflect the client's reluctance, mixed feelings, or reasons for not following through with the recommended exercises and therapy. For example, the clinician may respond to noncompliance with therapeutic tasks by wondering aloud: "I'm wondering if you are concerned about whether you will succeed on these exercises" or "I'm wondering if you are upset about not seeing faster improvement." This technique allows the clinician to side with the client's struggles while allowing him to maintain his dignity. Another approach is to assume that the client had good reasons for not doing something asked, for example, "You usually do most (some) of the exercises during the week that I give you. This week must have been extra hard for you not to do any of them. Are there any thoughts about the therapy you would like to talk about?" Once the client feels understood (rather than blamed), he will be much more likely to follow through on the tasks of therapy.

MAKING CLEAR STATEMENTS

An important principle when communicating with clients and their families is to use clear, unambiguous language so that there are no questions about your intent and message. Your effectiveness will be increased by eliminating vague words or statements. Such words and phrases as *I think*, *maybe*, and *sort of* convey uncertainty (Zaro, Barach, Nedelman, & Dreiblatt, 2000). There is considerable difference in impact between saying, "I think this might possibly help you," and saying, "I believe this will be helpful." Statements such as "I'm not really sure," "I don't have much experience with this, but it may possibly be helpful," or "I don't know about this, but let's try it out and see what happens" burden the client with the therapist's own insecurity and uncertainty. The clinician could be more effective by saying, "Research and experience show that this type of approach can be helpful and will likely be of assistance to you." Your confidence can help to instill hope in the client and her efforts to try new strategies.

COUNSELING WITH CHILDREN AND ADOLESCENTS

It is important to gauge our choice of words for the age of the individual with whom we are talking. We need to modify our interviewing and counseling techniques with children and adolescents (Novak, 2002; Ramig & Dodge, 2010; Zebrowski, 2006). A naturally warm, talkative clinician who likes and accepts children will be able to elicit more information than a rather cold, reserved clinician who does not particularly enjoy children and their characteristic behaviors. Clinicians should avoid looking down at children and should try to talk to them at eye level. This may mean getting down on one or both knees or sitting children in a higher chair than the one in which you are seated. It often helps to begin an interview or evaluation by sharing something fun or interesting, such as games or toys. Children usually like to do something with their hands while talking, and having them draw a picture during the conversation can often be useful and reveal salient events or feelings as well as keep the child's attention (Ivey et al., 2009; Ramig & Dodge, 2010; Reddy, Files-Hall, & Schaefer, 2005; Wachtel, 1993). Clinicians should use short sentences, simple words, and a concrete style of language, avoiding abstractions. Use names rather than pronouns because children often get confused with pronouns.

Young children generally respond better to a directive, structured style of interviewing with simple questions, rather than a nondirective, unstructured style with open-ended questions (Morrison & Anders, 2001). Our questions and messages to them need to be particularly clear, using words and language structures that match their language abilities.

Observing successful preschool and elementary school teachers' interactions with children can provide good models of how to talk with children at their levels.

Reflecting children's positive feelings seldom presents problems; reflecting their negative feelings often requires more skill. Clinicians should use words that cannot be misunderstood and that are not vague or evasive. When you are trying to identify the particular mood a child might be struggling with, try to be as specific and accurate as possible. Select the word that seems to describe what is going on with the child, the word that reflects the child's feelings at that moment. If a young child appears anxious you might say, "You look scared (or afraid)," because that is a word a child might use. The words *fearful, frightened, tense, anxious, nervous, edgy, jittery, alarmed, worried, uneasy,* or *apprehensive* may not fit because those are more adult words. Also, try to gauge the intensity of the affect as accurately as possible. If the child is very angry, "You seem annoyed" may underestimate the child's current feelings, whereas, "You seem hopping mad" or "really angry" may better capture the child's current emotional state. Adult words such as *incensed, infuriated, irate, outraged,* or *enraged* are not meaningful to many children. It is also important to remember that children do not need their feelings agreed with; they need them acknowledged. When you give words to children's and adolescents' feelings, they begin to trust that you understand them and are not judging them, only identifying what they are feeling and how deeply (Faber & Mazlish, 1995, 2005; Novak, 2002).

Ramig and Dodge (2010) and Zebrowski (2006) present many important points about building clinical relationships with teenagers who stutter, and these points are applicable to teenagers with other communication problems as well. Communicating with adolescents can be very challenging, and it is often even more challenging when the adolescent has a communication disorder. Teenagers frequently cannot or will not respond with a direct answer to a direct question. Zebrowski says that this may be because the adolescent may not know the answer, may be processing the question and the response slowly, and/or may be reticent to divulge information. Zebrowski recommends an "advance-retreat-advance" approach when trying to obtain information from adolescents. For example, when asking a direct question such as, "What are some of the things you would like to change about the way you talk?" (advance), the adolescent's response may be, "I don't know" or "I'm not sure." This may indicate the clinician needs to retreat by making a statement of acceptance such as, "That's okay" or "That's fine. It's something to think about." A general comment about either real or hypothetical clients may then be made, for example, "Sometimes teenagers want to learn how to talk more easily on the phone." This can be followed with an advance such as, "Is that true for you?" If the adolescent continues to be noncommittal, the clinician should move on to another topic (retreat), but return to the question later when it appears the adolescent will be more interested and responsive (advance). Using the adolescent's own comments as a bridge back to a previously asked but unanswered question helps the clinician obtain information when the adolescent is willing to share or divulge it. Conversely, pushing adolescents for responses or information that they are not willing to share can create power struggles that parallel relationships with their parents. These power struggles can usurp therapeutic efforts and lead to a stalemate in the therapeutic progress. In general, adolescents cannot be pushed, but they can be led.

Humor can be helpful in communicating with clients of all ages, but clinicians must be cautious about how it is employed (Manning, 2010; Ramig & Dodge, 2010; Zebrowski, 2002).

When clients are struggling with their symptoms and prone to shame or embarrassment about them, they may not yet have the critical emotional distance that will allow them to laugh at their own foibles. When clients are not ready to laugh at their own mistakes, it would be a therapeutic error for the clinician to do so. Even if done in a light-spirited manner, clients who are still very insecure about their symptoms may regard them as a no laughing matter and may (mis)interpret the clinician's laughter as cruel teasing. On the other hand, once the client begins to gain some self-confidence as well as trust in the clinician, the client may begin to laugh at some of his own communication errors or disfluencies. The clinician, at this point, may smile or laugh with the client as long as the client is laughing at the problem. This moment of humor and laughter may deepen the client-clinician relationship. Humor, though, is best occasionally interspersed through a therapy session and not necessarily a significant part of it.

Humor can reflect insight and perspective about a communication problem and indicate the realization that even with significant problems there can be a lighter side that may be appreciated (Manning, 2010; Ramig & Dodge, 2010; Zebrowski, 2002). Humor also reflects a person's ability to distance himself from the problem or current situation and indicates positive coping with a problem rather than avoiding or hiding from it. Stuttering therapy often involves helping the person desensitize himself to various aspects of stuttering and decrease emotional reactivity to his disfluencies. The child or adolescent's ability to use and accept humor that relates to the communication problem reflects development of insight and positive emotional distance. Some general cautions about using humor with clients are:

1. Be certain you are not laughing *at* your client or that you are not interpreted as doing so.

2. Do not use humor to avoid important topics related to the client's therapy.

3. Do not go overboard with laughter—use it sparingly.

4. Your manner of laughter needs to sound adult, not giggly or raucous.

5. Do not laugh at behavior or topics that you do not wish to reinforce, for example, an adolescent's sexual innuendoes or a young child's misbehavior.

When talking with adolescents it is generally best to avoid using the latest slang or jargon because teenagers often feel such language sounds artificial or phony when coming from an adult, particularly a professional. Also, avoid using profanity because you feel it might help you sound in tune with the young adult. In place of saying, "You look p-----off!" you might say, "You look *really* angry!" If you sense the adolescent is depressed, she would likely relate to the words *sad, unhappy,* or *miserable* more than *depressed, disconsolate, glum, gloomy, lugubrious, sorrowful,* or *melancholy.*

COUNSELING WITH ADULTS

When communicating with adults, consider their age, education, and professional background when known. Clear, concise, and precise wording, no matter what the person's background, is always appreciated. It is best to use ordinary and vivid words to express the mood you think the person is experiencing. When trying to identify an adult's mood, use adult words so that the person feels you are not talking down to her. For example, rather than saying, "You seem scared." you might say, "You look apprehensive." Most adults do not like their negative feelings to be exaggerated or amplified by someone else, for example, "You look *really* apprehensive!" It is usually best to understate an adult's feelings rather than overstate them (Brammer & MacDonald, 2002). Reflecting a client's feelings can help the client to bring subtle experiences and emotions into better focus.

COUNSELING WITH ELDERLY ADULTS

Gerontology is the study of four intertwined aspects of elderly or older people (i.e., usually considered 65+ years of age): chronological, biological, psychological, and sociological age. *Chronological age* is the number of years a person has lived. *Biological (health) age* refers to the physical changes (e.g., illness and disease processes) that diminish the efficiency of a person's organ systems (e.g., circulatory, renal, hearing, and vision). *Psychological age* includes changes in perceptual processes, mental functioning, adaptive capacity, personality, drives, and motivation. A person who is intellectually active and adapts well to new situations may be considered psychologically young. *Sociological age* refers to a person's changing roles and relationships in the social structure with family, friends, co-workers, and organizations. What determines older people's quality of life more than anything else are their biological and sociological ages (Hooyman & Kiyak, 2008).

When interviewing an older person, it is helpful to keep in mind that the person's psychological and sociological ages may be significantly different from the person's chronological or biological ages. These differences may affect how we communicate with an older person. For example, a patient who is 70 years old and has just had a stroke may have had a psychological and sociological age of someone in his 50s or 60s prior to the stroke. He may say that for the first time he is beginning to "feel his age," although he may still be thinking at much younger psychological and sociological ages. In contrast, a patient who is 65 years of age who has a history of serious illnesses, has smoked most of his life, and has been living with significantly decreased mental functioning, adaptive capacities, and motivation and little association with family, friends, and other people may seem more similar to a person chronologically 75 or 80 years of age.

For many elderly people there is an increase in emotional openness with age, a greater honesty and expressiveness regarding their feelings such as anger or sadness, and fewer attempts to conceal their emotions (Malatesta-Magal, Jonas, Shepard, & Culver, 1992; Shadden & Toner, 1997). Many people also tend to become more religious as they become elderly, and a person's religious faith may be an important contributor to her adjustment to the aging process and attitudes about death and dying (Eliopoulos, 2005; Hooyman & Kiyak, 2004; Wallace, 2007). Clinicians may sometimes have meaningful discussions about faith, death, and dying with their patients within the context of speech, language, and cognitive therapy. Once thought of as a sign of senility in elderly people, reminiscing about the past is now regarded as a way for elderly adults to seek social support, resolve the problems of the past, and seek integrity and serenity in the face of death (Woods et al., 2009).

Understanding the tendencies of elderly people can be helpful in determining how to communicate with them. For example, elderly people who have maintained vibrant social lives and are emotionally open and expressive regarding their feelings may, if their communication abilities allow, be very conversant and want to share their life experiences and wisdom with a young (relatively speaking) clinician who is there to help them. Such patients often want to "just talk" (reminisce) more than work on specific therapy tasks. In these cases, the clinician may suggest, "Let's work on your speech exercises for 20 minutes and then I would love to hear the story about your grandchildren that you began to tell me earlier." In other cases we may attempt to achieve our receptive and expressive language or cognitive therapy goals by incorporating them into the patient's stories. Some elderly people, however, have little energy, motivation, or interest in working and communicating with a speech-language pathologist (or most anyone else) and would rather be left alone.

COUNSELING SKILLS IN ACTION

Working in Skilled Nursing Facilities

In general, I have found most patients (residents) in skilled nursing facilities very motivated and happy to work with their speech therapist. I am not always certain if their motivation is to improve their communication, cognitive, or swallowing problems, or if they are just happy to have the undivided attention of a younger person who is willing to spend 30–50 minutes with them on a regular basis. These elderly people are often quite open about their physical concerns and are uninhibited about talking about their bowel and bladder problems and other such maladies that we, as SLPs, are unable to address.

CLINICAL QUESTIONS

1. If you are working with an elderly patient who would rather reminisce about his younger days than do speech, language, cognitive, or swallowing exercises, how might you approach the situation?

2. How would you respond and what would you say if an elderly patient began to tell you extremely intimate details about her marriage, her gynecological symptoms, or her children's financial difficulties?

Elderly people in convalescent hospitals often learn to be institutionalized and passively compliant. They feel that things are done to them rather than for them, with or without their consent. They are poked and prodded when examined; meals are provided with no say over whether they want the food offered; diapers are changed and other indignities occur; and so on. Patients also may feel as though they are passive participants in the rehabilitation process (Lubinski & Orange, 2000). Although professionals and caregivers rarely set out to disempower those under their care, this effect can be a sad and common reality for many elderly patients.

The attention and stimulation that an SLP provides may be the highlight of an elderly person's day. Patients commonly look forward to seeing their speech therapist and perk up as soon as the therapist appears. It is important for SLPs to maintain an upbeat demeanor when interacting with elderly people; an elderly patient may encounter other hospital staff who appear apathetic or exhibit few interpersonal skills as they go about their daily routines of managing the physical needs of the patient. Therefore, a warm smile and pleasant tone of voice are a welcome change to patients and may help draw them out of their doldrums and isolation.

Many elderly people have hearing losses, even though they do not have or use hearing amplification. It is helpful to follow aural rehabilitation techniques when communicating with the elderly, such as being in good lighting so the person can see your face easily, maintaining good eye contact with the person, and speaking clearly but not unduly loudly. Personal amplifiers (pocket talkers) may assist a person who is hearing impaired with her receptive language. Likewise, many elderly people have visual acuity problems even though they do not have or use eyeglasses. It is helpful to start speaking as you enter the person's line of sight; say the person's name and identify yourself (e.g., "I am Susan, your new speech therapist").

Patients who are unable to verbally communicate may not be able to reveal their personality or interests to medical staff and, therefore, may have difficulty establishing a relationship with their caregivers. A trusting relationship with caregivers is an important component of quality health care. Clinicians may want to help some patients construct a communication book with a portfolio of the person's life that can trigger conversations with staff and visitors (Bayles & Tomoeda, 2007; Code, Hemsley, & Herman, 1999).

There are a number of counseling challenges that are commonly encountered when working with older patients (Boles, 2002, 2006; Toner & Shadden, 2002). Older patients are often seen in medical settings in which there are time pressures and the clinician has insufficient time to conduct a thorough evaluation. Strict time limits can pose problems when working with older patients because of their often slowed response times, tendency to engage in tangential or unrelated conversation, attempts to extend conversation with the therapist in order to maintain social contact, and difficulty hearing which results in the need for frequent repetitions and rephrasing of statements and questions.

Many elderly people are most comfortable relating information in stories, which can be time-consuming and difficult to follow (Boles, 2002; Ryan, 1995; Toner & Shadden, 2002). Elderly people's narratives often have ambiguous references (e.g., using *him*, *her*, or *it* in place of a name or noun), which may be the result of word-finding difficulties. However, in order to obtain important information, clinicians need to be willing to listen to the form of communication the client prefers to use, which also may require the clinician teasing out the important information from an ongoing, ambiguous narrative. It is often helpful to begin an interview with informal conversation about casual or familiar topics. This encourages a more balanced, humanistic interaction with the clinician rather than a question-answer format that may seem abrupt or even rude to the elderly person. Elderly patients sometimes address professionals as "Dearie," "Honey," and so forth, especially if the clinician is much younger than the patient. Although the clinician may prefer to be addressed in a more professional manner, it may be prudent to accept such labels in order to maintain rapport. However, elderly people often appreciate being addressed as Mr., Mrs., or Dr. as a sign of respect.

COUNSELING SKILLS IN ACTION

Dr. M . . .

A resident I worked with in a skilled nursing facility had been a prominent physician in the community. After a CVA, he had a variety of speech, language, cognitive, and swallowing problems. Most of the nursing and rehabilitation staff spoke to him using his first name, however, I always addressed him as Dr. M . . . . He appeared to appreciate hearing his professional designation and responded quite favorably to what I asked of him.

CLINICAL QUESTIONS

1. What are some other ways of showing respect for elderly patients?

2. Consider your cultural or ethnic background and discuss some traditional ways of expressing respect for the elderly.

Many people adjust their style of speaking (accommodation) when talking to different age groups, for example young children, older children, adults, and older adults. However, over-accommodation occurs when individuals modify their speech style to a stereotypical pattern as a result of their perception of the person to whom they are talking, such as an older person (Toner & Shadden, 2002). Inappropriate speech registers or styles may be used, including oversimplification of language form and vocabulary, exaggerated suprasegmentals or intonational patterns, increased loudness, higher pitch, excessive slowing of speaking rate, and frequent repetitions or redundancy. Such over-accommodations are variously referred to as elderspeak, patronizing speech, or secondary baby talk (Caporael, 1981; Cohen & Faulkner, 1986; Ryan et al., 1991; Toner & Shadden, 2002). Ryan, Hummert, and Boisch (1995) and Toner and Shadden (2002) describe how many individuals use patronizing communication styles when "talking down" to older people while either caring for or controlling them. The following are examples of these communication styles.

Baby Talk

Baby talk may be considered both caring and controlling. In this communication style, elderspeak is used with generic terms of endearment (e.g., *Sweetie*, *Honey*, and even *Mama* or *Pops*). The younger person speaks in a tone (often with a high-pitched, saccharine voice) as though talking to an infant or very young child. A clinician may attempt to reinforce (control) desired behavior of an older person by saying, "You are working *so* hard today. I am *so* proud of you."

Overly Personal Talk

Overly personal talk is often accompanied by an endearing touch such as a pat on the shoulder, hand-holding, or a light hug. It is high in caring and low in controlling. The younger person may compliment the elderly person's appearance, such as, "You look *so* cute in that outfit" or "That color looks *so* good on you." It is important for SLPs and Auds to gauge their level of communication based on their familiarity and relationship with the client, and to avoid sounding patronizing or condescending

Directive Talk

Directive talk has the intent of having a person carry out a specific task, for example, taking medication, doing a specific exercise, or stopping a particular behavior such as moaning, crying, or using the nursing call button too frequently. This form of communication is primarily controlling with little or no caring. The speaker's goal is to obtain compliance from the person by being controlling while having minimum interaction (caring), for example, saying harshly, "You have already used the call button five times today. What do you want?"

Superficial Talk

Superficial talk is neither caring nor controlling; however, it can be considered rude. This may occur when an individual discusses a patient as though the person is not present, or when a professional discounts the person's expressions of feelings or needs by abruptly changing topics. Rather than seeing superficial talk as neutral (neither caring nor controlling), it may be perceived as uncaring and disrespectful.

Additional Guidelines for Working with Elderly Patients

Beyond the general guidelines of basic counseling skills, it is helpful when talking to elderly individuals to provide an environment that is communication friendly and age sensitive. Consider the arrangement of furniture to ensure safety, easy access, and comfort. Ensure adequate lighting, eliminate glare, and position yourself when possible to have light on your face to help the person better attend to your facial expressions and possibly help them with lip reading. Elderly people often have more difficulty hearing and understanding in noisy, distracting environments, and, therefore, working in a quiet room may facilitate interaction. Avoid a question-answer format (particularly closed questions) for obtaining information and allow adequate time for the person to respond to open-ended questions. Provide opportunities for the person to initiate topics and ask questions.

Elderly patients and caregivers appreciate being included in decision making about their care, which helps create a sense of partnership when planning goals, strategies, and therapy activities (Boles, 2006; Toner & Shadden, 2002). When clinicians make recommendations that elderly patients may not be ready to accept (e.g., an augmentative communication system or a hearing aid), they may appear to have not heard the recommendations or suggestions. Even when the clinician is confident that the recommendations have been heard, the patient may choose to ignore them by directing the conversation away from the clinician's focus. Seeking input from older patients rather than being directive helps them feel that they are still in control of their lives and that a younger professional is not determining what the patient must do.

Counseling with elderly patients and their caregivers often requires negotiating (Cohen, 2002; Toner & Shadden, 2002). In some cases the SLP and social service staff will need to work together to help patients and caregivers reach agreement about in-home care. What patients want may not be what caregivers in the home can provide. Sometimes a compromise must be negotiated with which neither person is completely satisfied, but where an agreement can be reached that is mutually acceptable (or tolerable). For example, an elderly patient may want to live with his children, but because of the patient's difficulty with communication and self-care, family members may not be able to provide the time and attention the person needs. Other living arrangements such as a board and care facility may be the best option for both the elderly person and family members.

Overall, communicating effectively with elderly individuals often requires greater than usual amounts of sensitivity and patience. By keeping in mind the changes in hearing, speech, language, and cognition that are part of the normal aging process, coupled with the impairments seen by SLPs and Auds, communication and counseling strategies can be optimized.

AVOIDING "PATHOLOGIZING" THE PERSON OR FAMILY

Although our scope of practice covers numerous diagnoses, it does not include emotional disorders. As discussed in Chapter 1, there is some overlap in disorders that psychologists and SLPs diagnose (e.g., receptive and expressive language disorders, phonological disorders, stuttering). We need to be cautious, though, about "pathologizing" a client by saying the person is depressed, anxious, paranoid, schizophrenic, narcissistic, histrionic, and so forth. Such labels and "diagnoses" are beyond our scope of practice. We also do not want to elevate symptoms to disorders. However, we do see clients who have such characteristics and symptoms, and some aspects of our observations may need to be included in our description of these individuals. In such cases it is prudent to use descriptions of behaviors that reflect our observations rather than global pathologizing terms.

SLPs and Auds can use **action language** (Moore, 1999; Schafer, 1983, 1992) to describe the behaviors of clients rather than drawing conclusions that objectify and pathologize clients. We can describe situation-specific behaviors but not label the complex of behaviors that may constitute a certain personality style (i.e., a trait) or a disorder. By providing behavioral descriptions of clinically relevant behaviors, we can document their occurrence in a professional manner and more easily write behavioral goals to increase or decrease certain behaviors. However, it is important to keep in mind that even though a client has a certain set of behaviors that we see in a particular situation, this does not mean that these are typical of the person. For example, rather than saying the child looked depressed, it is better to describe his behaviors, such as "he walked slowly with his head down, slumped in his chair, gave minimal verbal responses, frowned during many tasks, did not show pleasure or enjoyment during play activities, and did not give evidence of a sense of humor." The clinician may conclude based on these observations, plus collateral information from the parents, teachers, or other professionals (e.g., reading specialists, resource specialists, school nurse), that the child appears to be exhibiting depressive symptoms that may warrant further evaluation by another professional such as a counselor or psychologist. In the case of an adult, rather than saying a client or patient is anxious, the clinician might describe the person as having rapid speech, tense facial expressions, repetitive behaviors such as wringing hands or tearing paper into small pieces, or excessive perspiration. The clinician may conclude that the client exhibited symptoms of anxiety.

SLPs and Auds may note whether behaviors, characteristics, or symptoms are understandable reactions to a particular situation (e.g., during an evaluation), or whether they appear excessive and may be causing impairment in the client's functioning. By being careful to describe a person's behaviors rather than inferring the client's overall emotional state or disorder, SLPs and Auds can work within their scope of practice and avoid negative legal repercussions. Finally, it is important to keep in mind that many psychological symptoms mask medical disorders (Druss, 1995; Fava & Sonino, 2000; McBeth & Silman, 2001; Morrison, 1997, 2008). However, it is beyond the scope of practice for SLPs and Auds to make this determination. For example, patients showing symptoms of paranoia late in life may have acquired deafness. Clients who appear depressed or have poor attention and memory may have undiagnosed hypothyroidism. Morrison discusses the mental symptoms that accompany many physical disorders in his fascinating and helpful book.

NEGOTIATING

Negotiating is a skill that is used by all SLPs and Auds with clients, patients, family members, and even with other professionals (for example, clinicians with classroom teachers, clinicians with nursing staff, clinicians with administrators, clinicians with other clinicians) (Cohen, 2002). In all of our professional work it is helpful to present a negotiating posture. Negotiating connotes being empathic and understanding the other person's perspective. Clinicians who collaborate well with others may intuitively use negotiating skills, but even so, it is useful to have a framework to think about how to structure negotiation dialogues. The need for these skills becomes even more apparent when the client or family member demonstrates noncompliance or resistance (see Chapter 13). These challenging situations may be the result of the therapist dogmatically pursuing a therapy plan without considering the client's feelings, wishes, or desires. Noncompliance or resistance may occur when the SLP or Aud has not been sufficiently flexible and willing to negotiate with the client or family, or has failed to check with them to find out what they are interested and willing to do in therapy.

Katz and Pattarini (2008) state that it is only when negotiators (people attempting to resolve an impasse) are concerned about the interests of both parties that they have an opportunity to solve problems with some mutual satisfaction. The most productive posture is firm flexibility; that is, asserting one's own goals while being pragmatic about the means through which they are achieved (e.g., "I feel . . . when you do . . . . The next time, could you please do . . . ?"). It may then be possible to construct an agreement in which both parties make adjustments that allow them to receive more than they would have had they not cooperated. For example, when an SLP attempts to help a parent understand the importance of speech therapy for a child, the clinician needs to maintain a firm stance about the importance of therapy, but be flexible enough to help the parent feel that she has important input into the decision about whether the child will receive therapy. Another example is an audiologist who attempts to have a child begin wearing his first hearing aids. The child may recognize that they help him hear better, but be reluctant or unwilling to wear them because of embarrassment around his friends. The clinician may negotiate with the child about when he is comfortable wearing his new hearing aids.

Concepts and techniques from the Harvard Negotiation Project (Fisher & Ury, 1991; Fisher, Ury, & Patton, 2008) can be helpful to clinicians in their attempts to work with clients and their families. The Harvard Negotiation Project is an ongoing research project at Harvard University Law School that works on negotiation problems and develops and disseminates improved methods of negotiation and mediation. The principles and practices developed by the project are used at all levels of professional interaction as well as in state, national, and international negotiations. The following information is derived primarily from that source.

One of the basic principles of negotiating is that any method of negotiating may be fairly judged by three criteria: (1) it should produce a prudent agreement if agreement is possible; (2) it should be efficient; and (3) it should improve or at least not damage the relationship between parties. A prudent agreement can be defined as one that meets the legitimate interests of each side to the extent possible, resolves conflicting interests fairly, is durable, and takes into account all the people involved (Fisher et al., 2008).

When people (including clinicians and clients or family members) negotiate over positions, they tend to lock themselves into and defend those positions. Egos become identified with the position, and "saving face" makes it less likely that any agreement will reconcile the parties' interests. Any agreement reached may reflect a mechanical splitting of the difference, which may be less than satisfactory to either side. Position bargaining may become a contest of wills with an "I'm not going to give in" approach. As clinicians, we need to avoid viewing the other side as adversaries and use a more congenial style of negotiating. In the case of the mother who is reluctant to have her child in therapy or the child who does not want to wear his hearing aids, taking strong positions may include having feelings of winning ("I got my way!") or losing ("I gave in and the clinician got her way."). In either case, the parent, child, SLP, or Aud may feel that losing the argument means "losing face" or compromising self-esteem.

Fisher and colleagues (2008) stress "principled negotiation" or "negotiation on the merits" with the emphasis that the participants are problem solvers and the goal is a prudent outcome reached efficiently and amicably. Negotiating on the merits is based on four principles: (1) People—separate the people from the problem, that is, be soft on the people, firm on the problem; (2) Interests—focus on interests, not positions, that is, explore interests and avoid having a bottom line; (3) Options—consider as many as possible, that is, generate a variety of possibilities before deciding what to do; and (4) Criteria—evaluate the results based on some objective criteria, that is, try to reach an agreement based on criteria independent of will and personal feelings, and be open to reason but do not yield to pressure.

For example, some parents may doubt the value of speech therapy or may be reluctant to make the time commitment. Trying to understand parents from their perspectives can help the clinician be more empathic but at the same time maintain a firm position on the value of therapy. Both the parent and the clinician are interested in what is good for the child's speech and language development. The parent and clinician have options that can be explored to resolve the impasse, and objective criteria may be considered to determine the benefits of therapy for the child. The child who is reluctant or unwilling to wear her new hearing aids is understandably embarrassed about wearing them, but still needs to wear them to hear the teacher better and to improve communication with friends. Both the child and the audiologist are interested in the child having more positive experiences in the classroom and with friends. The child and audiologist have options that can be explored to achieve their mutual goals.

In all negotiating there are two kinds of interests: the substance (the problem) and the relationship with the people negotiating (i.e., the clinician and client or family). When negotiating with a client or family member, present the facts as each of you view them as well as the feelings behind the facts. In the long run, the facts may not be as important to the ongoing working relationship as the feelings. (*Note*: After I complete the evaluation of a client and finish explaining my findings and answering the client's and family's questions, I always ask, "How do you feel about the information I have just given you?" People usually remember the feelings they leave with more than the facts that were presented.) The mother who is reluctant for her child to receive therapy (the substance of the problem) may still be reluctant to alienate the therapist who may eventually provide therapy to her child. The child who does not want to wear her hearing aids may still want to stay on good terms with the audiologist who may test her hearing in the future.

No matter what the problem is that is being negotiated, we are always working with three basic categories: perceptions, emotions, and communication (Cohen, 2002). Understanding the client or family members' perceptions means understanding the problems as they view them. Trying to understand the problems from the other person's perspective can help us have a more empathic view of what the client is thinking and feeling. However, as objective and professional as we try to be when negotiating with a client or family, our own emotions may come into play. Anxiety, fear, and even anger are not uncommon emotions to feel in such circumstances. The client or family may be feeling similar emotions. It is helpful to ask ourselves what is causing these emotions. Why are we angry? Why are they angry? Are we feeling insecure? Is the client or family responding to past grievances (e.g., goals that were unmet, an insensitive comment)? Are emotions spilling over from one issue to another (e.g., difficulty with a teacher or physical therapist)? Are personal problems (on either side) interfering with "taking care of business"? Applying the principles and techniques presented in Chapter 13 may be helpful with several of the strong emotions people express when negotiating.

Underlying all fair and reasonable negotiations is participation and disclosure by both parties. Involving the client or family in the ultimate decision making is essential to their acceptance and treatment compliance. When a decision is made unilaterally by the clinician, it may be rejected by the client or family members who feel excluded from the decision-making process. Prior to entering a negotiation meeting, it is very helpful to carefully think through, "What do I want to come out of this meeting?" When communicating during your negotiations, try to sit on the same side of the table as the other person. A table between two people becomes both a physical and psychological barrier. Open body posture is very important, even if we are feeling somewhat anxious about the situation. Be aware that the other person may hear something quite different from what we are saying, and *we* may hear something quite different from what the other person is saying, particularly if our emotions are strong.

The basic problem in a negotiation process usually is not in conflicting positions; that is, the client, family, and clinician all want what is best for the client (e.g., the child to receive the help she needs to develop her speech and language, or the child to hear as well as possible in the classroom and with friends, or the adult to receive the maximum amount of therapy for which he will benefit). The conflict is likely between each person's needs, desires, concerns, and fears—ultimately, their interests (Fisher et al., 2008). For example, the mother may have concerns that her child already has too much time out of the classroom with the reading specialist and resource specialist, and that speech therapy will just be "too much." The child who does not want to wear his hearing aids has a desire to "look normal," even at the expense of hearing well, and is fearful that he will be teased by the other children.

Reconciling interests rather than positions is productive because both parties typically have many similar interests, although they may be taking opposite positions. Recognize what the common interests are, for example, wanting the child to have the best speech and language the child can develop, or having adequate hearing to have the best classroom and social experience. We can ask the child, client, or family members what their interests are and discuss ours openly with them as well. Be as specific as possible. Validate the other person's interests and follow up with a statement about your interest. For example, "Like you, I want Maria to do well in school and develop the best speech and language she can." Another example occurs when a patient or family member insists on the patient being discharged from the convalescent hospital (their interest). We can validate their interest by saying, "Like you, I am interested in Mr. Berger being discharged to his home when he is cognitively safe to be able to manage himself independently." These statements validate our client's interests while connecting them to your therapy goals. In this way, your respective positions can be viewed as compatible rather than as mutually exclusive.

If we want someone to listen and understand our reasoning, it helps to provide our goals and reasoning first, and our conclusions and recommendations later. For example, "Mr. Wilson, I want to help prevent you from having another episode of aspiration pneumonia by working on your swallowing. The pneumonia likely was caused by eating textures of foods that are not safe for you. For now I recommend that you be on a mechanical soft diet (include explanation and examples) and we can begin working on some exercises that will help you swallow safer. What are your thoughts and questions about what I have just said?" If we present our conclusions and recommendations initially, the other person may be thinking about arguments to counter them rather than listening to our reasoning. Many of our clients may not be well educated (at least in the areas of speech-language pathology or audiology) and may not fully understand or appreciate our reasoning about their problems. If the client or family feels threatened by our education and knowledge, they may become defensive and may cease listening to us. Our warmth and openness in sharing information and answering questions can help balance the strength of our statements. Successful negotiating requires being firm *and* open. When negotiating with clients, families, or other professionals, using the skills presented in the following chapter on Interviewing and Therapy Microskills can help foster a mutually successful outcome.

CONCLUDING COMMENTS

The therapeutic relationship and communication are intertwined and can enhance or diminish the potential effects of the SLP or Aud's treatment. The therapeutic relationship provides a basis for trust, motivation, and compliance in our professional work. Prerequisites for developing a therapeutic relationship are recognizing our clients' perceptions, needs, values, feelings, experiences, expectations, and expertise. Understanding and being attentive to transference and countertransference experiences can give clinicians tools with which to better manage therapeutic relationships. Attending and listening are foundational to the therapeutic relationship. Our tone of voice often conveys as much of the meaning as our choice of words. Empathy is central to the development of a therapeutic relationship and involves careful listening, understanding, and communicating that understanding to the client. Conveying empathy and respect for the person should affirm that the person is doing the best he can under the circumstances. The challenge is to convey acceptance of the person and still encourage change.

Therapeutic communication involves both verbal and nonverbal communication. Nonverbal communication includes our physical appearance, body language, proxemics, seating arrangements, eye contact, and touch. Consistency of communication helps create and maintain a therapeutic climate so that clients and patients can anticipate the way the clinician will present herself in dress and manner, attitude and behavior. Nonblaming language is an important element in therapeutic communication. Clinicians need to resist sounding disapproving or frustrated when clients do not do as much as we expect. Being clear in our communications will help clients and their families better understand our intentions and messages. Using descriptions of behaviors rather than pathologizing a person communicates respect and keeps us within our scope of practice. Negotiating is a skill that is used by all professionals with clients and patients, and sometimes even among ourselves. Principles from the Harvard Negotiation Project can be helpful in our professional work with challenging situations.

Discussion Questions

1. What does the following statement mean to you: "Technical expertise is necessary but not sufficient in order to be a competent SLP or Aud."

2. What are some of the feelings you have when you begin therapy with a new client? A type of client you have never worked with before? An adult client?

3. What expectations do you have of yourself when doing an evaluation? A therapy session?

4. How do you show clients that you are attending to them?

5. When talking with people, what behaviors do they exhibit that help you feel they are listening to you?

6. Practice your voice tone with another person to demonstrate how you convey empathy, friendliness, warmth, confidence, blame, belittling, and criticism.

7. How can communicating empathy help clients?

8. Provide examples of subtractive, basic, and additive empathy levels.

9. What do you think your physical appearance conveys to a client?

10. Show how you stand and sit when you are feeling comfortable with someone. Show how you stand and sit when you are feeling uncomfortable, guarded, or anxious with someone.

11. With various people in the room, practice establishing eye contact for about ten seconds before you begin to speak and maintain good eye contact even when you are uncertain of what you are saying (e.g., while discussing the anatomy and physiology of respiration).

12. Based on where and how you were raised, how comfortable are you with professionals touching your head, neck, and face? Inside your mouth?

13. How consistent are you in your communication and interaction with clients? How well do you think they can predict what mood you will be in and how you will respond to them?

14. How do you adjust your language when speaking to a child of six years old? 10 years old? 16 years old?

15. Discuss a clinical or work situation in which negotiation skills may facilitate your communication.

Role Plays

1. Divide into pairs of students and have one student play the role of an SLP or Aud and the other student play the role of a client. Conduct an initial interview of a hearing or speech problem in which the client expresses some emotion about her symptoms. The clinician's job is to practice good relationship-building

skills including therapeutic listening, expression of empathy, and making clear statements. After the interview (5–10 minutes), have the student who role played the client give feedback to the "clinician" about what skills were demonstrated and what skills may be improved.

2. Have students divide into pairs, and have one student in each pair play the role of the clinician and one student play the role of the client. The "client" expresses a combination of sadness, fear, and dependency during the interview. The clinician can role play providing therapeutic responses to the "client." Afterwards, the pair can discuss what transference and countertransference responses they found themselves having and how this affected the quality of their interactions with one another.

CHAPTER 4

Interviewing and Therapy Microskills

CHAPTER OUTLINE

INTRODUCTION

Interviewing is often a two-way street; as we are interviewing our clients, patients, and their family members they are often interviewing us. We want to know and understand our clients so we can help them with their communication problems; meanwhile, they want to know enough about us to feel confident that we can help them with their communication problem. The interviewing strategies described in this chapter can help clinicians to develop and refine their skills in conducting initial meetings and evaluations with clients and to enhance awareness of the potential, implicit meanings of various types of interview statements and questions. The initial contact may begin with a telephone call from a client or family member. During that brief exchange, both the clinician and the client or family member develop first impressions of one another. The first impression that the clinician makes may determine whether or not the client and his family select that clinician to be the therapist, or whether the client decides to look elsewhere. In medical, clinical, and rehabilitation settings, clinicians may receive a medical order or referral to see a particular patient and there is little choice as to who will be doing the evaluation and treatment. In such settings the first client–clinician interactions may influence or "color" future interactions. Our understanding of specific elements and skills that comprise the therapeutic relationship and therapeutic communication can help clients and their families develop positive first impressions of us and help get the interview off to a good start.

Clinicians typically gain most of their initial information from case history questionnaires (either tailored to the disorder or generic), interviews, and, when available, written reports from other professionals who have worked with the client (Shipley & McAfee, 2008). Further information and understanding of the client are obtained through direct observation and evaluation of the client's communication abilities.

The interview is a conversation conducted in order to develop a comprehensive picture of the client's communication problems and related contextual issues. Interviewing provides information and perceptions that help the clinician to generate hypotheses and interpretations about a client and his communication problems. Interviews are more than simple information-gathering operations; interviews are interactional social encounters in which knowledge is constructed. It is a time of, and occasion for, producing knowledge itself (Holstein & Gubrium, 2003). Therefore, the questions and style of interviewing that a clinician employs are critical in creating an accurate picture of the client's difficulties. The purposes of an interview may be primarily information gathering, information giving, or counseling (Stewart & Cash, 2003). Information-gathering interviews usually occur during the initial direct contact the clinician has with the client or family. During the information-gathering interview the clinician obtains objective information about the client and his description of the communication disorder, as well as the client's subjective feelings and attitudes about his impairment. Information-giving interviews focus on providing information to the client and family about the client's communication impairment, intended course of treatment, prognostic implications, and recommendations based on diagnostic findings. Counseling interviews may be designed to influence attitudes and/or behaviors of clients and their families, provide opportunities for them to discuss emotional issues related to the communication impairment, and provide support and encouragement (Luterman, 2008; Shipley & Roseberry-McKibbon, 2006). Throughout client interviews and during all counseling interactions, microskills are used.

Microskills is a term used in counseling psychology that refers to specific communication skills that help clinicians interact more intentionally with clients, that is, to thoughtfully but quickly choose responses to clients from a wide range of possibilities (Ivey et al., 2009). The assumption is that there is no one right therapeutic response to a person. The range of possible responses emerges from the clinician's assessment of the whole person and the situation. Microskills form the foundation of interviewing and obtaining information throughout our interactions with clients and family members. These skills are transtheoretical; that is, they are useful and necessary with any theoretical or therapeutic approach a therapist follows. Microskills have been considered technical skills used to understand how a client experiences and makes sense of his world. The intention is to gently enter the world of the client—seeking to understand the client through his perspective rather than our own. How is the client constructing his experiences and what sense is the client making of those experiences? From this understanding, the clinician and client can jointly search out new ways of helping the client think, feel, and behave with regard to the problems being experienced (Brock & Barnard, 1992; Corey, 2008; Ivey et al., 2009; Nystul, 2005).

Within the broad heading of microskills are several general and specific skills, including verbal and nonverbal encouragers, asking questions, paraphrasing and reflections, clarifications, reframing or relabeling, interpretations, suggestions, and the use of silence (Ivey et al., 2009). The clinician's process of learning and developing these skills follows much the same sequence that occurs in therapy with many of our clients. For example, a client who is disfluent and trying to become aware of, monitor, and then eliminate stuttering behaviors may follow this general sequence (Gregory, 2003; Guitar, 2006; Ward, 2006). The client:

1. Is made aware of a particular behavior by the therapist.
2. Becomes aware of the behavior *after* doing it.
3. Becomes aware of the behavior *while* doing it.
4. Becomes aware of the behavior before doing it but does it anyway.
5. Becomes aware of the behavior before doing it and intentionally does not do it.
6. Speaks naturally without the behavior.

As clinicians learn and develop microskills they often become self-conscious and aware of what they say, how they say it, and what they are doing with their bodies and voice while talking with clients. Being overly self-conscious of what you are doing can interfere with communicating naturally. However, the rehearsal and practice of these skills helps them become integrated into the way you communicate with clients (and everyone else) and they become natural strategies for communicating.

COUNSELING MICROSKILLS

The following interviewing and therapy microskills are integrated from a variety of sources, including Brammer and MacDonald (2002), Burnard (2005), Corey (2008), DeJong and Berg (2008), Evens, Hearn, Uhleman, and Ivey (2008), George and Cristiani (1995), Gladding (2009), Hackney and Cormier (1999), Ivey et al. (2009), Morrison (2008), Morrison and Anders (2001), Mosak and Maniacci (1998), Nystul (2005), Pipes and Davenport (1998), Shipley and McAfee (2008), Sommers-Flanagan and Sommers-Flanagan (1999), Wachtel (1993, 2007), and Zaro, Barach, Nedelman, and Dreiblatt (2000).

Verbal Encouragers

Verbal encouragers are prompts the therapist uses to try to elicit more information from the client, such as "Uh-huh," "Yes," "Ummm," and simple repetition of a word the client has said. When women are speaking with one another they tend to use many verbal encouragers, such as "OK" and "All right," which may help them feel they are being listened to and understood. Men, however, may feel that when a female clinician says "OK" or "All right" she has heard all she wants or needs to hear about that topic and he should move on to something else (Tannen, 2007). During interviews and therapy we need to consider adjusting our verbal encouragers to the gender with whom we are talking and to be alert for signs that we are being correctly understood.

 Nonverbal encouragers such as smiling, eye contact, leaning forward, open body posture, and nodding the head may be used alone or in conjunction with verbal encouragers. It is important to appreciate how much our verbal and nonverbal encouragers influence the direction of the conversation. What we encourage we will likely hear more about, and what we do not encourage we will likely hear less about. However, excessive verbal or nonverbal encouragers (e.g., excessive "Uh-huhs" or head nodding) can actually inhibit the client from talking. The use of too many encouragers can appear wooden and unnatural and the client may not see the clinician as genuine (Morrison, 2008).

"Therapist Noises"

"Therapist noises" is a term Wachtel (1993, 2007) discusses, and speech-language pathologists and audiologists need to be aware of these as well. One of the classic "noises" that clinicians might use when we do not know quite what to say (or do not want to say what we are really thinking) is, "That's interesting." *Interesting* is one of those words that, upon initial reflection, seems to convey the neutrality that is believed to be the proper stance for clinicians to maintain. By commenting that the client's behavior or thought is interesting, it may seem as if we are calling attention to the client's words and hoping that the client will examine the behavior or thought in more depth. However, many clients may detect a subtle form disapproval. Often there is a subliminal message in the phrase, such as "That's really weird," or "That's stupid." Therefore, we need to be cautious about what our complex interpersonal messages are when we make "therapist noises." Similarly, "huhm" is a noise that can have a variety of meanings depending on the context. There is usually some slight evaluative tone, either negative or positive, that goes with it. Our tone of voice, as well as our general attitude towards the client, will likely impact how the client hears us.

Counselors, psychologists, and psychotherapists sometimes use the word *sense* in place of *feel, feeling, thought, opinion,* or *idea.* For example, "I have the sense that you are . . . ," "It is my sense that . . . ," "I sense that you are angry with . . . ," and so forth. This way of framing a statement may be an effective or gentle method of proposing a tentative interpretation, which the client then has the opportunity to accept or reject. It is much less forceful, for instance, than saying, "You are really angry at your . . . ." Therefore, it may be less likely to raise the client's anger and resistance if the clinician is wrong. *Perhaps* is another word that therapists tend to use, for example, "Perhaps you're feeling a little . . . ." *Perhaps* also gives the client permission to disagree with the therapist's statement and to provide corrective information if needed.

When working with clients, some clinicians may frequently use responses and phrases such as "That's interesting," "How did that make you feel?" and "Perhaps." We need to be careful about not overusing such words and phrases because they can begin to sound stilted and nonproductive. They may boost the therapist's fragile sense of self-confidence but may not sound genuine to the client. If in doubt about what to say next, a moment of silence might sound more respectful than one of these overused phrases.

QUESTIONS

There are a variety of types of questions used in counseling that allow clinicians to understand clients and their families better. Clients, patients, and family members generally expect to be asked questions by a professional who is involved in helping them. Questions are essential tools in interviewing and counseling because they help focus the client or family member on issues that need clarification and understanding. Understanding the client assists the SLP or Aud to enter into the world of the client, that is, to understand the world through the client's perspective—how the client sees, hears, and feels the world. Understanding how the client makes sense of his experiences is one of the most important considerations for effective helping (Morrison, 2008; Ivey et al., 2009).

Asking questions of clients and families also can be therapeutic because it allows them to think about their situations and experiences in new or different ways, helps them look deeper into their own thoughts and feelings, and, we hope, helps them solve their own problems rather than expecting the clinician to solve them. Clinicians who have a more cognitive-behavioral orientation toward counseling are likely to use more questions than those with a person-centered orientation (Feltham & Dryden, 2005). Clinicians with a person-centered orientation also want to encourage clients to solve their difficulties but do not view the clinician's systematic questions as critical to this process. If the clinician feels that a client is becoming tangential with a response or moving in a direction that is not productive to the session, the clinician can use a question to redirect the focus and gain more control of the session.

It is important for the clinician's questions to be presented in an organized manner and for questions to be aimed towards identifying the client's strengths as well as their problems (Reiter, 2008). Questions should be presented in an open, direct manner. If clinicians present questions in a tentative, walking-on-eggshells manner, clients may not respond positively or gain confidence in the clinician. Inexperienced clinicians often overestimate how fragile or vulnerable clients are and may ask questions in a more timid manner. Instead of appearing sensitive, this style can simply appear less confident than a bolder, more assertive style. Clients typically respect clinicians who are more direct and honest with them.

Cautions When Asking Questions

The following section highlights additional cautions emphasized by Brammer and MacDonald (2002) and Ivey and colleagues (2009) that need to be considered when asking questions.

BOMBARDMENT OR GRILLING

Too many questions may overwhelm clients and put them on the defensive (Wachtel, 1993, 2007). The person asking the questions is usually in control of the interview or conversation. The questioner determines who talks, when, and about what. Too many questions may make clients feel controlled, manipulated, or criticized. "Why?" questions can be particularly intimidating and threatening to clients as they sound as though the client's reasoning and actions are being challenged. On the other hand, if a client is feeling uncertain about what to present and how, she may appreciate the structure provided by the clinician's questions. It is important to gauge what clients need to feel comfortable during the interview as you do your best job to gather the essential clinical information.

MULTIPLE QUESTIONS

If we ask several questions at once, clients may become confused and not know which one to answer or how. It is better to ask a single question and then wait patiently for the person to respond and, when the person appears to have finished responding, to wait a moment longer. This extra moment allows clients not to feel rushed and they may begin to add useful information that would not have been offered had the clinician rushed in too quickly with another question.

LEADING QUESTIONS (QUESTIONS AS STATEMENTS)

Clinicians sometimes try to make points or lead clients to different ways of thinking, feeling, or behaving by using a question rather than a declarative statement. Leading questions tend to encourage compliant responses, which may differ from what the client truly feels. For example, "Based on what we have discussed, don't you think therapy would be helpful?" "Don't you think practicing your oral-motor exercises would help your speech be more intelligible?" "Wouldn't working on listening skills help your son feel less rushed when he is talking and maybe help his fluency?" "Would wearing your hearing aid help you enjoy social situations more fully?" Such leading questions or indirect statements tend to sound condescending and manipulative; there are more direct and respectful ways to communicate with clients. A general rule of thumb is that if you are going to make a statement, it is best not to frame it as a question. Therefore, to extend the previous example, you could *ask* the client what benefits he may enjoy as a result of wearing his hearing aid or you could simply *suggest* that wearing his hearing aid may allow him to enjoy social events even more.

QUESTIONS AND GENDER DIFFERENCES

When posing questions, gender differences in communication (sometimes referred to as *intercultural differences*) also should be considered. The interaction of male–female cultures and gender differences in communication has been discussed by several authors (Burgoon et al., 2002; Dindia & Canary, 2006; Ivey, Ivey, & Zalaquett, 2009; Shipley & Roseberry-McKibbin, 2006; Tannen, 2007). Shipley and Roseberry-McKibbin (2006) summarize some common differences in male–female communication with the following points:

- In verbal communication, women tend to disclose more information about themselves, their families, and their friends than do men.
- Women tend to be generally outgoing, expressive, and open, whereas men are often more reserved and less verbal.
- Women tend to be more indirect than men and use more "softeners" such as "I could be wrong, but . . . ."
- Women tend to apologize more than men.
- Women tend to make eye contact, smile, and nod more than men.
- As a rule, men tend to interrupt women more than women interrupt men.
- Women tend to listen more than men.
- Men tend to provide content information while women tend to provide feeling information.
- Men are more likely to give information while women are more likely to seek information.

- Women tend to speak and hear a language of connection and intimacy, while men tend to speak and hear a language of status and independence.

- In general, men use language more for competition, to inform, persuade, and impress, whereas women use language more to establish rapport and connect with others and tend to emphasize feelings and attitudes.

Having stated these common gender differences, we are all aware that these differences are not uniformly found in any population. However, such communication differences may affect the way men and women conduct interviews and the way male or female clients interpret questions and the intentions of interviewers. Some female clients may perceive male clinicians who have an assertive style of communicating competence and authority as intimidating and insensitive. On the other hand, a female clinician who is striving to sound sensitive may be perceived by a male client as less competent than a female clinician who communicates in a more direct or assertive manner. Therefore, it is wise to consider the gender of the interviewer *and* the client in order to best calibrate your interviewing style with particular clients.

Closed Questions

Closed questions elicit a yes, no, or other very brief response and often include the words *is*, *are*, or *do*, for example, What *is* your name? How many children *do* you have? *Are* you able to be understood more easily now by your family? Closed questions are appropriate for gathering initial, basic facts about a client. However, too many closed questions can seem like an interrogation (Morrison, 2008). They also can inhibit the client from telling his story. We want to explore client experiences, not interrogate them (Wachtel, 1993, 2007).

Open Questions (Probes)

Open questions are generally preferable to closed questions because they encourage longer and more expansive responses (Brammer & MacDonald, 2002; Ivey et al., 2009; Shipley & McAfee, 2008). Open questions do not elicit a particular response; that is, the SLP or Aud cannot easily anticipate what the response will be. Open questions often use what are sometimes referred to as newspaper reporters' questions, that is, *who, what, when, where, how,* and *why*; SLPs tend to refer to them as "wh" questions. "*Why*" questions can be asked in a variety of ways without using the word "*why*," because that word often puts people on the defensive. *Can, will, could,* and *would* questions are special types of open-ended questions.

Frequently the first word of an open-ended question helps direct the type of information that is sought. For example:

- *Who* questions provide information about people involved in a situation, e.g., "Who do you think is the easiest for you to talk to at home?" "Who do you think might be able to help you when you get home from the hospital?"

- *What* questions most often lead to factual information or opinions, for example, "What are some of your concerns about your speech?" "What did you do when the kids made fun of your speech?" "What happened next?" "What do you think upset Samantha at school yesterday?"

■ *When* questions give information about time or sequences of events, for example, "When did you first notice your son's disfluencies?" "When are you supposed to give your oral book report in front of the class?" "When is your appointment scheduled to see the ENT doctor?"

■ *Where* questions provide information about locations, for example, "Where does Hector spend most of his time when he is at home?" "Where do you sit in the classroom?" "Where in the hospital are you now?"

■ *How* questions often give "method" responses, that is, the client's thinking processes that illustrate her problem-solving strategies, such as "How did you handle that situation with your teacher?" *How* questions also help us understand ways in which people's communication problems affect people's lives, such as "How is your speech (voice, hearing, etc.) problem affecting your job?"

■ *Why* questions lead to reasons or causes, for example, "Why do you feel you are having more difficulty talking today than usual?" "Why do you think you have more difficulty with chewy foods than other textures of foods?" The word *why* suggests interrogation and a sense of disapproval. *Why* questions often put people on the defensive and cause discomfort because they may feel they are being attacked or criticized. *Why* questions require people to justify their ideas, thoughts, opinions, or actions, with the uncertainty that their reasoning and justification will be satisfactory to the person asking *why*. We can avoid asking *why* by reframing the question. Often times *what* questions work well, for example, "You seem to be having a little extra trouble talking today. What do you think is going on for you?" "The exercises I gave you may have been a little too hard for you right now. What do you think made them so hard?" *What* questions are typically perceived as friendlier and less judgmental than *why* questions.

Wachtel (1993, 2007) discusses the "art of gentle inquiry," meaning the ability to inquire into aspects of the client's experience and motivations and to do so in a way that is minimally accusatory, judgmental, or damaging to the client's self-esteem. An example of a less-than-gentle inquiry is for a clinician to ask a client, "Why didn't you call to cancel our appointment?" while a more gentle inquiry would be, "You must have had a good reason for not calling to cancel our appointment" (spoken with an empathic tone). This statement invites the client to describe what is going on in his life without feeling pressured or accused.

During an interview you may ask each of the "wh" questions in a variety of ways to obtain information. For example, early in an interview you may ask who referred the client to you, and later in the interview you may ask who might be supportive of the client to help with the therapy exercises at home. You may use two "wh" questions within a single question, for example, "What do the other children do when you are stuttering?" or "When you are stuttering, what do the other children do?" You also can make a declarative statement rather than using an interrogative manner to obtain information. For example, rather than asking, "What kinds of speech problems does your child have?" you might say,

"Please describe your child's speech problems for me," or rather than asking, "What kinds of swallowing problems are you having?" you can say, "Tell me about the swallowing problems you are having."

During an interview or evaluation we want to gather answers to as many of the "wh" questions as possible (Ivey et al., 2009). For example, we want to learn:

- *Who* is the client? What is the client's background? Who may be part of the support system for the client?

- *What* are the client's problems? What happened or is happening to the client? What are the specific details of the client's problems? What helps or hurts the client?

- *When* do the problems occur? When did the problems first begin? What precedes or follows when the problems occur?

- *Where* do the problems occur? In what environments and situations do the problems occur?

- *How* does the client react to the problems? How does the client feel about her problems? How do family members feel about the client's problems?

- *Why* do the problems occur? Why is the client having problems with speech, language, cognition, or swallowing? (Once again, a *why* question may occur to the clinician, but it is usually preferable to ask a *what* question.)

When you have sufficient information from or about the client, patient, or family that answers the "wh" questions, then you have acquired much of the valuable information you need to help you understand the hearing, speech, language, cognitive, and swallowing problems of the people you are trying to help.

COUNSELING SKILLS IN ACTION

An Interview with Miguel's Mother and Father

Miguel is a seven-year-old boy whom his parents have brought to you to evaluate his speech and language. You can use open-ended questions during your interview with the parents to obtain important history that will help you understand Miguel and the direction you will take in your assessment of him. Some of the questions you may want to ask are listed below (not necessarily in the order you may ask).

- Please describe Miguel's speech for me.
- What are some of the concerns you have about his speech?
- When did you first become concerned about his speech development?
- Who first noticed or became concerned about Miguel's speech?
- Has he been evaluated by another SLP?
- Who evaluated him?
- When did the evaluation take place?
- What did you learn about the test results?

- How long was Miguel seen by the other SLP?
- What changes did you see in his speech while he was receiving therapy?
- Who referred Miguel to this clinic?
- What language is primarily spoken in the home?
- How has his speech changed over time?
- When does he have the most difficulty being understood?
- In your family, who do you think is easiest for Miguel to talk to?
- Whom do you think is hardest for him to talk to?
- In your family, who understands Miguel best?
- Who has the most difficulty understanding him?
- What do his brothers and sisters do when they cannot understand Miguel?
- Where does Miguel like to spend his time when he is at home?
- Where does he like to spend his time when he is not at school or home?
- What have you tried to do at home to help Miguel improve his speech?
- What do you hope will come out of my evaluation of Miguel?

(*Note:* Various questions about the child's language development, educational experience, and peer relationships also would be asked in an actual interview situation.)

During your interview and evaluation of Miguel, you also ask many open-ended questions to better understand how he understands and views his speech problem. When interviewing children, the questions are often interspersed throughout the evaluation and not necessarily in a formal interview format. Some of the questions you may want to ask are listed below (not necessarily in the order you may ask).

- Miguel, what do you think is the reason your parents brought you here today?
- What kinds of problems do you think you might have when talking?
- In your family, who is most concerned about your speech?
- Who talks to you the most about your speech?
- Tell me about what the other speech therapist did when she was working with you.
- What language do you speak most often when you are at home?
- Who at your home has the most difficulty understanding you?
- Who understands you the best?
- Where do you like to spend your time when you are at home?
- What do your brothers and sisters do when they can't understand you?
- Who do you like to play with the most when you are home?
- Who are your best friends in your neighborhood?
- Where do you like to spend your time when you are not at home or school?

- What does your teacher do if she can't understand you?
- What do the other kids at school do when they can't understand you?
- What do you think has helped you most with your speech?
- What would you like to change about the way you talk?

Can, *will*, *could*, and *would* questions are regarded as the most open-ended kind of questions because they may be considered by the person being questioned as either a closed question or a very open question. Because clients can respond either way they are sometimes called "swing questions" (Sommers-Flanagan & Sommers-Flanagan, 1999; Reiter, 2008). *Can* and *could* actually ask if the person has the ability to do something, although both the person asking the question and the person answering the question usually interpret it as a choice question, much like *will* or *would*. For example, "Could you tell me about the problems you are having with your speech?" A male therapist may want to ask, "Could you tell me a little about . . . ?" The "a little" is intended to soften the request and may sound less threatening than asking the person to tell you "all about" the problems: "Can you say more about that?" "Could you tell me (a little) about how people are responding to your new voice?" or "Would you tell me (a little) about how the kids at school are responding to your new hearing aids?" Depending on whether you are a female or male clinician, you may want to calibrate your style of questioning. Male clinicians may want to temper their questions to sound more gentle and less intimidating, while female clinicians may want to focus on being more direct and assertive.

As a closed question, a client may respond to a *can*, *will*, *could*, or *would* question with a "No, I don't want to talk about that." The better the rapport, though, the more likely the client will respond as if it were an open question and present a narrative or elaboration of her experiences. However, *can*, *will*, *could*, or *would* also may be used as an open question to obtain specific or concrete information, for example, "Can you give me a specific example of . . . ?" "Would you show me exactly what you do with your mouth when . . . ?"

We can use open questions about content (e.g., experiences) to understand the client's meanings. For example:

- "What does that mean to you?"
- "What sense do you make of it?"
- "That sounds very important to you. Can you tell me about that?"
- "What are some reasons you think that may be happening?"

Children may have difficulty with general open questions such as, "Could you tell me about your speech?" or "What do you think is causing your difficulty talking?" It is helpful to break down such general questions into concrete and situational language using a mixture of closed and open questions, for example, "When you are talking to your teacher, is your stuttering better or worse than when you are talking to other adults?" "Do any of the kids at school tease you about the way you talk?" or "What do you tell the other kids about why you can't yell on the playground like you used to?"

Open questions can be rephrased in a manner that produces a closed question (Sommers-Flanagan & Sommers-Flanagan, 1999; Reiter, 2008). However, when using an open question as a closed question it can sound confrontational (Burnard, 2005). Compare the four sets of questions below:

A. "How are you feeling about the therapy for your stuttering?"

B. "Are you feeling all right about the therapy for your stuttering?"

A. "What did you do when the kids made fun of your speech?"

B. "Did you get angry or embarrassed when the kids made fun of your speech?"

A. "What was it like to use your new lower voice pitch after having a higher voice for so long?"

B. "Did you feel more like a young man with your new lower voice pitch after having a higher voice for so long?"

A. "How do you feel?"

B. "Do you feel angry?"

With some clients, a closed question may facilitate a dialogue or the client's recollections of an experience. In other situations, clients may feel it is a forced-choice question and may be reluctant to respond, or respond with the answer they think we want to hear. For example, if an SLP asks a client whether the exercises are improving his speech, the client may feel compelled to answer in the affirmative to please the therapist and perhaps convey that the SLP is doing a good job. If the SLP senses that the client's response represents an effort to please, she may inquire further and ask for elaboration on the changes or improvements that the client is seeing. Clinicians should try not to ask closed or leading questions unless the client needs this level of specificity to produce a response. Clinicians can track client responses and modify their question style if they sense that the client is inhibited or fearful of displeasing the therapist.

Other questions may be used in order to encourage the client to think about the future and its possibilities. These questions can help clients to consider the consequences of beginning to make changes in their speech and communication patterns. The "miracle question" or "The question" is one example of a question used by counselors (Cade & O'Hanlon, 1993; de Shazer, 1988; de Shazer & Dolan, 2007), and it can be phrased many ways. For example, "Imagine that you wake up one morning and a miracle has happened; you no longer stutter. What would you do differently with your life if that happened?" "Pretend that I could wave a magic wand and make a miracle happen; your cleft lip is perfectly formed and your speech is perfect. How would your life be different?" The purpose of the miracle question is to see how the person would think, feel, or act if there were no problem. A follow-up question after the person has described how life would be if the miracle happened might be the following, "What can you do to start getting some of those things to make your life different?" The purpose of the follow-up question is to help the person focus on what she can begin to do that will make the differences happen, whether or not the problem is completely resolved.

The "What would you do if . . . ?" question is similar to the miracle question in that it attempts to have the client project, hypothetically, what he would do differently if circumstances were different or a particular situation arose. The question should be used to encourage the client to consider life if his symptoms were diminished or eliminated. This may plant a seed of hope or motivation to work on the current therapeutic tasks. For example, the following questions may help the client reflect on the current situation and how it may affect the future: "What will you do differently in your life once your stuttering is diminished?" "What would you do if your child was not able to function successfully in a regular classroom environment?" "What would you do if you were not able to return to your previous line of work?" It is helpful with some clients, patients, or family members to ask, "What wouldn't you change about yourself or the situation? What would you want to keep the same because you are happy with it?" Such questions help people focus on the positives in their lives. There is also a subtle secondary implication, that is, they *are* going to change. They are in control of what they want to work on and what they want to remain the same (Mosak & Maniacci, 1998; Reiter, 2008).

Funneling Questions

Funneling refers to using questions to guide the conversation from general to specific (Ivey et al., 2009). The conversation starts with broad, open questions and then, slowly, more specific questions are asked to focus the discussion. Open questions may be used throughout an interview, but the content is increasingly narrowed (funneled). Funneling questions are particularly helpful during an interview. For example,

> Clinician: "How can I help you?"
>
> Client: "I'm having trouble with my speech."
>
> Clinician: "What kind of trouble are you having?"
>
> Client: "My boss thinks I get tangled up with my words sometimes."
>
> Clinician: "What do you mean by tangled up?"
>
> Client: "I'm having more trouble talking to customers on the phone than I used to."
>
> Clinician: "What happens when you have trouble talking on the phone?"
>
> Client: "I have a hard time getting my words started."
>
> Clinician: "Can you show me what you do when you have a hard time getting your words started?"

Funneling questions may be used at any time in therapy to better understand specifics about a client's experience. For example, interviewing a fourth grade child who stutters:

> Clinician: "You seem a little upset at the moment. Can you tell me what's happening?"
>
> Client: "My teacher?"
>
> Clinician: "What about your teacher?"
>
> Client: "She made me read in front of the class again."
>
> Clinician: "How did you feel about that?"
>
> Client: "Embarrassed."
>
> Clinician: "Do you think working on your reading some in here will help so you are not so embarrassed in front of the class?"

Client: "If you think it'll help."

Clinician: "It could."

Another example, involving an elderly patient in a convalescent hospital:

Clinician: "Mr. Williams, you seem a little upset today. Can you tell me what's happening?"

Client: "My family."

Clinician: "What about your family?"

Client: "I feel like they have abandoned me."

Clinician: "How often are they visiting you now?"

Client: "Just a couple of times a month."

Clinician: "What do you think might be causing them to visit you less often?"

Client: "I don't think they like seeing me getting old."

Funneling questions can help the clinician and the client focus on specific problems rather than broad generalities. Counselors and psychotherapists sometimes use the concept of the abstraction ladder (Ivey et al., 2009). If you or the client are too high on the abstraction ladder, there is more difficulty finding solutions to problems. The funneling or narrowing of the focus can often help clients recognize that their communication problem is comprised of several or many smaller problems, and the smaller problems are less overwhelming and more manageable than a global problem. Funneling questions also allow the clinician to determine specific needs of the client and ways to provide therapy and measure progress using functional goals.

Requests for Clarification (Checking for Understanding)

Sometimes a client or family member provides a vague or circuitous response or sounds a little confused, and the clinician is left wondering what the person is trying to say. Asking for clarification at these times rather than guessing or making erroneous assumptions helps to show the client that you are sincere about your efforts to understand them and want to bring the information into sharper focus (Brammer & MacDonald, 2002). Requesting clarification or checking for understanding involves either: (1) asking the client if you understood him correctly, or (2) summarizing the conversation in order to clarify or confirm what has been said. It is wiser for a clinician to ask the client for clarification than to be confused or misinterpret the client's messages. The request for clarification asks the client to repeat or rephrase what she has said. For example:

- "Let me try to clarify. You're saying that . . ."
- "Could you try to describe what happened again? I'm not sure I'm understanding."
- "When you say that your throat feels funny, what does that mean?"
- "I think I got lost in that. Could you go through the sequence of events again?"
- "Let me see if I can sum up what we have talked about so far."

After you have summarized what you think the client has said, it is helpful to ask the client if what you have said is accurate.

Requests for clarification help the clinician increase her accuracy of information and understanding. If a clinician is not attending and verbally tracking the client well, requests for clarification will need to be more frequent. However, if requests for clarification occur too frequently, the client may sense that the clinician is not attending to what he is saying or is not particularly interested in the client's information. When frequent requests for clarification are needed, the clinician may wish to comment on this communication pattern, for instance by stating, "I apologize for my clarification questions; your story sounds complex." Such a statement can help to elicit a conversation about what is making the client's narrative difficult to follow without making him feel unduly criticized.

Comparison Questions

When clients complain about symptoms (e.g., vocal hoarseness, disfluency, difficulty being understood, swallowing), the clinician typically needs more specifics about times and conditions when the symptoms occur. Comparison questions can be very useful to discover the factors that either exacerbate or alleviate the client's symptoms (Brammer & MacDonald, 2002; de Shazer & Dolan, 2007). Comparison questions tend to use phrases such as *better or worse, more or less, hardest and easiest, this situation or that situation, with this person or that person*. The clinician is presenting forced-choice polarities that can, with additional questioning, be further refined. Obtaining this information can help the clinician discover the patterns of symptoms and behaviors and develop an appropriate therapy strategy, including a hierarchy of difficulty.

Some examples of comparison questions:

- "Is your speech more nasal when you are rested or when you are tired?"
- "Is it easier to talk to your mother or your father?"
- "Is your voice more hoarse in the morning or the afternoon?"
- "Do you choke more on regular foods or ground-up foods?"

Comparison questions are much like what an optometrist uses during an eye examination when he asks, "Can you see better with A or B, 1 or 2?" There is a refining of information to determine as closely as possible the client's experience. Ultimately, the comparison questions are trying to answer more specifically the "wh" questions of who, what, when, where, and how.

Counterquestions

When someone asks us a question, we are conditioned to answer it. However, in counseling it is often more revealing if we ask a question in return (Luterman, 2008). Luterman states that clients sometimes seek confirmation of a position or a decision they already have made, or they ask the clinician questions for which they already know the answers. They do not necessarily want the advice that their question indicates. Thus, the counterquestion encourages the client to reveal her position or decision so that the clinician and client can discuss this perspective. Illuminating the client's thoughts and feelings is often more productive and therapeutic than the clinician's providing answers or opinions. For example:

> Client (mother of an 8-year-old child): "Michael is starting to have a lot of trouble in school because the kids can't understand him. I'm not sure if talking to his teacher would help. What do you think?"
>
> Clinician: "What are your thoughts about approaching his teacher?" (The mother's "hidden agenda" was to have the therapist talk to her son's teacher.)

Another example:

> Adult voice client: "I am trying to decide how much longer I should continue therapy. What do you think?"
>
> Clinician: "How much longer would you like to continue therapy?" (The client clearly had some idea about when she wanted to terminate therapy.)

Counterquestions are important tools to understand a client's thoughts and feelings, and may help the clinician to avoid being "hooked" into answering a question that the client already may have made a decision about. Counterquestions, however, if used too frequently can become frustrating to a client; the clinician may appear to be playing therapy "games" or may at least appear to be giving stilted responses that avoid answering questions directly.

Keep in mind that clients may ask counterquestion themselves, and one we need to be particularly prepared for is, "Why did you ask that question?" or "Why do you need that information?" Clinicians' questions about client relationships (e.g., parenting styles and a child's disfluency, or co-workers and a client's voice disorder) may elicit a counterquestion from a client. The client may not understand the relevance of certain questions and the clinician needs to be prepared to explain the relevance in a calm, nondefensive manner. For example,

> Client: "Why are you asking me about my relationships at work?"
>
> Clinician: "I'm wondering when you are more stressed and if you notice a change in your voice when you are around your co-workers."

Counterquestions from a client may surprise an SLP and sound suspicious of the clinician's need to know certain information. Once again, responding in a calm, nondefensive manner to a client's counterquestion may not only provide the clinician with the information she is looking for, but also may strengthen the client–clinician relationship.

COUNSELING SKILLS IN ACTION

On several occasions over the past 30-plus years in private practice I have had clients who themselves have been counselors, psychologists, or family therapists or had a parent who was one of these professionals. During interviews and therapy with these professionals, counterquestions appeared to occur more frequently than with other clients. It was particularly important for me to maintain a nondefensive stance when responding to their questions.

CLINICAL QUESTIONS

Imagine in each case below that the clinician has asked a contextual question that is relevant to the client's symptoms. Provide nondefensive responses to the following client counterquestions:

1. Adult client: Why do you need to know about my work situation and how I get along with my co-workers?

2. Teen client: Why is it any of your business what my friends and I do after school?

3. Child client: I thought you were supposed to be helping me with my stuttering. What does it matter how my sister and I get along?

Broken Record

Broken record is a technique of repeating a word or statement until you get the person's attention, or asking the same question over (and over) again with the same loudness and voice tone until the person answers *that* question (Ivey et al., 2009). (Young children learn to use this technique automatically, like a four-year-old who says, "Mommy [pause] mommy [pause] mommy," and the mother says, "Huh? Did you say something?") Clinicians may use this technique when a client does not respond to a question that the clinician feels is important, for example:

> Clinician: "When are you going to schedule an appointment with the ENT doctor?"
> Client: "I'm really busy at work and have a lot of projects going."
> Clinician: "When are you going to schedule an appointment with the ENT doctor?"
> Client: "I can call this afternoon and try to get an appointment this week."

Broken record questions do not let the client off the hook until the clinician is satisfied that the question has been answered. This technique also may be useful if the client loses attention, concentration, and focus easily.

ACCURATE OBSERVATIONS AND LISTENING

In addition to asking questions, clinicians may employ other useful techniques in order to ensure that they have understood clients and their families. These techniques include paraphrasing, reflections, and the appropriate use of silence. These techniques can help clients to feel that you are interested in them, want to better understand their difficulties, and are treating them as individuals rather than as symptom or disease categories. They are particularly useful in encouraging clients to expand their story.

it to be after your accident." Other words and phrases may be used as well, for example, "It's common that . . ." or "It frequently happens that . . ." or "I have seen this occur other times." Helping people feel that their worst thoughts and feelings are normal and understandable allows them to begin accepting and managing their thoughts and feelings, rather than being embarrassed or feeling guilty about them as though they are shameful and reflect a possible character flaw. In short, normalizing strategies help clinicians to convey a nonjudgmental attitude toward clients, which is considered essential to the working alliance (Ivey et al., 2009).

Interpretations (Linking Statements)

Interpretations go beyond merely paraphrasing clients' statements and may present new information to them (Brammer & MacDonald, 2002). Interpretations are used by SLPs and Auds in an attempt to understand a person's thoughts, feelings, and experiences and to relay the interpretation back to the person. Interpretations are observations voiced by the clinician that make a connection or link between thoughts, feelings, and actions expressed by the client during the therapy. The goal of an interpretation is insight or increased client self-awareness and self-understanding. Clients sometimes report their stories as disjointed, meaningless, or confusing narratives, and one of the clinician's tasks is to remember statements, note significant themes, and reflect these back to clients for their consideration. Interpretations work best when we have correctly gauged the client's readiness to hear them and present them tentatively (Brammer & MacDonald, 2002). For example, it is sometimes helpful to use an introductory phrase such as, "I wonder if . . . ," "Is this a fair statement?" "Is it fair to say that . . . ?" or "The way I see it is . . . . Do you see it that way?" Some examples of interpretations follow:

> Client (adolescent boy who is disfluent and mentions occasionally in various therapy sessions his tendency to avoid talking to girls): "Usually I don't talk much to girls. I would just rather hang out with the guys."
>
> Clinician: "I wonder if you would be more comfortable talking with girls if you could reduce your stuttering."
>
> Client (adult woman with vocal nodules): "I get so angry with myself at work because my voice is so weak that it makes me sound like I'm uncertain of what I'm saying."
>
> Clinician: "Is it fair to say that you are concerned about how your co-workers and employer are perceiving you because of your voice?"

Interpretations require clinicians to be attentive to clients' comments and to hold them in mind, sometimes for days or weeks, to be able to later link together their thoughts, feelings, and experiences. Brief therapy notes about key points made by clients may help clinicians discover trends in client concerns and preoccupations that may later be interpreted and reflected back to the client.

The links made by the clinician can help the client develop stronger awareness of the links between their feelings and their actions. However, sometimes clinicians overestimate a client's willingness to hear certain interpretations, and the client may balk or protest that the interpretation is not correct.

The Beanie Baby Boy

I worked in the home of a six-year-old boy who stuttered. The boy had an extensive collection of Beanie Babies that he was very proud of and enjoyed showing them to me. After spending about half an hour with the boy in his room, I spent the rest of the time with the parents around the dining room table. Both parents were rather high-powered, no-nonsense business people. The mother began complaining about her son being "obsessed" with his Beanie Babies. I said that most everyone is obsessed with something and asked what she might be a little obsessed with. She said emphatically that she was an administrator of a residential care facility and had 200 elderly people she was responsible for. I said calmly, "Oh, you have 200 Beanie Babies." (Fortunately, in this case I had accurately gauged the mother's capacity to reflect on her own obsessive behavior.)

CLINICAL QUESTIONS

1. What could the therapeutic benefit be of this interpretation?

2. If the clinician does not gauge his client's reactions well, how can interpretations potentially misfire?

SLPs and Auds need to be extremely cautious about using interpretations and playing the role of "armchair psychologists" and attempting to go beyond our boundaries or training with psychological interpretations of clients' affects, cognitions, and behaviors. Shipley and Roseberry-McKibbon (2006) caution that interpretations can have powerful and sometimes negative effects on the clinician–client relationship, regardless of whether an interpretation is correct or incorrect. They may have negative effects because the client may not be ready to hear this information and may be upset or insulted by it. If the clinician's interpretation is incorrect or goes too far beyond the client's current understanding, the client may feel misunderstood or that the clinician is not "in sync" with him.

Suggestion Versus Direction or Instruction

Suggestion is a way of helping people see new ways of looking at old problems (Ivey et al., 2009; Mosak & Maniacci, 1998; Sommers-Flanagan & Sommers-Flanagan, 1993, 1999; Wachtel, 1993, 2007). Suggestions are not designed to be manipulative, but to open the person to possibilities he may have not fully considered, or may have been on the brink of considering but needed a little support from the clinician to know that it is all right to think about it. However, suggestion is an intervention that makes some clinicians uneasy because it raises concerns about the client's autonomy and the danger of the clinician imposing her values on the client. Providing a suggestion does not entail being authoritarian (Wachtel, 1993, 2007). A suggestion may be given to the client when the clinician wants to enhance the likelihood of maximum change or to encourage further change, especially when she notices a small amount of change that she wants to promote. Suggestion also may be used when the clinician notices inappropriate behavior to which she does not want to draw attention, and at the same time wants to attend to or reinforce positive behavior.

The client already may have tacit inclinations that parallel the suggestion. Suggestion can be viewed as a way of initiating a process, and the process then gets maintained by its effectiveness (the suggestion "works" for the person). However, a suggestion only works if it is within the person's frame of reference (almost a tip-of-the tongue experience) where the person may have come up with the thought on his own (a tacit inclination), but needed a little help. In a way, the clinician gives voice to a thought or solution that the client has already considered or may eventually consider without the help of the clinician. A suggestion only works if it "rings true" to the person, that is, the client can imagine that it could occur or work in his life.

Suggestions can be used to encourage compliance with an exercise or therapy procedure that we introduce to the client. For example, "When you use the chin-tuck technique, you will find that you don't choke as much when you are eating" or "When you improve your articulation of words, you will find that your speech does not sound as hypernasal." Suggestions should *never* be used as a veiled form of advice to encourage clients to take action in other parts of their lives, for example, work or family life, even if we think those areas of their lives have an impact on their speech symptoms.

There is an important distinction between a suggestion or advice on how a client's life should be lived and instruction about specific aspects of the therapeutic process. We should avoid offering both unsolicited and solicited advice (Luterman, 2008). If we suggest or advise a client to take some action on an area outside of our expertise and scope of practice, we have set the client up for potential failure and ourselves up for potential professional and legal entanglements if the client takes our suggestion or advice and it does not work out. Such suggestions step beyond our professional boundaries and could backfire if the outcome is not as positive as we or the client expected. If, for example, an SLP suggests that a client's current line of work is causing excessive stress that is affecting his voice, and the client quits his job and then has difficulty finding new employment, the client could potentially blame (or sue) the SLP because he followed the suggestion.

Some people can become very dependent very quickly on a clinician for advice on not only communication problems, but other personal problems as well. It is best to avoid the words *suggest* and *suggestion*, *advice* and *advise* when speaking with clients about their personal problems that are outside an SLP's or Aud's scope of practice. However, we can introduce thoughts and possible solutions without using these words. We can ask questions such as, "Have you considered . . . ?" "Have you thought about . . . ?" "What do you think would happen if . . . ?" "What do you think are the possibilities that . . . ?" "It's possible that . . . could work (happen). What do you think?" "I wonder how it would be if . . . . What do you think?" It is extremely important to emphasize to clients that we are not advising them to take action in areas outside our domain; otherwise, clients are likely to believe that our questions are actually suggestions.

Another form of suggestion that is used by counselors and psychologists frequently incorporates the phrase ". . . as you are . . ." (Wachtel, 1993). For example, to increase a positive behavior, the clinician might say, "It is very important for your child to feel she is listened to, and *as you are* listening to her more and more, you will probably find that . . ." Another example: "Using the chin-tuck position will help decrease your coughing and choking, and *as you are* using the chin-tuck position you will find that you will enjoy your meals more." This form of suggestion helps clients to imagine the future and the changes that may result from their positive behaviors.

Although suggestions can help to introduce a clinician's expectations (e.g., for the client to practice her speech exercises at home), clinicians typically must be direct and very clear about the exercises and tasks we want clients to complete. We do not want clients to experience ambiguity or uncertainty about what we feel will help them. Therefore, we must be explicit and sometimes adamant about what we want them to do. With some clients, a suggestion may not have the impact we feel is necessary to have the client follow through with an important behavior. For example, asking a seven-year-old child, "Have you considered starting to wear your hearing aids in the classroom?" may not be as therapeutic initially as instructing the child to start wearing his hearing aids in the classroom. Asking a child, "What do you think would happen if you stop yelling on the playground?" may not help him follow through with the behavioral changes needed. For children in particular, we often are initially direct about our instructions, expecting (hoping) that they will follow them. However, if we find that a child is not following our instructions, we may begin to inquire about his thoughts and feelings about our instructions to better understand why he is not following them. With all of the techniques we have discussed, clinicians must gauge what strategies will work best with each client.

Confronting

In common usage, confrontation is often seen as hostile or punitive. In counseling, confrontation is considered an advanced microskill (Evans, Hearn, Uhlemann, & Ivey, 2008; George & Cristiani, 1995; Ivey et al., 2009; Nystul, 2005). Confrontation may be briefly defined as noting discrepancies, incongruities, or mixed or conflicting messages in the client and presenting them back to the person. In general, the purpose of confrontation is to provoke an immediate response or action or to compel clients to take some desired action.

Confrontations can be used to facilitate change, and it is confrontation of discrepancies that may be the catalyst to change for some clients (Ivey et al., 2009). Often clients are stuck, experiencing internal conflict (e.g., opposing or discrepant wishes) and a solution may not be readily apparent to them. Confrontation can spur change when the clinician's observations of the client's thoughts, feelings, and behaviors are presented back to the client for her to reassess. The confrontation should invite the client to further explore thoughts, feelings, and behaviors and to go beyond usual explanations. Confronting a person is a delicate procedure requiring both a sense of timing and a sensitivity and awareness of the client's receptivity.

In counseling, confrontation is *not* a direct, harsh challenge, but rather a gentle skill that involves listening to clients carefully and respectfully and then attempting to help them examine a situation or their own thoughts, feelings, or actions. Confrontations should not include accusations, evaluations, or solutions to problems. Confrontation is not going against clients; it is going with them, seeking clarification and the possibility of a new resolution for their problems (Ivey, Ivey, & Zalaquett, 2009). Confrontation should be tentative and nonjudgmental, encouraging the client to explore the discrepancy. Tentative confrontations often begin with such phrases as "Could it be . . ." or "You seem to tend to . . . ."

Often, if the clinician notices discrepancies but does nothing about them, the therapy remains stuck at an impasse and the clinician's frustration over the situation builds. Discrepancies are fairly common in our work with clients and families, and there are several types of discrepancies that may be seen, for example (Ivey et al., 2009):

- **Discrepancies between what is said and what is done:** A parent may say how important her child's speech therapy is, but frequently cancels or is a no-show. Possible therapeutic confrontation: "You have mentioned how important your child's speech therapy is, yet there seems to be some difficulty getting him to therapy on a consistent basis." Or, a child who says she has difficulty hearing in class but frequently does not wear her hearing aids: "You have said a few times that you can't hear your teacher very well in class but you seem to avoid wearing your hearing aids."

- **Discrepancies between two or more statements:** "I agree with what you are saying, but I still think that telling my son to stop stuttering is just fine." Possible therapeutic confrontation: "You say you agree with what I'm saying, yet it doesn't seem to affect the way you talk to your son about his stuttering."

- **Discrepancies between verbal and nonverbal behaviors:** The patient says that his drooping mouth from the stroke does not bother him, but he often covers his mouth with his hand when speaking. A possible therapeutic confrontation: "You mentioned that the way your mouth droops doesn't really bother you, but I notice that you frequently cover it with your hand when talking. Could it be that you are more upset about your mouth than you may have realized?"

- **Discrepancies between nonverbal behaviors:** The client may display a pleasant "no problem" type of smile along with a furrowed, tensed forehead or clenched fists. A possible therapeutic confrontation: "You tend to give two messages with your facial expressions and body language. You have a smile that says everything is OK, but at the same time your tense forehead and clenched fists tell me that everything isn't OK. Would you like to share your thoughts and feelings about what we have been talking about?"

- **Discrepancies between the views of different people:** Parents disagree on the need for speech therapy for their daughter. A possible therapeutic confrontation: "Mr. Ferrero, you feel that speech therapy for your daughter's attention and auditory processing problems isn't really necessary because you had problems like those when you were young and that you are very successful now, yet both you and Mrs. Ferrero indicated that you struggled quite a bit in school and your struggles were caused by attention and processing problems that are similar to your daughter's" (Adapted from Ivey, Ivey, & Zalaquett, 2009).

As clinicians develop knowledge and skills in confrontation, Ivey and colleagues (2009) state that the following skills will develop as well:

- An increased ability to identify incongruities, discrepancies, or mixed messages in behaviors, thoughts, and feelings

- An ability to increase a client's willingness to discuss and possibly resolve discrepancies
- An ability to utilize confrontation skills as part of mediation and conflict resolution

Confronting a client or family member is likely to be uncomfortable to most clinicians, possibly because of the negative connotation of the term itself as well as the delicate nature of the technique. Confronting requires, like interpretations and linking statements, recalling what has been said or done in the past by the client that had some important discrepancies and then presenting them back to the person. Clinicians need to choose carefully those issues that may benefit from confrontation. Not every discrepancy or incongruity a client or family member presents warrants confrontation. Confrontation is likely to be needed most when clients are not sufficiently compliant with treatment recommendations and there is a need for the therapist to try an alternative method to activate them.

Once a client is confronted with a discrepancy, for instance, between what the person says and what he does, the clinician can encourage the client to talk about his feelings about the issue and then to problem solve how to handle the situation. For example, for the child who says she is motivated to hear better at school but then "forgets" to wear her hearing aids to school, the clinician can first explore the discrepancy and then help the child devise a plan that feels reasonably comfortable in order to acclimate to wearing hearing aids in the presence of her peers. In this way, confrontations frequently resolve what clinicians refer to as resistance.

CONCLUDING COMMENTS

This chapter provides a discussion of the numerous microskills used by mental health professionals during interviews and therapy. When SLPs and Auds have a variety of ways of eliciting information, thoughts, and feelings from clients and family members, a better understanding of the problems and the way they are being experienced is possible. Therapeutic microskills provide clinicians with a "toolbox" of specific ways to communicate with clients that can facilitate information gathering, rapport building, and the therapeutic process. While many of the microskills presented may feel artificial or unnatural when first attempted, clinicians may develop comfort and proficiency as they practice these skills.

Discussion Questions

1. Discuss why microskills are transtheoretical and what this means.

2. What verbal encouragers and "therapist noises" do you tend to use in conversations with clients?

3. Discuss how you feel when you are asked "why" questions by a professor or supervisor.

4. If you have ever been interviewed by a health professional, how did you feel about the experience? What aspects of the interview were conducted skillfully, and what aspects could have been improved?

5. What sensory system (auditory, visual, or kinesthetic) to you tend to prefer? What are some of the words or phrases you might use when describing something that reflects that sensory system?

6. Discuss a metaphor you used with a client that helped the client better understand a concept you were trying to explain.

7. Discuss a time when you had a long silence in therapy. What were you thinking about? How did you feel about the silence?

Role Plays

1. Divide into clinician–client pairs and role play an early therapy session. The client presents his feelings about himself or the therapy in sensory terms (e.g., using auditory, visual, or kinesthetic language). The clinician listens for the sensory modality used and practices responding therapeutically using the client's preferred sensory modality.

2. Still in client–clinician pairs, the client describes her stuttering problem and her anxious feelings about her speech problem. In response, the clinician practices using reflections, reframing, and normalizing in response to the client's worries and negative self-statements. Discuss afterwards whether the clinician statements felt helpful and validating or patronizing and unhelpful.

3. With a new client–clinician pair, practice an interview in which the client has difficulty giving responses to the clinician's questions. The clinician can experiment with asking different types of questions (including open and closed, comparison questions and counterquestions), and the effectiveness of these questions can be discussed afterwards.

Counseling in a Multicultural Society:
Implications for the Field of Communication Disorders

Marlene B. Salas-Provance, Ph.D., F-CCC-SLP
Associate Professor, New Mexico State University
Las Cruces, NM

CHAPTER OUTLINE

INTRODUCTION

Each person brings her own unique perspective and circumstances into the counseling process. This may be a reflection of diverse factors such as gender, age, education level, religion, sexual orientation, ethnicity, language, race, or socioeconomic background. All of these factors may have an impact on the outcome of counseling and should be thoroughly examined. Few programs in speech-language pathology and audiology provide clinical and/or classroom training in general counseling knowledge and skills (Kaderavek, Laux, & Mills, 2004), and fewer still provide training in effective counseling with culturally and linguistically diverse (CLD) clients (Horton-Ikard, Munoz, Thomas-Tate, & Keller-Bell, 2009; Vinson, 2009). Clinicians also can expand their knowledge in counseling CLD populations through readings found in several texts in the field of communication disorders (Langdon, 2008; Luterman, 2008; Shipley & Roseberry-McKibbin, 2006).

Considering the increase in numbers of CLD clients receiving services from speech-language pathologists and audiologists (U.S. Census Bureau, 2008), it is important to provide information that will assist professionals working in our culturally pluralistic society (Lee, Blando, Mizelle, & Orozco, 2007). This chapter considers the influence of cultural and ethnic diversity and its effect on the counseling process in the field of communication disorders. Although culture can be defined using ethnographic, demographic, and status variables (Pedersen, Draguns, Lonner, & Trimble, 2008), the focus here is on the ethnographic variables such as ethnicity, nationality, religion, and language.

The fact that the same counseling techniques are not applicable across all people was first identified almost 40 years ago (Pedersen, Lonner, & Draguns, 1976). A 1972 panel discussion on culturally competent counselors at a meeting of the American Psychological Association resulted in the first textbook on counseling across cultures, a textbook currently in its sixth edition (Pedersen, Draguns, Lonner, & Trimble, 2008). Many studies have found that the experiences of individuals vary as a result of their cultural, racial, and ethnic backgrounds and do, in fact, impact their response to the counseling process (Constantine, 2002; Pope-Davis, Toporek, Ortega-Villalobos, Ligiéro, Brittan-Powell, Liu, et al. 2002; Toress-Rivera, Phan, Maddux, Wilbur, & Arredondo, 2006; Twohey, 2004). Specifically, researchers have found that ethnically diverse groups use counseling services less often than other groups. One survey reported that "non-Caucasian people did not seek counseling because they believed counselors were not real . . . that counselors appeared too perfect, distant, and unable to understand non-Caucasian issues" (Marino, 1996, p. 1). Reportedly, counseling is limited to one session 50 percent of the time for ethnic groups compared to 30 percent for nonethnic groups (Gladding, 2009, Sue & Sue, 2003), suggesting a more negative experience with counseling for individuals from diverse cultures. Some of these negative experiences may be related to the fact that the counselor and the client may differ culturally and/or linguistically, resulting in cultural mistrust (Benkert, Peters, Clark & Keves-Foster, 2006; Terrell & Terrell, 1984). Other explanations given for the underutilization of counseling services by culturally diverse clients is that help-seeking behaviors and treatment expectations differ among these groups. For example, individuals from diverse groups may seek assistance within the family unit before formal counseling and may not expect counselors to fully understand or fix their problems (Kim, 2004; Lee, 2008).

The type of counseling that occurs when the counselor and client differ ethnically has been termed multicultural counseling (Locke, 1990, p. 18). The counselor and the client enter the "cross-cultural zone," a space where the counselor takes into consideration the multiple identities of her client (Lee & Diaz, 2009). Expanding our knowledge of the complexities of diverse populations is imperative. There is value in studying each racial and ethnic group from a narrow, culture-specific view. Equally important is the ability to view the broad differences between ethnic cultures and mainstream culture to address the myth of "sameness." The "theoretical myth of sameness" (TMOS) described in the counseling literature (Hardy, 1990, p. 17), puts forth a conventional notion that all individuals are the same. A more contemporary view asserts that there are differences among individual clients and it is important to recognize that some of the differences can be attributed to ethnicity and culture. Psychologists (Constantine, Warren, & Miville, 2005; Gushue, 2004) have discussed that adopting a color-blind perspective may actually have the opposite effect of that intended. In the process of ignoring that racism and prejudice exist, the counselor may in fact ignore that which makes the individual unique. The counselor may become less sensitive rather than more attuned to the client's experiences.

BROAD VIEW OF MULTICULTURAL COUNSELING

This view requires clinicians to make the assumption that there *are* cultural differences that go beyond those associated with socioeconomic level and there are a broader set of skills that can minimize those differences. One example is the use of the Practical Skills Model of Multicultural Engagement (Alberta & Wood, 2009) from the field of counseling psychology, which can be adapted for use in the field of communication disorders. This model incorporates information in five areas, including "basic skills, empathic communication, relationship building, diunital reasoning, and customs and practices" to develop culturally competent counselors (p. 564).

All the skills in the Practical Skills Model of Multicultural Engagement are commonly used counseling methods, but the strength in this model is the use of these skills in an integrated manner. This model allows practitioners to go beyond improving their culture-specific knowledge and awareness and move towards developing a set of behaviors and skills that can be generalized across cultures. First, basic counseling skills discussed throughout this text should be used with multicultural clients as well as with mainstream clients. Secondly, the use of empathic communication is an essential skill that can be used with all clients. When we empathize with our clients, we are able to understand their experiences from their unique frame of reference without making our view the priority. We can show empathy by allowing clients to share their experiences completely, without interjecting any of our own experiences, attempting to redirect the conversation towards topics that are comfortable for us, or trying to make them feel better by saying that the situation will improve (Brown, 2010). For example, the family may accept the birth of a child with Down Syndrome as "God's will" and may not be seeking a cure or treatment.

The third important skill from the Practical Skills Model is relationship building. Students in training are advised to maintain boundaries with their clients and to keep their professional and personal relationships separate. However, this may not be the best advice to meet the needs of the culturally diverse client. Rather, clinicians should consider developing relationships with diverse clients through the expansion of personal and professional boundaries. Development of stronger personal relationships may be the foundation for helping individuals from culturally diverse groups. A clinician may not necessarily accept an invitation to have dinner at a client's home, but could participate in community service or religious activities that include the client. Other relationship-building behaviors could include active listening, engaging in a level of self-disclosure, and sharing common experiences with the multicultural client (Alberta & Wood, 2009).

The fourth skill in the model that may improve counseling with multicultural clients is **diunital reasoning**, the act of validating and legitimizing other world views. We can reason that although the experience of another group is different from our own, we can still accept it as their truth. However, it is not necessary to abandon our own world view to accept another. For example, although we may solely use Western medicine, we respect others' wishes to use traditional or non-Western healing methods such as the use of herbs or a belief in the healing powers of prayer. For example, some Hispanic families may place a cotton ball with mentholatum into the ear canal to cure an ear ache.

In the final component of the Practical Skills Model, the clinician attempts to understand the customs and traditions of her clients. This can be done through observation. The first step is to identify the pattern of behavior that is unique. For example, in some cultures the oldest male son is the sole decision maker in the family and may independently decide whether the parent with a swallowing disorder is fed orally or by tube. We then try to understand why this is valued in the culture. This new knowledge and awareness allows clinicians to expand their world view. Observation allows the clinician to learn patterns of behavior, as well as the values and expectations that are the foundation of the behavior. For example, it is helpful to observe how different ethnic groups observe the use of space (proxemics). A comfortable distance between two people in American mainstream culture is almost 3 feet, whereas for Hispanics it can be as little as 18 inches. Observing how individuals touch each other during communication (haptics) is very instructive. Is it appropriate to touch a child's hair, an older woman's hand, a man's shoulder? Is a handshake appropriate and with whom, or is an embrace the culturally appropriate way to greet?

The use of body space (kinesics) can negatively impact the relationship with the client if not managed in a culturally sensitive manner. It is important to know if it is culturally appropriate for a woman to stand behind the man during conversations, whether the woman should enter a room first and take control, or whether the woman should be alone in the room with a male (prohibited in Middle Eastern cultures). Is it acceptable to maintain direct eye contact and lean towards the person to show interest? These details of nonverbal communication are probably unconscious and best learned through observation. If a clinician observes a behavior or situation that she does not understand, it is appropriate to ask for an explanation rather than place value on or make a judgment of that behavior. For example, if a clinician observes discoloration on a child's back, she may assume the child is being abused, whereas it may be the effects of *cao*, or coin rubbing, a traditional medical treatment for some illnesses used by some Asian ethnic groups (Cheng, 2002).

Another method of observation is to use **ethnography**, a method used in anthropology to gain information about a culture from the people who live in the culture. The ethnographic study of a Hmong child and her medical treatment is widely used for multicultural training (Fadiman, 1997). Mini-ethnographies can be used in our clinical practices to facilitate the development of a more culturally sensitive counseling process. A mini-ethnography could consist of a clinician attending a multiday religious ceremony for American Indian children. Observing this rich ceremonial event can increase the clinician's multicultural knowledge. The clinician can now be more sensitive to the importance of this native ceremony and can understand the reasons behind the child missing school and therapy on those days. Of course, these mini-ethnographies must be conducted within the boundaries of the culture. For example, there are some Native American ceremonies that are closed to the public.

When providing multicultural counseling there are some aspects that are applicable across all cultures. The counselor should have the following core skills:

- Be comfortable with issues of race, culture, and class
- Create an environment where the client is comfortable and can talk freely
- Build a trusting relationship

By possessing these core skills, the counselor can decrease the potential for the development of the following adverse behaviors in culturally diverse clients:

- Feelings that the counselor does not understand them
- Superficial self-disclosures rather than honest communication
- Poor follow-through resulting in unhelpful counseling interventions
- Premature termination of counseling due to misunderstandings or mistrust

Many ethnically diverse groups may be unfamiliar with the process and setting for counseling. Clinicians should explain the process and scope of counseling and ask their clients how they feel about the process. A common behavior of some ethnically diverse families is their wish to personalize the therapeutic relationship. For example, if the clinician rejects the offer of food (e.g., *empanadas*, "pies" from a Hispanic family) or gifts (e.g., Chinese New Year gifts from an Asian family), the family may view the clinician as uncaring and thus untrustworthy. Although some clinicians may feel that acceptance of a gift may be a breach of the therapeutic relationship and could compromise their ethical standards, this is an appropriate, socially sanctioned way to build rapport for some families and not a form of coercion for favor. These families also may attempt to incorporate the clinician into their own family by asking questions about the clinician's background. Clinicians are not expected to reveal in-depth details about their personal lives, but general information about themselves will help maintain and build rapport with the family. For some Hispanic and Native American families, there is an initial period of "small talk," specifically called "*la platica*" in Spanish-speaking homes, which occurs for only a brief period of time upon greeting. This conversation is crucial to providing a level of comfort and trust between the family and the clinician, which is the foundation for a successful counseling relationship.

Across all cultures, the counseling process begins with a successful greeting. There are common behaviors across ethnic groups that should occur to set up the counseling session. The majority of ethnic parents or adult clients may want to be called by their surname and may want the clinician to use their professional name, such as Mr., Mrs., or Dr. The client may feel it is disrespectful for the clinician to call them by their first name. It is appropriate for the clinician to say a few words of greeting in the language of the client, if possible. This will show clients that you respect their language and have taken the time to learn a few phrases. *Buenos dias* (good day) is a Spanish phrase that can be easily learned. Some Hispanic families may be comfortable with a slight embrace (*abrazo*) as a welcome gesture. It may not occur at the first visit, but if the client continues to see the clinician, the *abrazo* may be initiated by the client on arrival and departure. In the Asian culture, the handshake may be soft and brief. A strong handshake may show a lack of respect and seem overbearing. If the client does not maintain eye contact, it is not appropriate to force the eye contact, but attempt to make a connection with a slight touch on the arm to get the client's attention.

USE OF INTERPRETERS TO SUPPORT COUNSELING OF BILINGUAL CLIENTS

A counseling session should not be attempted if the clinician is not familiar with the language of the client. If the clinician does not know the client's language, an interpreter who is not a family member must be available. If the cost of the service being provided is reimbursed through a federal program such as Medicare, the use of an interpreter is mandated by Federal CLAS (Cultural and Linguistic Appropriate Service) Standards. Standards 4–7 mandate that language services must be provided in the dominant language of the client. Children should never be used to interpret; however, an adult family member may be used with permission from the client (U.S. Department of Health & Human Services, 2010).

The counseling process itself can be influenced by the language proficiency of the counselor. A bilingual counselor or an interpreter should be used with an English-language learner (ELL) client and can influence the outcome. Miscommunication and increased levels of discomfort can occur as a result of language differences. There is a great risk of misinterpreting cues when there is not a common language. The use of a trained interpreter could help alleviate these problems (Hwa-Froelich & Westby, 2003; Langdon, 2008; Wyatt, 2002).

An interpreter can be a cultural broker and provide a window into the culture. It is imperative to have access to trained interpreters for cross-cultural communication. The following case (Crawley, Marshall, Lo, & Koenig, 2002) reflects a conflict between the patient's culturally based medical understanding and her health care provider's emphasis on patient autonomy and informed consent.

CASE STUDY

Using Interpreters with the Culturally and Linguistically Diverse Patient

Wilma Martinez is a 67-year-old immigrant from El Salvador who moved to the United States to live with her daughter. Mrs. Martinez speaks only Spanish. Through her daughter's translations, the patient appears to comprehend details of her illness and treatment. When asked if she understands what the doctor is saying, she invariably nods affirmatively.

During a clinic visit when the patient's daughter is not present, the physician arranges for a trained medical interpreter to be present. When the physician discusses end-of-life preferences, the interpreter reports that Mrs. Martinez thought that ventilatory support and cardiopulmonary resuscitation would hasten her death. Later, the interpreter explains that Mrs. Martinez could not understand why staff were insistent that she, rather than her daughter, make decisions. Mrs. Martinez stated, "In my country, the family decides." Assuming that her daughter would make decisions for her, she saw no reason to sign forms. She worried that signing forms would cause legal problems because of her immigration status. The interpreter also suggests that Mrs. Martinez's nodding indicates politeness and respect for the physician, not assent (p. 674).

CLINICAL QUESTIONS

1. What is one advantage for using a family member as the interpreter?
2. What is one disadvantage for using a family member as the interpreter?
3. Can we expect the trained interpreter to know the cultural beliefs of the patients for whom they are interpreting? Why or why not?
4. Do you feel that the physician in this case had reliable medical information about his patient?

Trained medical interpreters can ensure effective, efficient, and reliable communication between providers and patients. However, interpreters themselves may influence the content of messages conveyed during translations. When professional interpreters are unavailable, physicians may need to use family members or bilingual health care workers for translation. Family members or untrained interpreters may misinterpret medical phrases, censor sensitive or taboo topics, or filter and summarize discussions rather than translating them completely. Mrs. Martinez's daughter may not have translated important information about mechanical ventilation and cardiopulmonary resuscitation accurately or may have been reluctant to tell the doctor that she or her mother did not understand the process, benefits, or risks.

CULTURE-SPECIFIC VIEWS OF MULTICULTURAL COUNSELING

The information that follows on culture specific populations is meant to serve as a framework or guide for decision making. It should not be used as a checklist for predicting how an individual from a particular ethnic background will behave. Clinicians are encouraged to complete further study specific to the ethnic groups in their practice. The goal is not to oversimplify the behaviors common to each ethnic group, but to understand and appreciate their values and common experiences. It is important to remember that although your client may be from a particular ethnic group, his cultural backgrounds may not be similar to other people of that ethnic group. For example, the information for the general group called Hispanics (who may also be called Latinos) may vary somewhat for Dominicans or Salvadorians, although they share the Spanish language and some cultural similarities. Likewise, Chinese Americans may have both similarities and differences with other Asian American groups.

One of the key aspects in multicultural counseling is to consider problems from the client's viewpoint and current situation. Not doing so can result in misunderstandings and problems in developing a trusting working relationship. Ethnically diverse families may have experienced disruptive conditions that go beyond a mismatch of the ethnicity of counselor and client and can multiply misunderstandings in the counseling process. These conditions include "stresses of migration, unsuccessful relocation, uneven cultural assimilation, inadequate schools, family separation, participation in unresponsive judicial and welfare systems, lack of job skills, relentless socio-economic obstacles and frustrated opportunities" (Montalvo & Guitierrez, 1990, p. 35). In situations such as these, a culturally sensitive counselor could do several things to alleviate some of these stressors for their client including: (a) sharing of self to establish an open and more humane interaction, (b) subordinating roles to eliminate a power relationship, (c) taking on the role of advocate to offer solutions and encouragement, (d) avoiding withdrawing from touch during greetings, which may alienate clients who value and initiate this ritual, (e) leaving behind the preconceived role of a counselor and making sessions more personable, (f) engaging in sessions within and outside of the structured environment, and (g) incorporating non-traditional customs to support the client's belief systems. Engaging in culturally sensitive counseling may require clinicians to expand their boundaries and comfort level in order to establish and maintain a positive treatment relationship with their multicultural clients (Pedersen, Draguns, Lonner & Trimble, 2008; Sue & Sue, 2003).

European Americans

Generally, there is no typical European American. They are a diverse group of people who represent a variety of ethnicities such as British, Dutch, or German, among others. Individuals from Spanish ancestry also are considered European Americans. However, there are likely different belief systems for those European Americans who have lived in the United States for generations versus those who are recent immigrants. A great deal of research supports the world view or mainstream characteristics that are associated with the European American (Trevifio, 1996; Williams, 2003). These include an individualistic versus group performance emphasis and a tendency to value "linear, analytical, empirical and task solutions" (Sue, 1992, p. 8). They may perceive the counseling process positively and approach the therapy in a very logical and rational manner.

No matter the ethnicity, when counseling the client who embraces mainstream culture, that is, white middle-class values, the clinician can expect a client who is assertive about her counseling needs, communicates well verbally, and will confront the clinician if their views are not in agreement (Sue & Sue, 2003). Mainstream cultural values and beliefs will impact the counseling process in other ways as well. For example: (a) a focus on the individual unit will result in the individual rather than the family taking responsibility in all areas of the care, (b) a competitive spirit may dictate that the counselor pursue and exhaust all avenues and methods to assure success in the therapeutic and counseling process, (c) the clinician will most likely engage in direct eye contact with these clients and have limited physical contact, (d) the client will probably be conscious of and adhere to time values such as coming on time and wanting to maximize his time in the session, (e) the client's focus on future orientation and the value placed on improvement may result in discontinuing the counseling session if improvement is not evident, and (f) the counselor may not fully understand the client's innermost feelings and problems, a consequence of the value placed on controlling the emotions (Gushue & Constantine, 2007).

African Americans

African Americans represent a diverse group of individuals including Black families from the North or from the South, many of whom came to this country as slaves and some who came as immigrants from the West Indies or Africa. Many African American families may enter the counseling process from a lens of experience with racism, discrimination, and prejudice. As with other ethnic groups, in order to be effective in the counseling of African Americans, clinicians should evaluate their personal belief system and any stereotypical attitudes they may hold. There may be a hesitancy among African Americans to voluntarily participate in counseling due to (a) their perception of unequal roles, which may evoke memories of unfair treatment as occurred in the Tuskegee experiments in which Black men with syphilis were intentionally misinformed and did not receive the treatments they were expecting (Brunner, 2010), (b) their unwillingness to "tell their business to a stranger" thus losing their independence, and (c) their discomfort in engaging in the unfamiliar process of resolving problems individually rather than in the group or collective manner common in the culture. The local minister may be chosen over the counselor to provide emotional support or resolve conflict.

The counselor also should consider five areas of strength identified within these families that may help in the counseling process, including: (1) strong bonds of extended families, (2) family roles that are adaptable, (3) religious focus and strength, (4) strong work ethic and belief in the value of education, and (5) skill in developing coping skills under socioeconomic hardship (Bean, Perry, & Bedell, 2007; Hill, 1972; Lewis & Looney, 1983). Counseling strategies that are appropriate to use with African American clients include, but are not limited to, increasing awareness of our own biases while avoiding stereotypes, developing a trusting bond with the client to counteract an African American's wariness of the motives of authority figures, and utilizing the strengths of the African American family to not only meet goals, but to retain the client in counseling as long as needed and assure good follow-up. Bean, Perry, and Bedell (2007) offer several guidelines for the non–African American family therapist working with an African American client that can be suitable for the speech and hearing clinician. For example, the counseling outcome can be improved by incorporating a religious leader or the father in the session, resisting the temptation to assume an intimate knowledge of the culture as familiarity will take time, addressing the issues of racism head-on as they arise, and using a problem-solving approach by utilizing the strengths of the family. Because counseling can be a foreign and uncomfortable situation, it is important to provide an orientation to the counseling process to maximize the client's comfort level.

The African American woman historically has been viewed as the person in the family who is the pillar of strength and the one who keeps the family together. Coker (2004) reports that some African American women may have a Superwoman Syndrome that can cause them to delay seeking therapeutic treatments and counseling, especially for themselves. In addition, they may not want the "intrusion" of the counselor in the life of their family, which may represent a residual effect of previous negative experiences with social workers or other social service providers. When they enter counseling, they may not fully disclose the depth of their difficulties to the counselor. It is important to identify the built-in supports and to identify and acknowledge the advice from these support systems as related to the communication disorder. Also, consider both external factors such as the socioeconomic status and internal factors such as personal fears should you meet with resistance to initiate or continue counseling. Especially in schools, however, African American mothers are highly likely to participate in counseling to assist their children with academic or behavioral problems (Coker, 2004).

Hispanic Americans

The majority of Hispanic people in the United States are bicultural, diverse in their beliefs, and have many within-group differences (Romero, Silva, & Romero, 1989). Depending on their level of acculturation, Hispanic individuals may view the counseling process along a continuum from great resistance to complete acceptance of the process. In many instances, however, Hispanic individuals are reluctant to use a counselor. This may be due to cultural traditions in which the Catholic priest supplants the role of the counselor, and where there is greater reliance on the family unit rather than on the individual professional to address problems. A strong sense of pride also may prevent Hispanic clients from seeking help, especially for men who have a high sense of *machismo*. Machismo is associated with behaviors such as a high sense of pride, superiority, strength, and masculinity. Opening up to the counselor could be seen as a sign of weakness; thus, some men in this culture may seem emotionless in their expression during counseling (Chavez, 2010). Machismo also is important to consider when directing attention during the counseling session. If a high degree of patriarchy is practiced in the family, decisions will be made by the male, and the male should receive the most attention as a sign of respect or *respeto*. The man also may be very protective of the family during counseling, showing pride, courage, respect, and honor for his family, which may represent signs of machismo.

There are attributes more closely associated with women in the Hispanic culture that may affect their attitudes toward counseling, For example, the Spanish term *aguantar* (suffer, tolerate) used in the Hispanic culture describes how women should manage difficulties in their lives. This feeling of withstanding difficulties comes from viewing life's inequities as "God's will" (Salas-Provance, Erickson, & Reed, 2002). This may result in acceptance of the disability and placing a lower value on "curing" the disorder through counseling or other means. However, Hispanic women may be more open to getting the help they need for their children before they seek support for themselves. For both Hispanic men and women, the counseling process, if entered, should proceed quickly. A counseling process that utilizes long-term talk therapy is foreign to Hispanic clients. Short-term, time-limited counseling that focuses on the current problem and the immediate future is recommended (Lee, 2008). Although the clinician may be focused on speech and hearing problems, it is important to remember that many members of the Hispanic culture may retain a view of counseling as an approach that is used only by those individuals who are crazy or *locos*. This understanding may create resistance to counseling. Accepting counseling services may be a sign to the world that they are unable to take care of their personal problems and are in the need of help from strangers for their most intimate affairs.

Asian and Pacific Islander Americans

Asian and Pacific Islander Americans represent a wide variety of individuals that includes Vietnamese, Koreans, Chinese, Japanese, Hmong, and Filipinos, among others. As a group they are referred to as Asian Americans. Like other minority groups in the United States, they have experienced bias and discrimination throughout history, expressed through denial of citizenship, relegation to concentration camps, denial of the ability to own land, and language bias. Similar to other ethnic groups, religious traditions should be considered when counseling. Many Asian Americans believe that "healing may take the form of invoking the help of some supernatural power or restoring the sufferer to a state of well being through prescribing right conduct and belief" (Das, 1987, p. 25). Sensitivity toward the unique characteristics of each group of Asian Americans can improve the counseling process. Kuo and Hu (2002) provide background information on Asian American cultures, describe their values, and recommend counseling strategies for the speech-language pathologists who work with these clients.

The following 10 points provide a basis for viewing appropriate communication skills during the counseling process with Asian American families. It is important to (1) form a social and cultural alliance with the family, (2) structure the initial sessions, (3) define the problem and set treatment goals, (4) employ a benevolent but authoritative attitude, (5) build an alliance with the family member with power, (6) use directive therapy, (7) assume multiple helping roles, (8) apply a psychoeducational approach, (9) reinforce culturally sanctioned coping mechanisms and cultural strengths, and (10) overcome language and cultural barriers (Omizo, Bryan, Kim, & Abel, 2008).

During the first encounter, the clinician should address the family in a formal manner that is warm and friendly, showing more interest in the person rather than the disorder or procedure to be conducted. Building the interpersonal relationship will be of paramount importance and put the client and family at ease. Clinicians should provide some level of personal (number of children, types of hobbies), professional (organizations they belong to), or academic (place where they went to college) disclosure to allow the family to make a judgment regarding the degree of trust and confidence they can place in the clinician. There are traditional age and gender hierarchies to be maintained with some Asian families, and it may be necessary to address general questions in the counseling process to the father first, then the mother, followed by older to younger children (Lee, 1996). Of course, it may be difficult to know these rules initially, but this information can be gleaned by becoming sensitive to cultural cues or simply asking the family for their input.

Asian Americans, like many ethnically diverse clients, may be apprehensive in the counseling process. They may be reluctant to publicize family concerns, worries, and problems in an environment where they may not trust the clinician or be suspicious about the clinician's motives. In particular, Chinese Americans have been called the "model minority" and the "silent minority"; thus, disclosing problems in counseling is contrary to this image and may be difficult for them to do (Cheng, 2002). A language barrier may compound the anxiety. Structuring the first counseling session so that the family understands their role and the expected length of the process is helpful.

Many families are in counseling because of the disorders of their children. A problem-focused rather than person-focused approach helps engage the family. Asian Americans expect their children to do well, and the parents may feel shame and personal failure if their child is having problems. Approaches that include generalization and normalization can help reduce blame and guilt. For example, you may say to the parents, "It is not your fault that your child has autism. The cause is unknown and there are many children who have this disorder. Your child can do . . . and . . . well, like other children his age." Goals are best stated in terms of external resolution or symptom reduction rather than from an abstract or emotional context. Continuing this example, the clinician may say to the parents, "The school has a special program for your child that will help him pay better attention."

A vertical approach to relationships is common in this culture and should be used in the counseling process. The family will expect the clinician to take on an authoritative role. An authoritative manner will help build confidence in the professional. Authority is claimed by the clinician through (1) firmly understanding the background information of the family, (2) explaining and providing causation for the problem, (3) making a cultural connection by showing evidence of alliance with the culture, (4) showing physical cues of authority such as displaying diplomas and other evidence of professional experience, and (5) providing some immediate solutions to the family's problem. The clinician should engage in careful listening, providing honest empathy and warmth. The family will respond with a sense of obligation to these positive traits of the clinician and "reward" the clinician by keeping appointments or following through on recommendations.

The clinician should assess the power structure within the family and communicate accordingly. The power can be role-described power given to the grandfather, father, eldest son, or sponsor, or psychological power given to the grandmother or mother. Permission to conduct an evaluation or carry out a specific treatment program must be obtained from the leader(s) to assure a successful outcome. The expectation for Asian Americans is to receive a directive during counseling rather than to engage in "talk therapy." Lack of directness from the clinician may lead the family to believe that the clinician is not interested, or at worst, incompetent. Traditionally, expressions of feelings are not encouraged in this ethnic group; thus, they may not express their dissatisfaction easily. Because education is placed in high regard by this ethnic group, using an education framework in the counseling process is helpful. Providing education about the disorder or problem, behavior management techniques, and problem-solving training can be useful strategies. Many Asian American families may live by the philosophies of Buddhism. The clinician may want to ask the client about her beliefs in the concepts of karma and fate as related to the disorder or impairment.

Native Americans

Similar to other ethnic groups, Native Americans have experienced hardships through loss of their ancestral lands, conflicts with mainstream values, and stereotyping that has resulted in confusion of self (Trimble & Gonzalez, 2008). They have high suicide rates, alcoholism, unemployment, and the highest school dropout rate of any ethnic group in the Unites States (Garrett & Pichette, 2000; Hawkins & Blume, 2002; Koss, Yuen, Dightman, Prince, Polacca, Sanderson, & Goldman, 2003). Effective counseling for Native Americans should consider three important aspects, including whether they live on a reservation, whether they receive assistance in the counseling process from other Native Americans, and whether their acculturation is traditional, bicultural, or assimilated (Garrett & Pichette, 2000). Acculturation is the degree to which they relate to their Native culture. Those who view themselves as traditional fully accept the values of their culture. With bicultural assimilation, they can relate to both their native culture and the main-stream culture. Those who have assimilated are completely integrated into the mainstream culture (Copeland, 2007). It remains a common practice today for some tribes to use a medicine man or woman or shaman and healing ceremonies to work through a variety of problems, thus bypassing professional counseling (Jilek, 1982).

Some characteristics of Native American traditional therapy have been used in family therapy interventions (Tafoya, 1989) and may be important to consider in general counsel-ing situations. One that applies to communication disorders is the use of directive ther-apy in which "homework" assignments are followed by the patient or families. These are expectations of many Native American clients and increase the likelihood of treatment compliance.

The differences in world views of illness and health held by Native Americans also may impact therapy and counseling. The primary world view (e.g., medical views of illness) and the secondary world view (e.g., cultural views of illness such as taboo breaking, witchcraft, spirit intervention, and harmony) may be in conflict for the Native American client and impact compliance with medical recommendations or understanding of treatment (Rybak, Eastin, & Robbins, 2004). For example, a Native American may believe in the concept of *wacunza* ("to cause to happen") where one person breaks a taboo and someone else suffers the consequences. In the case of Fetal Alcohol Syndrome, a mother can *wacunza* her child and not understand how her alcohol use caused the problem. The mother may not accept responsibility for the child's illness, not because she is in denial, but because she is simply following cultural beliefs (Medicine, 1982). A Native American patient also may use story-telling when facing difficult issues in therapy. Storytelling is a nonthreatening and indirect way of looking at a problem and can include the telling of legends or case histories of other patients. Through storytelling, a process of triangulation occurs by which the patient can develop a comfortable distance from the problem (Garrett, Garrett, Toress-Rivera, Wilbur, & Roberts-Wilbur, 2005).

When evaluating family support for treatment, it is important to understand that par-enting by grandparents is a time-honored tradition and is a typical Native American family style (Fuller-Thomson & Minkler, 2005). Historically, although not as common today, some Indian tribes practiced "fostering" in which children lived with various extended families and moved along to other extended families to alleviate stresses in living with any one family (Tafoya, 1982). This practice is less viable with the urbanization of Native people. It is important, however, to consider that children may have experienced various types of family units, and their upbringing may be nontraditional and dictated by their unique cul-tures and should not be considered as neglectful or abusive. More recently, Supplementary Survey 2000 data (Fuller-Thompson & Minkler, 2005) showed that of 53,000 American Indian/Alaskan Native grandparents, almost half were caring for grandchildren five years of age or younger. About one-third of these grandparent caregivers were living below the poverty level, and most were female. The clinician should investigate this possibility when counseling these children and consider that some of these grandparents are reported to be living with a functional disability of their own (Fuller-Thomson & Minkler, 2005). The implications for counseling are numerous in terms of ability to engage in counseling and compliance with recommendations.

There are other issues to consider when working with families from Native American cultures. There are many rituals associated with the body. In some tribes, the body is conceptualized as a seed that is planted whole into the ground at death. Because of this, they do not approve of amputation or cremation (Tafoya, 1982). It is important to consider these issues for patients who are amputees due to injuries or diabetes, or for end-of-life counseling. A similar belief is found in the Hmong, who believe that cutting open the body during surgery will cause the release of spirits, resulting in death (Cheng, 2002).

Native Americans have been found to have a high incidence of otitis media that may result in hearing impairments (Curns, Holman, Shay, et al., 2002; Stewart, 1986). It may be appropriate to position the client and family during counseling in a way that maximizes hearing ability for everyone. Increasing your vocal volume while maintaining a comfortable speaking level may be helpful as well. The client may not be able to hear what is being said but may feel that it is impolite to ask the clinician to repeat. There are implications for Native American students in a classroom who may underperform in school because of poor hearing. They may feel that it is impolite to ask the teacher to repeat herself. The student also may make the assumption that the teacher will provide information as needed and they should not request it.

Contact with Native American families may reveal differences in the use of power. In the mainstream culture, power may be constructed by a "take charge" attitude—a situation in which the problem is presented and the clinician takes care of the problem. In contrast, the Native American client may react in a passive and subordinate manner that is typical for some individuals in this culture, and this may be inappropriately interpreted by the clinician as being hostile, withdrawn, or having low affect. Passivity could prevent clients from asking the questions they wish, or silence may be used to challenge treatments with which they disagree. The counselor should attempt to understand the root of observed passive behavior. It also is important to remember that silences are a normal part of any therapeutic process (see Chapter 4, Interviewing and Therapy Microskills).

Arab or Muslim Americans

There is a growing body of literature about the cultural values and traditions of Arab and Muslim Americans that impact the counseling process. Increased knowledge of their culture and history will allow clinicians to develop a comfort level and knowledge base that can help to counteract negative views, avoid stereotyping, and ensure successful counseling outcomes. For counselors to best understand their Arab or Muslim clients, it is important to identify the level of acculturation or assimilation of the client. Identify whether your client embraces the Western values of the United States, the values of their Arab or Muslim country, or some combination (Dwairy, 2006). For an excellent overview of Arab and Muslim values and traditions see Battle (2002), who provides information on Arabic geographic diversity, religious beliefs, family patterns, dialects, languages, and clinical intervention strategies.

The Arab world is comprised of approximately 285 million people in 22 Arab countries and is bounded by northern Africa and southwestern Asia. Arabs are not identified by one racial group but represent a diverse group of people as a result of their nomadic nature (Gregg, 2005). Muslims account for approximately 1.2 billion people worldwide, with approximately 2.35 million Muslim immigrants in the United States who come from at least 68 countries and have different traditions, practices, doctrines, languages, and beliefs (Pew Research Center, 2007).

The greatest majority of Arabs are Muslims and a smaller number are Christian and Jews.

Arabs practice the Islamic religion and are connected by the Arabic language. As with the other cultures mentioned in this chapter, it is important to remember that Arabs have extensive within-group differences, but there is still value in understanding common cultural beliefs and attitudes. One of those beliefs is that those in the Islamic community who are "wealthy and able-bodied" should care for those who are not as fortunate. This is set forth in words that read, "none of you is a true believer until you wish for your brother what you wish for yourself" (Bradshaw, Tennant, & Lydiatt, 2004, p. 50). This knowledge can serve as a foundation to your counseling with the Arab client.

As with many other ethnic groups, and essentially most of the world population, the Arab or Muslim culture reflects a collective rather than an individualistic societal view. The counseling process that focuses on working on the needs of the individual and his disorder may be foreign to an Arab or Muslim client, who may be more concerned about the family and their external circumstances rather than internal and personal aspects. For example, when working with an Arab client who has experienced a stroke, it is recommended that the clinician identify the impact that the stroke has had on the entire family and restore the order in the family rather than focusing on the patient's individual problems. The counseling or treatment will be more indirect than the more Western symptom-directed treatment and will provide the client with more social coping mechanisms to solve her problems (Dwairy, 2006). Because of this focus on collectivism, the family, not the individual, makes most of life's decisions. There may be conflict when the clinician is expecting the client to take initiative for his treatment and the client is relying on some external force (i.e., family) to take care of his problem. Communication within this collective framework focuses on "values of respect (*Ihtiram*), fulfilling social duties (*wajib*), and pleasing others and avoiding confrontations (*mosayara*)" (Dwairy, 2008, p. 150).

There are some differences in the provision of special education services in the United Arab Emirates (UAE) (Bradshaw, Tennant, & Lydiatt, 2004) that may influence counseling the parent of a disabled child. In the UAE, children who are severely disabled may not receive any formalized schooling. Families are on their own to find special education services (with some centers having up to a two-year wait) or they may choose to simply keep their child at home. These beliefs and decision-making processes stand in contrast to American principles where the Individuals with Disabilities Education Act (IDEA) dictates the education of all handicapped children (U.S. Department of Education). Parents may need to receive information during counseling about their rights for education of their children in the United States. In terms of parenting, Dwairy (2008) revealed that Arab parents are accepting of teacher behaviors toward their children that may be regarded as abusive-aggressive. Authoritative parenting is common in this culture, and parents expect loyalty and high performance from their children. This authoritarian style may be

not be involved at this stage, it is important to be sensitive to the decisions that a family will be making.

A Hispanic Ritual for Death and Dying

I still remember my uncle being laid to rest in the parlor of my aunt's home. The parlor was in the direct line of traffic between the front door and the kitchen. I was about nine years old. The mourning extended for several days and nights and it seemed that there was always someone sitting next to my uncle's coffin praying and wailing. I do not remember being afraid. The crying and laughter, the joy and the sadness, were all of equal vigor. The mood was festive and there were lots of people coming and going; it seemed natural.

CLINICAL QUESTIONS

1. How do children view death in your culture?
2. What do you feel about home after-death care?
3. Do you feel that it is disrespectful for a funeral to have a festive mood?
4. What type of rituals for death and dying occur in your culture?

Loss of Self

Individuals with neurological disorders may experience a loss of self that reflects difficulty with comprehension, verbal expression, and cognitive functions such as reasoning and memory. In other words, these cognitive limitations can impact patients' sense of identity. They may have paresis or paralysis, swallowing disorders, or visual impairments, among other disabilities. Children and adults who stutter often feel a loss of self-confidence when they are disfluent, which may affect their ability to be as socially active as they might wish to be or to be economically independent. Their sense of loss may encompass multiple dimensions of loss. Clinicians should consider how such losses might affect their clients who are from culturally and linguistically diverse groups. For example, Native Americans have a "being" orientation and are more concerned with who they *are* and not with whom they will *become*. Their value as individuals is not diminished because of a disability. In fact, many terms such as *disability*, *handicap*, and *rehabilitation* do not have Native American language equivalents (Westby & Vining, 2002).

Loss of External Objects

When an elderly patient is moved to a skilled nursing facility, this loss includes the loss of tangible objects (e.g., the loss of proximity to friends and familiar possessions) as well as the symbolic loss of a familiar way of life and a sense of home. Individuals with communication disorders may experience multiple losses related to their treatments. For example, a child in a regular classroom who is moved to a special education classroom may experience the loss of her prior classroom space, friends, teacher, and schedule for class work, play, and lunch. This may have a greater effect on a culturally and linguistically diverse child who is a second language learner because these cumulative losses represent additional stressors to the language difference or disorder. When elderly individuals from an ethnically diverse culture are moved to a skilled nursing facility where they share a small room with a stranger, their sense of loss can be extreme. They are not only losing physical objects that may include extensive spiritual and religious artifacts, but there is the significant loss of home where extended family come and go freely and participate in the care of the elder. There also are changes of food choices from traditional ethnic foods to more bland and unfamiliar institutional foods.

Developmental Loss and Loss of Predictability of Reinforcement or Rewards

A young child may mourn the loss of secondary attention he received due to his articulation disorder once it is corrected. The child may have enjoyed leaving the classroom for speech therapy or may have developed a special relationship with his therapist. The speech problem may have been acceptable at a younger age, but not as a teenager. The child may now be bullied rather than considered special. The second language learner may partially or completely lose the ability to use the first language as she learns a new language. This may represent a significant loss to the grandparents, for example, who may only know the first language and thus are now unable to communicate with their grandchild. Elderly individuals may have changes associated with the aging process that they do not completely understand, such as loss of cognitive functions through dementia or loss of vocal quality as their voice changes due to the natural aging process. These individuals may go through the stages of grief similar to loss in other dimensions. The ability to express these types of losses may be more difficult for the new immigrant, for ethnically diverse clients who have not assimilated well, or for English-language learners.

Summary

By the year 2030, racial and ethnic minorities will represent approximately 25.4 percent of the elderly population in the United States, compared to 16.4 percent in 2000 (Jeffreys, 2005). It is critical to become familiar with the grieving rituals of individuals from the various CLD groups. Families will look to us for support, and we must be well informed and sensitive to their unique needs, being especially cognizant of the way in which their grief expression is connected to spiritual, mental, emotional, and physical aspects (Crawley, Marshall, Lo, & Koenig, 2002; Kitaoka, 2005; Koenig & Gate-William, 1995; Sue & Sue, 2003). Should grief counseling surpass our skills and comfort level, we must refer our patients to the appropriate mental health professional. Additional information on counseling children with communication disorders with an excellent review of grief and stress can be found in Friehe, Bloedow, and Hesse (2003).

END-OF-LIFE MULTICULTURAL COUNSELING

The way people think, feel, and react to death and dying are significantly influenced by their cultural background, perhaps more than other aspects of their lives. Yet most medical professionals are not trained in cross-cultural ways of addressing issues around death and dying. In America, individualism is celebrated and many physicians and caregivers tend to treat illness and death as a personal matter with little reaching out to community and other resources. However, community and cultural ties can provide a source of great comfort as patients and families prepare for death (Marshall, Koenig, Barnes, & Davis, 1998; Crawley, Marshall, Lo, & Koenig, 2002). Some clinicians may be a part of this end-of-life (EOL) community as they provide support services for swallowing disorders, cognitive disorders, or augmentative communication. Although we may have little direct clinical input, it is important to understand the EOL needs and views of ethnically diverse clients and their families and be able to offer culturally appropriate counseling at this crucial time.

In Asian and Latino communities, the family often determines what treatment should be administered to their loved one and even how a patient should be allowed to die. Some cultures, for example Korean families, expect the eldest son to make the decision about a parent's EOL care. Differences in beliefs, values, and traditional health care practices are of particular relevance at the end of life (Poulson, 1998).

Asian Family Hierarchy of Decision Making at the End of Life

I had been treating a Chinese American elderly man who was recovering from a stroke. The man's daughter accompanied him to all of the therapy sessions at the skilled nursing facility. The patient was improving and together, the daughter and I made the decision to remove the nasogastric feeding tube and to begin more advanced levels of oral feeding. The orders were approved by the physician on a Friday. On my return to work on Monday, my patient was back on the tube feeding and had regressed over the weekend. I was informed that his son was upset because he had not approved any changes in his father's care and demanded that the oral feedings be stopped. The father's health continued to decline and he passed away within the month.

CLINICAL QUESTIONS

1. As the speech-language pathologist, what would you have done in this case?
2. What do you think that the physician should have done in this case?
3. Should this decision have gone to an ethics board for review?

Some people plan EOL treatment in advanced directives, specifying choices about life support and hospice care. Caucasian and Asian Americans more often use advanced directives than other groups (Koenig & Gates-William, 1995). Cultural traditions that involve karma may be at odds with advanced directives. For Muslims, treatment that becomes futile is no longer mandatory. The sense of family may be so strong in some ethnic groups that they will not share the poor prognosis with the patient. They may fear that the patient cannot handle the information or that the patient will lose hope for the future and any possibility of getting well will be lost. Among the Zuni and Koreans, speaking of a person's death is taboo because it might bring sadness or hasten the demise. This is in contrast to mainstream care in which full disclosure is the norm (Poulson, 1998).

Hospice

Speech-language pathologists may be part of the initial stages of hospice care. Thus, they should understand the use of this care by their ethnically diverse clients in order to provide counseling as needed. Many European Americans choose to undergo the dying process in a more humane way through the assistance of hospice and palliative care. This type of care has its origins in European culture and is foreign to many other cultures, particularly Asian and Latino cultures. Hospice care is underutilized among ethnic minorities, with one study showing that of those who died in hospice care only 4 percent were Asian American, 6 percent were African American, and 15 percent were Latino, while the majority, 74 percent, were white (Poulson, 1998). African Americans believed that hospice and palliative care meant that medical care would cease, that physicians would give up on their care prematurely if they accepted hospice care.

The case of Mr. Byrd (Crawley, Marshall, Lo, & Koenig, 2002) addresses several of the EOL issues. Sometimes efforts to be culturally sensitive and culturally humble are as simple as using the given name of the elderly client as a sign of respect.

CASE STUDY

Mr. Byrd Demands Treatment at the End of Life

Communication between Lawrence Byrd, an African American, and his physician, a European American, has been difficult. In an effort to improve their relationship, the physician suggests using first names. Mr. Byrd does not use the doctor's first name, although the physician calls him "Lawrence." The doctor says, "Lawrence, I am worried about what happens when we reach the point where these interventions you are asking for will be costly and serve only to prolong your suffering." Mr. Byrd angrily demands that he receive "every medical test and procedure you've got—regardless of the cost" (p. 675).

CLINICAL QUESTIONS

1. Was Mr. Byrd being unrealistic about demanding such costly treatments at the end of life?

2. Discuss the level of trust that is given to doctors in your culture.

3. As a clinician, what are two key points that you have reflected upon based on this case?

In the case of Mr. Byrd, a subsequent discussion between the treating physician and an African American physician colleague revealed that the use of the patient's first name was a sign of disrespect and may have upset the patient. There may be residual memories of discrimination and withholding of treatment such as occurred with the Black men in the Tuskegee syphilis experiments. Crawley and colleagues (2002) note that "many patients seek aggressive treatment because they value the sanctity of life, not because they misunderstand the limitations of technology. Mr. Byrd may have perceived discussions of costs and the ineffectiveness of treatment as a devaluation of his life" (p. 675).

In people of some European backgrounds such as Bosnian Americans and Italian Americans, there is a belief among some individuals that direct disclosure of an illness is at minimum disrespectful and, more significantly, inhumane (Searright & Gafford, 2005). Native American, Filipino, and Bosnian cultures emphasize that words should be carefully spoken or they may become reality. A commonly held Navajo belief is that negative words and thoughts about health become self-fulfilling; thus, one should think and speak in a positive way. In Asian cultures, the elderly have a special status and thus these cultures feel that the elderly should not be burdened unnecessarily when they are ill. Filipino patients may not want to discuss end-of-life care because this would demonstrate a lack of respect for the belief that individual fate is determined by God. Religion plays a large role in many cultures when making end-of-life decisions. Carey and Cosgrove (2006) provide an excellent summary of attitudes towards death for Buddhist, Hindu, Islamic, Jewish, and Sikh faiths. The clinician can continue to be a source of social support at the final stages of life. The best practice is to wait for the family to request continuing services for swallowing, hearing, cognitive functioning, and augmentative communication needs. Maintaining open lines of communication is essential for the patient, family members, and professionals. The bilingual or bicultural speech-language pathologist or audiologist also may serve an important role as a translator and/or cultural broker during this time.

THE HIERARCHY OF CULTURAL KNOWLEDGE: A MODEL OF PROGRESSIVE LEARNING

To provide the best counseling to our clients, patients, and their families, we must be lifelong learners and continue to gain knowledge about our culturally diverse clients. The model of a Hierarchy of Cultural Knowledge shown in Figure 5-1 is a new model that shows the natural progression of cultural knowledge from a naïve knowledge of cultural

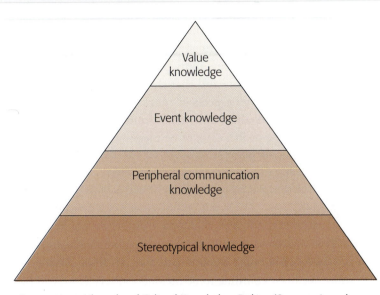

Figure 5-1 Hierarchy of Cultural Knowledge. *Delmar/Cengage Learning*

stereotypes level to the most mature value knowledge level. At the lowest *stereotype* level, we are influenced by and limited to the information provided from the media such as advertising, television, or movies. The information on ethnic diversity provided at this level may not only be biased, but untrue and hurtful. The majority of the time it represents stereotypes, defined as overgeneralizations of an individual trait to the entire group, such as the idea that Asian Americans are smart in mathematics and science but are not psychologically minded. While this may be true for some Asian Americans, it is not true for all individuals from this ethnic group.

At the *peripheral communication knowledge* level, the information we receive about individuals from diverse groups is based upon limited personal experiences, such as a passive acknowledgement of our ethnically diverse neighbors or co-workers. We do not make an effort to know them personally. For example, we may observe that the Filipino family that lives down the street has many family members who visit and they have many family gatherings on the outdoor patio. We can then interpret what we wish from this limited knowledge. We may decide that the family seems like a good family with strong family values, or that they are disruptive to the community with their frequent outdoor gatherings.

As we progress up the ladder of cultural knowledge we reach the *events knowledge* level. At this level, we have an appreciation of the ethnic group and their culture, but not a deep understanding. At the events stage we may attend a Native American dance, a Hispanic Day festival, or a Chinese New Year parade and truly enjoy the event. This is the stage where many well-meaning and culturally sensitive individuals remain.

The top level, the *value knowledge* level, is the highest stage of cultural competence, at which we are most equipped to meet the needs of our culturally and linguistically diverse clients. We value the diversity of clients and make a commitment to expanding our knowledge through additional training or readings. An organization that has reached this highest level of cultural knowledge may make monetary commitments to advance medical and educational research to decrease health care disparities or provide funding for training interpreters, for example. A government at this highest level passes laws and expands programs to improve the lives of these individuals. At this highest level it is understood that individuals are not all the same and that these differences are important and should be taken into consideration in all aspects of education, health care, and governmental policy. This level of awareness will allow individuals from diverse groups to maximize their ability to be educated, to access health care, to be meaningfully employed, and to be active participants in the country in which they live.

CONCLUDING COMMENTS

In closing, knowledge and skills for counseling ethnically and culturally diverse clients will best be developed through a combination of training, direct experience, and continuing education. We must continue to be lifelong learners as we will likely encounter clients in our practices from around the world who come from cultures of which we have little knowledge. Pedersen, in a forward for Dwairy (2006), speaks about three biases that we should consider in our final analysis when counseling culturally diverse clients from the United States, its territories, and worldwide. The alpha bias exaggerates the differences between cultures, the beta bias completely denies that there are differences between cultures, and finally, the generalization bias warns us about the pitfalls of stereotyping. It is not easy to move beyond our comfort zone and the bias we may possess at times, to be open to cultures different from our own. However, our counseling outcomes can improve through a concerted effort to learn more about the individuals we serve and to show respect for different values and beliefs. This chapter has provided you with some general values and behaviors that can be found among several ethnically diverse groups, both their similarities and differences. Foremost, it is critical to consider each client as an individual who presents his own unique set of beliefs and behaviors in the counseling process and to avoid biases that may negatively impact our counseling outcomes.

Discussion Questions

1. What are some of the reasons for underutilization of counseling services by some ethnically diverse groups?

2. Discuss the experience of different ethnic groups that may influence their mistrust of the counseling process.

3. How does the level of acculturation affect an individual's response to counseling?

4. Ten points were provided as a lens for viewing appropriate communication styles of Asian Americans. Use these 10 points and describe the communication styles of individuals from other ethnic groups.

5. Explain why it is important to a successful counseling outcome to develop rapport with the extended family of Hispanic and African American families.

6. What is meant by the term *cross-cultural zone* and how can this enhance your counseling session?

7. The professional should use a trained interpreter as needed to facilitate communication with clients. How would you differentiate between a trained and untrained interpreter?

8. What is meant by the term *wacunza* in the Native American culture? How can knowledge of this practice help you to understand views on disability of this ethnic group?

9. How is silence viewed by different cultures? Is this an aspect that should be considered in the counseling setting? If so, how?

10. Use the diunital model to show how you could develop your understanding of cultural differences. Describe a specific example.

11. How can you use the ethnographic interview style to improve your counseling skills?

12. The period of introduction during the counseling session may be longer for some ethnic groups. What may be the benefits to your counseling if you utilize these extended rapport periods?

13. How can you use the collective versus individualistic preference of certain ethnic groups to support your goals in counseling?

14. You are counseling a family whose young child has recently been diagnosed with a disability. How would knowledge of various family views on disability change your counseling methods?

15. Explain the statement "dying is culturally determined."

16. Why might a person from an ethnic culture reject the use of hospice care?

17. What is your most important role as a counselor at the end of life with families from diverse cultures?

18. Describe the model of the Hierarchy of Cultural Knowledge and how you can use this model to improve your understanding of ethnically diverse groups.

Role Plays

1. Have the students divide into client–clinician pairs. Have each client assume
    the role of an individual from a specific cultural background (e.g., Hispanic,
    Muslim) and have the clinician conduct a culturally sensitive interview in which
    information about the client's communication disorder and cultural background is
    obtained. Afterwards, discuss with the class which interview strategies felt *most* and
    least respectful and what cultural information was gleaned that could be used to
    facilitate the goals of therapy.

2. Divide into clinician–intern pairs and ask the clinician to provide culturally
    sensitive information to the intern who has just committed a *faux pas* in her
    interactions with a family from a culturally different group. The intern error could
    be giving insufficient respect to the family's role in the decision-making process,
    focusing too much on family factors that increase the client's sense of shame, or
    approaching the family in a manner that is too familiar and does not respect their
    cultural norms for social etiquette. Provide a constructive teaching moment to the
    intern who lacks sufficient training in multicultural issues.

References

Alberta, A. J., & Wood, A. H. (2009). A practical skills model for effectively engaging
clients in multicultural settings. *The Counseling Psychologist, 37,* 564–579.

Battle, D. E. (2002). Middle Eastern and Arab American cultures. In D. Battle (Ed.),
Communication disorders in multicultural populations (3rd ed.) (pp. 113–134).
Boston: Butterworth Heinemann.

Bean, R. A., Perry, B. J., & Bedell, T. M. (2007). Developing culturally competent
marriage and family therapists: Treatment guidelines for non-African-American
therapists working with African-American families. *Journal of Marital & Family
Therapy, 28*(2), 153–164.

Benkert, R., Peters, R., Clark, R., & Keves-Foster, K. (2006, September). Effects of
perceived racism, cultural mistrust and trust in providers on satisfaction of care.
Journal of the National Medical Association, 98(9), 1532–1540.

Bradshaw, K., Tennant, L. M., & Lydiatt, S. (2004). Special education in the United
Arab Emirates: Anxieties, attitudes and aspirations. *International Journal of Special
Education, 19*(1), 49–55.

Brown, J. (2010). Ten obstacles to empathic communication. Retrieved May 5, 2010,
from http://www.bloomington.in.us/~jwbrown/pdfs/obstacles.pdf.

Brunner, B. (2010). The Tuskeegee syphilis experiments. Retrieved from http://www.
tuskegee.edu/Global/Story.asp?s=1207586.

Canino, I. A., & Spurlock, J. (1994). *Culturally diverse children and adolescents:
Assessment, diagnosis and treatment.* New York: The Guildford Press.

Carey, S. M., & Cosgrove. (2006). Cultural issues surrounding end-of-life care. *Current Anaesthesia & Critical Care, 17,* 263–270.

Chavez, M. E. (2010, Spring). Emotional expression and machismo: Attitudes among second-generation Mexican-American and first generation Mexican-immigrant men. *The Berkley McNair Research Journal, 17,* 28–43.

Cheng, L. L. (2002). Asian and Pacific American cultures. In D. Battle (Ed.), *Communication disorders in multicultural populations* (3rd ed.) (pp. 71–111). Boston: Butterworth Heinemann.

Coker, A. D. (2004). Counseling African American women: Issues, challenges and interventions strategies. In G. R. Walz & R. Yep (Eds.), *VISTAS: Perspectives on Counseling 2004* (pp. 129–136). Alexandria, VA: American Counseling Association and Counseling Outfitters/CAPS Press.

Constantine, M. G. (2002). Predictors of satisfaction with counseling: Racial and ethnic minority clients' attitudes towards counseling and ratings of their counselors' general and multicultural counseling competence. *Journal of Counseling Psychology, 49,* 255–263.

Constantine, M. G., Warren, A. K., & Miville, M. L. (2005). White racial identify dyadic interactions in supervision: Implications for supervisees' multicultural counseling competence. *Journal of Counseling Psychology, 2*(4), 490–496.

Copeland, D. (2007). Being American: Traditional, bicultural, and assimilated: The American Indian dilemma. Unpublished master's thesis, Humboldt State University. Retrieved June 28, 2010, from http://humboldt-dspace.calstate.edu/xmlui/bitstream/handle/2148/239/Davita.pdf?sequence=1.

Crawley, L. M., Marshall, P. A., Lo, B., & Koenig, B. A. (2002). Strategies for culturally effective end-of-life-care. *Annuals of Internal Medicine, 136,* 673–679.

Curns, A. T., Holman, R. C., Shay, D. K., Cheek, J. E., Kaufman, S. F., Singleton, R. J., & Anderson, L. (2002). Outpatient and hospital visits associated with otitis media among American Indian and Alaska native children younger than 5 years. *Pediatrics, 3,* 109–111.

Das, A. K. (1987). Indigenous models of therapy in traditional Asian societies. *Journal of Multicultural Counseling & Development, 70,* 64–71.

Day-Vines, N. L., Patton, J. M., & Baytops, J. L. (2003, October). Counseling African American adolescents: The impact of race, culture and middle class status. *Professional School Counseling, 7*(1), 40–51.

Dwairy, M. (2006). *Counseling and psychotherapy with Arabs and Muslims: A culturally sensitive approach.* New York: Teachers College Press.

Dwairy, M. (2008). Counseling Arab and Muslim clients. In P. B. Pedersen, J. G. Draguns, W. J. Lonner, & J. E. Trimble (Eds.), *Counseling across cultures* (6th ed.) (pp. 147–160). Los Angeles, CA: Sage.

Fadiman, A. (1997). *The spirit catches you and you fall down: A Hmong child, her American doctors, and the collision of two cultures.* New York: Noonday Press.

Luterman, D. M. (2008). *Counseling persons with communication disorders and their families* (5th ed.). Austin, Texas: Pro-Ed.

Marino, T. W. (1996). The challenging task of making counseling service relevant to more populations: Reaching out to communities and increasing the cultural sensitivity of counselors-in-training seen as crucial. *Counselor Today, 8,* 1–6.

Marshall, P., Koenig, B., Barnes, D., & Davis, A. (1998). Multiculturalism, bioethics and end-of-life care: Case narratives of Latino cancer patients. In J. F. Monagle & D. C. Thomasma (Eds.), *Health care ethics: Critical issues for the 21st century* (pp. 421–432). Gaithersburg, MD: Aspen.

Medicine, B. (1982). New roads for coping: Siouxian sobriety. In S. Mason (Ed.), *New directions in prevention among American Indian and Alaskan Native communities* (pp. 189–212). Portland, OR: Oregon Health Services University.

Montalvo, B., & Gutierrez, M. J. (1990). Nine assumptions for working with ethnic minority families. In G. W. Saba, B. M. Karrer, & K. N. Hardy (Eds.), *Minorities and family therapy* (pp. 35–37). New York: The Haworth Press.

Omizo, M. M., Bryan, S., Kim, K., & Abel, N. R. (2008). Asian and European cultural values, bicultural competence, and attitudes toward seeking professional help among Asian American adolescents. *Journal of Multicultural Counseling and Development, 36,* 15–28.

Pedersen, P. B., Draguns, J. G., Lonner, W. J., & Trimble, J. E. (Eds.). (2008). *Counseling across cultures* (6th ed.). Thousand Oaks, CA: Sage Publications.

Pedersen, P. B., Lonner, W. J., & Draguns, J. G. (Eds.) (1976). *Counseling across cultures.* Honolulu: University Press of Hawaii.

Pew Research Center. (2007). Muslim Americans: Middle class and mostly mainstream. Retrieved July 10, 2010, from http://pewresearch.org/assets/pdf/muslim-americans.pdf.

Pope-Davis, D. B., Toporek, R. L., Ortega-Villalobos, L., Ligiéro, D. P., Brittan-Powell, C. S., Liu, W. M., Bashhur, M. R., Codrington, J. N., & Liang, C. T. (2002). Client perspectives of multicultural counseling competence: A qualitative examination. *The Counseling Psychologist, 30,* 355–393.

Poulson, J. (1998). *Impact of cultural difference in care of the terminally ill.* In N. MacDonald (Ed.), *Palliative medicine: A case-based manual* (pp. 244–252), New York: Oxford University Press.

Romero, D., Silva, S. M., & Romero, P. S. (1989). In memory: Rene A. Ruiz. *Journal of Counseling and Development, 67,* 489–505.

Rybak, C., Eastin, C. L., & Robbins, I. (2004). Native American healing practices and counseling. *Journal of Humanistic Counseling, Education and Development, 43*(1), 25–33.

Salas-Provance, M. B., Erickson, J., & Reed, J. (2002). Disabilities as viewed by four generations of one Hispanic family. *American Journal of Speech-Language Pathology: A Journal of Clinical Practice, 11,* 151–162.

Schneider, J. (1984). *Stress, loss, and grief: Understanding their origins and growth potential*. Baltimore: University Park Press.

Searright, H. R., & Gafford, J. (2005). Cultural diversity at the end of life: Issues and guidelines for family physicians. *American Family Physicians, 71*, 515–522.

Shipley, K. G., & Roseberry-McKibbin, C. (2006). *Interviewing and counseling in communication disorders: Principles and procedures* (3rd ed.). Austin, TX: Pro-Ed.

Stewart, J. (1986). Hearing disorders among the indigenous peoples of North America and the Pacific Basin. In O. Taylor (Ed.), *Nature of communication disorders in culturally and linguistically diverse populations* (pp. 237–239). San Diego, CA: College-Hill Press.

Sue, D. W. (1992, Winter). The challenge of multiculturalism. *American Counselor, 1*, 6–14.

Sue, D. W. & Sue, D. (2003). *Counseling the culturally diverse: Theory and practice*. New York: Wiley.

Tafoya, T. (1982, January). Native cognitive styles. *Journal of American Indian Education*, 24–36.

Tafoya, T. (1989). *Circles and cedar: Native American epistemology and clinical issues*. Durdich, Holland: Kluwer Academic Publisher.

Terrell, F., & Terrell, S. (1984). Race of counselor, client sex, cultural mistrust level, and premature termination from counseling among Black clients. *Journal of Counseling Psychology, 31*, 371–375.

Torres-Rivera, E., Phan, L. T., Maddux, C. D., Roberts-Wilbur, J., & Arredondo, P. (2006). Honesty in multicultural counseling: A pilot study of the counseling relationship. *Interamerican Journal of Psychology, 40*(1), 37–45.

Trevifio, J. G. (1996). Worldview and change in cross-cultural counseling. *The Counseling Psychologist, 23*(2), 198–215.

Trimble, J. E.. & Gonzalez, J. (2008). Cultural considerations and perspectives for providing counseling for Native American Indians. In P. B. Pedersen, J. G. Draguns, W. J. Lonner, & J. E. Trimble (Eds.), *Counseling across cultures* (6th ed., pp. 93–111). Los Angeles, CA: Sage.

Twohey, D. (2004). American Indian perspectives of Euro-American counseling behavior. *Journal of Multicultural Counseling and Development, 32*, 320–331.

U.S. Census Bureau. (2008). Press release CB08-123. Retrieved June 1, 2010, from www.census.gov/Press-Release/www/releases/archives/population/012496.html.

U.S. Department of Health & Human Services, Office of Minority Health. (n.d.). *National standards on culturally and linguistically appropriate services (CLAS)*. Retrieved June 1, 2010, from http://raceandhealth.hhs.gov/templates/browse.aspx?lvl=2&lvlID=15.

U.S. Department of Education. (n.d.). Building the legacy: IDEA 2004. Retrieved July 10, 2010, from http://idea.ed.gov/explore/view/p/,root,regs.

Vinson, B. P. (2009). *Workplace skills and professional issues in speech-language pathology.* San Diego, CA: Plural.

Westby, C., & Vining, C. B. (2002). Living in harmony: Providing services to Native American children and families. In D. Battle (Ed.), *Communication disorders in multicultural populations* (3rd ed., pp. 135–178). Boston: Butterworth Heinemann.

Williams, B. (2003). The worldview dimensions of individualism and collectivism: Implications for counseling. *Journal of Counseling and Development, 81,* 370–374.

Wilson, M. E. (1996). Arabic speakers: Language & culture, here and abroad. *Topics in Language Disorders, 16*(4), 65–80.

Wyatt, T. A. (2002). *Assessing the communicative abilities of clients from diverse cultural and language backgrounds.* In D. Battle (Ed.), *Communication disorders in multicultural populations* (3rd ed., pp. 415–460). Boston: Butterworth Heinemann.

CHAPTER 6

Working with Families

CHAPTER OUTLINE

- Introduction
- Traditional Therapist-Centered Model Versus Contemporary Family Involvement Model
- Rationale for Including Family Members
- Understanding Families: Common Family Patterns
- Working with Families in Assessment and Treatment
- Challenges and Cautions in Working with Families
- Concluding Comments
- Discussion Questions
- Role Plays

INTRODUCTION

Conducting speech and language assessments and therapy as well as audiological assessments and aural rehabilitation is often enhanced by working with family members rather than clients in isolation. A family-centered approach has become a common paradigm for providing holistic health care in allied health areas including psychology, nursing, pediatric and geriatric care, and physical, occupational, and speech therapy (e.g., Crisp & Taylor, 2008; Damboise & Cardin, 2003; Doherty & McDaniel, 2010; Hanna & Rodger, 2002; Watts Pappas & McLeod, 2009). Family-centered models have also grown in popularity in the speech-language arena where family involvement can lead to increased satisfaction with services and increased generalization of behaviors in authentic settings (Kashinath, Woods, & Goldstein, 2006; Luterman, 1984, 2008; Tye-Murray, 2009; Watts Pappas & McLeod, 2009). The inclusion of families in interventions initially received attention in the provision of services for young children (McWilliam, Synder, Harbin, Porter, & Munn, 2000) and in gerontology (e.g., see Gallagher-Thompson & Coon, 2007 for a recent review), in which a family member is often the practical and legal guardian. Including the family is no longer only an ideal to strive for, but the law when it comes to child services. Legislation in the United States during the past few decades has mandated the inclusion of families (i.e., family-centered practices) for children (Franck & Callery, 2004; Wehman, 1998). Further, the American Academy of Pediatrics (2002) has urged primary care providers to provide comprehensive, accessible, and coordinated family-centered care for children with special health care needs. Research conducted on this model thus far indicates that family-focused care not only improves family adjustment but also satisfaction with care, pain management, adherence to medical regimens, and health care utilization (Drotar, 2001; Kazak, 2001). Based upon these recent developments in models of health care, research, and law, a family-centered model is now a key component in the competent functioning of speech-language pathologists and audiologists. Further, given an imminent increase in our aging population, SLPs and Auds will be more likely to come into contact with adult caregivers for their older patients. Learning how to incorporate these valuable family members into our services and recognize their needs is essential.

TRADITIONAL THERAPIST-CENTERED MODEL VERSUS CONTEMPORARY FAMILY INVOLVEMENT MODEL

Watts Pappas and McLeod (2009) provide a succinct history of the shift from a traditional, therapist-centered model of care, in which the professional assumes control and a central role in professional decision making and intervention, to a more contemporary model of care that values family involvement. While Watts Pappas and McLeod describe the subtle differences between a family-centered and a family-friendly approach, this chapter does not distinguish between these models and instead presents a more over-arching notion of incorporating families into the planning and provision of services. Working with families, by definition, involves a collaborative counseling process in which the family is empowered (Dunst, 2002) rather than a process that is driven either by the family or the clinician. One basic premise in the family-oriented approach is that the family is the client rather than just the child or adult patient (Goetz, Gavin, & Lane, 2000). The model is driven by a philosophy of respecting family differences and showing flexibility to adapt interventions to meet the needs of different types of families, including families from diverse cultural and ethnic backgrounds. The belief that when one member of a family changes, the functioning of the other members of the family is also changed is a cornerstone of this perspective (Becvar & Becvar, 2009; Doherty & McDaniel, 2010; Minuchin, 1974; Minuchin et al., 2007). The client's problems as well as his adjustment inevitably alter the family's functioning.

There is research on the treatment efficacy of the participation of family members in speech-language therapy as well as on the increase in satisfaction of family members when there is parental involvement. Involving parents in speech-language therapy can be effective (Law, Garrett, & Nye, 2003; Watts Pappas & McLeod, 2009). While the findings are somewhat inconsistent in demonstrating the superiority of family-centered approaches over more traditional therapist-driven approaches (e.g., King, Rosenbaum, & King, 1997; White, Taylor, & Moss, 1992), these inconsistencies may reflect methodological differences and/or flaws; it is beyond the scope of this chapter to provide a detailed review of this research. Suffice it to say that speech-language pathologists and audiologists often find it useful and/or necessary to work with family members in order to promote speech and language development and rehabilitation. Recognizing the clinical benefits of including families, as well as the appeal this model has to families, various speech-language and audiology clinics around the United States advertise that they are "family friendly" or practice a "family-centered approach." Family members have many opportunities to work with clients in their natural environments and therefore can accelerate the rate of therapeutic gains. Including families can help clients to feel empowered in the midst of challenging circumstances. In situations with medically compromised patients, family members also may need to have strategies to ensure their loved one's safety in the home and community. Speech-language pathologists are often the professionals who educate and instruct family members about strategies for maximizing the patient's communication and cognitive abilities as well as providing the safest environment for these individuals (Bayles & Tomoeda, 2007; Fogle et al., 2008; Lubinski, Golper, & Frattali, 2007; Petersen, 2002). This chapter is intended to highlight the impact that a speech-language or hearing disorder may have on family members, some of the ways that families may participate in interventions, the strategies that promote family participation, and the barriers or obstacles to including family members in treatment.

In proceeding to discuss these issues, it is important to note that while Chapter 2 included a section on family therapy approaches, it focused more on providing a theoretical framework and central concepts in family therapy; meanwhile, this chapter focuses on a description of common family issues and the practical application of family-focused approaches for speech-language pathologists and audiologists. Further, while the recent text by Watts Pappas and McLeod (2009) addresses methods for involving families with particular kinds of childhood speech, language, and communicative disorders, this chapter focuses on common psychological and interpersonal effects on the family and strategies for addressing these family issues so that the clinician can foster the family's positive engagement, mutual problem solving, and resilience in the face of developmental challenges, illness, and health care issues.

RATIONALE FOR INCLUDING FAMILY MEMBERS

Hearing, speech, and language occur in an interpersonal context, and the client's communication patterns are inextricably intertwined with family communication patterns. Although clinicians did not always involve family members in assessment and treatment interventions for children (Bailey, McWilliam, & Winton, 1992), it is now widely recognized that our clients' interpersonal functioning provides a multitude of possibilities for incorporating treatment interventions into daily activities. Clinicians work with clients who operate in systems (e.g., family, school, work, and church) and we perform our work in systems as well (e.g., clinics, hospitals, schools, universities, and clients' homes). While this adds to the complexity and quantity of factors clinicians must take into account, it also highlights the interdependence of these domains of functioning and the areas addressed by each member of the educational and health care team. By including additional individuals in the client's assessment and intervention plan, the clinician can maximize the opportunities for new learning and capitalize on the therapeutic influence of family members and other individuals in the client's daily life.

Working with families is often "best practice" because speech, language, cognitive, hearing, and swallowing disorders do not occur in isolation but impact an individual's social and adaptive functioning within the family and extrafamilial relationships. While the client's disability inevitably impacts her role in the family, inclusion of the family in the provision of services can be empowering and can give family members an opportunity to work collaboratively on the problem. In many cases, the family can provide living strategies that minimize dependency (Luterman, 2008).

Further, the impact on the individual's psychological functioning and behavioral outcomes can be significant (Fogle, 2008). In fact, Fogle includes a section on "emotional and social effects" at the end of each of his chapters on speech, language, cognitive, and hearing impairments. Therefore, it is often not only the speech-language and hearing problems, but the cascade of associated mental health difficulties, that change the client's and, consequently, the family's functioning. To take a couple of clinical examples, a child with an articulation problem may be ridiculed by peers and consequently develop a lowered self-esteem and aggressive behavior (Gordon-Brannan & Weiss, 2007; Fogle, 2008). At home, the child may be irritable and withdrawn. While the SLP is not a psychologist or behavior management specialist, the SLP may note these possible links between the child's speech difficulties and his social difficulties. Suggesting this link or offering this hypothesis may change the way the parents view their child. Instead of viewing Sammy as "mean and aggressive" toward his peers, he may be seen more accurately as "frustrated and sensitive to peer rejection." This reframing of the problem may help his parents to better understand the relationships between his seemingly disparate symptoms (i.e., his speech and his aggressive behavior) and may place them in a better position to provide support and advocacy for their son in the school setting where he tends to be ridiculed for his speech impairments. Thus, the counseling skills that the SLP uses to communicate with parents may increase their empathy, understanding, and motivation to help their child to enhance his functioning in his daily activities. To better grasp the significance of these counseling interventions, just suppose for a moment that the SLP did *not* mention or address these links between the child's articulation problem, aggressive behavior, irritability, and withdrawal. The child may grow increasingly depressed and aggressive and may strike out and physically hurt a peer. Once this escalation of symptoms occurs, the child will probably be noticed (and labeled) for his behavioral problem. Then his aggressive behavior will likely become the target of treatment, and the underlying difficulties may be overlooked. By being cognizant of the links among common speech, behavioral, and psychological problems and employing counseling skills early on, the SLP may be able to intervene in a manner that prevents an escalation of behavioral and/or emotional symptoms.

Similarly, an elderly person whose cognitive skills are declining may develop word-retrieval difficulties and loss of working memory. She may begin to lose interest in some of her usual social connections as she cannot easily follow and remember her friends' conversations. She may begin to feel depressed due to increasing social isolation, and her husband may become angry because she forgets to pay some of their bills. She also may show less interest in cooking, complaining that the recipes are too difficult to follow. Her husband may accuse her of being irresponsible and inconsiderate because she does not perform her portion of the household responsibilities with the efficiency and reliability that she did in the past. Marital problems may develop as a consequence of these cognitive and language changes. On the other hand, an SLP who works with the family can help the husband to understand the connections among his wife's symptoms. The husband's better understanding may increase his empathy and support for his wife's cognitive and language decline. He then may be encouraged to learn tools for structuring their lives and schedules that increase his wife's general cognitive, language, and adaptive functioning. In this way, he can provide active support rather than being a helpless bystander. This inclusion of the husband in the SLP's therapy may help to prevent further decline in the marital relationship and could even help the couple to enhance their bond through the process of working together to overcome her memory problems. This last reframing strategy is known as "externalizing the symptom," a therapeutic tool made famous by the narrative therapists in psychotherapy (e.g., White, 2007), which will be discussed later in this chapter.

While the preceding two illustrations are hypothetical and based on an amalgam of various cases, they demonstrate the significant advantages and power that SLPs may harness by working with families instead of individual clients. A related theme (which also was illustrated in the vignettes above) is that SLPs can use psychoeducational strategies to help clients and their families better comprehend the interlocking impact of speech-language, cognitive, audiological, psychological, social, and behavioral issues. That is, they can educate clients and their families about these factors and their interplay. One caveat, however, is that this does not mean that SLPs are ultimately responsible for all of these social, psychological, and behavioral outcomes of clients. Sometimes a cascade of complicating factors has already emerged and has a powerful momentum, and psychoeducation alone is not effective, but rather a multidisciplinary approach to intervention must be considered (e.g., adding a behavioral management specialist, a psychologist, or marital therapist to the treatment team).

In addition to the multifaceted impact on the client's emotional and social status, the ripple effect that an individual client's functioning may have on the family can destabilize their functioning as well. Parents and other family members of patients of any age with chronic health conditions are at risk for emotional distress and adjustment problems (Cohen, 1999; Katz, 2002; Sharpe & Rossiter, 2002). Research to date suggests that it is not only the severity of the child's health condition, but the reciprocal interactions between child (including an adult child) and parent and the larger social context that affects the family's adjustment (Kazak, Segal-Andrews, & Johnson, 1995). In light of the stresses that families face in navigating medical systems, seeking associated social and academic services, and making adjustments to illness and disability, enhancing the scope of medical care to include the family has been shown to have a positive impact on family adjustment (Drotar, 2001; Kazak, 2001).

CASE STUDY

Haitham

Haitham was a 26-year-old man referred by a neuropsychologist in London, England to me for private therapy. He was a civil engineer who had been born and raised in Amman, Jordan, and his first language was Arabic. Haitham sustained a TBI when he was 23 years old during a motor vehicle accident in Jordan. Computed tomography (CT scan) and magnetic resonance imaging (MRI) of his head revealed multiple brain traumas with diffuse axonal damage and cerebral edema. Haitham was in a coma for eight months, and after recovering consciousness was transferred to a rehabilitation center in Amman where he received physical, occupational, and speech therapy. Eighteen months after the MVA he was flown to London where he was seen at a neurological rehabilitation center as an outpatient. A **mental status examination** by a **neuropsychologist** revealed that Haitham remained at considerable risk for emotional difficulties, particularly when the somewhat unrealistic goals he had set for himself could not be realized (i.e., returning to his work as a civil engineer).

Haitham came to California with his mother to live with his uncle and to continue receiving speech, language, and cognitive therapy. My evaluation of Haitham revealed severe dysarthria, mild to moderate receptive and expressive aphasia, and severe cognitive impairments that interfered with independent functioning in a consistently safe manner in the home and community. I worked with Haitham on a twice-weekly basis for several months in his uncle's home. Haitham and his mother and uncle wanted him to begin driving in order to be more independent; however, because of his cognitive impairments, lack of awareness of safety, and slowed reaction time, he would not be safe. It was important for me to discuss this emotional topic with Haitham as well as his mother and uncle. Although Haitham was somewhat angry with me for a while because I was not supportive of him driving, I maintained my stance and perhaps saved him or someone else from injury and his family from additional grief. He made significant gains in most all areas and then returned to his home in Amman, Jordan; however, he remained unrealistic about his potential to return to his previous work as a civil engineer and his potential to be a safe driver.

CLINICAL QUESTIONS

1. Why is it important to openly discuss with clients and their family members issues of client safety?

2. How would you have discussed your concern with this client and family about his wishes to begin driving when he was not cognitively capable of being safe?

3. How would you manage a client or patient's anger toward you and continue working with him in therapy?

First, let's examine the impact that speech-language and hearing disorders have on the family's psychological adjustment. Although there is only scant research in these specific areas to date, much can be learned from pediatric and behavioral medicine, in which a body of research has been conducted examining the effects of chronic illness on the family's perceived stress, functioning, and adjustment.

UNDERSTANDING FAMILIES: COMMON FAMILY PATTERNS

Unique Meanings and Previous Experiences with Loss

Families who have a member with a speech, language, cognitive, hearing, or swallowing disorder may undergo a period of shock, loss, and grief regarding their loved one's condition (Friehe, Bloedow, & Hesse, 2003). At times, the disorder is part of a larger medical condition, for instance a stroke, TBI, Alzheimer's, or Asperger's Disorder, and there is an abundance of information to process regarding the limitations in functioning that extend beyond speech, language, cognition, hearing, and swallowing. However, the severity of the illness may not be the main factor that determines the family's level of stress versus adjustment (Arpin, Fitch, Browne, & Corey, 1990). Research in health psychology supports the assertion that cognitive appraisal, or *how people think about illness*, is an important factor that determines caregiver adjustment and well-being (Trute & Hiebert-Murphy, 2002). For example, some families gain spiritual meaning or value from the experience of living with and caring for a family member who has an illness. Other families feel that family relationships are improved or more meaningful as a result of their shared experience with illness. Green (2007) found that most mothers of children with disabilities perceive valuable benefits of having a child with a disability. In a compelling book about a father's reflections on raising a child with a disability, Kappes (1995) articulates how the meaning and experience of loving is changed:

> The child with a disability enables, perhaps forces, the family to grow layers of unconditional love, selfless consideration and quiet strength around this unusual person. Peering into the crib of a child with a disability in the predawn moonlight can bring tears of truly unconditional love, love that will not be based on the report card performance, scores as a star quarterback, or excellent performance as a trial lawyer. This love is for who the person *is*, for their qualities, their trials, and for the inner strength they must develop to take their place (p. 25).

In a study of the meaning of disability expressed by Mexican-origin mothers (Larson, 1998), one researcher found that the mothers expressed apparently contradictory emotions of grief and joy that influenced their well-being and constituted a life metaphor, "the embrace of paradox." Larson explains that these mothers were able to embrace the disabled child while clinging to the desire for change. They both loved and accepted the child and yet wanted to eradicate the disability. She believes that the tension inherent in this thinking "became a driving force which energized the mothers to seek solutions, orchestrate daily routines, find programs, and search for answers for their child's sake" (p. 871). Larson cautions health care providers against making (false) assumptions regarding whether parents have a realistic notion about their child's future. Sometimes, opposing thoughts coexist and together create a new meaning.

Families can have different meanings and emotional valences associated with the client's symptoms. Some families may be very supportive and unembarrassed by their child's disorder, while other families suffer the anguish of wondering what they did to cause their child's disorder (e.g., a "bad gene" or retribution for past sins). Some families are concerned about the social implications of their family member's health condition. Another family may harbor feelings of shame about the client's difficulty with speaking clearly or loss of hearing. For example, a modest, upwardly mobile family may be reassured that their son has normal intelligence despite having a speech articulation problem. Meanwhile, an extremely achievement-oriented and status-conscious family may be overly anxious and fearful that others will view their son with a speech problem as "dumb." The different meanings families embrace may belie differences in a family's ability to tolerate differences and/or disabilities in their family members, and they also may reflect the amount of support they experience in their environments. In a 1997 study by Patterson and colleagues

different sense of loss and have difficulty reprioritizing their goals and energy to care for their adolescent son who sustained a TBI in a drunk-driving motor vehicle accident. Depending on the circumstances surrounding the incident, the accident itself may generate feelings of blame and animosity between the parents. It should be noted that single-parent or blended families as well as families from other cultures may be on a nontraditional schedule of growth and development. By asking families about their current roles, the clinician may get a sense of their current life stage and, in doing so, develop more empathy for the family's challenges.

Ken and Barbie

I received a call from a mother who sounded emotionally distraught and somewhat desperate. She had received my name from the parents of another child who stuttered whom I had worked with. The mother explained that Jonathan was 4 years old, and a sweet and bright little boy who was stuttering. The father was a fairly new police officer and the mother was a librarian with a degree in English. I scheduled an appointment to see the family in their home.

When first meeting the parents I got the impression that here were "Ken and Barbie" in person. Both parents looked perfect in every way with manners that seemed to have come from a manual on etiquette. The house was neat and clean (actually spotless) and there was a nicely circumscribed area in the family room for Jonathan's play area. Jonathan was very polite and well mannered. He shook my hand as though he had been well trained in this gesture. After I visited with the parents for a few minutes, the parents asked Jonathan to show his room to his "new friend." A very nice room it was: neat and orderly. When Jonathan finished playing with one toy he put it back in its place and took out another. Jonathan was definitely exhibiting some signs of disfluency (e.g., tense pauses when starting a word, repetitions of some sounds, tightly closing his eyes during moments of hard stuttering).

Over the next 2 1/2 months I met with the family once a week in the family home. Both parents were always present, and if one could not attend the session, they rescheduled. The parents and I sat around the formal dining room table each week to discuss stuttering in general, their child's stuttering in particular, and specific strategies the parents could use during the week to help Jonathan's speech. Never had parental perfectionism been so helpful. They did every assignment perfectly and began to see that the little changes they needed to make in their daily family lives could have big benefits for Jonathan. The parents eventually became less perfect (e.g., they became more relaxed and less demanding when talking and playing with their son, they allowed him to be a little messy, and they decreased their expectations for him to be "the perfect child") and, along with some direct work with the child, Jonathan's speech became more fluent.

Continues on next page

Continued from previous page

CLINICAL QUESTIONS

1. What are some examples of the language you might use to develop rapport with these parents while at the same time helping them to understand how their typical behaviors may exacerbate Jonathan's stuttering?

2. How would you handle it if you felt it would be most beneficial for the child to work with both parents but only one parent could attend (or would attend) the sessions regularly?

Medical family therapy has created a concept called "balanced coping" (Patterson, Budd, Goetz, & Warwick, 1993), which encourages families to meet medical and illness needs while still attending to and pursuing the life cycle activities and goals that are critical to the family's well-being. Thus, parents may need time to care for themselves and well siblings may need time to play with classmates, even as they also are dedicated to caring for an ill child or grandparent. One study (Haley, 1997) that supports this theory found that adult caregivers of Alzheimer's Disease patients who engage in social and recreational activities are less depressed than caregivers who are more socially isolated.

Additional Stresses and Unmet Needs

When a family visits an SLP or Aud, they may have additional stresses that impinge upon their ability to devote time or energy to the clinician's recommendations. The family may not spontaneously disclose these other stresses because they do not fall directly within the SLP's or Aud's professional purview. However, these stresses and unmet needs may emerge during the course of therapy when the family member is unable to devote the time you have prescribed to a family-focused intervention. Some needs may be related to the condition you are treating, including information about services for the patient, respite care, dental care, family support services, and financial need (Farmer, Marien, Clark, Sherman, & Selva, 2004). Divorce, other special-needs children, unemployment, and medical needs of elderly parents may be among the additional stressors in the family. While it is often beyond the professional scope of the SLP or Aud to address these areas therapeutically, it can often help to understand what other stresses, challenges, and demands a family is currently experiencing. This understanding can help the client to feel understood (e.g., the client may feel that the SLP understands that she was not able to do the language exercises with her son for the past two weeks because she was tending to her own elderly mother's medical needs). This can help to protect the alliance with the SLP, as family members can be assured that the professional knows how much they are "juggling" and how hard they are trying. Meanwhile, when the unmet needs are related to the SLP or Aud, then a dialogue with the family member may help to illuminate these needs, and the professional may be able to offer suggestions for educational or psychological resources to support the family.

"That's—That's My Wife!"

I had been working in a skilled nursing facility during the summer and one of my patients was Mr. McAdams, an 84-year-old man with cognitive-linguistic impairments. I had worked with him for several sessions when I learned from another staff member that his wife was in the residential care facility across the parking lot from the facility we were in. I also learned that Mr. McAdams had probably not seen his wife in at least two months because no staff member had taken the time or effort to bring her over to the nursing facility.

After working through the normal nursing and administrative channels to no avail to try to arrange a visit of Mrs. McAdams to see her husband, I took it upon myself to make all of the arrangements. The following day at 2:00 I rolled Mr. McAdams in his wheelchair into the empty dining room that was light and cheery and had little vases of flowers on the tables. I placed Mr. McAdams beside a table with two glasses of water on it and turned his chair to face the open door. I told him I would be back in a few minutes. I walked across the parking lot, found Mrs. McAdams in her room where she had put on her best dress and had her hair and make-up done. She was beaming as I rolled her across the parking lot to the convalescent hospital where she would see her husband for the first time in over two months.

When we got to the door of the dining room Mrs. McAdams sat up straight and had a big smile on her face. I wheeled her directly to her husband and she had tears in her eyes. When Mr. McAdams could clearly see her, he said, "That's—that's my wife!" I placed Mr. and Mrs. McAdams beside one another in their wheelchairs. They started to hug and cry. I left the room and closed the door.

After that day I brought Mrs. McAdams over to see her husband twice a week, sometimes during craft time so they could work on crafts together. When it was time for me to leave the hospital at the end of the summer to return to teaching, I wrote in the Patient Care Plan in Mr. McAdam's medical chart that his wife was to be brought over twice a week for visits. By having this officially written in his medical chart it was then nursing's professional obligation to carry out all that was written in the resident's care plan.

CLINICAL QUESTIONS

1. How could helping this patient reconnect with his wife on a more regular basis help him with his cognitive and communication abilities and his emotional health?

2. Why is it important for clinicians to sometimes go the "extra mile" to help their clients and patients?

What the Client Brings to the Family "Table"

Clients with speech, language, cognitive, hearing, and swallowing disorders often have complex clinical pictures that significantly impact family harmony and functioning. Psychological and behavioral problems associated with communication and swallowing disorders can range from low self-esteem to anxiety and depression, impaired social competence, and social rejection or isolation (Beitchman, Wilson, Brownlie, Walters, Inglis, & Lancee, 1996). Follow-up studies of children with speech and language impairments show an increased prevalence of learning disorders and ADHD (Cantwell & Baker, 1991; Gordon-Brannan & Weiss, 2007; Ramig & Dodge, 2010; Rock, Fessler, & Church, 1997). Forensic clinical studies have revealed correlations between speech-language impairments and dropping out of school, juvenile delinquency, and other forms of crime and violence (Brownlie, Beitchman, Escobar, et al., 2004; Bryan, 2004; Castrogiovanni, 2002; Crowe, Walton, & Burnett, 1990; Zingeser, 1999; Sanger, Hux, & Belau, 1997). In cases of adults with neurological and speech-language impairments, their maladaptive and confused, repetitive behavior can be extremely disruptive and distressing to family members (Mitrani & Czaja, 2000; Sanders, 2007).

The SLP or Aud may be part of a medical or allied health team of experts who assess the breadth of the problems in order to determine the best ways to provide support to the families. As the treatment team develops a conceptual understanding of the relationships among the patient's various communication and mental health difficulties, they can present this formulation to the family so that the family can be in a better position to develop a supportive attitude and to prioritize needed areas for change. Depending upon the underlying psychiatric, cognitive, communication, or medical issue (e.g., Pervasive Developmental Disorder, TBI, or Alzheimer's) and the subsequent adaptive, social, and emotional functioning, family support and inclusion in assessment and therapy are often needed.

Effects on Parents and Adult Caregivers

INCREASED RISK OF PSYCHOLOGICAL DISORDERS

The stresses of dealing with a child or an adult with a serious or chronic illness or impairment can take an emotional toll on families, especially on the parents and caregivers who bear the majority of the burden of care. Parents and caregivers of family members with medical disorders and rehabilitation needs are at increased risk of psychological disturbance. While some families manage to traverse the journey of having a family member who requires significant care with psychological balance and grace, many families experience stresses and strains that render them vulnerable to depression and marital discord (Cohen, 1999; Ievers & Drotar, 1996). Adult caregivers may experience many negative consequences as well, including anxiety, depression, and increased use of psychotropic medications, as well as immunological dysfunction (Mitrani & Czaja, 2000).

GRIEVING AT DIFFERENT PACES

When parents or caregivers receive a diagnosis of a medical, developmental, hearing, or speech-language diagnosis, this news can trigger a wide range of responses. Some parents go through a process of grieving the "perfect child" they hoped for, and the grieving process can isolate them from each other and cause them to feel alone in their suffering. If one parent tends to progress through phases of grief at a different pace than the other parent, this also can be a source of stress and can cause difficulty in parental communication and problem solving. Through a psychoeducational process, clinicians can encourage parents to be tolerant of each other's emotional states as it is natural to go through the process of adjusting to diagnostic news and concomitant life changes at different rates. In this way, the clinician models the tolerance and acceptance that the couple can develop for one another.

For some parents and couples, a diagnosis or the caregiving process can trigger psychological growth or the consolidation of the couple relationship through a common effort. In other families, discordant views of the caregiving situation can exacerbate the stress they already feel (Hasselkus, 1988). Trute and Hiebert-Murphy (2002) emphasize that it is the subjective interpretation that affects the family's level of perceived stress and coping. Does the family view the experience as a tragic loss, or are they able to find benefits in adversity (Hefferon, Grealy, & Mutrie, 2010; Katz, Flasher, Cacciapaglia, & Nelson, 2001; Miller, 2010; Tennen & Affleck, 1999)? Finding benefits in adversity may promote resilience and recovery in the functioning of a family.

PARENTING STYLES

Additional variables to take into consideration when interviewing and working with a family include parenting styles: authoritarian, authoritative, and permissive. Baumrind (1967) developed this typology of parenting styles based on the constructs of parental control and parental support. These parenting styles have implications for how parents are likely to treat their children in different circumstances, and it may illuminate challenges that some families face in following clinician recommendations. Based upon a particular family's ingrained parenting practices, clinician recommendations may be congruent or highly incongruent with their existing parenting practices.

Bailey (2005) has provided an updated overview of these parenting styles. An **authoritarian parenting style** is very high in control and low in support. These parents may use physical, emotional, and verbal means to force their child to comply. Rules tend to be rigidly enforced and children do not have much decision-making power. These parents may put their child down and may not listen to what their child has to say; they may respond in a critical way more often than a validating way to their child's communications. They may use threats or guilt induction to control the child. Authoritarian parents may therefore have difficulty with clinician recommendations that emphasize validation of what their child says or providing frequent praise for positive efforts at communication. They may find it easier to follow highly structured homework assignments, such as "Practice reading for 20 minutes each night, and give Judy a 'star' sticker on her calendar for each (target behavior) she attempts." The clinician may need to work on building an alliance with such parents by making recommendations that are client focused and behavior oriented (e.g., "You can help your daughter increase her language comprehension in these ways") before confronting them with their nonproductive parenting strategies. However, if you notice that harsh and inhibiting parenting strategies continue to impede the child's progress, you may address the issue by first "siding with" their positive intentions.

For example, "I know you want Judy to try her best. Let's see if she responds more posi-tively when you are gentler with her" or "If you were going to sound more encouraging, what would you say?" Alternatively, the clinician can model the praise and positive feed-back in a parent-child session that she wants the parents to deliver at home.

An **authoritative parenting style** is high in control and high in support. These par-ents balance control and warmth. They set clear expectations and limits for their child's behavior but also have a give-and-take system for communicating with their children and allowing increasing autonomy and independence that is developmentally appropriate. They are accustomed to validating their child's behaviors and communications and usually do not have difficulty following through on clinician recommendations. In fact, they may appreciate recommendations that help them to be more focused and targeted in selecting behaviors they wish to encourage and reinforce.

A **permissive parenting style** is low in control and high in support. These parents avoid exerting their authority and believe that their children will thrive with few limits and restrictions. They are uncomfortable setting limits and may balk at or simply ignore a clinician's attempts to set up a regular schedule of exercises. They may say that they are "not good at" keeping reward charts, although they are typically comfortable giving spon-taneous praise. Depending on the amount of adult structure needed to enhance the thera-peutic benefits, the therapy may falter if these parents are unable to provide the structure that is needed. They may need more modeling or "hand-holding" to develop and imple-ment a structured system at home. For example, the clinician may wish to sit down and work out the exercise schedule with them and help them create the chart for recording the home exercises. This is structure that they are not likely to impose without your specific guidance and help.

Effects on Sibling Relationships

DISPLACEMENT AND EXCESSIVE RESPONSIBILITIES

In the psychological and medical literature, there is substantial evidence that sibling adjustment is negatively impacted by a child's chronic illness (Cohen, 1999; Sharpe & Rossiter, 2002). However, there is evidence that the family's open communication and problem solving can be stronger predictors of the sibling adjustment than the siblings' experiences of stress and coping (Giallo & Gavidia-Payne, 2006). There is also some in-dication that parents' ability to cope with illness may impact their ability to parent well siblings (Cadman, Boyle, & Offord, 1988). Therefore, while we should remain aware of how siblings adjust to having a disability, it is important to remember that the parents and family play a critical role in helping siblings to be more resilient. One study showed, for example, that siblings of chronically ill children may develop adaptive strategies for coping including choosing a career in the helping professions (Simons Michelson, 1985).

A well sibling who is struggling with her behavioral and emotional adjustment may be feeling either displaced in the family or may have new responsibilities that she was not pre-pared to assume. Often, when there is a chronically ill or impaired child, the healthy sibling may have more caregiving demands than her counterparts with healthy siblings (Sharpe & Rossiter, 2002). This **"parentified" role** can take a toll on the healthy sibling, and some-times behavioral (externalizing) or internalizing problems can occur in children who are recruited into this quasi-parent role. For example, a child who is forced prematurely to care for her younger, deaf sibling may develop irritability and aggression. An older sibling who has taken a caregiver role for her brother with a developmental disability may develop signs of withdrawal and depression as a consequence of feeling isolated from friends and burdened by family responsibilities. Clinicians working with families can investigate the impact of a child's condition on his siblings to see whether a causal relationship exists. The family may need encouragement to reorient some of their nurturing attention to the well sibling. Often, the clinician can be an advocate for the well sibling who is unable to voice her emotional needs directly.

Sibling relationships can also be negatively impacted if one is in a parentified role. Often, the parentified sibling has the responsibilities for caring for her sibling but not the authority. This can lead to conflicts *between* the siblings because the healthy sibling is trying to parent her sibling, while the sibling with a disability is not typically eager to have three "parents." A brief observation of the sibling interactions can often illuminate this family pattern. When this dynamic is operating, we frequently observe the older child behaving in a protective albeit controlling manner with her younger sibling who has a disability. The younger child may "play along" with his older sibling's guidance for a while, and then rebel when he no longer wants to be controlled by a mere brother or sister. When parents complain that their children fight excessively with each other, this is one viable hypothesis the clinician can investigate.

The healthy sibling's responses always need to be understood within the context of the individual's level of physical, mental, and emotional development. The impact of having a sibling with a disability is likely to vary depending upon the healthy child's developmental needs and how much the sibling's needs impinge on her developmental needs. For example, a 7-year-old who is naturally egocentric may have greater negative emotional responses to a younger sibling who has cerebral palsy than an older child. The younger sibling's cerebral palsy and its impact on the family may mean that the 7-year-old feels neglected and does not have the "special time" with mommy that she desires. However, let's imagine that a 7-year-old with a language delay has a 16-year-old sibling. This teen sibling may experience fewer emotional complications (e.g., less jealousy) due to enjoying more independence (and, concomitantly, fewer expectations for parental attention) unless, of course, a large burden of care for the younger sibling falls on her. While younger healthy siblings may be more distressed about unmet emotional needs (i.e., for parental attention), older healthy siblings may be more concerned about caregiving demands that impinge on social time with peers. Older healthy siblings also may worry about their parents and the toll taken on their health by the child with a disability.

The development of behavioral or other symptoms in the healthy sibling can be a way of trying to garner attention from parents who are preoccupied with a child with a disability. Unequal time and attention from parents may be mistakenly perceived to mean that the parents love the disabled child more. This does not suggest that the healthy child is malingering or even consciously "faking" symptoms, but rather that the healthy sibling may unconsciously seek the attention and nurturance that she observes her sibling receiving. In a poignant letter to Dr. Luterman (2008), an adult who grew up with a sibling with deafness writes that as a child she felt jealous of her brother and neglected by her parents. She recalls wishing she could be deaf so she could get more of her parents' attention, and even tried to fall out of her treehouse in an effort to break her arm so that she could secure the attention her brother enjoyed. Children can be quite creative and effective in redirecting their parent's attention toward them.

Peer Relationships

As children reach elementary school age, their peer relationships influence their developing identity and self-esteem. Having a sibling with a disability can sometimes threaten that process. One common stressor can occur when classmates compare the siblings and tease the healthy sibling by asking questions such as, "Are you autistic like your sister?" or "Are you 'retarded' like your brother?" Healthy siblings may struggle with conflicts regarding family loyalty while attempting to gain acceptance by peers. In addition to the potential stresses of having a sibling with a disability, there is some evidence that healthy siblings may learn greater compassion and acceptance by growing up in these families (Simons Michelson, 1985).

Autonomy vs. Dependency Conflicts

Speech, language, hearing, and swallowing problems can impact the social adjustment of the client, whether it is a child or an adult (Fogle, 2008). Within the family, one consequence can be that the disability turns developmental trajectories upside down. In a normal developmental trajectory, children evolve from more dependent states in their early or young childhood years to increasing autonomy and self-reliance as they get older. Adults typically have many years of self-reliance before illness or a tragedy such as a stroke or cardiac problems diminishes their ability to live and function independently. When normal, expected developmental trajectories are interrupted or thwarted by a person's illness or injury, it can place a strain on the entire family.

Disabilities and illness also can reverse the usual hierarchy within a family so that individual roles within the family are forced to change. The caregiver becomes the recipient of caregiving and the one who formerly received care now has to "step into the shoes" of the caregiver. In families where an adult family member has a stroke that results in aphasia or cognitive impairments, the couple's roles may change drastically. The spouse who had the stroke may have been the one who took care of the family financial affairs and was the overall "leader" in the family. The well spouse may need to quickly assume a new leadership and caregiving role in the family. Some families make these adaptations more easily than others.

The client may be relieved to have family members who can care for him, but distressed to have to rely upon others for basic needs and functioning. Thus, the client may be ambivalent about his new role in the family; he may enjoy the attention and nurturing he receives but resent the impingement upon his self-direction and autonomy. Meanwhile, family members may rapidly come to an acutely ill family member's aid but have quite a different response when the situation is chronic and lifelong adjustments and sacrifices have to be made in the family (Luterman, 1995). Illness can derail family plans and dreams.

Illness can create increased interdependence, which both strengthens the bonds within families and creates strain as family members do not enjoy the freedom that they otherwise would have. A mother may spend long hours helping her son who has autism with language stimulation, or an adult couple may spend hours each week taking an elderly parent to speech therapy and managing the business that the elderly parent was formerly capable of handling. Upon initial glance, we may see a family that is loyally providing its family members with the practical and emotional support it needs. But once we look beyond the surface, we may discover that there are strained relationships, ambivalent feelings of appreciation and resentment, or exhausted family members who need to take care of themselves for a while.

WORKING WITH FAMILIES IN ASSESSMENT AND TREATMENT

Research on working with families, especially in medical settings (e.g., Eggenberger & Nelms, 2007) indicates that in addition to the instrumental function family members may provide (e.g., facilitating social communication or providing appropriate foods to a family member with a swallowing disorder), family members often want to be included in the treatment process in order to show support for a family member. The inclusion of family members can enhance their connection to one another as they share the challenges, experience a sense of togetherness, and create stories and shared meanings regarding what is happening in their lives. Families appreciate it when health care professionals take the time to interact with them and treat them as integral members of the treatment team.

Specific Purposes of Including Families

The inclusion of family members in assessment and treatment can be to provide part of the supportive network for the client. To summarize some of the major reasons for including family members, they can be included in order to:

- Provide collateral information about the client's functioning.

- Share an understanding of the client's difficulties and learn what the disorder means and encompasses and the reasonable expectations given the diagnosis.

- Provide acceptance. Understanding increases the likelihood of acceptance.

- Support the client. Emotional support is enhanced when family members have an accurate understanding of the client's condition.

- Provide opportunities for generalizing skills and enhancing communication. What can family members do to help the client develop or correct his speech or language patterns? Who is in the client's environment that can help to implement these strategies on a daily basis?

- Employ safety measures. What can family members do to ensure that the patient has safe eating and swallowing habits, or that the patient is not allowed to drive until she is cognitively ready?

- Advocate for the client and seek needed ancillary services. What can the family do to advocate for the client in the health care or educational system?

In order to include families in the SLP's and Aud's work, a "road map" should be developed by the clinician that specifies how to include a particular family in the provision of rehabilitation services. This plan should not be adhered to rigidly, but can be used to give the clinician a tentative map as she develops an intervention strategy with a particular case.

The Therapeutic Relationship with the Family

When working with a family, as when providing professional services to an individual, the therapeutic relationship is the fulcrum for producing change. It is not only the technical skills of the clinician that matter but the interpersonal skills of the clinician and the relationship she develops with the family that are important (Thompson, 1998; Van Riper, 1999). Family members are more likely to provide important information and follow through on treatment plans if they have been part of the process of their creation (Crais, 2009). What are the factors that can help clinicians to develop a facilitative and positive relationship with families? Parents are satisfied with services when they feel that the care is provided in a supportive and respectful manner (Carrigan et al., 2001; King, Cathers, King, & Rosenbaum, 2001; Watts Pappas et al., 2008). Additional clinician factors that clinicians and parents perceive as important when establishing relationships with families are well summarized by Watts Pappas and McLeod (2009) in their review of the relevant literature:

- Interpersonal skills: being friendly, caring, and sensitive to the family's feelings
- Respect for family members' ideas and opinions: feeling that their input and knowledge of their family is valued; valuing the family's expertise
- Communication skills: taking time to explain and answer questions and use language that family members understand
- Professional competence and commitment to providing services of a high standard
- Acknowledgement of the family's individuality: being willing to adjust interventions so that they are feasible and meaningful for a particular family

Thus, creating an atmosphere of trust, listening, and respect for families' individual differences provides a foundation for a positive and collaborative working relationship with families. At least one study that examined factors affecting service delivery for children with disabilities found that satisfaction was linked to the parents' perceptions of "family-centeredness" of the service (Law, Hanna, Hurley, King, Kertoy, & Rosenbaum, 2003).

Some studies (e.g., Watts Pappas et al., 2008) have found that clinician variables and employment settings can influence the tendency to include families in interventions. These factors can include the clinician's confidence in including family members effectively and the workplace setting. SLPs who work in schools and who endorse a family-centered service philosophy paradoxically are less likely to include families than SLPs working in private practice or health settings. Perhaps many parents are less likely to understand or collaborate intensively when school-based services are provided. There also may be workplace models and pressures that contribute to the exclusion of families in school settings. Despite these trends, SLPs can include parents and family members as much as possible through phone calls as well as in-person conferences in order to maximize the effectiveness of their evaluations and treatment.

Assessing the Client's Functioning in Different Settings

Family members can often provide essential information regarding how the client functions across different settings. From the initial appointment onward, clinicians can show that they value multiple perspectives and inquire about the major social settings and community activities where a client functions. Furthermore, informants do not need to be limited to the immediate family members. It is wise to inquire about additional family members who also may have a caregiving role. For example, if grandparents or an aunt are caregivers for a child after school, clinicians can gather information from their perspectives as well.

Does the client speak without stuttering in the home setting but stutters at school? Are the parents relatively unaware of the child's language deficits, but these deficits are more evident in the school setting where more highly developed language skills are expected? What is the quality of the language and social performance in each of these settings? Which relative is going to care for the adult who had a TBI or stroke? Will this family member also be available to coordinate speech-language care as well as other aspects of the patient's medical treatment? Understanding the client's functioning in different settings may help to provide clues about the social factors that facilitate versus hinder effective communication.

Seeking a Contextual Understanding

Speech, language, and hearing are social behaviors at the core. Thus, clinicians are not simply seeking an outsider's objective view about the symptoms but are seeking a contextual understanding of what happens in various social contexts and how the client and others reciprocally influence each other. For example, when a grandfather who recently suffered a stroke tries to speak, do other family members say his words for him? The next time he tries to express a want, need, thought, or feeling, does he just point rather than try to produce his imperfectly articulated words? When adolescent Marie is at home, her parents are frustrated because she does not speak to them very much, and when she does, she frequently uses profanity. At school, she tends to give teachers short, concrete answers and she does not appear to enjoy spending time with her peers. Her speech and language evaluations indicate that she has very weak expressive language skills. Marie's behavior in different contexts "pulls for" unique interpersonal responses. At home, she tends to be punished for her poor expressive language, while at school, she avoids speaking whenever possible for fear that her speech and language deficits will elicit teasing or bullying. From these examples, we can see how critical it is to take a systems approach and to include the family in helping to understand Marie's struggles. Language and social behavior are intertwined.

Family Roles in Provision of Services

The various roles that family members may take are summarized by Watts Pappas and McLeod (2009), who note that parents and caregivers can serve as:

■ **Informants**   Each family member may be able to offer unique information about the client's functioning. As in family therapy, oftentimes one member of the family has a unique vantage point to observe how the client functions. A very accepting parent, for example, may experience her child's language functioning very differently from the parent who is very critical. Therefore, including both parents in the assessment process enables the clinician to gain information about the client's functioning in different settings and from different perspectives.

- **Therapist aides** Once a general intervention plan is developed, the clinician can collaborate with key family members in order to include them in providing structure, support, and opportunities for practice of therapy exercises or naturalistic communication.

- **Models** Family members can provide examples and coaching in the kind of communication skills that are desired. For example, parents may say to a young child, "Please give me a glass of milk" to provide an example of what is expected and to encourage a young child to speak in sentences.

- **Reinforcers** Family members can provide encouragement and rewards for achieving targeted communication goals. For example, parents can respond to a child's correct speech patterns with praise and by providing a treat, such as allowing the child to choose a favorite book to read.

Granlund, Bjork-Akesson, & Alant (2005) also note additional roles that family members may take while involved in the process of assessment and treatment of their loved one:

- **Decision maker** Sometimes parents or adult children of elderly clients are the major decision makers in the family, and clinicians should respect this family hierarchy and role designation.

- **Consumers** Clients and family members are consumers who pay for our services and have a right to be informed in clear terms of our conclusions and recommendations.

- **Crisis Managers** Parents or caregivers may be in charge of managing the client's acute medical or behavioral situations.

These roles make it clear that the clinician needs to be aware of the roles in the family, what is needed at a particular time, and who is likely to be able to serve in that role.

Involving the Family in Assessments

Studies conducted by Crais and colleagues (Crais & Belardi, 1999; Crais, Roy, & Free, 2006) have examined the beliefs and perceptions of both parents and professionals regarding the inclusion of families in the assessment process, contrasting actual versus ideal practices. They found that families do want to have more input and control over decisions made during the assessment process. They discovered that there are many ways in which professionals already include families in the assessment process, but there are also ways in which parents would like to have even more input and participation. Results of these studies indicate that ways in which families are being included in the assessment process include: (1) finding out the family's most important concerns, (2) explaining the tests to the family before they are used, (3) summarizing assessment results with the family, (4) asking what the child does well, and (5) identifying next steps for the family and the professional. Practices that were identified as being ideal but happening less often included having a family meeting with the whole team before the assessment, asking the family to comment on the assessment tool they completed, asking them if they agreed with the diagnosis, and asking the family to help identify future goals for their child.

Clearly, there is room to improve and expand the roles that families play in the assessment process. Family inclusion in the assessment process is not only regarded as helpful to gaining a comprehensive evaluation and increasing family satisfaction, but also as helping to align the family with the service provider in order to pave the way for collaborative intervention planning (Crais, 2009). In fact, the assessment process should be viewed as a series of consensus-building activities that increase the likelihood that families will understand and follow through with treatment recommendations (Boone & Crais, 1999; Dunst, Trivette, & Deal, 1988; McLean & Crais, 2004).

When conducting interviews with families, the first task is to gain everyone's respect and confidence. Asking systematic questions about the problem and its history conveys a professional, information-gathering stance. When speaking with families, clinicians should not appear aloof or distant and should take care not to criticize or confront family members before developing a foundational alliance. Thus the clinician should convey an attitude of nonjudgmental curiosity (Cecchin, 1987) about the particularities of the problem and the family members' experiences.

Clinicians should take care to address each individual family member and to inquire about each person's unique views and experiences. Clinicians may attempt to "side with" family members' concerns and to find some positive aspect of each family member's behavior to comment on (de Shazer, 1988). For example, a clinician may provide positive feedback on one family member's patience, another's acceptance and support, and another's steadfast dedication to seeking appropriate treatment. The final statement during the session can emphasize the way in which each family member can contribute to the teamwork that lies ahead.

When conducting assessments, parent involvement is critical in developing the historical background and functional analysis of a client's speech and language difficulties. While some difficulties may seem straightforward and less subject to interpretation or emotional factors, the presentation of some disorders such as stuttering may differ depending on the setting or social context. In these cases, it is best to gather information from multiple family perspectives to determine variations in the symptomatology across settings and among individuals. For example, you may ask each parent separately what they notice about their child's speech behaviors in different contexts. Perhaps the mother can comment on how easily Susie speaks when at home with other family members. Perhaps the father who coaches his daughter's soccer team is better able to inform you about his daughter's speech when she is interacting with her peers. With adult clients and patients, it may be a sibling, spouse, or adult child who can provide vital information.

Extending the Invitation to the Family

While the clinician often has a clear idea about how incorporating the family into assessment and/or treatment sessions may facilitate the therapeutic process, often the family needs to hear a rationale, which may be given over the telephone and again in person once all members of the family whom you wish to interview are present. The rationale may be something like, "I would like both parents (caregivers) to attend the initial interview so I can find out more about each parent's (caregiver's) perspective. Often, each parent (caregiver) sees something a little different." Or, you may ask a sibling of the client to attend, suggesting that, "Sally and (the client) play together every day so I would like to find out a little about Sally's perspective so that we can explore how we may include her in helping her sister." Parental concerns about drawing attention to the family member with the problem can be countered by asking if other family members already know about the problem and suggesting that the client may appreciate how much everyone in the family cares and the opportunity to engage in teamwork.

Often, by providing a rationale over the telephone, the client's family members will readily agree to bring whomever you recommend to the first session. If they are still not persuaded, however, you may want to move ahead with the family members who agree to attend so that you do not start the process with a power struggle. Later, you may renegotiate with the family members if you feel that you are still missing important family perspectives. At that point, you will probably be able to be even more specific about why you would like to include the additional family members (e.g., siblings or grandparents) in the interview.

While clinicians typically prefer both parents to attend sessions, some families make this scenario a challenging feat to accomplish. Let us first consider some factors that may be affecting families in our culture. Despite many changes to the traditional family roles during the last few decades (e.g., an increase in working mothers, more stay-at-home fathers), families still strive to develop a division of labor and responsibilities that works for them. In some traditional families, the mother is still in charge of child-rearing matters and the father is the breadwinner. In these families, the mother may be the one who typically takes the child to school and medical appointments. Even when you ask for both parents to attend an evaluation or treatment session, only one parent may attend. While this is usually the parent who spends the greatest amount of time with the child and therefore is the one who is most likely to implement your recommendations on a regular basis, the clinician need not simply accept the absence of the second parent. Excusing the absent family member may mean that only one parent benefits from getting a better, more empathic understanding of their child, while the absent member is deprived of that opportunity.

There are strategies for reaching out to a reluctant parent or caregiver to encourage his participation, such as requiring both parents to attend a feedback session or calling the absent parent and specifically inviting him to attend the next session. It is vital to stay emotionally neutral as you discuss these strategies and not to neglect or villainize the absent parent. As Luterman (2008) wisely states, it is typically poor case management to enter into an "unholy alliance" with the mother against the father who is distant and reluctant to attend sessions. This can only make matters worse, and it will likely be more challenging to develop a working alliance with the absent family member at a later date.

Often, a time element is introduced as the barrier to the second parent's attendance. The clinician can be politely persistent and respond with, "I understand that your husband tends to work long hours. Let's try to find a time that would be best for him under the circumstances." If you are conducting an assessment, you can emphasize the importance of hearing *both* parents' perspectives and concerns. If you are providing feedback, you can emphasize the importance of providing feedback that is critical to accurately understanding their parent or child's needs and the best ways of helping her. If you are conducting treatment, you can emphasize the theme that both parents need to understand how to support the client, which can in turn relieve some of their stress. You may offer to call the second parent directly to invite him to the session rather than relying on the first parent's report that the spouse cannot attend. In some cases, the first parent is acting to shield and protect her spouse's time, but her statement may not reflect the spouse's actual wishes.

In more dramatic cases of the "absent parent syndrome," these parents may lack a strong bond or attachment with their children. However, once these parents begin to participate in the assessment and/or treatment of their child, they can develop a better appreciation of the physiological, neurological, and emotional bases of their child's behavior. Understanding the child's genuine areas of weakness helps parents to understand that the child's problematic behavior (e.g., "not listening" or "forgetting what he is told") is not always willful. This increased understanding allows parents to soften their views and judgments of their children with communication disorders and to better accept the child with his impairment. From the clinician's perspective, this experience can illuminate the fact that there are seldom "bad" parents, but more often ones who struggle with misconceptions and painful emotional feelings about their children's symptoms and disorders.

Gathering Information from Multiple Sources and Interpreting Different Reports

Before conducting the first diagnostic or background interview, the clinician may consider what sources of information are needed. If you believe that it is possible that certain family members may provide useful input, then you may encourage them to attend the initial information-gathering interview. During this interview, be sure to ask each caregiver parallel (i.e., similar) questions about the client's symptoms. Sometimes, two parents may have different ideas about a child or family member's communication abilities in the same environment. The two perspectives may reflect different cognitive styles, for example, a tendency toward greater hope and optimism in one family member and a more pessimistic style in another family member. In one family, the daughter-in-law tells you that she has seen "great gains" in her elderly father-in-law's recovery of speech since his stoke while the patient's son reports that "not much has changed" since his father came home from the hospital. Differing perspectives also may reflect different relationships between family members. For example, it may be that the daughter-in-law interacts more and makes consistent efforts to engage her father-in-law in daily conversation. Meanwhile, her husband works long hours and is more introverted when he is at home; hence he has less exposure to his father's speech improvements. In a second illustration of divergent reports, a father whose adolescent son had a vehicular accident and a resulting TBI may have a close relationship with his son. Thus, the father is prone to speak for his son and overrates his son's communication abilities. Meanwhile, other family members who were less close to the young man prior to the accident may view the young man as fairly quiet and relatively noncommunicative with others.

If parents or family members express disagreement about the frequency of certain communication behavior (e.g., stuttering), you may ask them to log or journal their observations so that you can review their observations in an upcoming session. This strategy may help you to test various hypotheses regarding what makes speaking easier or more difficult for the client. In this case, family members can be recruited as co-therapists to help uncover what factors inhibit or promote the client's speech. While this strategy can help the clinician "join" with family members, it is also important to consider the impact upon the client. The client should not feel like the subject of an experiment. Therefore, it is important to gauge the client's responses to such a strategy and to consider asking her to log her behavior also in order to gather some helpful information about situations that promote versus inhibit fluent speech. This process can be encouraged by letting family members know that each member has a unique and important vantage point. For example, while the mother is home with the children after school, she may observe certain behaviors, while the father may observe other important behaviors when he takes his children to their music and sports activities. By asking each parent or family member for their observations, the clinician honors each family member's perspective.

Hypothesis Testing

As clinicians conducting family-based assessments, you inevitably begin to generate hypotheses about a family's problem-maintaining behaviors (Minuchin, Nichols, & Lee, 2007; Palazzoli et al., 1980). A father who speaks in a gruff and sharp manner may inhibit his child's speech or contribute to her disfluencies. A very nurturing and protective spouse may say words prematurely for her husband (who recently had a stroke) instead of giving him clues that will aid him in his word-finding efforts. This does not mean that the family member caused the symptoms or disorder but that their responses may inadvertently exacerbate symptoms or interfere with rehabilitative efforts.

Family-Oriented Questions: Assessing Interactional Effects

In interviewing family members, there are many types of questions that clinicians can ask. Some types of questions will elicit more historical or linear (i.e., cause-and-effect) information, such as, "When did you first notice that Tammy had difficulties remembering words she wants to say?" or "What accommodations or interventions are in place at school to help Randy with his language difficulties?" Tomm (1988) refers to these as orienting questions; they have an investigative intent and they help the clinician to understand what is happening in a particular case. Tomm points out that these types of questions help clinicians to "join" with clients as clients often have linear assumptions about the nature of the symptoms.

Additional types of questions that have been developed by family therapists can elicit more information about the family's interactions and meanings around a particular symptom or disorder (Boscolo, Cecchin, Hoffman, & Penn, 1987; Cecchin, 1987; Penn, 1992; Tomm, 1987, 1988). These questions draw attention to the social context in which the symptoms occur and the family's repetitive patterns around the symptoms. "Who notices Mary's stuttering the most?" "What does your father do when he hears you getting stuck on a word?" "Who gives Mary the most positive feedback?" "Who worries about Mary the most?" "What does he do to try to be helpful?" "What does Mary do next?" This line of questioning helps the family to reflect upon their communication and interaction patterns so that they can start to generate solutions. In line with the therapeutic approach of Boscolo and Cecchin, questions can become a key staple of the clinician's "tool box," thus helping the family to experience the process as collaborative and one in which they find unique solutions to old problems (Sprenkle, 2005). In other words, while linear or orienting questions serve the primary purpose of information gathering, **circular questions** can help clients to see themselves in a new light and begin to create solutions for themselves. Thus, this category of questions serves to mobilize clients to change their patterns of interaction with each other.

To extend this solution-oriented function of questioning, clinicians can help family members to become more self-aware of their impact on the client's symptoms by asking them about their interactions with the client and what they have found that helps. For example, "Does it help if you give Amanda a moment to think about your question and formulate her answer before you repeat the question?" or "Have you noticed that your tone of voice can have an effect on how much your son stutters?" This type of question helps family members to consider the *interactional* nature of the client's symptoms (Doherty & McDaniel, 2010), and also embeds a suggestion in a question (Tomm, 1987), for instance, that the parent may be able to help by delaying his response rather than giving a quick or impatient verbal response. Thus we can see that questions are not simply linear, information-gathering tools but can serve to investigate different hypotheses and better understand family patterns that help to alleviate versus exacerbate symptoms, and can serve to influence family member's behavior so that they change how they interact with the client.

Strength-Based Questions

Finally, important areas to assess with family members are the strengths that they possess (de Shazer, 1988; Wetchler & Gutenkunst, 2005). The clinician may ask, "What would you say is best about your family?" or "What are Susan's strengths?" These questions serve multiple purposes. First, as you reach the end of the session in which the focus has been on defining the problem, this shifts the focus to the positive aspects of the family's functioning, which can help family members to leave the session with a feeling of hope and encouragement. Second, by asking this question, you are communicating that clients are more than a list of symptoms and problems; they have strengths that can help them overcome their current challenges. Third, the client's and family's strengths can become clues to how you will choose to work with the family. For instance if a family describes themselves as fiercely loyal, hard-working, or one that can "pull together to overcome big problems," you can begin to incorporate this language into your recommendations.

Often, families arrive at initial sessions ready to list all the problems they have observed in the client. They may even enumerate the problems that the client *creates* for them. Whether clients are visiting a physician, a psychologist, a speech-language pathologist, an audiologist, or another allied health professional, they are often already trained to enumerate symptoms rather than strengths. A guiding principle for many brief therapists and solution-focused therapists, however, is to discover the family's strengths and to help them build upon their competencies rather than fixating on the problems. There are a number of strategies for achieving this goal. The first is to ask clients and their family members about their strengths and resources. In their words, once they articulate their goals, you may ask them, "What are you already doing to try to achieve this?" or "What have you already tried?" By identifying what families are already doing, you can draw upon their expertise and experiences with their unique family situation and find opportunities to compliment them for their creative strategies, emotional attunement to a family member, and commitment to helping a family member. Thus, you may start at a place of identifying competencies in the family rather than a focus upon problems. This focus on what the family is already doing well can enhance your rapport building with the family, but more importantly may help to instill a sense of hope in the family and their efforts to help a family member.

The Family's Story

As families describe their history, experiences, and meanings, one process that unfolds is that the family tells you their "story" (White, 2007). That is, they share with you what has happened from a chronological perspective. This story, you may notice, has certain themes. You can pay attention to the themes implicit in the client's story. Is it a story of hope, of pessimism, of family sacrifice, or of the family's ability to find renewal in loss (Burack-Weiss, 2006; Schultz & Carnevale, 1996; Schultz & Flasher, in press, 2011)? While it is not the SLP's or Aud's job to provide time to allow the *complete* unfolding of a client's story, you inevitably will be exposed to aspects of your clients' stories. It is important to recognize that stories may help clients organize their experiences. Stories provide "flesh" to the "bones" of the meanings that clients embrace. In other words, the family's story provides the temporal context through which the meanings are lived.

Listening to the story means listening to *themes*, not only to the content. For example, when a parent describes a history of seeking interventions from previous professionals, you can listen not only to the list of professionals who were seen, what interventions were tried, and so forth, but also to the message "in between the lines." Is the parent telling you that he trusts professionals because they have always been helpful? Or is he telling you that he doubts if you can help because other professionals have "wasted (his) time"? Is a wife describing her husband who was in a motor vehicle accident as someone who was "always in the wrong place at the wrong time" (i.e., innocent but unlucky) or as someone who is finally getting his comeuppance for his carousing, reckless ways? The way the client tells the story may "offer a means of containing wild, threatening and unpredictable experiences, and re-establishing some kind of order and relationship" (Roberts, 1999, p.13). When parents have a child with a disability, adults suffer a medical event such as a stroke, and so forth, people understandably look for ways to find meaning in those events. The client's story may offer "a defense against futility, emptiness, and formless terror" (Roberts, 1999, p.13). In the neuropsychologist Luria's (1973) account of a man with a TBI, *The Man with a Shattered World*, he explains that the man struggled to rediscover his identity by writing the story of his life. This exercise not only contributed to his cognitive rehabilitation but gave him reason to live. Stories may be ways for clients and family members to create meaning and order or to regain their humanity.

Clinicians can gain insight into what motivates clients and their family members based upon their stories. One story may suggest that the adult caregivers are seeking atonement for their past conflicts with their elderly parents; therefore, they are trying to do all that they can to support them. In another client story, you may learn that a young adult who stutters has a lifelong dream to have a girlfriend and to become active in politics. You can try listening to your next clients with the intention of discovering what motivates them. Understanding each client's story can help you to anticipate what will be motivating and then to frame exercises in terms of what is meaningful to a particular client. For the last client described above, you may devise speech assignments that will help him to speak to girls and in public situations in spite of his fears of stuttering. As well as striving to understand your client's story and what motivates him, your therapeutic role may include helping a client transform his narrative from a tragic story to one of hope. Sometimes, the family's initial story is one that is problem saturated and seems to contain insurmountable obstacles (Haggen, 2002). The impact of a chronic illness or the ramifications of an acute accident may set the family reeling and feeling helpless and hopeless. Further, suffering is magnified when the problem (e.g., the child's communication disorder or the adult's medical condition) is interpreted to mean something negative about the family's identity. Families may suffer not only from the illness or disability but from the belief that its existence proves that they are inadequate, bad, dumb, or negligent (Freeman, Epston, & Lobovits, 1997).

It is important to listen carefully to the family's perspective and not to try to put a "happy face" on the situation too quickly. This can cause families to feel that the clinician is minimizing their problems and does not appreciate their struggle. However, you may start to ask the family what things were like when they did not have these problems, or what they do to "work as a team," what strategies have worked in the past, and what strategies have helped even a little, such as when they have encountered challenges. By taking a methodical, step-by-step approach, you may help to transform the family's story from one of tragic proportions to one of hope and agency. Thus, a family's narrative can be reconstructed or "restoried" to incorporate the family's strengths. Even in families who have suffered from adversity and have been impacted by illness and disability, "resilience continually emerges in small ways" (Becvar, 2007, p. 76). By helping families to identify resources and strengths that they possess, they become better able to withstand stress (Patterson, 2002; Schwartz, 2002) and more able to activate themselves to engage in productive actions.

Never Take "Always" at Face Value: Finding Exceptions to the Rule

In creating **case formulations** and when writing clinical reports, it is good to avoid using *always* or *never* even if these were the client's or family member's words. Many clients and their family members who are feeling frustrated by their problems use extreme language that may not be entirely accurate and may in fact perpetuate a sense of discouragement with the problem's existence. Specifically, some clients or families begin their description of problems by saying something "always" or "never" happens; for example, "She always stutters when she talks to her father," "Since his stroke, he always chokes on his food," or "She can never remember the word she wants to say." Most of the time, this kind of extreme statement is not literally true and instead reflects frustration and the emotionally charged feelings around the symptoms. While challenging or debating this kind of statement directly may not be productive, an alternative strategy is to challenge the statement in a positive manner by asking the client if she recalls any exceptions to this rule. For example, you may ask, "When is the last time that you did not stutter when you spoke with a classmate?" or "During the last week, when did your stuttering occur less often than usual?"

This principle is referred to by **solution-focused therapists** as finding the exceptions to the rule (Cade & O'Hanlon, 1993; de Shazer & Dolan, 2007; Freeman, Epston, & Lobovits, 1997). Thus, you may first ask, "When does X happen the most?" After finding out when the symptom occurs most frequently, for example, 7-year-old Frank has the most difficulty with his receptive language skills both on the playground and in Mrs. Smith's fast-paced classroom, the next challenge is to discover when the symptoms occur less often. That is, what are the exceptions to the rule? Perhaps Frank understands his math teacher best because she speaks slowly and clearly and provides Frank with a visual outline of her lesson. In another case, perhaps Mr. Quincy notices that his wife does not tend to have a choking episode if he takes care in advance (of feeding her) to help prop her up in bed with her special pillow. In a third case, Sally notices that her elderly mother who has Alzheimer's Disease remembers her daily routines better when Sally provides her with a visual list of her routines and reminds her mother to read her list every morning. Upon learning about the family's successful strategies, you can affirm what they are already doing well and compliment them for their caring and efforts. This approach can help families to feel that you are tailoring the treatment to them as unique individuals; you are not just giving them a prefabricated list of strategies (some of which they may have already tried to no avail).

It is interesting to notice that this approach to working with families focuses on solutions and on affirming the family's strengths. It does not focus or fixate on the problem itself, blame the family members, or spend time searching for answers about why the problem exists. Thus, it may initially seem the opposite of a psychologically informed approach; however, it is a psychologically informed approach that is focused on the present and the future and the resources that a family brings to helping to solve a challenging situation. By employing this strategy with family members, clinicians can begin the process of transforming the family's frustration into hope.

Summing Up the Assessment Session

At the end of the assessment session, the clinician cannot only summarize the results and overall treatment plan but can incorporate specific feedback about how each family member can add an important element to the treatment approach. One family member may bring "patience in working on speech exercises," another may bring "persistence" in not allowing the client to give up, and another may bring "creative ways" to integrate speech exercises into naturalistic activities for the client. If these attributes resonate with family members, it can help to highlight the valuable roles they each play in helping the client. In this way, the clinician can build upon not only the client's strengths but the family's strengths and contributions as well to tailor an intervention plan for a particular family.

Clinicians who present a therapeutic imperative for parents to be involved in treatment may see parents as noncompliant when they do not wish to be involved (Leiter, 2004). In some cases, families simply wish for the clinicians to take the main role in intervention services. Labeling the parents or other family members without understanding their point of view is likely to cause a schism in the therapeutic relationship and minimize the likelihood of further collaboration.

Family Underinvolvement in Services

Sometimes family members are dealing with multiple stressors (although they may not have disclosed these with the clinician) and competing demands that make it difficult for them to devote the optimal amount of time and energy to your intervention plan. For example, some families have multiple children with special needs, or they have additional family members who have health care needs. A parent may be in the "sandwich generation," caring for an elderly parent and his health care needs at the same time she is caring for her school-aged child's needs. Families may be struggling with anxieties about health care costs or other issues such as moves, marital strain, or any of a multitude of stresses and/or losses. During the last few years, the economic recession has caused many families to fear job loss, and consequently they are reluctant to leave work early or to take time off work. Family members may already feel guilty about their inability to "do it all"; therefore, clinicians need to try to understand them and provide support, not make them feel more guilt.

To better understand what is going on in a particular family and the possible causes of underinvolvement or noncompliance with homework exercises, the clinician may offer, "I know you care about Freddy and want to do everything you can for him. It seems you have a hard time keeping up with the language exercises I have recommended. There must be a good reason why you have not been able to carry out these recommendations." This statement is supportive rather than blaming and invites the family members to tell you what else is going on in their lives that may be creating obstacles to the current therapy. You may add, "Perhaps if you tell me more about your daily schedule, we can come up with a strategy for working in some language exercises for Freddy." This last statement asks for additional specificity about daily schedule issues and stressors that may interfere with getting SLP homework completed.

In addition to family stressors and scheduling issues, caregiver mental health issues sometimes play a role in the ability to comply with treatment recommendations. The burden of care can have negative consequences for the caregiver's mental health. The clinician can attend to the caregiver's affect and general presentation (e.g., physical appearance, fatigue) to stay alert for signs of depression. Individuals who are depressed may suffer from fatigue, lack of energy and focus, and inability to assemble and follow an organized schedule. Sometimes recommending that the caregiver take time to engage in self-care activities is enough to get them back on the right track, while sometimes a referral to a mental health professional may be needed if the caregiver's symptoms appear severe, interfere with caretaking responsibilities, and do not remit.

Through this review of family stressors, scheduling challenges, parenting styles, and parent mental health issues, we see that there are many possible reasons why a family may

Counseling Skills for Working with Speech, Language, Fluency, Voice, and Cleft Lip and Palate Disorders

CHAPTER OUTLINE

- Introduction
- Articulation and Phonological Disorders
- Language Disorders in Children
- Stuttering and Fluency Disorders
- Voice Disorders
- Cleft Lip and Palate
- Concluding Comments
- Discussion Questions
- Role Plays

INTRODUCTION

While Chapter 6 discusses general family issues, this chapter discusses particular family issues that are unique to and often accompany specific disorders. For each of the speech, language, fluency, voice, and resonance disorders discussed in this chapter, some attention is devoted to discussing the common experiences of clients, often specifying age group responses and strategies with the specific disorders, and these discussions are followed by suggestions for relevant counseling skills. It is hoped that the descriptions of common experiences associated with each disorder will not be interpreted as stereotyping but will enhance the clinician's ability to anticipate some common scenarios for each type of client and to generate more empathy for these clients' experiences. In other words, possessing tentative hypotheses about what clients with certain disorders may be experiencing can provide a foundation for exploring particular client experiences and meanings and exercising highly attuned and sensitive counseling skills.

ARTICULATION AND PHONOLOGICAL DISORDERS

Clinicians may not consider that they are using counseling skills with children with articulation and phonological disorders, but even the most typical therapy session requires considerable counseling skills, whether or not the clinician is aware of using them. An emphasis throughout this chapter is that clinicians need to increase their awareness and intentional use of counseling skills when working with clients of all kinds and at all times. However, before we discuss counseling skill that are specific to these disorders it is helpful first to consider the emotional and social effects of a communication disorder on the individual, as well as the emotional and social effects of the communication disorder on the family, particularly the parents.

The Emotional and Social Effects of Articulation and Phonological Disorders on Children and Families

Children of all ages with mild or moderate articulation and/or phonological disorders may hear negative comments about their speech and may be the target of teasing, ridiculing, mocking imitation, labeling ("He talks like a baby."), and even exclusion and ostracism from conversations, games, parties, and clubs (Van Riper & Erickson, 1996). Not surprisingly, children who have such experiences are likely to feel emotionally distressed, embarrassed, and/or frustrated about not being able to speak normally. They often suffer in silence and feel misunderstood by others. They may develop negative attitudes about themselves, such as feeling different, inadequate, disliked, and/or socially incompetent. Children with more severe articulation and phonological disorders, as well as apraxia of speech and dysarthria, likely experience the most severe emotional and social consequences. Debout and Bradford (1992) found that normal speaking children are less likely to initiate conversations with children who have speech impairments. Trapp and Evans (1960) found that children with articulation disorders demonstrate anxiety levels commensurate with the severity of their speech disorder; that is, in general, children whose speech was more difficult to understand tended to have more anxiety about talking. Frustration about difficulty being understood easily and anxiety about social interactions due to impaired articulation may be more common in children than clinicians (and families) recognize. It is therefore important to notice what behaviors a child may exhibit that may be indicators of anxiety. Psychosomatic symptoms (e.g., headaches and stomach aches) may plague a child who is anxious about speaking clearly. Other children may develop avoidance symptoms and attempt to avoid social and/or academic situations in which their speech difficulties may be noticed and attract negative attention.

Many children with moderate to severe speech disorders experience socialization and interpersonal difficulties (Gordon-Brannan & Weiss, 2007; Rice, Hadley, & Alexander, 1993). When children have difficulty acquiring intelligible speech, they are limited in their abilities to communicate their wants, needs, thoughts, and feelings. When these children are difficult to understand, or they choose to remain silent or to speak only minimally, they may have difficulty developing normal social skills. Parents report that approximately 55 percent of their children with speech disorders also exhibit social competence problems, and 70 percent of the children have behavioral problems 10 years after they were initially diagnosed in preschool as having communication impairments (Aram & Hall, 1989). In order to help children become better communicators and more successful in academic and social domains, speech-language pathologists need to be aware of a child's potential academic, social, and emotional struggles rather than viewing speech-language disorders in a narrow context. Communication is important in the development of self-concept, self-image, and self-esteem. Children with communication disorders are at risk for developing impaired emotional well-being (Prizant & Meyer, 1993). Poor **self-concept**, **self-image**, and **self-esteem** that may be partly attributed to speech disorders may also have secondary effects on behavior, such as withdrawal or aggression (Gordon-Brannan & Weiss, 2007). Speech intelligibility that is below what is expected for a child's age level may have subtle if not significant consequences. Therefore, it is important to consider the possible links between a child's communication difficulties, self-esteem, emotional well-being, and behavior.

Teachers perceive students with speech and language disorders (including articulation and phonological disorders) as poorer performers in the classroom than their normal peers (Ebert & Prelock, 1994; Gordon-Brannan & Weiss, 2007). Teachers also may show impatience at not being able to understand a child with a moderate to severe speech problem. Early detection and therapy for articulation and phonological disorders may prevent children's peers and teachers from developing negative perceptions of them, which in turn can help to prevent negative self-perceptions for children with speech disorders.

Children with Articulation and Phonological Disorders

Depending on the work setting, clinicians may have little contact with parents of children with articulation or phonological disorders, particularly in the public schools (except for Individual Education Plan [IEP] meetings). In university clinics, however, student clinicians typically are involved in the initial interview process when the clinician and parent meet, as well as seeing the parent who brings the child to each therapy session.

CASE STUDY

Hunter

Hunter was a 7-year-old boy whom I saw for private therapy because of his difficulty being understood by friends, family, and even his parents. The parents had resorted to using a simple sign language system to better understand his communications. An evaluation of his speech systems revealed that his respiratory, phonatory, and resonatory systems functioned within normal limits for the development of normal speech. His articulatory system was within normal limits in structure and symmetry, as well as for function (i.e., range of motion, strength, coordination, and rate of movement). Analysis of his speech errors did not reveal a phonological disorder. Neurologically, Hunter appeared intact; he was an excellent student with no apparent attention or behavioral problems, and he was very motivated to improve his speech. The cause of his articulation problems could not be determined. However, following a traditional articulation therapy approach, Hunter became 95–100 percent intelligible to his family and friends.

CLINICAL QUESTIONS

1. What interview strategies might you use to discover how Hunter interacts with various family members?

2. What strategy might you use with Hunter's parents to help them change their approach to communication with Hunter from sign language to verbal communication? How would you do this in a way that maximizes the likelihood that the parents will not be offended and will be compliant with your approach?

Typically undergraduate or graduate students' first clients are children with articulation and phonological disorders. The first concerns of students are usually, "Will the child like me?" and, "Will I embarrass myself in front of my supervisor?" Less thought may go into the counseling skills that will be an omnipresent part of the interaction with the child and the child's parents. The student may be concerned mainly with getting and keeping the child's attention and interest, managing behavior if necessary, and having sufficient activities planned to fill up the entire hour of therapy.

Students may not realize that every moment of interaction and therapy with the parents and child (or any client) involves a combination of good interpersonal communication skills that set the stage for an effective counseling relationship, counseling skills, and microskills, for example, the clinician's manner of dressing; her body language and facial expression (including good eye contact) when approaching the parents and child; her choice of words and tone of voice when introducing herself to the parents and child; the way she invites the child to come into the therapy room; the arrangement of the table and chairs in the therapy room, where she has the child sit, and where she sits; (e.g., placing the chairs so that only the corner of the table is a physical barrier between the clinician and child, rather than having the chairs on opposite sides of a table, which suggests confrontation instead of collaboration); the items she chooses to be in view when the child enters the room to show warmth and interest rather than sterile, empty walls; how she begins interacting with the child; how she transitions from "visiting" with the child into the assessment or therapy; the congruity of the words she chooses and her tone of voice, facial expressions, and body language during each moment of therapy; how she reinforces the child's behaviors; when and how she transitions from one task to another; how she ends the therapy session; how she takes the child back to the parents and tells them how well their child did, again with congruity in her words, voice, facial expressions, and body language so the parents will believe her; and how the clinician says goodbye to the family and that she looks forward to seeing the child for the next session.

For most young children with articulation and phonological disorders, the basic personal qualities (attributes) of effective helpers that the clinician has (and is further developing), such as congruency, empathic understanding, unconditional positive regard, encouraging, and patience are likely sufficient for good interactions with children and their parents. However, there are challenging situations when more sophisticated counseling skills need to be used, particularly when the child is resistant to therapy or presents behavioral difficulties.

Mike's Apraxia

During the first three years after earning my master's degree I worked in what was then called an aphasia classroom with adolescents who had "childhood aphasia" (a term no longer used). The class was limited to eight students. One student was Mike, who had normal cognitive abilities and speech prior to a sledding accident at age 13 when he was on a snow trip with his Boy Scout troop. Mike had been a successful student and a good Scout, and he loved playing Little League baseball. During the sledding accident he hit his head on a tree and received a traumatic brain injury.

The results of Mike's TBI were moderate to severe receptive and expressive aphasia, mild-moderate cognitive impairments (memory, organization of information, reasoning, and problem solving), and profound apraxia. He was extremely frustrated and angry with his impairments and newly acquired limitations. He tried to play baseball but no longer had the motor skills to play well. He now had learning disabilities, although learning used to come easy for him. His greatest frustration, however, was not being able to speak intelligibly. In the classroom my job was to teach academic subjects at the level that each child could learn and to provide speech, language, and cognitive therapy. Mike continued being as active in Boy Scouts as he could, but he was sometimes teased by the other boys. His mother asked if I would be willing to come to one of his evening Scout meetings to talk to the Scout Master and the other Scouts about Mike's acquired difficulties. I was happy to do that. On the evening of the meeting Mike proudly wore his full Scout uniform. He knew I was going to be talking about him. The Scout Master and other Scouts listened attentively and asked some good questions as I tried to explain Mike's complex problems in layperson's terms. I could see that they were beginning to understand Mike's problems and were developing some empathy. The mother and Scout Master felt that the evening was a success.

CLINICAL QUESTIONS

1. What skills do you feel you would need to develop (or demonstrate) in order to be able to address this child's Boy Scout troop?

2. What might you say to the child if he tearfully told you that he was being teased by kids outside of the school environment? (Keep in mind that the child has some limitations in receptive language, severe limitations in expressive language and speech, and some cognitive problems.)

LANGUAGE DISORDERS IN CHILDREN

Children of all ages with language disorders often do not recognize that they have a problem, or they do not want to admit to it. Children who have difficulty understanding what their parents tell them to do and difficulty understanding their teacher's instructions often feel that it is because they are "dumb" or "stupid." For a moment, consider how much education and studying it has taken you to begin to understand language and language disorders in your own college education, and compare that to a young child who has a language disorder and how much more difficult it must be for him to understand his own problem. It is often important to provide feedback and education to children as well as to their parents about childhood language disorders so that they can begin to grasp that they are not "stupid" and their self-esteem can begin to improve.

The Emotional and Social Effects of Language Disorders on Children and Families

The emotional and social effects of language disorders on children and their families are important for speech-language pathologists to be aware of, although these effects are seldom discussed in the literature. It is not easy to separate language (especially pragmatic problems) from psychosocial problems because of their considerable overlap. While some language disorders occur in the absence of emotional disturbances, there is a clear relationship between some degree of psychosocial involvement and language impairment. Research also shows that psychosocial involvement will likely continue throughout children's education and into (or through) adulthood (Beitchman, Wilson, Johnson, et al., 2001; Prizant, Audet, Burke, et al., 1990).

The research on the overlap or comorbidity of speech-language difficulties and psychosocial problems in children dates back to the 1980s. For example:

- Of approximately 300 consecutive intakes of children to a community-based speech and language clinic, 95 percent of the children with expressive language problems had some form of psychosocial difficulties according to 1980 criteria used by the American Psychiatric Association (Baker & Cantwell, 1982).

- Of 40 consecutive admissions to a child psychiatric unit, 50 percent of the children had language problems (Gualtieri, Koriath, Van Bourgondien, & Saleeby, 1983).

- Of the children consecutively admitted to an inpatient facility because of behavioral or emotional problems, 67 percent failed a speech and language screening (Prizant et al., 1990).

Thus, clinicians need to be aware that some children with language disorders may have psychosocial problems as a result of or in concurrence with the language problems we are treating. However, before we discuss the emotional and social problems of the children, we first will consider the parents.

Parents of Children with Specific Language Impairments and Language Disorders

Beyond the child with a communication disorder there is a family that may well be having its own emotional and social struggles related to their child's communication problems. Research focusing on mother–child interactions has shown that mothers of children with language development disorders tend to make adjustments in their interactions with these children. When compared to mothers of children developing normal language, the mothers of children with language impairments tend to (1) initiate more interactions (perhaps to compensate for their children who tend to be less able or willing to initiate conversations); (2) use more interrogatives, especially *who, what, when, where, why,* and *how* questions as well as other "quiz" questions; (3) use fewer utterances per turn, which may help the children more easily understand and follow their mothers' messages; and (4) respond or comment less to their children, especially with respect to the description of objects (Conti-Ramsden & Dykins, 1991; Conti-Ramsden & Friel-Pattie, 1984; Kaye & Charney, 1981; Paul, 2006; Reed, 2010; Tiegerman & Siperstein, 1984).

Parents report that, like their children with speech and language impairments, they sometimes feel stigmatized (i.e., negatively evaluated and given less respect) by other adults, family members, and even other children because of their child's problems. Macharey and von Suchodoletz (2008) found that 50 percent of parents reported negative labeling of their child and approximately 40 percent felt they were also stigmatized. Parents whose children also had behavioral problems more often reported negative labeling than the parents whose children did not. In counseling such families, clinicians should, therefore, address the possibility of stigmatization and its consequences as separate and important issues. More specifically, parents may benefit from open discussions with a speech-language pathologist about their feelings of being stigmatized and how it affects their parenting skills, interactions with their children, and interactions with other family members and family friends.

Sometimes parents benefit simply from a patient, nonjudgmental listener, and at other times what seems to be most useful is to provide the parent with specific intervention skills to counter their negative feelings. For example, parents may be encouraged to educate their family members and friends about their child's difficulties (e.g., Johnny has a language difficulty; it does not mean he is "stupid." We all have things that are hard for us; for Johnny, it is understanding what others say and expressing himself). This strategy can not only help the parent to feel empowered but simultaneously provides support for the child. If parents appear to be having an extreme emotional reaction to a child's communication problems, the clinician may decide that the parents could benefit from more specific assistance from mental health professionals and make appropriate referrals.

When considering their involvement in their child's intervention, parents often speak about a desire to do the right thing for their child and state that it is their responsibility to seek out sources of professional assistance and interventions to help their child. However, for some parents, being involved in their child's intervention is perceived as a burden or unhelpful, particularly when a child has a pervasive disability (Brady, Skinner, Roberts, & Hennen, 2006; Rollin, 2000; Watts Pappas & McLeod, 2009). We need to appreciate that a child we are working with for an hour or two a week represents only a ripple in the clinician's week, but the child's problems may create a significant burden to the child, parents, and sometimes the entire family on a daily basis (Holland, 2007). Furthermore, parents do not automatically have complete trust in a clinician's professional expertise, and many parents recognize that young or newly educated clinicians have not developed expertise through years of additional education, training, and professional and life experiences. Although young professionals may try to present a façade of confidence, many savvy parents can see through their insecurities (and *all* clinicians have insecurities—even experienced clinicians).

Toddlers and Preschoolers with Specific Language Impairments

Rescorla and Achenbach (2002), a speech-language pathologist and a psychiatrist, studied toddlers who were identified as "at risk" for specific language impairments. They found no significant association between toddlers with slow expressive language development (i.e., fewer than 50 single words or no two-word combinations) and elevated scores (i.e., in the problematic range) on a parent-rating protocol of their child's behavior (Achenbach's 1992 *Child Behavior Checklist for Ages 2–3*). Rescorla and Achenbach believe their research suggests that "significant behavioral/emotional problems may be more likely when children have been delayed in language for many months (i.e., after 36 months [of age])" (2002, p. 742). This hypothesis was confirmed by studies that found preschool children with specific language impairments were perceived negatively by other preschool children because of their poor communication and social skills (Conti-Ramsden & Botting, 2004; Segebert-DeThorne & Watkins, 2001). Rescorla and Achenbach's hypothesis also has been confirmed by a variety of studies that followed up on preschool and kindergarten children 12 to 19 years after their language impairments were first identified; that is, significant behavioral and emotional problems may be more likely when children have been delayed in language for many months.

Most young children with specific language impairments are not identified, diagnosed, and treated before age 3 or 4 years, and by that time many have had some negative experiences because of their communication delays or disorders. "Counseling" for these young children typically includes being supportive, empathic, and caring when they want to share negative, frustrating, or embarrassing experiences they have had due to their communication problems. The clinician's good listening skills, warmth, and enthusiasm help affirm to these children that they are important communicators and that adults are interested in what they want to say. A few specific microskills that are helpful with preschoolers are verbal encouragers and closed questions. Young children often can answer closed or simple comparison (e.g., "Do you like A or B better?") questions easier than open questions, particularly when they have language problems.

School-Age Children with Language Disorders

Early elementary school children (6 to 9 years of age) with language disorders are often less accepted by their peers when working or playing because of their "different" verbal interactions and behaviors. For example, children with language disorders are less likely to take the lead, stay on task, or persuade others to agree with them and are less tactful in their word selection. They often appear boring, passive, or inappropriate to other children (Bryan, Donahue & Pearl, 1981; Vaughn, Elbaum, & Broadman, 2001).

By 10 to 13 years of age, children with language disorders often perceive themselves more negatively than their peers. Children with language disorders tend to avoid social interactions (talking and playing) with school peers and feel rejected, neglected, and lonely throughout their school experience (Jerome, Fujiki, Brinton, & James, 2002). Camarata, Hughes, and Ruhl (1988) found that 71 percent of students 8 to 13 years of age who had language scores between one or two standard deviations below the norm were identified as having mild to moderate behavior disorders.

Children with communication problems often are unable to manage their emotions as well as children with normal language and learning abilities, which may affect their inter-personal relationships. They may, for example, lack a "feeling vocabulary" similar to their same-age peers and have difficulty expressing their emotions other than through crying and acting out behaviors. By early adolescence, children with language disorders rate themselves lower on measures of scholastic competence, behavioral conduct, and overall self-worth. Most children show some adaptation and response (sometimes positive and sometimes negative) to their language disorders as they try to overcome or work around their disabilities (Camarata, Hughes, and Ruhl, 1988; Jerome et al., 2002). However, many children with language disorders experience negative effects to their self-esteem and social relationships. Counseling the school-age child with a language disorder does not imply that an emotional disturbance must be a prerequisite condition (Rollin, 2000). Counseling can help children develop insights and understanding of their communication difficulties as well as coping and problem-solving skills to address those difficulties and the interpersonal problems they may be experiencing with peers, teachers, and parents (Wiig & Semel, 1984).

The initial counseling with a child should include **informational counseling**; that is, explaining to the child, at the level the child can understand, the nature of his problems "using words" (language) and your role in helping him. Many children have attended therapy for months or semesters without really understanding the purpose; they often just think they are with the "speech teacher" to play games. For young children it is usually wise to not emphasize that they have a problem with language, but to emphasize that you are going to help the child understand and talk to adults better (children usually feel that they understand and talk to their peers fine because their peers speak at more of a child-like level than adults). Many clinicians like to tell children that they are going to play games together in the "speech room." However, placing the emphasis on games rather than work sets the child up for expecting to play games and to be entertained rather than the real purpose of a productive therapy session. Parents also may be invited to observe the clinician doing therapy. This may help to teach parents what they can do at home with the child and may increase the sense of parent-child satisfaction and reward if a parent can congratulate the child after the session for a job well done. However, direct discussions with the parents about what they can do at home to help their child are often more productive than hoping the parents get out of the observation general and specific adult-child interaction techniques the clinician demonstrates.

Perhaps most beneficial to the working relationship is the child's recognition of the clinician's openness, acceptance, awareness, and empathy for the child and his communication difficulties. Clinicians also learn to take advantage of "counseling moments" (Holland, 2007); that is, the unplanned and usually brief opportunities to provide insights and observations that may help a child understand something about himself and his communication problem.

Rollin (2000) believes that the counseling process may actually enhance the form and content of a child's language. Helping children understand their problems and develop the language to talk about language (metalanguage) is an element of language therapy. Clinicians can help children learn how to express their negative feelings (frustration, anger, fear, embarrassment, etc.) in ways that communicate without alienating their listeners. One method of teaching a child to communicate a strong feeling is to help her describe it in terms that she and other people can understand, using metaphors such as "My frustration is bigger than a house," "I am so angry that I'm burning up," "I'm so afraid that I can't even move," and "I'm so embarrassed I want to crawl in a hole and hide." Teaching the child to use metaphors can help her realize that she can use words to express her thoughts and feelings rather than using inappropriate and sometimes harmful behaviors.

When a child realizes that the clinician is really listening to her and is able to help her describe how she is feeling, the child develops trust in the clinician—that he truly is "on her side" and understands her. The child may not have many adults in her life who genuinely listen to her, provide meaningful feedback and insights, and do not make her feel guilty or punish her because of her thoughts and feelings. Carl Rogers' (1957) concept of unconditional positive regard can provide a foundation for a meaningful approach to working with any child.

Sometimes children do not recognize that adults and sometimes even their peers do not understand them easily or well. By letting the child know that you, the clinician, do not understand her, even though you are trying, may help her realize that other adults also may not understand her messages. For most young children the adults in their lives who they are concerned about are their parents, grandparents, and teachers, and these are the adults who should be emphasized. We can emphasize that good speech and language helps communicate what the child wants or needs and her important thoughts and feelings.

When children become aware of their difficulties understanding others and communicating their messages, they sometimes react to their difficulties with frustration, which may result in angry outbursts or signs of depression and withdrawal. We can help children understand their frustration using empathic language (e.g., "I understand why you are frustrated with not being able to tell me just what you want."), and maintaining a posture of acceptance and patience so children feel that we are accepting of their difficulties and are happy to remain patient and willing to help them communicate. Parents, teachers, and other important people in a child's life can be educated about this positive approach to a child's frustration and angry outbursts. The clinician's responses to a child's difficulty communicating may be very different from what she is accustomed to in her home environment and among many of her peers. The clinician's acceptance of the child's feelings and of the child herself are ways to show unconditional positive regard (Rogers, 1957), which can be helpful in diminishing a child's frustration about her communication difficulties.

We can talk with a child about her feelings by using reflections of feeling words and nonjudgmental language to help her make links between what she is feeling and her communication difficulties. It is clear that counseling and therapy interventions are not two separate and distinct entities, but are often intertwined. One moment the clinician may be doing speech therapy and the next moment talking with the child about her feelings and then continuing on with therapy, often with a seamless transition between the two components of therapy.

Children who are nonverbal or minimally verbal because of neurological or developmental impairments are particularly challenging to counsel. They may use elementary nonverbal communication as their primary means of communicating. The clinician often needs to decipher their messages, using his best interpretation skills and sometimes just educated guesses. These children may understand the clinician's nonverbal language better than his verbal language. Most importantly, we need to keep in mind that children with neurological and developmental impairments have emotional and social reactions to their communication problems, including feelings of rejection, anxiety, and embarrassment, just like any other child. These children also may have emotional attachments to classmates and other such normal emotional experiences that need to be respected. Sometimes, because we are good listeners who try to have unconditional positive regard toward all people, we may be the only people with whom these children will share their heart-felt feelings toward others and themselves. We need to avoid, of course, ever sounding condescending or patronizing to these children.

Adolescents with Language Disorders

Emotional and social difficulties increase for adolescents with language disorders (Ehren & Lenz, 1989; Nippold, 2001; Reed, 2010; Snow & Powell, 2004). Mental health issues may develop in some adolescents, such as mood disorders (e.g., depression, dysthymia [low-grade chronic depression], and bipolar disorders [alternating manic and depressive episodes]). Anxiety disorders are seen in these children (e.g., generalized anxiety disorder, social or specific phobias such as school phobia, and panic attacks). Boys are more likely than girls to react with frustration and externalizing behaviors (i.e., behavioral problems). However, it is sometimes difficult to delineate normal preadolescent and adolescent mood and anxiety problems from those that language disorders may contribute to or create (Beitchman et al., 1996; Wiig, 1995).

When children are identified as early as preschool or early elementary school and do not receive sufficient therapy to remediate their communication problems, they are at risk for developing emotional, social, and behavioral problems during their formal education years, with significant problems clearly occurring in adolescence. These problems do not necessarily go away when a person reaches adulthood. Various studies (Aram, Ekelman, & Nation, 1984; Beitchman et al., 1996; Johnson et al., 1999) that followed up on preschool and kindergarten children 12 to 19 years after their language impairments were first identified found they:

- Were rated as less socially competent than their peers
- Participated less in extracurricular non-sports activities and organizations
- Had elevated rates of anxiety disorders, with social phobia the most common
- Had a greater prevalence of behavior problems
- Were more likely to have antisocial personality disorders than their peers
- Had an increased risk or presence of psychiatric disorders in adolescence

When speaking with adolescents, as with children, our questions and statements to them need to be clear, using words and language structures that match their language abilities rather than their chronological age. However, adolescents are very sensitive to adults talking down to them. We need to keep in mind that adolescents do not need us to agree with their feelings; they need us to acknowledge them. Adolescents, like younger children, sometimes do not have words to describe their feelings, but when clinicians can identify their feelings and give them words that help describe them, they begin to see their feelings are validated. Microskills that are essential when working with adolescents include verbal encouragers, open questions, funneling questions, requests for clarification, comparison questions, counterquestions, paraphrasing, reflection, selective reflection (restatement), reflection of feeling, and silence. Many of these same principles apply to working with young adults with language disorders.

Stephanie

Stephanie was a 23-year-old woman whom I supervised in a university clinic. Stephanie had spastic quadriplegic cerebral palsy and developmental delays, and functioned linguistically and emotionally at an early adolescent level. On most days Stephanie attended a program for adults with developmental delays. She had severe communication impairments but could communicate most of her thoughts and feelings to a patient, careful listener. As the semester progressed, Stephanie's clinician, Ellen, found that Stephanie sometimes wanted to talk about her boyfriend who was in the same program for adults with developmental delays. One day Stephanie asked Ellen, "What is love?" Considering her professional boundaries, but also attentive to the working relationship with this young woman and her developing expressive language abilities, Ellen gave her best answer to this profound question.

CLINICAL QUESTIONS

1. How would you have handled this situation? What might you do differently?
2. What would you do if an adolescent or young adult wanted to talk about personal issues?
3. How might you make this an opportunity for helping the client to develop her language and interpersonal skills?

STUTTERING AND FLUENCY DISORDERS

Since the earliest work with children and adults who stutter it has been recognized that there are important emotional and social effects of the disorder on the person (Ainsworth, 1945; Darley, 1955; Johnson, 1939; Sheehan, 1953; Travis, 1931; Van Riper, 1957; West, 1942). The more recent literature continues to emphasize such emotional and social effects (Bloodstein & Bernstein Ratner, 2008; Contour, 2001; Gregory, 2003; Guitar, 2006; Manning, 2010; Ramig & Dodge, 2010; Ward, 2006; Zebrowski, 2002; Zebrowski & Kelly, 2002).

The emotional adjustment of individuals who stutter was investigated extensively between the 1930s and 1980s. The findings of most studies indicated that people who stutter are about as well adjusted as people who do not stutter (Bloodstein & Bernstein Ratner, 2008; Semans & Cox, 1982; Van Riper, 1982). Early research did not indicate any particular personality traits that are typical of individuals who stutter (Bloodstein, 1995; Silverman, 1996). However, recent research conducted in Australia by Iverach, Jones, O'Brian, and colleagues (2009) used the *International Personality Disorders Examination Questionnaire* to screen 92 adults seeking treatment for stuttering with 920 age- and gender-matched controls from the Australian National Survey of Mental Health and Well-Being. Based on first-stage screening, the presence of any personality disorder was significantly higher for adults in the stuttering group than matched controls, demonstrating almost threefold increased odds. This difference between groups remained significant for all specific personality disorders, with four- to sevenfold increased odds found for Borderline, Dependent, and Paranoid Personality Disorders, and two- to threefold increased odds for Histrionic, Impulsive, Schizoid, and Anakastic (a lack of adaptability to new situations) Personality Disorders. The authors concluded that stuttering appears to be associated with a heightened risk for the development of personality disorders. There are also certain behaviors of people who stutter that tend to be fairly common; that is, being reticent to speak and avoiding social situations in which they expect people will react negatively to their stuttering (Guitar, 2006; Manning, 2010; Manning, Dailey, & Wallace, 1984; Turnbaugh, Guitar, & Hoffman, 1981). Children and adults who stutter have tendencies toward low self-esteem and reluctance to take risks (Bloodstein & Bernstein Ratner, 2008; Mast, 1952; Sheehan, 1979; Trombly, 1965).

The literature on stuttering and psychological symptoms such as anxiety shows some inconsistent results, which reminds us that all individuals who stutter are not alike: (1) some of these individuals may have significant psychological symptoms; (2) some parent behaviors may contribute to their child's stuttering; (3) anxiety may contribute to the development of stuttering; and (4) counseling is an important part of therapy, even when children and adults who stutter are generally well-adjusted.

Some parents of children who stutter are dominating, overanxious, striving, or set high standards of behavior for their child's language and communication. Likewise, many children who stutter have tendencies to be anxious, sensitive, perfectionistic, and have excessive needs for approval; however, these characteristics only become a clinical concern to speech pathologists when they contribute to or maintain stuttering behaviors. How much anxiety children and adults have about their stuttering may be partly dependent on their levels of sensitivity and their general temperament (Lewis & Goldberg, 1997). Anderson, Pellowski, Conture, and Kelley (2003), using parent responses to the *Behavioral*

Style Questionnaire (McDevitt & Carey, 1978), which investigates temperamental characteristics of young children 3 to 5 years of age, found that children who stutter, when compared with children who do not stutter, exhibit temperamental profiles consistent with hypervigilance (i.e., exhibit minimal distractibility), are slow to adapt to changes in their environment (e.g., have difficulty separating from parents, making initial adjustments to preschool, and making new friends), and have irregular biological functions (e.g., sleep and hunger patterns). Oyler and Ramig (1996), using the *Parent Perception Scale* (PPS), assessed parents' perceptions of personality characteristics as related to sensitivity of their school-aged children who stuttered. Compared to the control group, the children who stuttered were significantly more sensitive (e.g., more reactive to environmental stimuli, anxious, introverted, or withdrawn). SLPs should not make assumptions about a child's or adult's adjustment or personality but should simply remain open to information that indicates good adjustment (e.g., the child or adult has friends and does not experience limitations at school or work due to his stuttering), or that indicates otherwise (e.g., the child or adult is afraid to speak to others because he fears being disfluent, and has few friends and social interactions).

Considering the number of possible psychological and behavioral issues that may be involved with a child or adult who stutters, why are speech-language pathologists qualified to work with children and adults who stutter? Our education and training, more than that of any mental health professional, includes all aspects of speech and language development and disorders, which gives us a holistic view of communication disorders, including stuttering. Also, we are the only profession that includes in our education one or more full semesters of course work on theories, assessment, and treatment of stuttering. Our clinical training also, whenever possible, includes direct hands-on experience working with individuals who stutter. Psychologists who treat individuals who stutter operate on *psychological* and *behavioral theories*; however, speech pathologists operate on *theories of stuttering*, which far more specifically target the problem. Speech-language pathologists also have produced the largest body of literature of any profession on this disorder. Although speech clinicians typically feel insecure and even inadequate to help individuals who stutter, there is really no other professional who is better qualified.

Emotional Effects of Stuttering on the Person

There are a variety of emotional effects of stuttering, but it is sometimes difficult to know which comes first—the stuttering or the emotional effects. It is the classic "chicken or the egg" question; however, stuttering and emotional symptoms may occur simultaneously. For example, a child or adult who stutters may have anxiety about stuttering, and the stuttering can create anxiety about speaking situations and speaking (Bloodstein & Bernstein Ratner, 2008; Guitar, 2006; Manning, 2010).

ANXIETY

As children become aware of their stuttering they may develop mild feelings of anxiety, but if their stuttering becomes increasingly severe they may develop stronger feelings of anxiety (Guitar, 2006; Manning, 2010). Anxiety has been recognized as an important emotional characteristic of individuals who stutter. Anxiety is a distressing feeling of uneasiness, apprehension, or dread. Anxiety may be rational and based on actual events, or irrational and based on anticipated events that likely will not occur. Anxiety and fear are on a continuum and, therefore, it is difficult to determine when a person passes anxiety and moves into fear. The terms *anxiety* and *fear* may be used interchangeably, or a client may feel more comfortable with one term rather than another. In therapy, though, we tend to talk about *feared* words, people, situations, and so on, rather than *anxiety-producing* words, people, and situations. (See Chapter 11 for a more complete discussion of anxiety and fear). SLPs may recognize and describe the symptoms we see in both children and adults that reflect or indicate anxiety. It is important to note that an individual may have symptoms of anxiety but may not have the constellation of symptoms or severity of symptoms needed to diagnose a disorder.

For many people who stutter, it is their constant anxiety and fear of stuttering that motivates them to seek therapy. People who come for therapy are typically unaware of many of their stuttering behaviors, even their worst and most obvious behaviors to listeners. But they are aware of how they feel before and during speaking, and it is their feelings about their stuttering that are most distressing. Some of the stressors that may trigger anxiety in people who stutter are embarrassment, humiliation, and fear of loss of self-esteem and self-image when stuttering (Conture & Curlee, 2007; Guitar, 2006).

Eventually, the trepidation associated with speaking may produce chronic anxiety and a host of avoidant behaviors; for example, avoiding speaking situations, particular people, topics, words, and even sounds. These avoidances become a significant part of the participation restrictions of people who stutter; that is, they participate less in the social, educational, and work-related opportunities to communicate. Therapy for adolescents and adults who stutter often includes learning how to be more open about their stuttering (i.e., not trying to hide it) and forms of desensitization that help to decrease anxiety about disfluencies.

Counseling skills are so thoroughly intertwined with therapy when working with children and adults who stutter that both are taking place simultaneously. Several general counseling approaches may help decrease anxiety in people who stutter (see Chapter 11). *Hierarchy analysis* can be used, for example, to help clients determine who are the easiest and the hardest people they talk to, and then the people in between. An important component of many therapy programs for older children and adults includes a form of *desensitization* in which the individuals are asked to talk openly and honestly about their stuttering to family and friends, and to stutter openly rather than using "tricks" or "crutches" to try to hide it (Gregory, 2003; Guitar, 2006; Manning, 2010; Ramig & Dodge, 2010; Zebrowski & Kelly, 2002). The client can work on systematic desensitization while doing therapy tasks presented by the clinician. Guitar (2006) says that most listeners are not half as bothered by a person's stuttering as the person who stutters thinks they are. The clinician can have the client test his hypothesis about the concern listeners have about his stuttering by asking family and friends to talk honestly about how much his stuttering affects them in conversations. By seeing that most people are far less concerned about the person's stuttering than he could have imagined, he can begin to talk and stutter more freely. The less he tries to hide his stuttering, the fewer tricks, crutches, and avoidances he will need to use to be fluent (Bloodstein & Bernstein Ratner, 2008; Conture & Curlee, 2007;

Gregory, 2003; Guitar, 2006; Manning, 2010). *Cognitive approaches* are commonly used to help people identify their dysfunctional and distorted thoughts about their stuttering that produce negative feelings and maladaptive behaviors; to self-monitor their negative thoughts and self-talk; to identify the relationship between their thoughts and their underlying beliefs and feelings; to identify alternatives and more productive thinking; and to test their hypotheses (e.g., listeners' [observers'] perceptions of stuttering) regarding the validity of their basic assumptions about themselves.

PERFECTIONISM AND EXCESSIVE NEED FOR APPROVAL

Two other emotional and social characteristics of children and adults who stutter may be related: perfectionism and the excessive need for approval. Individuals who are perfectionistic may be concerned about how others view them as well as how they evaluate themselves. People who stutter often want perfectly fluent speech, not normally fluent speech. By placing this perfectionistic weight on themselves, they create pressure to speak (perform) better than they are capable, often causing them to be more disfluent. Thus, perfectionism may impede rather than aid fluent speech. Therapeutically, clinicians try to show children how disfluencies are quite acceptable in both children's and adults' speech by modeling easy disfluencies. Children learn that the goal of therapy is not perfectly fluent speech but normally fluent speech (Dell, 2002; Conture & Curlee, 2007; Guitar, 2006; Manning, 2010; Ramig & Dodge, 2010; Zebrowski & Kelly, 2002).

As children begin to learn that they can have disfluencies in their speech without feeling like failures, and as they learn to speak more easily through various therapy techniques, their self-esteem tends to improve. They begin to approach speaking situations with less trepidation and with more confidence. When they do have some difficulty stuttering they learn that it is not "the end of the world" and that they can turn their failures into successes. They can speak and be understood despite some stuttering and imperfections in their speech.

Self-esteem is partly dependent on how honest people feel they are with themselves. When adolescents and adults who stutter try to hide their stuttering they are taking on a false role; that is, the role of being a normally fluent person. However, the person who stutters knows he stutters, and his hiding and dishonesty with herself can create a sense of being an "imposter" and that others do not truly know him. As clients become more open about their stuttering, they feel they are being more honest with themselves and their self-esteem tends to improve.

LEARNING TO TAKE RISKS

Through classical conditioning in the person's daily environment, people who stutter feel punished by their stuttering, which results in reluctance to take risks (Guitar, 2006). For these individuals, risks may include the fear of being disfluent and the negative consequences related to particularly feared words, people, and speaking situations. Therapy encourages clients to take risks: to go ahead and say words they fear; to talk to people they are afraid of; and to approach speaking situations that cause anxiety. However, they are not expected to take risks without tools—therapeutic tools. In therapy, clients learn how to manage their speech so that they can take risks with a reasonable expectation of being successful. But even if the outcome is not what they wanted (i.e., they are disfluent), they realize that they will survive and they can take the risk again and likely do better.

When clients are increasingly willing to take risks, they often develop more self-esteem. One of the secondary benefits of therapy for many individuals is an overall increase in self-confidence, a feeling that, "If I can take on this problem, I can take on any problem." Clients who stay with therapy and practice the challenging assignments often feel stronger as individuals and feel more capable of realizing other goals in their lives.

Emotional Effects of a Child's Stuttering on the Family

Parents often wonder whether they may have caused or contributed to their child's stuttering problem. As Ramig and Dodge (2010) state, "Parents do not cause stuttering, but they may contribute to its development and maintenance" (p. 10). Parents often feel some guilt and even embarrassment and shame about their child who stutters. Clinicians should avoid implying or suggesting that the parents were the cause of their child's stuttering because this can create more guilt and resistance. A statement such as, "We don't know what caused your child's problem, but you can be part of the solution for it," may help parents feel that the clinician is not placing blame on the parents but that they can be important in helping their child develop better speech.

Guilt may have motivated the parents to seek therapy for their child, but guilt is not helpful to the child–parent relationship or clinician–parent interaction. We should do our best to assuage parental guilt and channel it into productive energy to do specific assignments that parents can work on to improve their listening skills with their child; to talk *with* rather than *at* their child; to express and accept their emotions in order to make changes in their behaviors; to adopt realistic expectations for change in their child; to show unconditional love, acceptance, and support of their child; to spend quality time with their child; to model interactive behaviors conducive to fluency development; and to consider the effects of various life events, activities, school placement, and scheduling on the child's speech and overall well-being (Hill, 2006).

When working with adults who stutter, clinicians often encourage them to talk openly to other people about their stuttering, including the client's parents. Parents at any age may feel guilt about possibly having caused their child's stuttering. A client may need to be encouraged to talk openly with his parents about the work he is doing in therapy to overcome his stuttering problem. People who stutter benefit from having their parents as supporters and allies in their treatment.

A Swedish Client

Lorraine was an adult who stuttered. She was born and raised in Sweden. During her school years she received some speech therapy for her stuttering, but it was only minimally effective. As a young woman she came to the United States, where

Continues on next page

Continued from previous page

she worked and received her college education, married, and had a family. While a college student, she received more therapy for her stuttering but still had significant problems. In her mid-30s she came to me for further therapy. She made significant gains in her speech fluency and self-acceptance as a person who stutters. In a later session with her mother and stepfather, Lorraine's mother talked about all that she did to try to get appropriate help for her young daughter's stuttering. I had the feeling that the mother continued to feel some guilt that she may have in some way caused or contributed to her daughter's stuttering. For many parents, guilt for their child's problems never ends.

CLINICAL QUESTIONS

1. What might you say to assuage the mother's guilt about possibly causing or contributing to her daughter's stuttering?

2. What might you say to an adult client who blames her parents for her stuttering problem?

COUNSELING PARENTS OF CHILDREN WHO STUTTER

Hill (2006) and Ramig and Dodge (2010) state that parent counseling should be a key element of any approach to treating children who stutter. The way parents think, feel, and behave contributes to the child's environment and influences treatment progress. The severity of stuttering exhibited by a child often influences the degree of parental concern. The four main goals of counseling parents of children who stutter are to help them: (1) express their feelings, thoughts, and beliefs about the problem; (2) make the connection between their emotions and actions (e.g., fears of sounds, words, individuals, and their stuttering behaviors); (3) manage their emotions through activities that transform or "bind" free-floating emotions into positive actions (e.g., transforming fear that they will say or do the wrong thing when they see their child stuttering into productive behavior such as learning how to listen patiently and attentively and providing comforting feedback); and (4) provide educational information about the problem of stuttering and how the parents can make changes to support the therapy process. The long-term goals of counseling are to assist parents in coming to accept their child's stuttering and their feelings about the problem and to cope positively with their child and her stuttering.

Ramig and Dodge (2010) explain that there are a number of things parents need to know that can be helpful in achieving fluency for their child, and these are areas that clinicians can discuss with parents, such as minimizing interruptions; speaking slower; respecting silence; minimizing rushing and hurrying; asking one question at a time; avoiding "show and tell"; talking about meaningful topics; reading to the child; talking about stuttering; lessening conversations when the child is more disfluent; inserting short, easy, stutter-like mistakes in their own speech; teaching turn taking; and building self-esteem. Helping parents talk about stuttering to a young child is a delicate process, but parents may show their young child support by making nonchalant comments such as, "That's okay, Jimmie, everyone gets bumpy speech sometimes. Mommy does, Daddy does, everyone does sometimes. It's okay." This can be followed up with, "Mommy (Daddy) will wait for you to finish" (p. 15).

In my private practice, when I am working with a school-age child I give both the child and the parents their own assignments to work on during the week. Part of the child's assignment is to talk to the parents about his assignment and part of the parents' assignment is to talk to the child about their assignment. This opens weekly dialogs between the child and parents and lets the child know that the parents have some things to work on and that it is not just the child who is trying to make changes. The child and parents learn to be supportive of one another in their efforts to improve.

Familiarity with family systems theory and common family dynamics in families of children who stutter is particularly helpful when working with parents of a child who stutters (Gregory, 2003; Guitar, 2006; Ramig & Dodge, 2010; Zebrowski, 2002). Including both parents in the therapy often enhances and may even determine the success of the child's therapy. Too often clinicians in public schools have little or no direct interaction with the parents, and when they do it is typically only briefly with the mother. Family systems theory, however, extends beyond the triangle of the child who stutters and the parents. For therapy to be most successful, grandparents, aunts and uncles, and siblings who are significantly involved in the child's life can be useful allies in the therapeutic process. The child's entire family can be part of the "team" who are there to help and support the child in therapy. They may even participate in specific therapy exercises designed for the family, which also may help the child who stutters feel less alone or that the burden of change is not solely on him. It is important for clinicians to listen to, value, and understand the unique perspectives, emotions, and beliefs that each family member reveals because these determine the overt and covert behaviors each person displays toward the child who stutters.

Nelson (2006) emphasizes a variety of recommendations for family members that can be incorporated into our counseling:

- A child who stutters should be treated as a "regular kid"—a child who happens to stutter.
- Children who stutter take more time to talk and, therefore, need patient listeners.
- Children who stutter benefit from extra attention and listening time from the parents and not being interrupted by siblings when they are talking.
- Do not let brothers or sisters imitate or tease the child about his stuttering.
- People involved in the child's life (e.g., all family members, family friends, teachers, and babysitters) should be instructed to listen to what the child says, not how he says it.
- When children who stutter feel pressured to live up to all of their parents' expectations, their stuttering can be aggravated.
- If fatigue increases a child's stuttering, make sure he gets plenty of rest.

- Many children who stutter benefit from a slowing down of the family's pace.
- Parents should avoid arguing in front of their children because they can become alarmed, and the child who stutters may have increased disfluency.
- Children who stutter, like all children, benefit from regular bedtime hours and some general daily routines and mealtimes.
- Avoid having the television or radio on during meal times because it requires the child who stutters (as well as all family members) to compete with excessive background noise and distractions.
- If pressuring him to keep his room neat increases his stuttering, it is probably better to decrease that pressure for now—strive for a middle ground.
- Family members should avoid correcting the child's stuttering—it does not help (if it did help, there probably would not be any children who stutter).

Parents benefit from meeting other parents of children who stutter and attending a support group for parents of children who stutter. Most parents have never met or talked to another parent of a child who stutters and they often feel as though they must have done something terribly wrong to cause their child to stutter. When parents meet other parents of children who stutter, they begin to recognize that they are not alone in their feelings and fears. Parent support groups allow parents to hear how other parents are working on similar problems and the struggles they are having making changes that could benefit their child's speech. This gives parents hope that they can make changes too.

Counseling Children Who Stutter

The form and style of counseling children who stutter varies significantly with the age of the child: preschool, school-age, and adolescent. Williams (2006), whose Ph.D. is in psychology, states that there is general agreement among most speech-language pathologists that some form of counseling is appropriate for adolescents and adults who stutter. However, there is not similar agreement for the appropriateness of counseling children of elementary school-age, much less preschool-age children. We will discuss principles of counseling for each of these three general age groups, followed by counseling principles for adults who stutter.

PRESCHOOL CHILDREN WHO STUTTER

Most evaluations and therapy with preschool-age children are done in a play atmosphere, usually without the young child knowing the purpose of the presence of his new adult playmate. The parents, as discussed above, are key players in any therapy for young children who stutter. The child's psychosocial abilities and ease with a stranger are observed. It is helpful for the parents to observe the clinician's interactions with the child so the clinician can model techniques of listening and interacting that parents can use to enhance their child's fluency. Most of the direct therapy to help a preschool-age child is with the parents, and as the therapy progresses the time the clinician spends with the child is mainly to monitor his progress in developing normal fluency.

SCHOOL-AGE CHILDREN WHO STUTTER

Essentially all of our therapy with children who stutter requires the most subtle and sophisticated counseling techniques that clinicians can use. Our choice of words, tone of voice, timing, body language, and facial expressions (as well as our knowledge of stuttering) can determine the success of therapy. Explaining complex concepts to young children can be a challenge to any clinician. For example, Chmela and Reardon (2005) state that *learning about talking* helps children develop an understanding of what happens when they stutter and that it lays the foundation for learning specific tools to make talking easier. These authors emphasize three concepts: (1) the body parts involved in creating speech, (2) the process or order by which speech is produced, and (3) the choices we have when producing speech. These explanations help children understand why they stutter, what they are *doing* when talking becomes harder, and that there are choices they have to make talking easier. The concepts of "I know, I understand, and I have choices" prepares the foundation for developing a positive attitude and helps motivate the child to change.

Williams (2006) and Ramig and Dodge (2010) emphasize that the purpose of talking with a child who stutters is to discuss frankly and openly what he believes is wrong, what he believes helps him talk better, and what his feelings are about talking. However, before the clinician can talk to a child about his feelings, the clinician must first earn the child's trust. This can best be accomplished by using Rogers' (1953) principles of acceptance, unconditional positive regard, genuineness, and congruence in the clinician's words, voice, facial expressions, and body language. Children are masters at detecting phoniness in adults.

The primary feelings many children have about their stuttering is that it makes them feel "bad" or "sad" and frustrated. Embarrassment, shame, and guilt about their stuttering and fear of talking often begin in the late preschool years when children become cognitively mature enough to compare themselves to others. These feelings can increase if they remain concealed and unexamined (Guitar & Reville, 2006). Eventually feelings of helplessness and hopelessness may develop. Our microskills and ability to ask questions in a nonthreatening manner are essential in helping children reveal their feelings about their stuttering.

CHILDREN'S BELIEFS ABOUT STUTTERING   School-age children who stutter have been told by parents, other family, and well-meaning adult friends what to do or what not to do to stop stuttering (e.g., slow down, relax, think before you talk, take a deep breath). Most of these suggestions are confusing and misleading and can actually add to the child's problem. Using various questioning techniques, it is important for the clinician to find out from the child what he has been taught and what he believes about his stuttering. Regardless of the beliefs the child has about his stuttering, they deserve respectful discussion, and the clinician should not imply that they are silly, wrong, or unimportant. Without understanding the child's beliefs, the child will likely interpret what the clinician says from a distorted and erroneous foundation of information (Ramig & Dodge, 2010; Williams, 2006).

The clinician needs to help the child build a new, more accurate, and healthier foundation of information and beliefs. In order to do this effectively, the child must trust the clinician's experience and expertise with this problem. The clinician has to be careful about how she presents information that may be diametrically opposed to what the child's parents have taught the child. It is, of course, essential that the clinician also is teaching the parents during their sessions the same new information and helping the parents develop a new understanding and new beliefs about stuttering. When a child has erroneous beliefs about what is causing or making him stutter (e.g., words get caught on fishhooks in his throat) then he may do things with his throat, voice, and mouth to help get the words off of the hooks.

Helping a child develop new and healthier beliefs and the ability to be aware of what he is physically doing when he stutters helps reduce the mystery of his stuttering. Further, better understanding of stuttering leads to realistic expectations about increasing normal fluency. This process takes time. There are no long-lasting quick fixes for stuttering. The clinician's empathic responses to the child help him understand that this is not an easy problem that they are working on and that it will take some time to see gradual improvement; for example, "It's confusing, isn't it?" or "It's kind of scary when you don't know what to do to talk easy," or "I know you want to take care of your problem right away, but it's going to take some time to work on this. We both need to be patient here."

CHILDREN'S FEELINGS ABOUT STUTTERING   Clinicians need to be aware that stuttering is a very sensitive, emotional issue for children (as well as for adolescents and adults), and painful emotions may surface. It is essential that children develop trust in their clinician in order to be willing to talk honestly and openly about their feelings. Trust of children is built by being sensitive, nonjudgmental, honest, and congruent during all interactions. As Van Riper (2006) emphasizes, "These children [particularly those who stutter severely] hurt badly, and they show it" (p. 66). The clinician needs to handle emotions and responses of these children with sensitivity and caring, but not appear patronizing or condescending. The old, "There, there, everything is going to be all right." is never acceptable to a person of any age who has no idea if everything will ever be all right—and how can you predict the future? "All right" to the child who stutters probably means totally fluent speech on every word, in every situation, and with every person. Chmela and Reardon (2005) emphasize that it is essential to validate children's feelings by accepting them without judgment. This acceptance helps diminish tension and may result in positive changes in how the child learns to cope with the stuttering problem.

Van Riper (2006) describes a treatment technique in which he tries to mirror the child's feelings. The child must trust that the clinician genuinely wants to understand and accept the child's feelings as natural and justified, and even to experience the same feelings as the child. Van Riper introduced this technique by saying something like, "I think I've now pretty well learned what you do when you stutter, and maybe you have too. Now let's see if I can understand how you feel at the time you stutter or just before or afterwards. I'll try to act out what I think your feeling is and if I'm wrong, let me know." Van Riper spontaneously might droop his body or whimper when he thought a child was feeling helpless, or bang the table if the child seemed hostile, or cover his face as a gesture of shame, or show a fearful face if that is what he thought the child was feeling. When Van Riper failed to mirror the actual feelings of the child because he misinterpreted them, the child was encouraged to correct him. This technique also helped the child learn how to verbally describe her feelings and talk openly about them.

Another procedure that Van Riper used involved projective drawings of the feelings evoked by stuttering. Both the child and Van Riper drew and labeled their own pictures representing anger, fear, helplessness, sadness, shame, and others. After the drawings on the cards were made, they were laid on the table. Then while the child was talking and had a moment of stuttering, she picked up the card that she felt best reflected her feelings at the moment, and Van Riper picked up a card that he had drawn that he thought represented the child's feelings. They compared cards to see if the child and Van Riper picked up the same card. The procedure stimulated discussion of the child's feelings when there were discrepancies. The child felt compelled to explain why she chose a particular card and often in the process revealed many of the rejections and penalties she had received at home and school.

GROUP THERAPY FOR CHILDREN WHO STUTTER   Guitar and Reville (2006) and Ramig and Dodge (2010) discuss the purposes and benefits of group therapy for school-aged children who stutter. They feel that children treated in groups (as small as two children) are guides and models for each other. For example, when children share their experiences and feelings about stuttering, the other members of the group feel supported and understood. Children can identify with other children in the group. Group therapy is a safe environment where the children feel free to be themselves and to talk freely despite their stuttering. They can practice and improve their fluency and communication skills by watching, listening, and talking to each other. The role of the clinician in a children's group is to plan and guide activities that children enjoy (i.e., promote skill building) and to give them a chance to talk about their stuttering (i.e., provide support) and learn that they are not the only one in their school or community with this difficulty. A clinician's counseling skills are particularly challenged when working with groups. She has to be aware and tuned into the nuances of every child in the group and realize that what she says to one child may be interpreted differently by each child.

ADOLESCENTS WHO STUTTER

Zebrowski (2006) discusses the challenges that adults (including parents, teachers, and others in the helping professions) face when attempting to teach, guide, instruct, and advise adolescents. Speech-language clinicians are inevitably in the same position as other adults—the position of an authority figure, which automatically sets the stage for potential conflicts between clinicians and adolescents. Adolescents are undergoing many cognitive, emotional, and physical changes. A major developmental task during the teenage years is individuation, or becoming more independent from parents and developing a separate identity. Consequently, teens are frequently resistant to or uninterested in what adults have to teach them. An additional challenge arises when the emotions that typically accompany stuttering collide with the emotional upheavals and changes of the teen years. Thus, the way that teens present themselves to clinicians can result in appearing unmotivated, and they may be prematurely dismissed from therapy. Zebrowski, however, feels that the apparent lack of motivation reflects the surface attitudes and behaviors, and that being "unmotivated" is actually a place to start, not to end attempts to help adolescents. That is, being unmotivated to improve their speech may be an important topic of discussion to understand what feelings (e.g., anxiety and fear) are contributing to the adolescent feeling unmotivated.

There is a possibility that the adolescent had some speech therapy in his preteen years; previous therapy may have been unsuccessful, or the adolescent may have stuttering that has reoccurred after a period of more fluent speech. If the adolescent had an experience with previous unsuccessful therapy, the new clinician may not have the automatic credibility with the adolescent that she would like to have. Credibility is not earned by expounding on all of the knowledge about stuttering the clinician has learned. Credibility is earned by listening to and valuing what the adolescent is willing to share with the clinician, along with having the skills to help with the stuttering problem. The clinician needs to provide a safe and accepting environment in which the adolescent can tell his story. Based upon the adolescent's narrative, he can begin to understand how his thoughts, feelings, and stuttering behaviors may be linked.

When working with adolescents, it is important to ask them about their experiences and to "treat them as the expert" rather than to "preach" to them. Clinicians have a better chance of successfully engaging adolescents if they attempt to collaborate with them rather than flaunting their authority. If we do not listen carefully to the adolescent's point of view, we run the risk that the adolescent will feel that he is not being heard and understood. Luterman (2008) encourages clinicians to *listen and value* the adolescent and view him as competent to make good decisions.

LISTENING AND VALUING: FEELINGS ASSOCIATED WITH STUTTERING

Since the adolescent may have lived with his stuttering for 10 or more years, he has thought about it and experienced feelings related to his problem more than any other person around him. His perceptions about his stuttering may be based on what he has figured out for himself coupled with what he has been told by family and friends (see the section titled "Counseling School-Age Children Who Stutter"). The emotions that accompany stuttering in school-age children, such as feelings of isolation, anxiety, confusion, guilt, shame, fear, embarrassment, and helplessness, persist and are often magnified during adolescence.

Zebrowski (2002, 2006) employs a cognitive therapy approach that incorporates listening and valuing and then questioning to better understand the person's perceptions of himself, others, and the world, and the influence these perceptions have on his emotions and behaviors (see "Cognitive Therapy" in Chapter 2 for more information about this theory and therapy). Following Beck's (1995) cognitive theory, there is a relationship between beliefs and behaviors. A person's core beliefs develop in childhood and are part of his world view; for example, that adults are generally good and can be trusted or that adults are generally bad and cannot be trusted, or that people make fun of children who cannot talk normally. Although the child cannot clearly articulate these beliefs to himself or others, they influence his automatic thoughts, perceptions, emotions, and behaviors. If questioned, however, an adolescent may be able to articulate the core beliefs which underlie his automatic thoughts and actions. Automatic thoughts tend to be fleeting; they can influence behavior and feelings as though we are on "automatic pilot." As such, they are often unexamined thoughts and beliefs. Core beliefs may be momentarily brought into awareness and then may resubmerge, leaving behind the emotions that they trigger. These emotions then may trigger specific and sometimes general autonomic system responses that reflect anxiety, such as dry mouth, increased heart rate, and "butterflies" in the stomach. These "automatics" for the person may result in cognitive distortions such as catastrophizing, "I should" statements, dichotomous thinking, and overgeneralization (see Chapter 2 for further discussion of cognitive distortions).

Zebrowski (2002) describes a technique that she refers to as "advance-retreat-advance" when talking to teens about their stuttering. While listening to a teenager's stories, she might ask an open-ended or closed-ended question and then look for an "affect shift" (Beck, 1995), such as a change in facial expression, eye gaze, or posture, or a verbal cue such as a pitch, tone, or volume change while talking. When such shifts are observed she might ask, "What was going through your mind just then?" If the teen says, "nothing" or "I don't know," she nods and moves on. The clinician has "advanced" (i.e., asked a question) and then "retreated" when the teen was noncommittal. However, when the teen later makes a comment that the clinician can bridge back to an earlier comment that he had made or a question she had asked, she advances again with another question, trying to elicit his "hot cognitions" (i.e., important automatic thoughts and images that arise in the therapy session and are associated with a change or increase in emotion) (Beck, 1995). This technique can help the teen recognize how his automatic thoughts trigger automatic emotions, which in turn can trigger habitual stuttering behaviors.

Curlee (2008) talks about self-defeating thoughts and behaviors that teenagers who stutter often use; for example, "If I felt more secure, I wouldn't stutter," "I stutter because I lack self-confidence," or "I just can't keep from stuttering in front of strangers." People who stutter need to recognize their automatic beliefs, thoughts, emotions, and behaviors. This provides a basis for rational examination. This process does not mean they will be "cured" from stuttering; it means that they are free to talk and enjoy communicating and being themselves in spite of their stuttering.

People can change their beliefs by changing their behaviors, and they can change their behaviors by changing their beliefs. Adolescents may believe that they cannot do something, but once they work on it they discover they can do it and they change their beliefs about it. Many people need to believe that they can accomplish something long before they ever accomplish it. For example, students have to believe they can finish school and graduate long before they ever graduate. The behavior ("I graduated") follows the belief. A person taking charge of his own life means taking charge of his beliefs, thoughts, feelings, and behaviors. This taking charge is a lifelong commitment and project, not just for those who stutter, but for everyone who is trying to better himself in some way.

When a person stutters severely, most people—after they get over the surprise of seeing the person in the middle of a stuttering block—do not notice it as much as the person might think (Guitar, 2008). What they notice, instead, is how distressed the person is about his stuttering. In our therapy and counseling work we can encourage clients to "test their hypotheses" by asking listeners about what they notice and think about their stuttering. Most clients are surprised that people do not think nearly as much about the person's stuttering as they do about what they are thinking and feeling about themselves.

On the basis of over four decades of clinical experience with children, adolescents, and adults who stutter, Williams (2008a) concludes that many parents do not talk to their children about their stuttering because: (1) they are afraid it would upset their child if they showed disappointment in the way their child talks; (2) they feel their child's stuttering is not a big issue to them; (3) their child does not like to talk about personal things; and (4) they just do not know enough about stuttering and they do not know what to say. Overall, parents do not talk to their children about their stuttering because they believe that the child does not want to talk about it; meanwhile, the child does not talk to her parents about her stuttering because she believes that her parents do not want to talk about it. Hence, a cycle of communication avoidance is created.

In therapy, however, Williams puts the ball in the teen's court by saying that there is "no way" that parents can know what their teenager is thinking and feeling unless the teenager is willing to tell them. He says, "You're unhappy because you stutter. Your parents are unhappy because they don't know what to do or say to be helpful. It's time to talk with each other" (p. 31). Williams says that the "toughest" part for teenagers is to summon up the courage to begin the conversation. Most adolescents have talked to friends and other people about issues when they were scared or anxious, and the teen should expect to feel uncomfortable and even a little scared when he begins to talk to his parents about a problem that is as personal as his stuttering.

In order to help teens and their parents initiate conversations about stuttering, Williams offers a few suggestions. First, select a good time and place to talk. Find a time when there is time to talk and when no one is in a hurry, such as when riding in the car together or at the dinner table. Take the responsibility to find the time or make the time. Second, be aware that parents are likely to feel awkward, too, and maybe even embarrassed. Teenagers can try to accept their parents' feelings, just as they would like their parents to accept their feelings. Third, remember that it is the teen's responsibility to start the conversation and to set the tone for it. This strategy can be empowering to teens who may ordinarily feel that they are at the mercy of parental decisions and behaviors. Being straightforward and direct is the best approach, and it may help if teens acknowledge their own discomfort while being willing to tolerate it in order to discuss the issue with their parents. The teen does not have to talk about every issue around her stuttering during the first conversation, but it is essential to open a dialogue so that further conversations can take place. The door can be opened and both the teen and the parents will need to work at it to maintain their dialog.

Overall, the reality for many adolescents is that their stuttering may improve but seldom ever completely be eliminated; that is, they will likely enter adulthood with some level of stuttering and will need to work on it throughout their lives. One of the goals of therapy is to help teens learn that their speech problem does not have to dictate their future education, occupation or profession, and relationships with people; they have control over the lives they lead, and their quality of life depends on their good choices and decisions—and not on their stuttering.

Counseling Adults Who Stutter

Most of the best counseling skills and strategies for clinicians working with adults who stutter come from speech-language pathologists who themselves stutter, and many got into the profession because of their stuttering problem. Their insights come from their education, training, and personal experiences of living the life of a person who stutters. The counseling principles and techniques vary in their emphasis, but there are overall common themes of taking responsibility for the success or failure of therapy, not hiding their stuttering, and not allowing stuttering to control their lives.

Most authorities on stuttering emphasize that therapy with adults who stutter is a step-by-step process involving both attitude and speech changes (Aten, 2008; Bloodstein & Bernstein Ratner, 2008; Conture & Curlee, 2007; Gregory, 2003; Guitar, 2006; Luper, 2008; Manning, 2010; Murray, 2008; Ramig, 2008; St. Louis, 2008; Van Riper, 2008; Ward, 2006; Williams, 2008b). Breitenfeldt (2008) discusses "managing your stuttering versus your stuttering managing you." He states that severe chronic stuttering remains a problem at some level for most adults and, therefore, they need to learn to live successful, fulfilling lives in spite of this constant, unwanted companion. Because stuttering is both a communication problem and a problem of living, it needs to be attacked from all angles, and the clinician needs to work with the *person who stutters*, not just the stuttering. Breitenfeldt says that experience has demonstrated that people who stutter and who continue to manage their stuttering also make major lifestyle changes, such as admitting openly that they stutter and not avoiding sounds, words, people, and situations in which they may stutter.

ADULT STUTTERING CAN COEXIST WITH PSYCHOLOGICAL DISORDERS

Adults who enter therapy for their stuttering problem may have other problems that become apparent as therapy progresses. Stuttering and anxiety are commonly intertwined and interrelated. On the other hand, a person who appears anxious may have aspects of his anxiety that are not related to his stuttering problem, and a person who appears depressed may have depressive etiology that is not related to the stuttering. When a clinician becomes aware of such symptoms or other significant psychological or emotional concerns that are outside of our scope of practice or beyond what we can reasonably address in the context of the stuttering therapy, it is appropriate and ethically responsible for the clinician to suggest or recommend that the person seek help from a mental health professional, although not all clients will follow through with such a suggestion or recommendation. This does not prevent the speech-language pathologist from continuing to provide therapy to the person; it means that we recognize and adhere to our scope of practice. The following example illustrates how profoundly stuttering can affect an adult.

Jacob

Jacob was a very fluent man who stuttered and had "successfully" hidden his stuttering from everyone, including his wife and employer, by using countless subtle tricks and crutches. Jacob was also a veteran police officer who preferred to work the night shift in the roughest high-crime areas of a large city. He had done plenty of "take downs" and had "taken men out." During one therapy session he told me about an experience he had just the night before. He was in hot pursuit on foot of an armed robber. He knew the robber could turn at any moment and shoot at him.

Continues on next page

Continued from previous page

Jacob admitted that his greatest fear was not whether he might be shot by the man he was chasing, but whether he would stutter badly at the moment he caught him.

CLINICAL QUESTIONS

1. How would you respond to Jacob in order to communicate empathy and understanding for his ability to hide his stuttering?

2. How would Jacob's story affect your selection of treatment interventions?

PRINCIPLES OF COUNSELING FOR ADULTS WHO STUTTER

Cooper (1997) describes stuttering in adults as a syndrome that consists of multiple, coexisting and interactive affective, behavioral, and cognitive components coalescing over a period of years. Each of these three major components of stuttering needs to be addressed in therapy, and counseling is an essential part of any therapy that works with the entire person and not just the stuttering behaviors.

Sheehan (2008) offered several principles for counseling people who stutter, with emphasis on the feeling level:

■ Create a relationship and an atmosphere in which the person is able to express whatever he feels, without prior censorship. Help him understand that he is never wrong on the feeling level, and never tell a client, "You shouldn't feel that way." However, on the "doing level" (i.e., *how* he stutters), he has responsibilities and choices.

■ Make the person who stutters the focus of therapy, not just the immediate suppression of stuttering. Help the person realize his potential for growth and development and self-realization.

■ Begin where the client is, not where the clinician is. Give him room to feel comfortable about the way he feels. For example, if he is not yet ready to admit certain fears and feelings, do not force him to talk about them.

■ Respect the person's feelings of frustration, fear, anger, shame, guilt, and so on as being valid. The person has had decades of conditioning in his life to these feelings.

■ Help him discover that the more guilt, shame, and hatred he attaches to his stuttering, the more he will hold back and try to hide his stuttering, which will result in even more stuttering.

■ Deal with the here and now. Emphasize the possibilities of the future, not the mistakes of the past. Some questions that lead to a positive future are, "Where do I go from here?" "What behavior choices do I have?" and "What can I do at this point?"

- Let the person know that you are interested in more than just the stuttering, that you are interested in him as a person, what he thinks and feels, and that you have unconditional positive regard.

- Be watchful for signs that the client is pretending more progress than he is actually experiencing, just to please you and maintain your support.

- As the client reduces his frustration, shame, and guilt, help prepare him for the possibility that he may become more aware of other problems that he must face or address.

- Every client should be encouraged to develop initiative and independence of the therapist by learning how to recognize which assignments he needs to work on for the maintenance of his improved speech. Fostering independence means that the client should always feel free to return to the clinician if he needs some refresher work or if new problems arise. Stabilization is needed for a considerable amount of time to maintain the fluency that the client has developed.

In summary, therapy for children, adolescents, and adults who stutter involves a team approach in which the clinician is not only working with the individual who stutters but important family members as well. Counseling is interwoven throughout the therapy process, and clinicians who work with individuals who stutter will find that they must develop their counseling skills to a high level of sophistication in order to be most effective.

VOICE DISORDERS

The voice has long been considered a mirror of the person—the inner self. Shakespeare's Hamlet asserts, "Tears in his eyes, distraction in his aspect, a broken voice" (*Hamlet*, II, 2:557–558). The voice is a reflection of the individual's personality and is a sensitive indicator of emotions, attitudes, and the roles we play. The voice serves as an emotional outlet. We can recognize the typical voice of intense, hard-driving people and the nasal singsong voice of the constant whiner. We detect a depressed or withdrawn person's monotone, de-energized voice and know the voice of the outgoing, charismatic, happy person. People use their voices to attract others and to repel them. A soft, soothing voice tends to calm an agitated person, and a tense, strident voice tends to be discomforting (Andrews, 2006; Aronson, 1990; Boone, McFarlane, & Von Berg, 2009; Colton, Casper, & Leonard, 2006; Rammage, Morrison, & Nichol, 2001; Roy, Bless, & Heisey, 2000a, 2000b; Rubin, Sataloff, & Korovin, 2006; Sataloff, 2005; Stemple, Glaze, & Kleben, 2009). Boone (1997) asks the question, "Is your voice telling on you?" Probably for most people the answer is "yes," even though we may not want it to.

Certain personality styles and voice characteristics may develop together as reactions to situations involving social communication. A person's facial expressions and voice are the two most important ways of communicating emotions. The human voice simultaneously conveys semantic content, momentary emotional states, and personality characteristics of the speaker, all of which are interdependent and contingent upon the social context. Our voices also can reflect our emotions related to events long ago, such as

- Help the child communicate more congruently and more directly when he needs attention from his parents in order to help eliminate the habit of loud talking or yelling.

- Transfer the new vocal behaviors and communication skills from the therapy environment to the child's home, school, and community.

- Take permanent responsibility for using appropriate vocal hygiene and voice therapy techniques in daily communication.

There are several general and specific counseling concepts and principles from therapy with children who stutter that apply to children who have voice disorders. For example, three concepts that Chmela and Reardon (2005) emphasize with children who stutter—the body parts involved in creating speech, the process or order by which speech happens, and the choices we have when producing speech, that is, "I know, I understand, and I have choices"—also apply to children working to improve their voices. Clinicians help children who stutter see and feel their behaviors by using a mirror and the sensations of tactile and proprioceptive feedback, as well as verbal feedback from the clinician (Ramig & Dodge, 2010; Williams, 2006). This same technique applies to children with voice problems, that is, helping them hear and feel what they are doing with their voices that causes or maintains their problems. The clinician tries to help the child become aware of vocal abuses and misuses so that the child can then learn and practice alternatives to these behaviors. The clinician must use terms and descriptions that the child can clearly understand, and should avoid professional jargon, criticism, and negative judgment. It is only when the child is aware of what he is doing when he is using unhealthy vocal behaviors that he can learn to do things differently.

Overall, voice therapy is initially a period of self-discovery: discovering what the child believes about his voice and voice problem and what he does with his voice. Therapy then moves into a period of learning: learning new and healthier attitudes about using the voice, learning what he does (his behaviors) when he is abusing and misusing his voice, and then learning what he can do differently to improve his voice. These are structured experiences designed to guide the observations and insights the child is making about himself and his current vocal behaviors.

Parents

Various authors discuss the psychological, behavioral, and etiological considerations of voice disorders of children and the possible contribution of emotional conflict between children and their parents as contributing to voice disorders of various kinds (Andrews, 2006; Aronson, 1990; Barker & Wilson, 1967; Miller & Madison, 1984; Rollin, 2000). However, there is no one psychological common denominator that explains the occurrence of somatic voice disorders in children (Rollin, 2000).

Like young children with voice problems, parents usually are not particularly aware or concerned about their children's vocal hoarseness. Often it is only when a child loses his voice completely that parents decide there is a problem that must be addressed. If the parents take the child to the pediatrician, the doctor may not necessarily make a referral to an otolaryngologist for a closer look at the vocal folds. If the child is seen by an ENT, the physician may not refer the child to an SLP for voice therapy. Just telling the child to "take it easy" on his voice and telling the parents to try to keep him from yelling and screaming may not provide sufficient assistance for the voice problem for either the child or parents to eliminate the vocal abuses and misuses and to achieve healthy vocal folds and a better sounding voice.

If the child is to be helped to eliminate the vocal abuses and misuses that cause and maintain most childhood voice disorders, it is necessary to have the full cooperation of the parents to ensure carryover in the home and community environments. Therefore, a primary goal in voice therapy is to provide the parents with information about what causes and maintains their child's voice problem and to involve family members in helping to encourage and reinforce more appropriate voice use.

Adolescents

It is usually during adolescence, when children begin focusing on their every little imperfection, that they begin to be concerned about their voices. Adolescent boys and girls may "yell their voices away" while cheering at football, soccer, or rugby games. In a way, the acute laryngitis they develop is a badge of honor—they cheered for and supported their team. It is only when adolescents develop chronic voice problems that interfere with verbal communication that they may be sufficiently motivated to follow a voice therapy regimen. However, adolescents are able to do much of their communicating now without their voices, using social networking sites such as Facebook, instant messages (IMs) on their computers, and text messages on their mobile phones, which may have a secondary benefit of providing some voice rest.

In conducting voice therapy with teens a critical factor is the partnership between the speech pathologist and the client, which is quite different than with younger children (Andrews, 2006). Adolescents, because of their emerging autonomy and more advanced cognitive skills, benefit significantly from co-managing and becoming collaborators in their voice therapy program. Along these lines, asking the teen how much her hoarseness bothers her and what kind of voice she would like to have helps to establish a shared understanding of the teen's perspective and her potential motivation to try various strategies to improve her vocal hygiene.

FALSETTO VOICE

Adolescent males with (mutational) falsetto (puberphonia) voices may have strong emotional reactions to their voice quality or disorder. (Most individuals with falsetto voices have sought professional help by early adulthood). A male's falsetto voice may be perceived by others as feminine or immature. The social penalties can be significant for adolescent boys and men who sound effeminate or child-like. They typically feel rejected and isolated and are ridiculed by their peers. Because of the social penalties, most individuals with falsetto voices are highly motivated to make an effort in voice therapy and have good prognoses for change (Andrews, 2006; Boone et al., 2010; Peppard, 2000).

The parents of an adolescent or young adult male with a falsetto voice are often very concerned about their child. Some parents may be embarrassed by their son's voice while others are primarily concerned about how their son is feeling about himself and how it is affecting his friendships and other social relationships. Parents may be concerned about whether their teen is socially isolated and feels rejected. Often the parents of an adolescent with a falsetto voice are as relieved and pleased with the voice change as the young man.

Voice therapy techniques to achieve a more natural and mature-sounding voice for individuals with a falsetto voice are discussed by various authors (Andrews, 2006; Aronson, 1990; Boone et al., 2010; Case, 2002; Colton et al., 2006; Rammage et al., 2001; Stemple et al., 2009). As with other voice disorders, good counseling skills are essential. The clinician does not want to place the cause of the problem on the person but on the vocal folds, for example, "It sounds like your vocal folds are not working the way you want them to. Let's see what we can do to make them work properly." Once the more natural, mature-sounding voice is achieved (which often occurs during the first session), the clinician can support the adolescent by saying something like, "It sounds like you have the option now of choosing one of two voices—your old one or your new one." It is important for the clinician to appreciate that the adolescent's new voice also means a new identity and one that will require adjustment. When resistance to voice therapy or habituation of the new voice becomes evident, the clinician can explore the teen's beliefs and perceptions regarding identity development and how he would like to be viewed by others. When the clinician feels that the adolescent's beliefs and perceptions of identity are beyond the scope of practice of the SLP, a referral to a counselor may be appropriate.

Adults

Many adults with hyperfunctional voice disorders have considerable stress and tension in their lives. While most people spend the majority of their waking time in two places, home and work, many people have considerable stress in one or both places. Ideally, people have a place of "sanctuary" where they can generally feel relaxed and good about themselves, whether it is home or work (preferably both). However, when there are significant stresses in both environments, there is little opportunity to be renewed and refreshed and, for some people, a voice disorder may reflect this chronic tension.

Having learned from an otolaryngologist who takes a **holistic** approach toward medicine, I tell many of my clients that "The bad news is you have a voice problem. And the good news is you have a voice problem." I go on to say that our bodies give us "messages" and if we don't listen to the first message, it will give us another message (maybe headaches), and then another (maybe stomach problems), until we finally listen and say, "I need to do some things differently." Fortunately, many voice problems are relatively benign messages that usually do not have serious medical complications. The voice often mirrors what is going on in a person's life. As clinicians, our understanding of voice problems allows us to help people regain their voices and then maintain them by learning strategies to better cope with life's vicissitudes.

Andrews (2006) discusses the role of the speech pathologist with adults who have voice disorders. She says that although mental health counselors can help clients understand the psychosocial dimensions of voice problems, the speech pathologist can help clients produce and habituate more appropriate vocal behaviors. When clients exhibit significant emotional problems, the treatment plan should involve a team approach that includes a mental health professional who provides counseling to the client. However, with most voice clients the counseling goals can be addressed by the speech pathologist as part of the voice treatment program, including consultation with mental health professionals as needed. The counseling goal for the speech pathologist is not to discover or to resolve the emotional issues in a person's life, but to understand how the person's feelings about those issues may be affecting the way the person uses her voice. Counseling is a part of the fabric of voice therapy. We use counseling skills to help our clients learn to examine themselves and to develop and enhance confidence in their own problem-solving abilities.

Individuals who seek voice therapy frequently disclose personal information to the clinician during the initial interview. It is not uncommon for a client to say something like "I have never told anyone this before, but. . . ." Adults are often comfortable talking to speech pathologists about issues that they may be reluctant to seek counseling for from a mental health professional. As therapy progresses and greater trust is developed in the speech pathologist, the client may openly discuss interpersonal conflicts or life stresses that underlie the voice problem. It is important for the speech pathologist to help the client notice the links between her voice symptoms and certain life or interpersonal stresses, but it is not within the speech pathologist's purview to give the patient advice to eliminate certain stresses. It is more appropriate to help the patient think through how she can cope better in those situations so that she can maintain better control over her voice, such as when she gets angry, counting to 10 and then concentrating on using her soft voice.

BENIGN LESIONS ON THE VOCAL FOLDS

The nature of voice disorders with benign lesions or masses on the vocal folds (e.g., vocal nodules, vocal polyps, contact ulcers) is that they are often triggered by stress and overuse of the voice. They frequently have psychosocial factors associated with them, such as personality type, tension, stress, and inefficient coping strategies. In general, individuals with vocal nodules tend toward extroversion (Roy, Bless, & Heisey, 2000b) and individuals with contact ulcers tend to be ambitious, rather aggressive, competitive males (Andrews, 2006).

Andrews (2006) recommends that the existence of unresolved conflicts and the lifestyle of such clients should be considered by the clinician designing the treatment plan. More specifically, attention should be given to the client's perceptions of daily stresses and the coping strategies used; education about the relationship between emotional stress and voice; modification of the client's perceptions of certain situations and any inefficient coping strategies that are used; and expression of feelings concerning unresolved conflicts to acknowledge and resolve emotional stresses.

CASE STUDY

Beverly

Beverly was a 45-year-old woman who was an elementary school teacher for 20 years. She loved teaching and she loved the children. She was a single mother struggling financially to support 14- and 17-year-old daughters. She was active in her church and sang in the choir. She was, in many ways, typical of many adults with vocal nodules: she had a job that required excessive use of her voice, sometimes with vocal abuses such as yelling to children on the playground, and she had a variety of stresses in her life from financial pressures to trying to raise teenage children. Beverly tried to reach the extremes of her vocal range during choir practice, choir performances, and singing around the house, and she had little time to take care of herself and relax. She felt guilty when she tried to do something for herself even though she felt chronically tense.

Besides symptomatic voice therapy and vocal hygiene (conservation) education, the clinician tried to encourage Beverly to learn how to take care of herself. She eventually began to appreciate that if she "used herself up and burned herself out" she would not be able to continue teaching or singing, and she may have difficulty using her voice when trying to communicate with her family and friends, while teaching, and in all other environments. As she learned to balance her life a little better, some of her generalized tension as well as her vocal fold tension began to diminish.

CLINICAL QUESTIONS

1. How would you educate this client about the links between her voice and her lifestyle patterns?

2. What would you say if the client asked you for specific advice, for instance, "Should I stop singing in the choir so I can take better care of my voice?" or "How can I juggle all of my daily demands and still work on my voice?"

DISORDERS RELATED TO PSYCHOSOCIAL FACTORS

Aphonia and dysphonia may be behavioral responses to emotional stress and unconscious attempts to avoid dealing with distressing situations or interpersonal conflicts and, with some clients, may be considered a **conversion reaction** (Andrews, 2006; Aronson, 1990; Boone et al., 2010; Case, 2002; Rammage et al., 2001; Rosen & Sataloff, 1997; Stemple et al., 2009). Aronson (1990) cautions against premature referral to a psychologist and instead advocates the following steps in the treatment sequence.

1. Laryngeal evaluation by an otolaryngologist to rule out organic disease and systemic illness

2. Symptomatic voice therapy to achieve a functional voice

3. Exploring psychosocial problems that may have contributed to the loss or dysfunction of voice and suggestion that stress and tension can interfere with voluntary muscle action, including the vocal folds. The clinician needs to anticipate that emotions such as crying and anger may occur when the patient is discussing related life circumstances and events

4. Referral to a mental health professional if necessary to achieve a more enduring stabilization of the client's life adjustment and the benefit of a comprehensive, coordinated treatment plan

CASE STUDY

Irene

Irene had suffered with intermittent functional aphonia for several years and now the aphonia was becoming more persistent. When her lack of voice began to threaten her job security, she sought help from a speech-language pathologist who specialized in voice disorders. The therapist saw Irene for one session, and she was able to achieve some phonation during various non-speech tasks. However, before proceeding further the therapist requested that Irene be seen by an ENT. She scheduled an appointment with an ENT at a time when the voice therapist could be present. The physician, therapist, and client were all able to view her vocal folds clearly with videostroboscopy. There was no apparent organic or neurological basis for her aphonia. Within two more therapy sessions, Irene was able to achieve and sustain good phonation but with intermittent phonation breaks when talking about certain job stresses. The therapist recognized that she needed to work with a mental health professional to help her manage some of the personal stresses in her life, and that the improvements in her voice functioning would enable her to better communicate with a mental health professional. Sometimes voice therapists can help prepare clients to work with mental health professionals who can work with areas outside of our scope of practice. However, it is difficult for mental health professionals to provide "talk" therapy when an individual does not have a voice for communicating. Speech-language pathologists can help clients achieve a satisfactory voice so that they can more fully participate in and benefit from verbally mediated therapies with mental health professionals.

CLINICAL QUESTIONS

1. How might you explain to a client that you feel she may benefit from mental health services?
2. How would you manage the situation if the client became visibly upset and angry that "you could even think of such a thing"?

PATIENTS WITH LARYNGECTOMIES

There are few physical losses that can have a more devastating effect on a person than the loss of the larynx—the primary source of communication. The initial shock of being diagnosed with laryngeal cancer and the need to have laryngectomy surgery inevitably has a major impact on a person's life, and many patients initially consider it to be a disaster. Whatever counseling is provided by the physician (often it is simply "informational counseling"—telling the person the diagnosis and the need for surgery) is never sufficient for the patient and the family. This condition can catapult the patient into a state of shock, grief, and fear.

When the diagnosis of laryngeal cancer is made, the laryngectomy surgery is usually scheduled as soon as possible. This leaves little time for the patient to meet with a speech pathologist to discuss the physical changes that will take place from the surgery, teaching the person what alternate communication techniques may be used immediately after the surgery (i.e., writing, communication board, and use of an electrolarynx—many patients do not fully understand that they will not have a functional voice immediately after the surgery). An even greater concern is that there is little if any time available for counseling with the patient and family about the fears and anxieties associated with cancer (e.g., will the surgeon get all the cancer by removing the larynx?), and the psychological and social adjustments the patient and family will need to make.

Because voice is a critical component of a person's identity, the loss of voice causes profound changes in a person's self-identity, self-worth, independence, and perceptions of self as a "normal" social being. In addition to the psychosocial effects of the laryngectomy, there are possible (and likely) effects on employment and the ability to produce income, which can result in loss of status in the family and community; that is, the person may no longer have the capacity to function as a primary "bread winner."

Following laryngectomy surgery, the patient (and sometimes close family members) will likely experience some fear, embarrassment, and depression relating to his loss of voice and adjusting to an alternative method of vocalizing (e.g., tracheoesophageal puncture, esophageal speech, or electrolarynx). In addition, they are concerned about their hygiene and physical appearance related to their stoma or the appearance of their radical neck dissection. These feelings and concerns are exacerbated by the emotional and social isolation experienced by the complete loss of voice (e.g., friends often stop visiting when they realize the patient cannot talk). The patient and even close family members will likely go through the stages of grief (as discussed in Chapter 11). For many, if not most, patients and families this is a crisis, and the information on managing a crisis discussed in Chapter 14 can be helpful.

Changed attitudes and behaviors of the patient are to be expected following the laryngectomy surgery, including depression, irritability, emotional lability, resentment, reassignment of family duties, and anticipated rejection (Andrews, 2006). Providing educational reading material to the patient and family can help them realize that these are common feelings among patients. Encouraging the patient to join a support group for people who have had a laryngectomy can help him and his family relate to others who are experiencing similar life changes.

■ Support from family and friends is essential in the rehabilitation stages of the patient as he learns to use his method of choice (or what works best for him) for oral communication. Providing reading material to the spouse and other interested family members can be helpful because they can reread, think about, share, and discuss what they learn from the material. Andrews (2006) discusses issues that the patient and family members may deal with, including changes in status and dependency. It is essential that the patient is not inadvertently treated as a child because he cannot talk. In areas involving personal and family decision making, the patient should be expected and encouraged to continue his usual role. He has lost his voice, not his cognitive functioning.

- The patient should be encouraged to feel confident and competent to carry out normal family business.

- Opportunities for stimulation and socialization are restricted. The patient's embarrassment and fear about social contact and the family's natural protectiveness can limit opportunities for learning how to adjust to and compensate for changed conditions. Recognition and open discussion with the patient and family about goals and strategies to address these areas, and sensitivity about not pushing the patient beyond comfortable levels too quickly, are important. The patient and family should be provided with online support networks such as the International Association of Laryngectomees (www.theial.com) and Web Whispers (www. webwhispers.org).

Most people who have had a laryngectomy make remarkably good adjustments to the changes in their lives; however, the speech pathologist must be alert to signs of serious adjustment difficulties, prolonged depression, withdrawal, and serious deteriorations in family relationships. When problems of this magnitude occur, referral to a mental health professional should be made.

CLEFT LIP AND PALATE

An infant born with a serious facial disfigurement sets in motion a wide array of emotional responses in everyone related to or involved with the newborn. Even the attending medical staff who must maintain their professional posture may have a momentary, controlled startle with widened eyes when they see a complete bilateral cleft lip and palate. Their first concerns are for the physical well-being of both the infant and mother, but they also know that there will be emotionally trying times for the family who will be taking home a less-than-perfect baby (Fallowfield & Jenkins, 2004). Ultimately, though, it is the parents who first must adjust to their disappointments and fears. Later, the children develop increasing awareness that they look and sound different from everyone in their family and, likely, all of their playmates.

Parents' Initial Shock and Adjustment

Probably all soon-to-be-parents have said, "I don't care if it's a boy or girl; I just want my baby to be healthy." In some cases, because of increasingly refined ultrasound techniques, a cleft lip or other craniofacial anomaly may be detected in utero. The parents' initial response to learning about their baby's cleft at this stage of development is often accompanied by emotional shock, and from that point on they need to receive information and counseling from the obstetrician and pediatrician (Strauss, Sharp, Lorch, & Kachalia, 1995). The knowledge that the unborn child is not perfect—that it has a cleft—allows the parents some time for learning about the problem and perhaps developing some adjustment to the reality of the child's condition.

Most parents, however, have no advance warning and opportunity to prepare for the birth of a child with a cleft; the baby is born and the parents' first awareness of the facial anomaly is when they are shown their new baby (Strauss, Sharp, Lorch, & Kachalia, 1995). Many parents of babies with clefts have never heard of or seen pictures of clefts (*harelip* is usually the term adults have heard) before their child's birth (Koepp-Baker & Harkins, 1936; Middleton, Lass, Starr, & Pannbacker, 1986; Peterson-Falzone, Hardin-Jones, & Karnell, 2010). Parents may find it very difficult to admit their unspoken feelings about the child they created. These self-directed or outer-directed recriminations add to the difficulty and frustration parents have in facing the reality before them (Rollin, 2000). Additional emotional reactions and concerns often occur when the cleft is part of a larger syndrome, such as Pierre Robin syndrome (Barnett, Clements, & Kaplan-Estrin, 2003).

Drotar, Baskiewicz, Irwin, Kennel, and Klans (1975) describe five stages of adaptation by parents to the birth of a child with a deformity or visible handicap, including: (1) the initial shock and disbelief, (2) denial, (3) anger, (4) adaptation, and (5) acceptance. These stages are similar to Kubler-Ross's (1969) stages of grief discussed in Chapter 11. Rollin (2000) says that how successfully parents move through stages of adaptation and what effects they have on the child depends on several interrelated factors, including:

- The mental health of individual family members
- The nature of the marital relationship
- The ability to cope with stress
- The kind and degree of the child's deformity
- The nature and degree to which the family receives information about the deformity and its possible sequelae
- The effectiveness of the rehabilitation team

Parental reactions to first seeing their baby's birth defect include disbelief, shock, anger, guilt, depression, inadequacy, resentment, grief, frustration, anxiety, fear, and protectiveness—all common reactions to any serious physical defect in newborns (Bradbury & Hewison, 1994; Dolger-Hafner, Bartsch, Trimbach, Zobel, & Witt, 1997; Speltz, Armsden, & Clarren, 1990; van Staden & Gerhardt, 1995). Further, these emotional reactions may not be simply fleeting feelings. Because a cleft is a chronic problem, parental reactions may become long-lasting and cyclical; that is, they may recur during different stages and ages in their child's life, such as infancy, preschool, school age, junior high school, and so forth, when new encounters with groups of people and their questions may be expected. Sometimes the emotional reactions of parents may be externalized (e.g., by frustration and anger) toward the spouse or team of professionals who are involved in trying to help the infant and family. Realizing that this might occur, it is wise to not take parental frustration and anger personally, but to appreciate the profound loss and all of the stressors around it that are anxiety producing for the parents.

Parents of newborns with clefts report that they want more information from the physician at the time of the birth, as well as compassion and greater opportunity to discuss their fears (Strauss, Sharp, Lorch, & Kachalia, 1995; Young, O'Riordan, Goldstein, & Robin, 2001). New parents of a child with a cleft have many serious concerns and fears: "How will we feed and care for the baby?" "Can the cleft be repaired and how soon can it be repaired?" "Will the baby eventually look all right?" "Will she be able to talk normally?"

"If we have more children, will they have clefts?" and perhaps the greatest fear, "Is my baby going to be retarded?" Health care professionals (primarily nurses and pediatricians) can be important sources of support and information for parents in the early months. In addition, parents who are able to talk to other parents of children with clefts are comforted by learning that they are not alone and that there are solutions to problems and daily care challenges (Broder, 2001; Byrnes, Berk, Cooper, & Marazita, 2003; Peterson-Falzone et al., 2010). It is important for parents, as much as possible, to maintain a positive attitude and not impart negative feelings onto their children during the long and complicated process of management of the child's cleft and its secondary effects.

In addition to the concerns about the appearance of an infant with a cleft, parent–infant attachment and bonding have been a concern for many years (Koepp-Baker & Harkins, 1936; Peterson-Falzone, Hardin-Jones, & Karnell, 2010). In general, the more severe the cleft, the more likely parents are to perceive their infants as irritable and having less pleasing personality characteristics; mothers delay in touching their babies and are less interactive (e.g., less playful, less responsive, and less facially expressive) with their babies (Coy, Speltz, & Jones, 2002; Slade, Emerson, & Freedlander, 1999). Clinicians can notice whether this seems to be the case and provide gentle encouragement to parents to provide the infant with the love, security, and social interaction he needs. If this encouragement does not seem to be sufficient, a referral to a psychologist who specializes in young children and parent–child attachment may be warranted.

It is interesting to note that the numerous studies and reviews of literature on parental reactions to newborns with clefts or other physical abnormalities are almost exclusively in reference to mothers' reactions, with a few notable exceptions. Clifford's (1969) study on parental ratings of infants with cleft palate included perceptions of fathers, and Pelchat, Lefebrie, and Perreault's (2003) study examined the similarities and differences between mothers' and fathers' experiences of parenting a child with a disability. Collett and Speltz (2006) discuss parent coping and parent–child relationships but do not distinguish differences between mothers and fathers. A 2009 questionnaire study by Umweni and Okeigbemen of 25 mothers and 25 fathers of newborns with cleft lip and/or palate found that 23 (92%) of the mothers reacted with shock and grief compared to seven (28%) of the fathers. Fifteen (60%) of the fathers were calm or apparently indifferent to their child's cleft, and three (12%) reacted negatively, ranging from anger to outright rejection. Concern about financial burdens was common to both parents. Overall, this study indicates that the birth of a child with a cleft lip and/or palate typically has more adverse effects on the mother than the father. However, understanding the emotional reactions of fathers is important too. Most fathers are not just passive, unconcerned parents. There is a good chance that they are feeling many of the same things the mothers are, but perhaps trying to be more stoic about it ("Take it like a man").

Research into grieving men has shown that they tend to focus on problem solving more than expressions of feelings; their internal adjustments to loss are usually expressed through activity; intense feelings may only be expressed privately; and they have a general reluctance to discuss their feelings (Martin & Doka, 1996; Perlmann & Berko-Gleason, 1994; Sanders, 1998). Therefore, it is important for clinicians not to mistake stoicism for lack of feelings. It is important to recognize as well that individuals from different cultural backgrounds may be more or less expressive with their feelings.

We do not want to forget that the newborn may have older brothers and sisters who also will be reacting to the baby's physical appearance. The grieving behavior of a sibling may be similar to that of the same-gender parent. For example, a son may try to be stoic and "strong," much as he sees his father trying to be (Sanders, 1998). Likewise, grand-parents have their own reactions but do the best they can to be supportive of the new parents and the other grandchildren. Therefore, it may be helpful to include siblings and other family members in informational sessions so that they can ask questions, express their fears, and develop a process of sharing and supporting each other through this challenging process.

COUNSELING PARENTS WHEN ANTENATAL DIAGNOSIS OF A CLEFT IS PROVIDED THROUGH ULTRASOUND

Facial clefts as a group represent one of the most frequently occurring congenital ab-normalities detectable on prenatal mid-trimester ultrasound scans (Wayne, Cook, Sairam, Hollis, & Thilaganathan, 2002). The opportunity for forewarning the parents is now pos-sible with antenatal ultrasound diagnosis of the cleft. This has opened up a new area of an-tenatal counseling by obstetricians, pediatricians, speech pathologists, psychologists, and other members of cleft palate teams. Davalbhakta and Hall (2000) presented in the *British Journal of Plastic Surgery* the results of their study in which the parents of 124 infants with cleft lip and/or palate responded to a questionnaire. In the study 30 percent of the infants were diagnosed antenatally through ultrasound and the parents received antenatal counseling, and the rest of the parents received postnatal counseling because a cleft had not been detected. Of the parents who had an antenatal diagnosis of a cleft, 85 percent felt that the diagnosis and subsequent counseling from the cleft palate team prepared them psychologically for the birth of their child with a cleft. Members of the cleft palate team can provide important information to parents that can prepare them for the birth of a child with a cleft.

COUNSELING BEFORE THE INITIAL LIP AND PALATE REPAIR

The initial information about clefts is usually provided by pediatricians who contact the nearest cleft palate team. Depending on the structure and procedures of a hospital's cleft palate team, speech-language pathologists may do much of the counseling with the family of a newborn with a cleft. SLPs may be the designated counselors for the families because of their education and training in many of the areas of concern parents typically present and their skills in communicating sensitive information. It may be helpful for other team members, such as the pediatrician and plastic surgeon, to inform the parents that the SLP will be able to answer most of the parents' questions so that the parents know early on that there is a "go-to person" for many of their questions. The role of the SLP is to provide information to the parents about the nature of cleft lip and/or palate; feeding problems of infants with clefts; developmental aspects of language, cognition, and phonology; reso-nance disorders and velopharyngeal dysfunction; dental anomalies that may accompany the cleft; and middle ear and hearing problems that are commonly associated with the cleft. The SLP needs to be prepared to answer the numerous questions most parents have and to be sensitive to the emotional reactions they may present. When necessary, the SLP needs to refer the parents to a psychologist or other mental health professional. The SLP is usually one of the most important cleft palate team members who provides counseling to the parents and other family members because we see the parents and child on a consistent and long-term basis (Kummer, 2008).

Most infants with clefts are born without parents having any preexisting information, and 96 percent of the time it is the physician who has to present the bad news. An interdisciplinary team (physicians, dentists, and social workers) study was conducted by Strauss, Sharp, Lorch, and Kachalia (1995) on the biological parents of 100 children born with cleft lip and/or palate who answered a questionnaire about their actual experiences with the physician's communication of the diagnosis (the bad news) compared with their desired experiences with the information interview. The results showed that the parents wanted more opportunity to talk and express their feelings and they wanted the physician to try harder to make them feel better. The parents wanted more information and more of a discussion about the possibility of their child being mentally retarded. They wanted the physician to show more caring and confidence, and wanted referrals to other parents who have children with clefts. In a related study, Young, O'Riordan, Goldstein, and Robin (2001) found that the critical information parents wanted about their new baby with a cleft lip or palate was how to feed the newborn and to learn how to identify illnesses in their baby. Ninety-five percent of the parents wanted to be shown all normal aspects of their baby's examination (i.e., the ways in which their babies were normal and healthy), and 87 percent wanted to be told that the cleft was not their fault. It was also important to the parents that the presenters of the information use proper terminology to describe the infant's problems, and to receive assurance that their baby was not in pain. The parents answering the questionnaire reported that the physicians who presented the information about the clefts in the children did not address these concerns.

These studies are relevant to speech-language pathologists because they point out the need for parents that we counsel not only to be presented information using the appropriate terminology, but for parents to have the opportunity to discuss their concerns and be in an atmosphere where sharing feelings is accepted. We also may want to provide more hope for the parents in discussing the strengths of the cleft palate team, particularly the excellence of the surgeon. Discussions should include the fact that their baby is not in any pain that is related to the cleft and to emphasize the normal areas in the appearance and other aspects of the child. The parents need to be informed that there is little likelihood that the child will be cognitively impaired (this information may need to be altered if the cleft is a part of a syndrome in which cognitive impairment is a known co-occurrence). The parents also need to hear that the cleft was not their fault; there was nothing they could have done to cause or prevent the cleft. When possible, providing contact information of other parents who have children with clefts could be helpful. Throughout interactions with parents, clinicians need to maintain a posture of confidence and caring. The clinician should realize that the amount and kind of information that parents want, and their need for us to listen to their concerns, may take one or more hours of the clinician's time. However, the cost–benefit ratio certainly is weighted toward taking the time and providing the information that the parents want and need.

In addition to the above areas of discussion, research conducted by SLPs indicates several other areas that need to be addressed and information provided to the parents; for example, what the parents need to do at the present time; information about the likely surgical intervention; prognosis related to survival, cosmetic, and physical aspects of the cleft; how to explain the child's cleft to family and friends; the possible speech and language problems, hearing impairments, personality, and social adjustment of the child; and educational problems (Kummer, 2008; Rollin, 2000). The area that the SLP is least qualified to discuss with the parents is the surgical intervention; however, the parents are normally put in contact with the plastic surgeon for information related to surgical options.

It is important for the parents to understand that even though the infant may have a bilateral cleft lip and clefts of the hard and soft palate, there is no pain involved in having a cleft because there are no raw surfaces. Also, of course, the infant does not know how he looks and is not concerned about his appearance. It needs to be emphasized to the parents and other family members that the child with a cleft needs to be treated the same as any other newborn.

Although SLPs try to answer all of the questions that the parents may have, the initial concern is feeding the infant and providing good nutrition because the newborn's weight gain (usually to 10 pounds [4.5 kg]) is essential before the cleft lip can be closed (Smedegaard, Marxen, Moes, Glassou, & Scientsan, 2008). SLPs on cleft palate teams typically develop considerable expertise in infant feeding and, along with a nurse who is specially trained in this area, will provide important information to the parents.

The second major area to address with parents (after they understand their baby's condition) is language development and making certain that the parents are providing rich stimulation to the infant by talking to and reading to their new baby, just as any other parent would. Typically, it will be approximately 10 weeks before the cleft lip is closed and 12 to 18 months before the palate is closed, and those are important weeks and months in infant–parent bonding. Although some parents may not want to show off their new baby to everyone, they still need to provide all of the stimulation they would provide an infant without a cleft. As Hahn (1989) states, "Parents are going to teach speech and language consciously or unconsciously, whether or not they are advised; they need direction, information on normal language development, and specific suggestions on practical ways to start" (p. 313). Parents need to know early on that the goal for the child is normal speech and language and that their participation is needed to meet that goal (Peterson-Falzone et al., 2010). In addition, parents should be informed of the potential for middle ear infections their child will likely develop, the early and subtle signs of hearing and middle ear problems, and the need for immediate medical management.

The third area to address with parents is speech or articulation development. Brochures that address the infant's inability to achieve velopharyngeal closure for adequate production of pressure consonants before surgical repair of the palate are sometimes misleading to parents who interpret that information to mean that their baby will not talk before palatal surgery. Parents may assume that there is little to be gained by stimulating their child's vocalizations before surgical repair of the palate. It is important for the SLP to identify any inaccurate, preconceived notions that parents may have about the relationship between the infant's cleft and speech, and then to provide accurate information and encouragement of vocalizations and sound productions (Peterson-Falzone et al., 2010). The parents need to encourage vocal play and babbling games. The parents should be informed that nasal consonants and glides will be more easily produced than pressure consonants; however approximations of pressure consonants should always be accepted despite any distortions that may be present. It is important for parents to learn what sounds the infant may be able to produce (i.e., /m/, /n/, and /ng/), and that the vowels and consonants will be hypernasal. Compensatory articulations, particularly aberrant glottal behaviors, should be described and the parents counseled to avoid reinforcing them (e.g., by repeating them back to the baby). Rather than repeating the "cute" growl to the baby, parents should be encouraged to simply ignore these undesired behaviors when they are produced but reinforce the baby's efforts to vocalize by producing a babble or word that contains desired consonant sounds (e.g., "mamma") (Peterson-Falzone, Hardin-Jones, & Karnell, 2010).

Daddy Wanted to Hear "Daddy"

I was conducting a research study on the speech sound development of 11-month-old babies with cleft palate. One of the babies produced many glottal stops. The parents were very proud of their daughter because she produced this sound to communicate in a very expressive manner. The sound sounded like "uh uh uh." She was a "daddy's girl" and daddy was happy with the glottal stops but was very emotionally hurt because the baby had only one recognizable word, "mamma." No matter how hard the father worked with her, she could not say "daddy." When I explained to him that it was physically impossible at this time for her to make a /d/ sound, he was so relieved he just squeezed his little girl and said, "You do love daddy, I knew you did!" In addition, I took the opportunity to tell the parents not to reinforce the glottal stop sounds and taught them how to help their daughter make other speech sounds with her lips and tongue.

Source: Marlene B. Salas-Provance, Ph.D., F-CCC-SLP.

CLINICAL QUESTIONS

1. How can providing "academic" information (e.g., the physical impossibility of producing a /d/ sound) to parents be helpful in the parents' emotional adjustment to their child's problem?

2. What is another situation in which the parents' improved understanding of their child's limitations might lead to greater parent acceptance?

3. What would you say to parents of an infant born with a cleft palate if the parents did not seem to spend time talking to and enjoying their infant?

Parents and Their Toddlers

The initial challenges of parent–infant bonding may persist and continue to impact the next stage of development—toddlerhood. Studies have revealed that some mothers of

CONCLUDING COMMENTS

This chapter focuses on some of the unique challenges that individuals with specific types of speech, language, voice and cleft disorders may face and the counseling issues that may arise when working with these clients and patients. For each disorder, attention was devoted to discussing the common psychological and emotional experiences of clients and, when appropriate, their families, followed by suggestions for relevant counseling skills.

Discussion Questions

1. Why is it important to understand the common psychological and emotional issues that may occur with various types of clients?

2. Why is it important to appreciate that various psychological and emotional issues may change as a client grows older and that different counseling strategies may be necessary with different ages of clients?

3. Why would a "cookbook" approach to counseling not be effective with clients or their families?

4. What psychological and emotional issues might you find most challenging with children who have articulation or phonological disorders?

5. What psychological and emotional issues might you find most challenging with children who have language disorders?

6. What psychological and emotional issues might you find most challenging with children who have fluency disorders? With the parents of a child who has a fluency disorder? With adults who have fluency disorders?

7. What psychological and emotional issues might you find most challenging with children who have voice disorders? With adults who have voice disorders?

8. What psychological and emotional issues might you find most challenging with children who have craniofacial anomalies? With the parents of children who have craniofacial anomalies?

9. Of the various kinds of clients you have had experience with, which ones do you feel are the most challenging in terms of counseling? What makes them more challenging than other kinds of clients?

10. How much do you think your self-confidence plays a role in your ability to counsel clients and their families effectively? What can you do to increase your self-confidence in this area?

Role Plays

1. Divide into groups of three; in each group one person can role play the SLP while the other two students play the parents. The parents tell the SLP that their child has a stuttering problem but they are afraid to mention it to him. Role play a conversation in which the SLP attempts to explore with the parents their fears and concerns as well as provide some guidance for appropriate interventions.

2. Again, using groups of three, have the SLP counsel a pair of parents who have just learned that their baby has a cleft palate. The parents exhibit different emotional reactions and personalities, making it more challenging for the SLP to counsel them. The SLP can draw upon her knowledge of common male versus female responses to problems in crafting responses to each parent.

3. An adult client and an SLP are working on strategies to minimize the client's stuttering, and the client confesses to the SLP that she always stuttered more around her father who had a very harsh, authoritarian manner. She reports that her current boss has some similarities to her father and she feels very nervous and anxious around him. Engage in a role play around this dialogue and the interventions appropriate for the SLP. Afterwards, discuss with the class how each student would determine the professional boundaries in this situation and what each would say to the client.

Counseling Skills for Adult Neurological Disorders and Dysphagia

CHAPTER OUTLINE

- Introduction
- Neurological Disorders in Adults
- Swallowing Disorders/Dysphagia
- Concluding Comments
- Discussion Questions
- Role Plays

INTRODUCTION

This chapter is a continuation of the discussion of counseling skills for working with specific disorders, that is, neurological disorders in adults and swallowing disorders/dysphagia. Good counseling skills are essential when working with all types of clients, patients, and their families; however, they are particularly crucial when working with individuals and their families when a sudden neurological impairment has occurred, as well as when patients and families are struggling with chronic neurological disorders. The patient's dramatic changes often create "ripple effects" (i.e., additional changes) in the family.

NEUROLOGICAL DISORDERS IN ADULTS

Beyond the communication and cognitive impairments of individuals with neurological impairments, there are inevitable emotional and social effects for both the patient and family. The classic phrase "a stroke in the family" suggests that, although one person may have had the stroke (TBI, etc.), the entire family is affected. For this reason, a family systems approach to counseling is particularly helpful with these patients (see Chapters 2 and 6). As clinicians, we always need to keep in mind the entire person (and the family) with whom we are working, and not just the patient's disorder(s) (LaPointe, 2005). Parkinson and Rae (1996), of the School of Psychology and Counseling in London, England, emphasize the need for SLPs to focus on a holistic view of the person. Viewing patients holistically includes using person-first language that reflects that the impairments individuals experience do not define who they are; that is, people are not their problems, but problems are something people experience. The language clinicians use may, in some way, affect how they view and treat some patients; for example, "I'm working with a new stroke patient" versus "I'm working with a new patient who had a stroke last week." As clinicians, we need to be careful to not dehumanize our clients and patients, no matter how severe their injury or impairment.

The Spiraling Effects of Stress

Over time, **stressors** (i.e., conditions or external events that create emotional strain or challenge an individual's coping resources) can result in hypertension and stress responses such as neurochemical and structural changes in the brain, which can increase the risk of strokes (Surtee, Wainwright, Luben, Wareham, Bingham, & Khaw, 2008). Furthermore, Tanner (2003) says that stress plays two important roles in individuals with neurogenic communication disorders, including those in which stress may have contributed to the neurological event. First, stress places demands on coping skills. The patient's previously learned and automatic psychological adjustment strategies are taxed to the maximum as he attempts to cope with a myriad of stressful events immediately following the stroke; for example, experiencing a medical emergency; being physically separated from loved ones while in the hospital and psychologically separated from them because of the communication disorder; new relationships with doctors, nurses, and therapists; undergoing extensive medical testing; impairments in walking, communicating, and self-care; and financial concerns, to name just a few. Second, coping deficits themselves can exacerbate stress. The patient's slowed and impaired cognitive functioning, as well as difficulty communicating his thoughts and feelings, can create a perception that the brain injury has eliminated previously successful coping abilities. These perceptions and fears can lead to overwhelming feelings of helplessness and hopelessness.

Patient and Family Responses to Strokes and Neurological Injuries

When an individual has a neurological injury it often sets into motion a chain of events for the patient and family. The patient is rushed to the hospital and from that moment his life will be changed. For the immediate future, his life will be in the hands of other people. The person is often helpless to communicate his feelings of fear (terror) and confusion, or to decide what will be done to keep him alive. A formerly strong, independent person now may become a physically weak, dependent person with limited communication abilities. This rapid change in status can have a profound effect on how the person views himself and his relations with all of the people he cares about. Likewise, the family has immediate changes in their status and role in the life of the person. They initially must "take a back seat" in the life of their loved one and spend their time waiting, hoping, and praying that he will be all right.

SELF-IMAGE AND SELF-CONCEPT

Initially, after a neurological insult, a person may be comatose or semicomatose and, therefore, not aware of significant changes in his communication and cognitive functioning. However, when awareness emerges and the person begins to realize that not only is he having difficulty communicating, remembering, and recognizing other people, he may have obvious bandages and scars on his body, face, and head from a motor vehicle accident or neurosurgery. His self-image takes a blow, and mental confusion may add to his lack of understanding regarding his hospitalization and the medical procedures he is experiencing.

Not only does the person with the neurological impairment have an immediate alteration of his self-image, the family does also. The family may view themselves in a passive role during the immediate phase of medical treatment to keep their loved one alive and to minimize the brain damage. Like the person with neurological damage, the family often experiences a level of fear and confusion that is different from anything the family has undergone before. Often families have not had experience in problem-solving situations of this magnitude. The family endures a series of anxiety-provoking and life-altering events including anxious waiting in an emergency room; admission of their loved one to the hospital, possibly to a critical care unit; possible neurosurgery and wondering if it will be successful and their loved one will survive and recover; weeks to months of rehabilitation; and often having a loved one's levels of functioning altered forever.

Stages of Grief for the Patient and Family

Tanner (2003) discusses the tangible and symbolic losses that accompany neurological injuries and points out that the result of significant loss is grief. A tangible loss occurs when a person loses an important object, an ability or skill, or something or someone who is loved (such as through death); that is, the person is separated from a valued part of his life. However, when there is a tangible loss such as an ability or important skill, there is often also a symbolic loss that involves a person's self-concept. It is the change and diminishment of the self-concept that often is the most difficult for a person to adjust to.

Family members, particularly the healthy spouse, often feel the profound pain of loss. It is the loss of the dream of the expected future. At unexpected times the sense of loss can be overwhelming, and the healthy spouse grieves. If it is an acute illness or neurological insult, once the patient is medically stable, rehabilitation begins and there are signs of hope for everyone that the patient will improve. However, not all neurological disorders have an acute onset and then a long period of recovery and rehabilitation. Some neurological disorders are diseases, such as multiple sclerosis, muscular dystrophy, and Alzheimer's Disease, that may take a slow and insidious course and may more gradually impact the patient and his family. Family experiences can differ widely; some live with fear and a sense of emotional devastation while some families live with hope and faith in the midst of illness and loss. It is critical not to make assumptions about a particular family's responses but to engage them in discussions to learn how they are coping and understanding the situation.

Luterman (1995) describes his wife's chronic illness in his book *In the Shadows: Living and Coping with a Loved One's Chronic Illness*. The early symptoms of many progressive neurological diseases may be easy to ignore, deny, misdiagnose, and mistreat. For such chronic illnesses the patient may go through several physicians and diagnoses before the disease is diagnosed accurately. For the patient and family it is a roller coaster ride with no end in sight. There may be elation when there is an optimistic diagnosis and prognosis,

inadequate insurance, and time off work; and fear of the possibility that the injured spouse may never be able to help support the family again.

BARGAINING

In the bargaining stage family members may try to bargain with the medical staff, hoping there is something more the staff can do to make their loved one recover sooner. Family members bargain with rehabilitation therapists for extra physical therapy, occupational therapy, or speech therapy, wanting to know what the family can do to accelerate the patient's rehabilitation. Family members often bargain with God, committing their money and time to the church if only God will make their loved one all better. Some patients bargain with themselves saying they will never drive fast again or drink and drive. However, when bargaining does not change anything, patients and families usually move on to the depression stage.

DEPRESSION

Approximately 70 to 80 percent of patients survive a stroke, with major depression occurring in about 20 percent of patients and minor depression occurring in about another 20 percent of patients (some studies estimate depression post-stroke at nearly twice that amount). Most depression occurs within the acute period after the stroke; however, 10 to 20 percent of survivors develop either major or minor depression some months or even a year after the onset of the stroke. Depression is one of the major impediments to full physical and mental recovery from stroke (Canadian Stroke Network, 2006; Jia, Damush, Qin, et al., 2006; Dundas, 2006; Goodwin & Devanand, 2008; Williams, 2005). Patients who are depressed often have difficulty mustering the energy to participate fully in rehabilitation. They often "go through the motions" without appearing engaged in the therapy tasks. Clinicians need to be extra encouraging and reinforcing during this time to motivate patients to "try one more time," "stay with it," and "hang in there—you can do it."

Because depression is an expected stage of grief for patients with neurological disorders, physicians may let them "work through it" rather than prescribe antidepressant medications. However, depression during this stage of grief can be treated pharmacologically. Tricyclic antidepressants (TCAs) and selective serotonin reuptake inhibitors (SSRIs) have been shown to be particularly effective with stroke survivors (Davidson & Zhang, 2008; Holland, 2007). Because of the cognitive and communication problems of patients with neurological disorders, traditional "talk therapies" with mental health professionals may not be particularly effective. Typically, counseling with patients who have some degree of depression is often left to the SLP during individual therapy sessions. SLPs also have been conducting group therapy with patients and their families for decades, and group therapy is often helpful to patients (and their family members) who are depressed.

Group therapy allows new and old survivors to feel as though they are not alone with their problems, that others have experienced the same or similar difficulties and are working to manage their lives. Groups provide members a sense of community, and membership in communities has been shown to impact overall health and well-being. In addition, groups provide an excellent environment for language improvisation, which is important for creative language use. Group therapy can be beneficial to stroke and TBI survivors for many years following the termination of formal speech, language, and cognitive therapy

(Avent, 2004; Bernstein-Ellis & Elman, 2007; Elman, 2005, 2007; Ross, Winslow, & Marchant, 2006; Shadden & Agan, 2004).

Social isolation, not only of the person with a neurological disorder, but also the healthy spouse, is often the most devastating consequence of aphasia and a leading cause of depression after discharge from rehabilitation. Alarcon and Rogers (2007) discuss the supported communication intervention (SCI) approach to aphasia rehabilitation, which emphasizes the need for multimodality communication, partner training, and opportunities for social interaction. The three essential elements of the supported communication intervention approach include (1) incorporating augmentative and alternative communication, (2) training communication partners, and (3) promoting social communication, including participating in an aphasia group.

Family members often become depressed when they realize how long and slow the course of rehabilitation is going to be. When the acute phase is over and all but the core family members have returned home to resume their lives, the remaining family may feel abandoned and that an unmanageable weight has been placed on their shoulders. The family may try to hide their concerns and fears from the injured loved one, but often the person senses something is wrong.

Commonly, patients are discharged from the acute care hospital to return home before the family members have advanced to the acceptance level. Therefore, when the person returns home with all of his many needs for patience and loving care from family members, the family may not have the emotional energy to be good caregivers. They may go through the needed motions to provide for his basic needs, but they are still dealing with too many of their own emotions to be fully giving to a person who seems to never get enough.

Family members, like individuals who have sustained strokes or head injuries, benefit from the supportive environment present in group therapy. Family members often experience feelings of isolation, as though they are the only ones who have someone in their family who has ever had a stroke or TBI. When family members participate in group therapy with their loved one, they naturally make comparisons of their family member with the other people who have survived strokes or TBIs. If their family member is a fairly new survivor and still has relatively severe impairments, listening to and observing some of the other survivors who are longer post-onset and less severely affected may give family members hope that their loved one can continue to improve. Family members are likely to "connect" with certain other family members of survivors, and friendships may form that provide a new social outlet. As with the survivors, group therapy can help family members for many years after the onset of the stroke or TBI (Avent, 2004; Bernstein-Ellis & Elman, 2007; Elman, 2005, 2007; Ross, Winslow, & Marchant, 2006; Shadden & Agan, 2004). Groups also are excellent environments for families to develop self-advocacy projects to help their community better understand and appreciate the needs of individuals with neurological disorders (Pound, Parr, Lindsay, & Woolf, 2000).

Working with a Client Who Is Depressed

I supervised a man for several semesters who had been a successful automobile mechanic and taught automotive mechanics at a community college. He was also

Continues on next page

Continued from previous page

a stockcar race driver. He sustained a TBI in an accident during a practice run—the one time he did not wear his helmet. He was diagnosed with moderate to severe receptive and expressive aphasia, cognitive impairments, and apraxia. He often appeared depressed when he attempted to speak about his former work, his racing, and his family (his wife left him and he had little, if any, contact with his young daughter). The students working with the client were encouraged to use strategies that are discussed in Chapter 11 under Depression; however, I felt that his depressive symptoms also needed professional attention and referred him to the counseling psychology clinic at the university.

CLINICAL QUESTIONS

1. Would you refer a patient for a psychological evaluation or consultation who: (1) said he lost "everything" but he had a strong religious faith to help him cope, (2) said she could not think of a good reason to continue living, or (3) said he was having trouble getting out of his house (i.e., social withdrawal) since his accident?

2. The case example above illustrates that clinicians may use some counseling skills while also referring a patient for psychological services. What counseling skills would you use with the client above?

ACCEPTANCE

Acceptance involves an acknowledgement of the medical condition and its ramifications, including the symptoms, likely course of change over time, and functional impairments. Some patients with significant neurological losses and their families may struggle to achieve a state of acceptance, and may instead settle into a quiet *resignation* or *adaptation* to the way things are and the changes in their lives. Eventually, many stroke survivors and their families find an acceptable adjustment, but it is a different life than they had envisioned before the stroke.

Most patients learn to stop complaining about their losses, which give family and friends the impression that they have accepted their losses. They have learned that others tire of their complaints and that they get less sympathy and more angry responses from complaining as time goes on. Eventually, many patients try to make the most of what they have and are thankful that they are still alive and have people who care for them.

What may be more difficult for stroke survivors to accept are the changes in their lives, such as changes in the family structure and position within the family; changes in marital relations; decreased ability to be involved in their children's lives; loss of job or diminished responsibilities and job status; decreased energy level and increased fatigue; decreased social life and status in the community; embarrassment about their impairments; and so on. The rehabilitation phase involves not only acceptance of having a stroke or aphasia; it involves acceptance of the "new self" and its concomitant functional limitations.

In a 2002 Canadian study of well-being in 5,395 community-dwelling seniors after experiencing strokes, Clarke, Marshall, Black, and Colantonio found that, compared with community-dwelling seniors who had not experienced a stroke, stroke survivors reported a lower sense of well-being. Stroke survivors also were more likely to be restricted in their physical and cognitive functions, to report poorer mental health, and to be living with a greater number of comorbid health conditions. Overall, mental health and physical and cognitive disabilities were associated with a reduced sense of well-being in stroke survivors, but social supports and educational resources moderated the impact of functional status on well-being.

SLPs working with patients with all types of neurological disorders may be able to help their patients increase their sense of well-being by working on coping strategies and emphasizing their strengths more than their weaknesses. "Life coaching" principles and practices provide a pertinent model that clinicians could use in conjunction with more traditional counseling-based approaches (Holland, 2007). Coaching is a process grounded in wellness, and its emphasis is on normalcy and health, on correctly identifying sources of problems and teaching problem-solving skills to apply to them, and on developing and implementing relevant action plans. Coaching also focuses on differentiating those problems that are within a person's ability to control from those that are beyond their control. In a way, life coaching follows the principles of The Serenity Prayer: "God, grant me the serenity to accept the things I cannot change, the courage to change the things I can, and the wisdom to know the difference" (attributed to Reinhold Niebuhr, 1934, a Protestant theologian [Niebuhr, 1987]).

SLPs in medical and rehabilitation settings have limited time with most patients to accomplish their communication and swallowing goals. However, adjusting the emphasis to a wellness perspective may be a reasonable redirection from the more common medical model focus on treating the disorder. The emphasis on a wellness approach can begin early on and extend throughout therapy with patients. Teaching problem solving is commonly a part of therapy for cognitive impairments, and many clinicians incorporate problem-solving tasks into work with patients who have aphasia and swallowing disorders (see *The Source for Safety: Cognitive Retraining for Independent Living* [Fogle, Reece, & White, 2008]). It should be noted that this wellness perspective and the more traditional medical approach to patients are not mutually exclusive approaches. Clinicians may emphasize issues related to each model depending on the phase of treatment and what is required at the time.

Many patients with neurological impairments are discharged from rehabilitation services before they have fully worked through the depression stage and are moving into the acceptance stage. However, the groundwork may be laid during rehabilitation sessions for patients to focus more on what they can do rather than what they cannot do, identify sources of problems and the skills to solve them, and develop and implement action plans to solve or better cope with their limitations. Group therapy is one setting for continued focus on wellness as well as receiving some life coaching.

A Nurse's Aphasia

A male nurse in his early 40s had a CVA that resulted in receptive and expressive aphasia, cognitive impairments, and right-side hemiparesis. He received physical therapy, occupational therapy, and speech therapy at the acute-care hospital and in the rehabilitation unit. After being discharged from rehabilitation he learned that because of his impairments he had lost his job at the skilled nursing facility where he had worked for several years as a nurse. He was unmarried and had difficulty taking care of himself in his small apartment, but he was determined to be as independent as possible.

He began speech therapy at a university speech-language clinic and worked diligently and consistently for several semesters. His goal and motivation were always to return to nursing. He even brought in nursing textbooks to use as part of his therapy. The client made significant improvement during his semesters in the clinic, although he continued having difficulty with auditory comprehension, verbal expression, and cognition, as well as right-side hemiparesis and balance problems. He eventually became more realistic about returning to nursing work. He stopped attending therapy when he reached an acceptance and adjusted to his communication problems and his new self. As SLPs, we need to keep in mind that clients and patients will sometimes remain in therapy only until they reach their personal goals or have accepted their limitations, even though they may have potential for further improvement.

CLINICAL QUESTIONS

1. What kind of conversation might you have with a patient to encourage him to continue speech therapy even as he is reaching an acceptance of his new limitations?

2. What behavioral or cognitive signs might you expect to see if a mental health issue is affecting a patient's acceptance of his impairments?

The Family's Adjustment

Family members, like the person with the impairment, have many areas in which they must adjust or accept. The person returning home from the hospital may not be the same person who was taken to the hospital. (As the wife of one of my private clients said to her husband, "*You* never came home from the hospital.") The person returning home may seem somewhat like a stranger in his own home. He may look mostly the same, but he thinks, feels, and acts differently. Like the person with neurological damage, the family is thankful that their loved one survived and has made some recovery.

Acceptance of or resignation to the patient's current state is not a synonym for giving up. It is recognizing the reality of the person's condition, making room for changes, and moving on with life (Holland, 2007). Luterman (1995) describes the time when his wife used a wheelchair for the first time in an airport. He had wheeled her to an area to the side of the departure gate where there was another couple with a wife standing by her husband's wheelchair. As the wife and he exchanged glances he realized at a gut level that he was no longer like everyone else; he had joined a new fraternity and the other spouse was welcoming him to the "club"—a club neither of them wanted to join.

The spouses of patients who have had strokes typically function as caregivers in the home and community and provide informal care ranging from physical assistance to psychosocial support, all of which can be stressful and physically exhausting. As a result, these caregivers may experience high levels of burden that can result in anxiety, depression, and deterioration of health, social life, and well-being. Family physicians can be helpful in recognizing the signs and symptoms of caregivers who are overburdened, assessing as needed, and providing practical counseling about common caregiver stresses and about resources that benefit caregivers (Parks & Novielli, 2000).

Marital relationships are often affected, particularly when there is frontal lobe damage or a traumatic brain injury and there are significant personality changes. It is difficult to love a stranger, even if the person is the parent of your children. In many families the person who comes home from the hospital is never really accepted, and there is a high divorce rate among these couples (Leys, Bandu, Henon, Lucas, et al., 2002; Teasell, McRae, & Finestone, 2000). In a Swedish study of 121 couples on the psychosocial functioning of spouses of patients with strokes from the initial inpatient rehabilitation to three years post-stroke, Visser-Meily, Post, Meijer, and colleagues (2009) found that burden on the spouse decreased over time, but harmony in the relationship and social relations also decreased, and there was an overall long-term increase in depression of the healthy spouse. The authors concluded that follow-up of spouses of patients with stroke requires not only assessment of burden, but also other aspects of psychosocial functioning such as harmony in the relationship, depression, and social relations because of possible long-term negative consequences of stroke for these aspects of caregiver quality of life. SLPs need to be alert for signs of changes in adjustment in family members so that they can make appropriate referrals when needed.

Sometimes a stroke in the family represents the final stressor for a marriage that was already in trouble and the choice becomes fight or flight (*fight* may mean either continuing an unacceptable marriage relationship or fighting the increasing burden of the spouse's impairment). Luterman (1995) noted that when the healthy spouse feels continually and totally overwhelmed, flight (divorce or abandonment) is a possible response. However, fleeing can create feelings of guilt and loss of self-esteem. Therefore, many healthy spouses remain married but feel increasingly emotionally detached.

On the other hand, some spouses may opt for a divorce. As clinicians, we need to be careful not to be judgmental if the healthy spouse decides to leave or divorce the patient. We never know what the marital relationship was like before the person had the stroke, and this may be the "straw that broke the camel's back." However, for many couples (especially older couples), the illness experience brings them closer together, knowing that some parts of their lives will be changed forever. The bond remains strong, and the healthy spouse cares for the injured spouse as she would want to be cared for herself (Michallet, Tetreault, & Dorze, 2003).

Beyond feelings of concern for the loved one, family members may have some unexpected negative feelings, including anger that the person had the stroke or TBI. One man who had a stroke and needed neurosurgery woke up in the recovery room with his wife standing over him, not with an expression of gratitude that he had survived the stroke, but an expression of anger because, as she said, "You damn fool! You never took your blood pressure medicine and now look at you—you had a stroke!" Survivors of strokes may have strong feelings of guilt: they did not take care of their health properly and now they can no longer support their family and will be a burden to them. Family members also may have mixed feelings toward a motor vehicle accident survivor: gratitude that the person survived; anger for having gotten in the accident because of speeding; and resentment because the burden of care of the patient eventually will be on the family. MVA survivors may experience strong feelings of guilt, particularly if they were driving and a passenger in the car was injured or killed.

When the survivor of a stroke or TBI returns home, the caregiver may face many days, weeks, months and years of confusion, fear, isolation, loneliness, fatigue (exhaustion), sleeplessness, and other mentally and physically demanding stresses. They may feel trapped and hopeless. They may love the person but hate the burden placed on their lives. It is not uncommon for caregivers to become angry and resentful toward the person for whom they are caring. In addition, they may become greatly distressed that they could have such appalling reactions to the person they love and to whom they are dedicated. Anger and resentment are honest and frequent feelings of the unwanted, unplanned, and unwelcomed changes in the lives of caregivers. How these feelings are handled can affect the lives of all concerned (Broida, 1979; Lafond, DeGiovani, Joanette, Ponzio, & Sarno, 1993; Luterman, 1995; Tanner, 2008).

It helps many family members to learn that this anger and resentment toward their loved one is normal. It is helpful for family to understand the true nature of their feelings and not to deny them, bury them, or pretend they do not exist. Buried resentment and anger may emerge later in a disguised form, or be directed toward other people or towards oneself, resulting in depression, self-loathing, and hopelessness (Broida, 1979).

For some spouses there even may be the unthinkable fantasy of ultimate release from the painful situation—the death of the spouse. It is difficult for the healthy spouse to admit this death wish, but it is due to wanting to make this problem go away—not the spouse necessarily, but the stress of the situation. As would be expected, such thoughts generate enormous amounts of guilt. Death fantasies also may be helpful in preparing for the actual death of the spouse, an anticipatory mourning or something of a "dress rehearsal" (Luterman, 1995).

Out of guilt related to unexpected negative feelings, family members may overcompensate in their caregiving activities, doing for the person what the person really could do for himself. This may be become apparent when a family member tells the clinician that another family member is taking on a "martyr" role. The overcompensation assuages the family member's guilt, but it is also problematic. The more the well family member does for the impaired family member, the more the resentment builds, and then the more the guilt increases, and so on. Also, from the patient's perspective, the more that is done for him, the more he becomes dependent on others and the more they *have to* do for him. When such a vicious cycle begins, the caregiver and other family members could benefit from family therapy that is beyond the scope of practice of SLPs.

EFFECTS ON PARENT–CHILD RELATIONSHIPS AND INTERACTIONS

Brain injury can affect a person's energy and stamina, and the person may not have the same resources and patience to play with and enjoy his children. Both quantity and quality time with children are diminished, which in turn impacts the child's contact with the parent who has suffered a brain injury. Children in families in which a stroke occurs may be severely affected by the changes, not only in the parent who had the stroke but by changes in the entire dynamics of the family. A study conducted in the Netherlands by Visser-Meily, Post, Meijer, Maas, Ketelaar, & Lindeman (2005) investigated the clinical course and prediction of mood, behavior problems, and health status of children during the first year after a parent's stroke. The researchers interviewed 82 children (4 to 18 years of age) and their parents ($n = 55$) shortly after admission to a rehabilitation center, two months after discharge from inpatient rehabilitation, and one year later. Adjustment of the children was measured with the *Child Behavior Check List*, the *Child Depression Inventory*, and the *Functional Status II*. The results revealed that at the start of rehabilitation of the parent, 54 percent of the children had subclinical or clinical problems, which decreased to 29 percent one year after the parent's stroke. Children's functioning one year after the parent's stroke could best be predicted by their functioning at the start of rehabilitation. Spousal depression and perception of the marital relationship were also significant predictors of the child's adjustment. The authors emphasized that the results of their study demonstrate the need for a family-centered approach in stroke rehabilitation.

CASE STUDY

Dr. Johns—"An Easier Man to Live With Now"

Dr. Johns was a dentist by profession and a perfectionist by nature. He was not only demanding of himself but of others around him, especially his family. He had alienated his daughter, and his wife had recently divorced him. Following these family events, Dr. Johns had a severe stroke in his left hemisphere resulting in global aphasia, cognitive impairments, and significant changes in his personality. Dr. Johns' former wife (Marilyn), because she still cared for him, chose to move back into the family home to take care of him.

Marilyn brought Dr. Johns for therapy at a university clinic. She explained to the clinical supervisor that following the stroke, her husband began to have some personality changes. He began to "mellow" (normally, strokes do not improve a person's disposition; more commonly they exacerbate the worst of an individual's personality traits). Dr. Johns began functioning somewhat like an individual who had a frontal lobotomy. Marilyn stated "He is an easier man to live with now." They got along better; he was more appreciative of her and less demanding. His adult children also began to enjoy their father more, even though he could not verbally communicate his thoughts and feelings very well. From his family's perspective, Dr. Johns appeared to have become a better person.

Social Effects

Neurological disorders affect individuals and their families in many ways that extend beyond the home. When the person returns home, old friends may initially visit fairly frequently. However, because casual conversation with the injured person may be difficult and strained, visits become more irregular. Friends start making excuses for not visiting regularly, and then their visits may eventually end. The patient may find that he spends most of his time alone, often bored, which may turn into depression and even despair. The person with speech, language, or cognitive impairments may just want to have a quiet evening at home—every evening, while the healthy spouse may still want an active social life. One of the most difficult experiences people with neurological damage are confronted with is "reintroducing" themselves to friends and colleagues. Many people who have been very successful in their occupations and professions and have lived active social lives find that even their best and truest old friends begin to drop away. Families are expected to accept and love the person no matter what has happened to the person. However, as the old saying goes, "Blood is thicker than water." Many couples, on the other hand, find ways to meet the needs of both individuals and, although they may not do everything as a couple like they used to do, they still find ways to have enjoyable lives.

Most people who have sustained neurological damage are not able to return to their former jobs, or at least not at the level they once performed. Financial stresses as a result of not being employed, with only worker's compensation or disability insurance to contribute to the family budget, adds to the feelings of loss as a family provider. For most people, the work they do is an important part of their identity. When a person no longer has some place to be and something to do, he has lost two of the three necessities to feel life still has excitement, challenge, and meaning. The third necessity is someone to love.

Another common stressor for families who have a family member who has experienced a stroke is financial strain. The financial effects of having a brain injury can be devastating. Even with the best of insurance, there are still many expenses that come out of the pockets of the family. Time taken off work for the healthy spouse to care for the injured spouse during the acute stage may put an immediate strain on the family income. Insurance may pay for much of the medical care, but not all of it, and families often leave the hospital with extraordinary medical debts. The injured person's worker's compensation or disability insurance may not begin for several weeks or a few months after discharge from the hospital, and family savings may be drained. The family may need to borrow money from other family members or other sources, creating more strain within the entire family and putting the couple deeper in debt.

When the person who has neurological damage cannot return to work for months (or ever) a readjustment of family lifestyle is needed. Children's schooling may be affected and family vacations may be put on hold. The family has to "tighten its belt" and learn to live with a smaller portion of the income that they previously depended upon or enjoyed. However, many people make the adjustments, struggle through, and remain happy, cohesive families.

Quality of Life

The overall significance of a neurological disorder of any degree of severity becomes evident in the effect it has on the person's quality of life (QOL or QoL), or as is now used in medical literature, *health-related quality of life* (HRQOL) (Colwell, Mathias, Pasta, Henning, & Hunt, 1999). For many patients, the psychological reactions to their neurological impairments can be so prevalent that they can be considered part of the syndrome of these disorders. Agitation, fear, anxiety, confusion, panic attacks, depression, withdrawal, and crying can be as much a part of their disorders as the comprehension problems, word-finding difficulties, memory problems, and reading deficits (Tanner, 2003).

Concern for HRQOL emphasizes that intervention and treatment of illnesses and diseases has been expanded to include the person, not just the disease. Concern for quality of life represents a movement away from the traditional belief that the purpose of health care is solely to treat or cure specific impairments (e.g., hypertension, anxiety, aphasia) to a belief that the purposes of health care include helping the person adapt to or compensate for physical, psychological, and social effects of disease or physical impairments, as well as helping the person resume a productive and rewarding role in daily life (Brookshire, 2007).

Judgments of quality of life are typically rated based upon an individual's perceptions of life across various domains (e.g., *Stroke-Specific Quality of Life Scale*, Williams, Weinberg, Harris, Clark, & Biller, 1999; *Centers for Disease Control and Prevention Health-Related Quality-of-Life 14-Item Measure*, Centers for Disease Control and Prevention, 1995; *World Health Organization Quality of Life-BREF*, World Health Organization, 1998). There are individual differences regarding what is considered a good quality of life. What is considered an impoverished existence for some may be considered rich and rewarding by others (Tanner, 2003). However, because obtaining information from those who have communication disorders is often difficult, collateral sources (e.g., spouses, parents, children) may help professionals to assess a patient's quality of life.

In addition to general quality-of-life scales, the ASHA *Quality of Communication Life Scale* (QCL), developed by Paul, Frattali, Holland, and associates (2004), was designed to permit individuals who have significant language impairments to rate their quality of communicative life. The ASHA QCL provides information about the impact of a communication disorder on an adult's relationships; communication interactions; participation in social, leisure, work, and educational activities; and overall quality of life. It is intended to provide information about the psychosocial, vocational, and educational effects of having a communication impairment. The average time it takes to complete the scale is 15 minutes. The QCL is considered a valid measure of the quality of communication life as a distinct, but related, aspect of general quality of life, and is valid for adults with neurogenic

Continued from previous page

rather than just physically. Had the patient received a G-tube months before, he could have had the comfort of his wife's hand on his, meeting both of their emotional needs. Sometimes we can only watch in sadness as medical decisions are made that we may not feel take into consideration the patient as a whole person.

CLINICAL QUESTIONS

1. How might you use quality-of-life considerations as a rationale to tactfully discuss with a physician your recommendations that are in disagreement with the medical recommendations?

2. How would you (or would you) present your recommendations (as discussed above) to a family member?

ANXIETIES, FEARS, AND FRUSTRATIONS

Anxiety and fear are discussed in some detail in Chapter 11. However, for patients who have swallowing problems the anxiety and fear are around a biological function rather than a communication function (Ekberg, Hamdy, Woisard, Wuttge-Hannig, & Ortega, 2002). We all know what it is like to cough and choke on some food or liquid, and we know that we will be OK and are not going to choke to death. Patients with dysphagia may not always have that same assurance. If they are not silent aspirators, they may have experienced severe episodes of choking and difficulty "catching their breath." This is very frightening. People have choked to death.

Patients may experience a variety of fears around eating, for example, fear of embarrassment in front of family and friends who visit during meal time; fear of an acute or chronic illness (aspiration pneumonia) or even death because of aspiration; fear of the discomfort of suctioning food or liquid out of the oral cavity, trachea and lungs; fear that they may never be able to eat their favorite foods (at least with a normal texture) and have normal thin liquids again; and other fears. It is strange to think that what people do for enjoyment (i.e., eating) could become such a source of anxiety and fear. One of the symptoms of dysphagia is weight loss. Patients who are having difficulty swallowing foods and liquids tend to eat and drink less, which results in malnutrition and dehydration.

Patients also may experience frustrations as a result of being hospitalized because of being away from family, being off work, experiencing dramatic changes in daily routines, not having favorite personal items easily available, and so on. These normal hospital frustrations are added to food or liquid consistency restrictions, not being able to eat their favorite foods, being told how to eat and drink and follow specific safe-eating instructions, and others. We sometimes wonder why patients are irritable or grumpy and not happy to see us, but if we consider their losses we can be more empathetic toward our patients.

LOSS OF ENJOYMENT AND INDEPENDENCE

People who lose their ability to swallow normally have a sense of loss of an important part of their lives—the enjoyment of a relaxed meal. It is difficult, if not impossible, to have a relaxed meal when a person is concerned about what she has to do with every bite of food and sip of liquid to prevent herself from coughing, choking, and aspirating. Many patients have an imposed change of diet to mechanical soft or even puree textures with thickened liquids. There is a sense of loss of independence—not being able to eat "what I want when I want it." Patients are advised that when they return home alcoholic drinks may affect their ability to consciously and methodically swallow in the prescribed manner. A glass of wine or a beer may have little or no effect on swallow-safety procedures, but beyond that there is no guarantee. For some patients there is the loss of having a glass (or more) of wine, beer, or a cocktail as a way of relaxing (Ekberg, Hamdy, Woisard, Wuttge-Hannig, & Ortega, 2002).

When people lose lifelong natural abilities, they can lose a secure sense of self. They have to readjust their self-images and self-concepts, and that takes time. Very few, if any, patients receive counseling from any professional (including SLPs) about the emotional struggles they are dealing with around their swallowing problems (Ekberg, Hamdy, Woisard, Wuttge-Hannig, & Ortega, 2002). Many patients struggle in silence, complaining and grumbling sometimes, but never "talking through" their sense of loss of who they were as a person.

Emotional and Social Effects on Family

The husband or wife of a patient has vowed to care for the person "in sickness and in health." However, even after years of loving and caring for the person, seeing a spouse struggle with one of the simplest—and most public—functions can be confusing and disturbing. Spouses and family members who are empathic recognize and understand their loved one's emotional struggles of anxiety, fear, depression, grief, and embarrassment. Nevertheless, the spouses or family members may face their own fears. For example, they may feed the person meals and try to carefully follow the directions of the SLP or nurse. They may feel nervous about doing it "just right" and fear that if a mistake is made, it could cause their loved one to aspirate. The one feeding the person with dysphagia will likely feel some guilt if the person coughs and chokes on a bite of food or sip of liquid. The fear of injuring a loved one and the guilt that accompanies the times when the person aspirates and coughs and chokes can discourage the spouse and family from trying to help. Feeding the person may be a loving gesture, but it can be fraught with distressing emotions. As clinicians, we need to be both instructive and supportive of family members who are trying to help their loved ones. Most people are doing the best they can with the resources (time, energy, patience, tolerance, etc.) they have. Taking care of a sick or injured family member is wearing and usually "gets old" very fast.

Quality of Life Issues

The quality of life of the patient is always the most important concern in all aspects of patient care (Bruni, Mosconi, Boeri, et al., 2000; Chen, Frankowski, Bishop-Leone, et al., 2001;

Cox, Fitzpatrick, Fletcher, et al., 1992; Stephens, Hopwood, Girling, & Machin, 1997; Watt & Whyte, 2003), and dysphagia can have a significant impact on a person's quality of life (Bennett & Steele, 2006). When a person cannot eat regular textured foods or drink thin liquids, or has to be concerned about the possibility of coughing and choking on each bite of food and sip of liquid, the enjoyment of food and drink are significantly reduced and, thereby, the quality of life. The 44-item *Swallowing-Related Quality of Life* (SWAL-QOL) (Langmore, 2000; McHorney, Robbins, Lomax, et al., 2002; McHorney, Martin-Harris, Robbins, & Rosenbek, 2006; Daniels, Schroeder, DeGeorge, Corey, Foundas, & Rosenbek, 2009) was developed to assess patients' self-reports of their quality of life with dysphagia. The SWAL-QOL has been translated into other languages, such as French and Dutch. By monitoring functional outcomes with tools like the SWAL-QOL in clinical practice, physicians, SLPs, and other health care and rehabilitation providers may be able to better assess and adjust their treatment of dysphagia. Data addressing patient perceptions of social dining, food selection, and burden of help document the effectiveness of any given treatment on quality of life.

CONCLUDING COMMENTS

It is important to view and work holistically with patients who have neurological disorders and recognize the inevitable emotional and social reactions to their impairments. Because many of these patients have complex problems, good counseling skills are crucial when working with them and their families. Patients and families are under tremendous stress when there is a sudden neurological insult and are confused about all that is happening. Both the patient and family may begin going through the stages of grief, each in their own way. The need for and focus of counseling changes as the patient progresses in rehabilitation. Following most any kind of significant neurological injury there are effects on the quality of life of both the patient and family.

Patients with swallowing disorders often have emotional reactions to their problems, and most would benefit from an open discussion with their SLP about their concerns. Patients often develop anxieties, fears, and frustrations around eating and drinking. Some patients also may go through the stages of grief when they realize that they will have a chronic swallowing disorder. Quality-of-life issues are also important for people who have swallowing disorders and clinicians can be sensitive to these issues as they discuss interventions and realistic expectations with their patients.

Discussion Questions

1. What is meant by the phrase "a stroke in the family"?

2. Why would a family systems counseling approach be particularly helpful with patients who have neurological disorders?

3. What are some of the stresses that may be placed on patients who have neurological impairments?

4. How could denial of impairments be dangerous for some patients?

5. What kind of information do family members need when they are in the denial stage of grieving?

6. What are some of the underlying feelings of patients who are angry?

7. What are some things you need to be aware of with family members who are in the bargaining stage of grief?

8. What would you try to do to help a patient who is depressed to keep her working in therapy?

9. Discuss the benefits of group therapy for individuals who have neurological disorders and their families.

10. Why might some patients with significant neurological losses struggle to achieve a state of acceptance? Why might their families struggle with acceptance?

11. What are some of the emotional and social effects of swallowing disorders that patients may experience?

12. What are some of the emotional and social effects on the family that may occur with a person who has a swallowing disorder?

13. Why is the quality of life of the patient an important concern in all aspects of patient care?

Role Plays

1. Ask two students to role play a couple in which one of them recently has had a stroke. Two additional students can role play the SLPs. The well spouse complains to the SLPs that her husband is not getting out of bed, prefers to sleep most of the day, and wants the well spouse to do everything for him. Have a clinical discussion in which the SLPs explore the patient's symptoms, help the couple to understand what may be happening, and discuss what adjustments to their schedule and routine may be feasible.

2. Have student pairs role play a patient with a swallowing disorder and an SLP. The patient reports that she has canceled all of her usual weekly luncheons with her friends. The SLP is concerned because this is the main social activity the patient has during the week. Role play a clinical discussion in which the SLP explores the patient's recent changes to her social routine and makes suggestions for strategies that will help the patient stay socially engaged.

Counseling for Adults and Children Who Have Hearing Loss

Nancy Tye-Murray, Ph.D., CCC-A
Professor, Washington University School of Medicine
Department of Otolaryngology
St. Louis, MO

CHAPTER OUTLINE

INTRODUCTION

Hearing loss often has pernicious and pervasive consequences for adults. In the home, casual conversation may diminish or even disappear, and familial relationships may lose some of the nuanced intimacy that stems from talking about everyday life occurrences. In the workplace, hearing loss may erode an adult's effectiveness and sense of self-efficacy and might result in lost opportunities and fewer conversational interactions between colleagues and clients. Social interactions for the adult with hearing loss may become more effortful and less rewarding, and the temptation to avoid them altogether may become increasingly attractive. Counseling, in conjunction with traditional audiological services such as a hearing aid fitting, can serve to alleviate some of these consequences. In the first part of this chapter, we review counseling for adults.

The consequences of hearing loss for children are perhaps even more far reaching. Hearing loss incurred at an early age may affect children's acquisition of speech and language, as well as impede their everyday listening. It may also hinder children's development of social skills and world knowledge and their later academic achievement. Hearing-related counseling is often directed towards the family, especially when the hearing loss is identified in infancy or early childhood. About 90 percent of parents of babies who have hearing loss have normal hearing themselves, and so they are typically unfamiliar with the ramifications of significant hearing loss and are uninformed about potential interventions. In the latter part of this chapter, we review counseling for children and families of children who have hearing loss.

ADULTS WHO HAVE HEARLING LOSS

We are social creatures, and spoken language is how we most readily connect with one another. When one of the communication partners has a hearing loss, conversational fluency becomes impaired. Conversational fluency pertains to how readily we can exchange information and ideas through spoken language and is reflected by the ease in which we can select and discuss topics, the occurrence of communication breakdowns, and the sharing of speaking time. In a conversation in which one communication partner has a significant hearing loss, the communication partner with normal hearing may have to repeat and restructure messages many times and may have to tailor remarks so that they are more readily received. The communication partner with normal hearing may have to speak with only commonly used words and simple syntax and may be limited to speaking about commonplace topics, such as the weather or a popular sports team. The communication partner with hearing loss may often request communication repair ("Huh?" "Can you say that again?" "Jane is going to do what?") and/or may bluff and pretend to understand. By doing so, the communication partner with hearing loss breaks at least one of two implicit maxims of conversation, *receive readily* and *recognize genuinely* (Tye-Murray, Mauzé, & Schroy, 2010). These maxims stipulate that when we engage in conversation, we will understand the gist of what our communication partner is saying (i.e., *recognize genuinely*) and that we will not require our communication partner to expend undue effort in conveying the intended message (i.e., *receive readily*). A conversational maxim is a general rule of conduct during conversation (Grice, 1975). Unfortunately, the net result is that the conversations may sometimes not be very rewarding for either the communication partner with normal hearing or the one with impaired hearing, as the conversations may be marred by poor conversational fluency and by violation of socially accepted conversational maxims and conventions. A major goal of aural rehabilitation is to promote conversational fluency.

Receive Readily, Recognize Genuinely

At least two maxims govern the conduct of listeners during casual conversations:

■ Receive readily

■ Recognize genuinely

When we engage in a conversation, we enter into an implicit agreement with our conversational partners that we care about what they are saying and that we are willing to expend the necessary effort to ensure that we understand their intended messages. For listeners with normal hearing, the first maxim governing listening behavior stipulates that they pay attention to what their conversational partner is saying and not be distracted by other activities, such as reading text messages while simultaneously listening. The second maxim stipulates that they seek clarification when they do

Continues on next page

Continued from previous page

not grasp a spoken message. When a conversational partner has a hearing loss, these maxims may present an either/or situation. For example, Tye-Murray and colleagues (2010) analyzed the videotaped conversations of two cochlear implant users, "Frank" and "Roger," as they each spoke with a woman who had normal hearing, "Liz." Frank followed the first maxim at the expense of the second, whereas Roger followed the second maxim at the expense of the first. Frank frequently bluffed and pretended to understand so he appeared to receive readily but he did not recognize genuinely. His conversation progressed smoothly until Liz realized that he had not recognized a name she had mentioned, but he had gone along with the conversation, acting as if he knew this named person. When a panel of judges viewed this conversation, one noted that Frank was not very "honest" about not understanding, and another noted, "I'd rather repeat myself multiple times than have someone pretend to understand me." In contrast to Frank, Roger was determined to recognize genuinely, and as a result, he did not receive readily. His conversation with Liz was marred by a communication breakdown that lasted over a quarter of the conversation, and was belabored by extensive attempts at repair (e.g., "Please repeat" "Would you run it by me again?" "Studies? Did I get that part right?" "I'm still not getting that. Just what does that involve?"). In a 10-minute conversation, he used 31 repair strategies in an attempt to repair communication breakdowns, as compared to Frank's use of eight. Some of the judges from the viewing panel noted that Roger was not very easy to have a conversation with, and that his conversation with Liz lacked "flow." As these two examples illustrate, sometimes individuals with hearing loss are in a no-win situation, in which they have to choose between adhering to one conversational maxim at the expense of violating another. Being unable to follow widely accepted maxims of conversation, as well as the inordinate effort and anxiety sometimes involved in trying to listen, lip-read, and repair breakdowns in communication no doubt exercise a psychoemotional cost and may be reasons that some persons with hearing loss avoid engaging in casual conversations.

Types of Counseling

The counseling that is provided during the course of aural rehabilitation is largely *informational counseling*, which concerns the nature of the hearing loss and the use of the hearing aid. Typically, the patient learns about the degree of hearing loss, the configuration of the loss, and the effects of this loss on his or her ability to understand speech. The patient receives information about treatment options and then, once a hearing aid or other listening device has been fitted, the patient receives information about the device itself.

Less often, the patient receives *personal adjustment counseling*, where the focus is on the patient's psychological, social, and emotional acceptance of the hearing loss and its concomitant consequences. Topics that might be included during personal adjustment counseling include how to increase one's self-esteem, how to manage communication interactions assertively, how to deal with feelings of isolation, and how to deal with negative feelings related to hearing loss, such as anger and isolation. During personal adjustment counseling, the patient may be asked about his or her reactions to hearing loss, motivations for seeking audiological help, and willingness to try using a hearing aid or to consider other aural rehabilitation interventions. One reason for its rarity may be that many speech and hearing professionals are uncomfortable or may not feel adequately trained in providing this kind of counseling. Another may simply be that the time constraints associated with a busy audiological practice limit the topics that can be discussed.

Although there may be distinct times when the audiologist provides solely informational counseling, as when describing how to insert a battery into a hearing aid, and times when the audiologist provides solely personal adjustment counseling, as when discussing a patient's hearing-related insecurities, ideally, informational counseling and personal adjustment counseling are interwoven such that the audiologist provides information but is also responsive to and supportive of the patient's mental and emotional states. The following two exchanges illustrate the difference between providing informational counseling alone and interweaving informational counseling with personal adjustment counseling. The audiologist has just finished summarizing the audiology test results to a first-time patient.

> Audiologist: "Ms. Watkins, people with a moderate-to-severe bilateral hearing loss often do well with two hearing aids."
>
> Ms. Watkins: "A hearing aid? I didn't realize that my hearing was that bad. After all, I hear all right most of the time."
>
> Audiologist: "The test results suggest that you are only recognizing about 50 percent of the test words. Your hearing loss is probably causing you communication problems throughout your day. Once you try using hearing aids, you may realize just how much you've been missing all this time."

The audiologist is providing information and probably too much of it: the hearing loss is significant, the patient could benefit from wearing not only one but *two* hearing aids, and the patient is missing out on daily conversation unawares. The possible result here is an impasse, with the patient asserting that her hearing loss isn't problematic and the audiologist implying that Ms. Watkins isn't taking ownership of her listening problems. The patient hasn't entertained the idea of wearing one hearing aid and yet here is the audiologist recommending two. The stage has been set for frustration and dissatisfaction for both audiologist and patient.

In this alternative exchange, the audiologist interweaves both informational and personal adjustment counseling.

> Audiologist: "The test results seem to confirm what you shared with me, Ms. Watkins. People with this kind of hearing loss often have difficulty understanding when there is noise in the background."
>
> Ms. Watkins: "That's why I'm eating at my desk these days instead of trying to join everyone in our cafeteria. It's so loud there."
>
> Audiologist: "Sounds like you might be missing socializing and relaxing with your co-workers at lunch."
>
> Ms. Watkins: "Yeah (smiles ruefully), but I get to skim the newspaper while I'm eating, so it's not all bad. But I do miss being a part of things."

Audiologist: "With the kind of hearing loss that you have, Ms. Watkins, we might be able to improve your ability to hear in the cafeteria. Would you be interested in exploring the possibilities?"

Ms. Watkins: "I'd certainly like to learn about my options."

In this alternative exchange, the audiologist provides information, but does so in the context of the patient's perspective. The audiologist acknowledges that the patient is likely having problems in understanding speech and verbally acknowledges and sympathizes with the patient's reactions to these problems. The audiologist does not assume that Ms. Watkins is ready to consider hearing aids, but instead initiates a dialogue so that the two of them can begin to consider various interventions.

Sometimes patients ask for more in-depth counseling in order to deal with some of the psychological and social consequences of hearing loss and to hearing-related stress. *Hearing-related stress* includes the stress of adjusting to a new self-concept (e.g., "I used to be able-bodied and now I'm not"), the stress of living with reduced conversational fluency, and the stress of living with the reactions of society to people who have communication difficulties and a physical disability. Psychosocial support is a kind of counseling that helps patients acquire long-term self-sufficiency in managing the social and psychological challenges associated with hearing-related communication difficulties. It typically is provided in a group-session format (e.g., Hogan, 2001), although it is rarely provided in most audiological clinic settings.

Solution-Centered Interventions

Aural rehabilitation for adults is often considered a "solution-centered intervention process" (e.g., Gagné & Jennings, 2000). The patient arrives at an audiological clinic and reports a problem—"I'm not hearing on the telephone like I used to," or "The wife tells me I'm not listening right"—and the audiologist sets about devising a solution, ideally with the patient acting in willing partnership. For example, the patient reports difficulty in conversing with business clients over the telephone. The solution might be a telephone amplifier. The patient's wife complains that he does not hear well during their weekly neighborhood bridge games. The solution may be binaural hearing aids with directional microphones for him and a pamphlet describing repair strategies for rectifying communication breakdowns for her.

This solution-centered approach is described in more detail in Table 9-1. It entails a precise identification of the problem and then specific objectives to be achieved. For instance, for the patient who cannot hear well in background noise, an objective might be "Mr. Hanley will understand his friends' remarks during their weekly bridge game and Mrs. Hanley will assist in communication repair in those instances when communication breakdowns occur." The counseling that occurs during a comprehensive audiological examination can best be described as informational counseling, and its progression is represented in Table 9-1. Hearing-related difficulties are identified and prioritized, desired outcomes are clearly articulated, and possible solutions are reviewed. A number of instruments have been designed to accommodate the progression depicted in Table 9-2. For example, the *Client Oriented Scale of Improvement* (COSI; Dillon, James, & Ginis, 1997) asks the patient to nominate up to five situations where he would like to improve communication, in order of importance. At the end of the intervention, the patient reviews the list and indicates how much better or worse the situation is as a result of the audiological intervention. The *Glasgow Hearing Aid Benefit Profile* (GHAP; Gatehouse, 1999) is another instrument that offers a similarly structured approach. Taken together, the approach described in Table 9-1 and the informational counseling depicted in Table 9-2 characterize the experience that many patients receive when they interact with audiologists and other speech and hearing professionals.

TABLE 9-1 The Sequence of Events Stipulated in a Solution-Centered Approach to Aural Rehabilitation

Solution-Centered Intervention Process	
Parameterize the Problem	Acknowledge that a real problem exists.
	Identify the problem that needs to be addressed.
	Analyze and define components of the problem.
	Determine goals to achieve desired outcome.
Explore Solutions	Brainstorm and identify as many different solutions as possible.
	For each solution identified, evaluate pros and cons associated with the solution.
Evaluate	Select one (or more) acceptable solution(s) from possibilities.
	Implement the solution(s) one at a time or together.
	Evaluate the success or failure of the solution(s).
	Identify the factors that helped or hindered the application of the solution(s).
	Repeat steps until desired outcome is achieved.

Source: Based on the work of Gagné & Jennings, 2000, p. 569.

TABLE 9-2 Setting Priorities within a Solution-Centered Approach

Hearing-Related Difficulty	Priority	Expectation	Possible Solution(s)
Understanding speech at a business meeting	2	Patient will follow and understand flow of conversation 95% of the time	• Hearing aid • Assertiveness training • Communication Strategies training • Environmental accommodations
Understanding speech on a cell phone	3	Patient will be able to understand clients' orders and requests via cell phone	• Hearing aid • Neck loop for cell phone or hands-free device • Speaker phone
Listening to speech in the car	1	Conversation with wife or client in car will be successful 100% of the time	• Hearing aid • Communication strategies training • Environmental accommodations • Assistive listening device/FM system

Source: *Delmar/Cengage Learning*

There is much merit in the solution-centered intervention approach. Treatment outcome is assessed in terms of how well the presenting complaint(s) is alleviated, so there is real accountability in terms of success and failure. Counseling is focused on managing communication-related problems, and patients often gain a sense of empowerment and self-efficacy as they overcome these problems. Moreover, the approach pragmatically accommodates the fiscal realities of today's audiological clinics, where patient visits are often tightly scheduled and where getting to the business of addressing complaints straightaway ensures that time is spent most efficiently.

In the real world of providing services to persons with hearing loss and their family members, the service delivery model described in Tables 9–1 and 9–2 is less formulaic and less contingent on patient report and test results than would appear, and is more pliant and reliant upon the personal adjustment counseling skills of the speech and hearing professional than either would suggest. For example, an older patient might state that his number one priority is to enhance his ability to enjoy his television-viewing experience. This patient spends most of his day watching hourly news broadcast shows, and his wife complains that he keeps the volume set at too loud a setting. Upon careful questioning and insightful commenting, his audiologist discovers that the patient watches an inordinate amount of television because he cannot communicate easily with his family members. The patient believes that his wife mumbles when she talks to him, that his grandchildren don't enjoy his company, and that his own children leave him out of their conversations. While discussing his audiogram, the patient reveals that at the last Thanksgiving dinner gathering, family members talked about him behind his back (he was sure of this!), and that this was most disconcerting. In short, his present means of staying connected to the world is through news broadcasts and not through human contact. In this instance, hearing loss is affecting this man's emotional well-being and self-perception and is interfering with his ability to play the roles of husband, father, and grandfather and perhaps the roles of neighbor and community member. The man may not realize that he is withdrawing from daily life, and he may not associate his feelings of despondency and low-grade anxiety to his loss of everyday conversation. Superficially, a solution-centered approach might point to the provision of a television-related assistive listening device. However, because the audiologist interwove informational counseling with personal adjustment counseling and took the time to listen to the patient and draw the patient out by sharing insightful comments and questions, a different, more appropriate treatment plan is devised, one that is targeted towards enhancing conversational fluency between the patient and his family members. The desired outcome is that the patient will begin to spend more time interacting with his family members and less time watching television news. An example such as this points to the importance of both types of counseling and to the importance of a patient-centered orientation.

A Patient-Centered Orientation

The most effective way to effect a solution-based intervention is to implement it within the context of a patient-centered orientation. A patient-centered orientation will help ensure that the appropriate problems are targeted in the intervention plan and that realistic solutions are considered. In the course of establishing a patient orientation the speech and hearing professional will identify hearing-related difficulties, probe the significance of each one for the patient, and learn about the patient's expectations and attitudes about interventions such as a hearing aid.

A patient orientation stipulates that services provided be based on the patient's background, current status, needs, and wants. Two counseling skills are crucial for actualizing this orientation. The first skill is an ability to assess how hearing loss might be affecting a patient as a person and as a member of a family and a society. The second skill is to help the patient identify and articulate those inchoate or difficult-to-admit hearing-related difficulties.

One means to assess who the patient is as a person is to consider the factors reviewed in Table 9-3. These factors include the patient's age; stage of life; life factors; gender; socioeconomic status; ethnicity and culture; social, vocational, and home communication difficulties; and psychological well-being. The center column of Table 9-3 provides a description of each factor and the right column provides examples of how each factor might affect the intervention plan. Because of these factors, patients will vary greatly in the services and support they need. To illustrate, we can contrast two patients, a mid-career sales associate who has a wife and three teenage children and an older woman who is a housewife, mother, and grandmother. The sales associate has lost his job in a down economy. His audiogram reveals a bilateral mild to moderate hearing loss. He is bedeviled with doubts about whether to use hearing aids: Will their use make him look old as he applies for a new job? Can he afford it with college tuition bills looming ahead? Is this yet another sign that he is losing competency? He knows that he must communicate easily with co-workers and clients if he is to succeed as a salesman, but he is having difficulty accepting ownership of his hearing problems, much less agreeing to purchase and wear a hearing aid. In contrast, the grandmother with a similar mild to moderate hearing loss is unconcerned about the implications of wearing hearing aids—she is quite comfortable with her senior citizen status—but she worries whether she can handle the device, given her arthritic hands and her ignorance of technology. The counseling needs for these two patients will likely be quite different.

TABLE 9-3	Variables to Consider when Adopting a Patient-Centered Orientation	
Variable	**Description**	**Influence on AR Plan**
Age	Chronologic and/or cognitive age of patient	Types of activities used may vary for different ages and abilities.
Socioeconomic Status	Status in society based on income, occupation, education, and dwelling type	This can influence patient's ability to afford hearing aids or other assistive devices, ability to attend scheduled classes due to work commitments, transportation availability, etc.
Stage of Life	Age ranges in which a hearing loss may have a different impact	The needs of a young person just starting his or her career are vastly different from someone established in a profession or nearing the end of his or her work life.

Continues on next page

Continued from previous page

Variable	Description	Influence on AR Plan
Race, Ethnicity, and Culture	A confluence of biological factors, geographic origins, economic, political, and legal factors, thoughts, communications, actions, customs, values, and beliefs	These may impact how a person interacts with health care professionals and may involve the need of an interpreter.
Life Factors	Conditions that help define one's life such as relationships, family, and vocation	A person whose job involves lots of communication on the phone or in person has different needs from someone who works on a computer most of the day. In the same way, a person with a spouse, children, and extended family will have different needs than someone who lives alone and does not have much family.
Degree of Hearing Loss	Amount of hearing loss, ranging from mild to profound in degree	The more significant the patient's hearing loss, the more difficulty he or she may have and the more need for intervention. Milder losses may need more training in noise while more severe losses may need more lip-reading practice.
Social, Vocational, and Home Communication Difficulties	Where and how patients spend their day	How active a person is in society and what types of situations they are in most of the day impacts their needs for rehabilitation. Some may need more communication strategies, while others may need training in noise.
Psychological Well-Being	Psychological and emotional state	Hearing loss can compound or exacerbate loneliness, depression, and other psychological issues. These patients may need more psychosocial components included in their intervention plan and may need a referral to a professional counselor to help deal with these issues.
Other Hearing-Related Complaints	Impairments related to hearing loss such as tinnitus	Tinnitus retraining therapy may become part of an intervention program if this is debilitating to the person.

Source: Based on Tye-Murray, 2009.

The second counseling skill is to help patients identify and articulate problems and to encourage them to pursue solutions. Many of the interviewing techniques and therapy microskills discussed in earlier chapters of this text review communication skills that will encourage patients to verbalize their concerns and thoughts. When interacting with adults who have hearing loss, it is important to listen without interruption and to talk openly. Open-ended questions may reveal issues that would not have been revealed with simple *yes-no* questions. Empathy can be a powerful tool. One empathy-related technique is to introduce hypothetical situations or people. For example, when reviewing the audiogram with an older patient, one audiologist said, "Many people who have this kind of hearing loss tell me that they can't understand their grandchildren, especially if they are in a noisy room. Can you recall similar situations, Ms. Moore?" Initiating questions with phrases such as, "Do you recall . . . ?" and "Do you think of . . . ?" encourages a patient to give thoughtful, detailed answers, and there is no implication that there is a right or wrong response.

Aural Rehabilitation Intervention

An aural rehabilitation plan for an adult patient usually unfolds sequentially, beginning with an audiological evaluation and consultation, followed by an intervention such as a hearing-aid fitting or cochlear implant surgery, and sometimes including other interventions such as group sessions or psychosocial support.

During the audiological evaluation, the audiologist collects a case history, conducts audiological testing, shares the test results with the patient and possibly a patient's family member, and then discusses what happens next. The case history entails listening carefully to why the patient has decided to come for the evaluation and often begins with the question, "What brought you here today?" The case history affords an opportunity to address those two questions we just considered, "Who is the patient?" and "What are the patient's listening difficulties?". Sometimes the patient will complete a self-report survey or questionnaire that will assess activity limitations and participation restrictions and indicate communication challenges in home, work, and social environments. Examples of these questionnaires include *The Hearing Handicap Inventory for the Elderly* (HHIE; Ventry & Weinstein, 1982) and *The Communication Profile for the Hearing Impaired* (CPHI; Demorest & Erdman, 1987).

Audiological testing determines degree and type (i.e., sensorineural, conductive, mixed) of hearing loss. The assessment entails collecting a pure-tone audiogram and performing speech testing. Speech testing usually determines the softest level at which patients can recognize spondees with 50 percent accuracy (called the *speech reception threshold*) and how well the patient can recognize monosyllabic words that are loud enough for the patient to hear (called *speech recognition*). How test results are described will depend on the background and emotional state of the patients. For instance, the language used to describe an audiogram to an electrical engineer will be very different than that used to describe an audiogram to an adult who has a seventh-grade education. The language used with someone who has long suspected a hearing loss will differ from that used for someone who is only at the appointment in order to prove a family member is wrong in asserting that a hearing loss exists. Table 9-4 presents some general *Do's* and *Don't's* for describing test results to patients. These are guidelines only, and should be followed with flexibility as the situation warrants.

TABLE 9-4	Do's and Don't's for Describing an Audiogram to a Patient		
	DO	**DON'T**	**Example**
Describing the audiogram	DO: Include significant other or family member in the session if they are at the appointment. Two sets of ears are better than one when it comes to listening to the results.	DON'T: Exclude people at the appointment who may be in the waiting room unless the patient requests that they be excluded. The family members can provide a wealth of information.	
	DO: Keep it simple. Try and relate everything to what the patient knows.	DON'T: Use a lot of jargon. Even words audiologists use daily like *frequency* and *decibel* may seem confusing to some people.	"You heard lots of different beeps. Some were low pitched like a foghorn and some were higher pitched like a bird chirping. This graph tells us how loud we need to turn things up for you to just barely hear these sounds that are important for speech."
	DO: Write information down so the patient can remember what you said later.	DON'T: Assume the patient understands everything you tell him or her. It is a lot of information to take in, especially for a new patient. Often people are coming in for an audiological evaluation because family members think there is a problem and you are the first person to confirm that fact.	Make a copy of the audiogram and make notes on it or let the patient or family member take notes on it as you talk so they have something to take with them.
	DO: Describe what type of hearing loss (sensorineural, conductive, or mixed) the patient has. Focus on what this type of loss means for him or her more than the label.	DON'T: When describing the type of hearing loss, don't get too detailed and confuse matters.	"When you heard the beeps through the headband we put behind your ear, we found the hearing loss is in the nerve, or what we call sensorineural. This means that we can't 'fix' the hearing loss with surgery or medication."

Continues on next page

Table 9-4. *Continued from previous page*

	DO	DON'T	Example
	DO: Relate the hearing loss back to the problems the patient reported having in the case history.	DON'T: Explain the hearing loss and audiogram without any referent that the patient can understand. Telling a patient that he or she has a 50 dB HL loss at 4000 Hz will not mean much. It is a lot more useful to give them examples of speech sounds or noises that they may be missing. A familiar-sounds audiogram or an audiogram with the speech sounds on it can be very helpful, even when counseling adults.	"You told me that you have trouble hearing the microwave beep when you aren't standing right next to it. Because your hearing loss is in the high pitches, that is one of the sounds you are missing. The further away you stand, the less likely you are to hear it."
Describing Word Recognition	DO: Be careful when describing word recognition scores. Some patients think if this score is good, they do not have a problem, even if it was presented at a very loud level.	DON'T: Focus too much on the percent correct of the word recognition test. Often people walk away thinking this is their percent hearing or hearing loss. Many times people come into an office and say "My last test showed a 20 percent loss" when what really happened is they scored 80 percent on a word recognition test. These are *not* synonymous.	"When I turned up those words you heard loud enough so you could hear them, you understood most of them. This means if we *amplify* speech for you, you may understand quite well in quiet situations. However, we had to turn the volume up louder than normal conversational levels for you to hear that well."
Psychological Reactions	DO: Pay attention to how patients react to the description of their hearing loss. Are they confused? Do they understand what you are saying? Are they getting upset? You are often the first one breaking the news or telling them how significant the problem may be. Be sensitive to that when talking to patients.	DON'T: Assume that if patients have no questions now, they won't have any questions when they get home. Sometimes they need to process the information before knowing what they want to ask. Make sure to give them a way to contact you if questions come up later.	

Continues on next page

Continued from previous page

	DO	**DON'T**	**Example**
Planning the Next Steps	DO: Give the patient and his or her family *all* the options available, including doing nothing. Hearing aids aren't always the right answer or even the best solution. Be sure you have taken a thorough enough case history to really understand what the patient's goals are when the test is finished.	DON'T: Tell the patient what to do. It is his or her decision whether to follow your recommendations or not. You need to give him or her a list of options and pros and cons for these options, but the ultimate decision is the patient's.	"You told me when we started today that you really want to be able to hear your grandchildren on the telephone. One thing that could help you do that is an amplified telephone. Another option may be hearing aids. Here are some pros and cons to each . . . ."

Source: Based on Catherine Schroy, personal communication, March 1, 2010.

Psychological reactions to a diagnosis of hearing loss range from relief ("I'm not losing my memory, I'm simply not hearing what's being said") to denial ("It's not me, it's everybody who can't talk clearly") to depression ("I really am getting old, this just proves it"). Time may be required before acceptance of hearing loss and its permanency occurs. Discussion about possible solutions may begin right after the test results are presented, or might be delayed until the patient has had time to absorb the diagnostic news. In order to move forward, the patient has to have a state of psychological readiness to explore solutions, and this readiness may take time to evolve.

The most common intervention to treat hearing loss is the provision of hearing aids. Hearing aid candidacy is defined not only by a patient's degree of hearing loss and potential to benefit from amplification, but also by the patient's motivation and willingness to become a hearing aid user. Only about 24 percent of the 31.5 million potential candidates in the United States own hearing instruments (Kochkin, 2005). Although many of these candidates opt not to buy hearing aids because of their cost, about 20 percent are concerned about vanity and the stigma attached to wearing a hearing aid (National Council on Aging, 1999). Common beliefs are, "My hearing is not bad enough," and, "I can get along without one." Unfortunately, for many, use of hearing aids is associated with a perceived stigma of aging and disability.

Factors That Influence a Professional's Determination to Perform and Advance in the Workplace

Many working professionals who incur hearing loss grow concerned that their hearing loss may limit their ability to perform their responsibilities competently and/or might affect their competitiveness. After conducting a series of focus groups with professionals who have hearing loss, Tye-Murray, Spry, and Mauzé (2009)

Continues on next page

Continued from previous page

identified five factors that influence an adult's determination to perform and compete in the workplace, as opposed to seeking early retirement or a change in job position. These factors are as follows:

- Self-concept and locus of control. *Self-concept* relates to how a person views himself, and *locus of control* pertains to one's sense of control over events and control over one's behaviors. A businessman in one of our focus groups exemplified a strong self-concept and locus of control, saying, "Get in there and go for it," and insisted that hearing loss should never be a deterrent from performing a job effectively.

- Use of hearing assistive technology. Hearing assistive technology includes listening devices such as hearing aids and other instruments that help to improve awareness or identification of environmental sounds and speech, such as a telephone amplifier. Use of hearing assistive technology often relates to an adult's determination to perform and compete in the workplace. For example, a bank collection manager opted to obtain hearing aids only after realizing that his chances for promotion depended upon his ability to talk easily with clients.

- Supervisors' and co-workers' perceptions and provisions of accommodations. The behaviors of supervisors and co-workers influence whether adults with hearing loss decide to remain in the workplace or whether they become resigned to the limitations imposed by hearing loss and even consider early retirement or a career move. For example, one of the focus group participants described how his supervisor allowed him to arrange the office furniture so as to maximize his listening capabilities. Conversely, another participant spoke about a boss who "was always uncomfortable because he didn't want to deal with [my hearing loss]."

- Use of effective coping strategies. Many of the participants who had experienced continued success in the workplace despite hearing loss spoke about using strategies to circumvent or marginalize communication breakdowns. A state hearing officer said, "When I conducted my hearings [during a trial], I made a point of telling people, 'I have trouble hearing. I want you to speak up, speak slowly, because I want to hear what you have to say.' "

- Communication difficulties and problematic situations. The final factor that influences an adult's determination to remain in the workplace relates to communication difficulties and problematic situations that exist in the workplace. One frustrated participant noted, "I work in an office that's filled with cubicles. A lot of times, people will come over and they'll almost whisper to have a conversation and I can't hear them!" Many of the participants in this gentleman's focus group nodded in empathic agreement.

There is some evidence that adults with hearing loss may feel less stigma in today's world than they have previously. For instance, Hétu, Getty, and Waridel (1994) found that male factory workers often reported being ostracized by their peers, minimized in the workplace, and forced to accept changes and limitations in their everyday roles. Self-stigmatization, negative self-image, and feelings of shame and inadequacy were common experiences. Roughly 15 years later, Tye-Murray and colleagues (2009) conducted focus groups to determine how hearing loss affects the psychoemotional status and job performance of office professionals. Results indicated that although most participants believed that hearing loss had negatively affected their job performance, and some believed that they had lost their "competitive edge" as a result, they did not appear to experience an inordinate degree of stigmatization. About 70 percent of the 48 participants in the study reported having told co-workers about their hearing loss, and many did not hesitate to remind others to speak clearly or to use repair strategies. This is a different era than the era of only a few decades ago. The baby boom generation has aged, and many more people have hearing loss. The ubiquity of ear-mounted technology, such as Bluetooth devices, has probably made using hearing aids less of a signpost of a disability. The Americans with Disabilities Act (ADA), a law enacted in 1990 to provide equal access to persons with disabilities, has helped to ensure that accommodations are made in the workplace, and so persons with hearing loss may be able to function more effectively as a result. In sum, having a hearing loss may carry a lesser stigma in today's world than in previous generations.

Even though stigmatization may have lessened, it still exists in varying degrees in many sectors of today's society, and as a result, many adults are reluctant to use a hearing aid. A fine balance may have to be attained, where patients' self-concepts and normal vanity are respected, yet their preconceptions about hearing aid use and associated connotations are challenged and revised. A five-stage process may be involved in developing motivation to use hearing aids, including the following steps (Tye-Murray, 2009):

1. Education. The patient understands the nature of the hearing loss and what a hearing aid can and can't do. The establishment of realistic expectations early on is crucial if the patient is to become a satisfied hearing aid user.

2. A change of values. The patient comes to realize that use of hearing aids does not necessarily connote aging and disability. Pointing out the ubiquity of ear-level hearing technology and the aging of the U.S. population may alleviate some of a patient's perceptions of stigmatization.

3. A change of attitudes. The patient considers different styles of hearing aids and realizes that the benefits of using a hearing aid supersede the monetary and psychosocial costs. Improved communication may outweigh a life with untreated hearing loss.

4. Impetus to act. The patient learns about the steps involved in obtaining a hearing aid and acquires one. This will entail a hearing aid evaluation and a hearing aid fitting.

5. Establishment of a use pattern. The patient is encouraged to use the hearing aids. A successful user is a user who wears the device full time or at least in all situations in which a device would be helpful. Initially, the patient may feel self-conscious

about wearing hearing aids and may be unaccustomed to hearing everyday sounds such as paper rustling and plumbing noises. It is important that the patient is aware that there is a learning curve associated with adjustment.

Some adults experience hearing loss that is severe to profound, and hence they may become candidates for a cochlear implant, especially if they have had trial periods with hearing aids. Counseling for cochlear implant candidates usually entails developing realistic expectations about what a cochlear implant can and cannot do both before and after cochlear implant surgery. For instance, most patients can communicate more effectively in an audiovisual condition (i.e., when they can see and hear the talker) with a cochlear implant than without one, but most cannot appreciate listening to music as it sounds quite different than their memories of it. Following implantation, patients may need counseling as they re-identify themselves as persons with some or even much hearing capability. Sometimes this may require that family members participate in counseling, as they may have to realize that the patient is no longer dependent upon them for verbally communicating with the outside world.

Both hearing aid users and cochlear implant users may seek other counseling support, including group follow-up sessions and psychosocial support (sometimes these two services coincide). During group follow-up sessions, patients receive informational counseling about the use and care of their devices. They may also have an opportunity to share their experiences with hearing loss, device use, and psychosocial adjustment. The speech and hearing professional typically serves as a facilitator during these sessions, which often follow a solution-centered format. For instance, a group may identify "talking with my spouse without communication breakdowns at the dinner table" as a primary goal. The group can explore possible solutions (e.g., turn off the television during dinner, refuse to take phone calls during the dinner hour), and then members can select amongst the alternatives and test them out in a role-playing scenario within the group and then at home.

Desire for Counseling

A number of studies suggest the importance of good counseling. As just one of several examples, Sweetow and Barrager (1980) found that many patients wish they had received more emotional support and counseling from their audiologists. Patients who receive counseling are more likely to use their hearing aids than patients who do not receive counseling, and counseling reduces the number of hearing-related difficulties (Brooks, 1979; Taylor & Jurma, 1999).

CASE STUDY

Sometimes the Spouse Is the Person Who Needs Counseling

When Martha Kennedy called the office to speak to an audiologist about her husband's hearing loss, she was clearly at her wits' end. With little preamble, she declared that George had lost his hearing 96 days previously and if things didn't turn around, she was going to leave him. According to Martha, George's job was in jeopardy, they were fighting constantly, and their 8-year-old son was miserable and confused. George had received hearing aids from another audiologist, and the aids were often not working. The audiologist scheduled an appointment and asked that both husband and wife attend. George arrived first, and reported that he had incurred a sudden mild-to-moderate hearing loss and was fitted with binaural completely-in-the-canal hearing aids. Although adjustment was ongoing, he expressed realistic expectations about what he would and would not be able to hear. He was a tenured teacher (so job security was not actually an issue) and the middle school students in his class knew that when he was not wearing his hearing aids, they needed to speak louder or wait until he approached them. His major concerns were that his hearing aids often stopped working due to moisture and that his wife expected him to hear as if he had normal hearing. When Martha arrived, the audiologist and the couple continued this discussion. The audiologist listened carefully and noted that George appeared to be accepting of his hearing loss and his communication difficulties, and she acknowledged that Martha seemed justifiably anxious about his new limitations. The audiologist addressed the problem about the hearing aids not working by suggesting a hearing aid drying system to be used at night. She then described realistic expectations for George's degree and type of hearing loss and acknowledged that the resultant communication difficulties were understandably frustrating for the couple. This was the first time that anyone had talked to Martha about George's hearing loss and how it affected her. The audiologist recommended further counseling by a professional as well as membership in a support group comprised of couples dealing with similar hearing-related issues. The couple appeared to be more at ease as they left, appreciative of the audiologist for taking the time to listen and acknowledge their feelings and concerns. Often times, family members are left languishing in the waiting room as speech and hearing professionals attend to the patient. It is better to let the patient's significant communication partners tell their stories, and provide them with informational and personal adjustment counseling when appropriate.

CHILDREN AND THEIR FAMILIES

Hearing loss in children is sometimes categorized according to four types: (1) *congenital*, meaning that the hearing loss was present at birth; (2) *prelingual*, meaning that the hearing loss had an onset before the age of 3 years; (3) *perilingual*, meaning that the hearing loss had an onset between the ages of 3 and 5 years; and (4) *postlingual*, meaning that the loss was incurred after the age of 5 years. Figure 9-1 presents an overview of the course of events that typically happens when a child is suspected of having a hearing loss. First, the hearing loss is detected. Detection often occurs when the child fails a universal newborn screening test (UNHS) or a school screening test. UNHS, which is mandated in almost every state in the United States and the District of Columbia, requires that newborn infants be screened for hearing loss before they leave their birthing hospital. Pure-tone hearing screening programs exist in most schools in the United States, beginning with kindergarten or first grade. Sometimes detection occurs when a parent

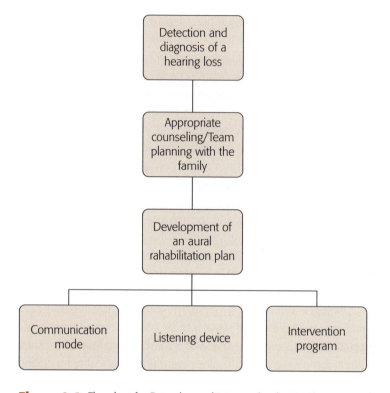

Figure 9-1 Flowchart for Detection and Intervention for Hearing Loss. *Delmar/Cengage Learning*

or guardian notices that the child does not respond to sound in the way that other children do. Following detection, a child will receive a comprehensive audiological examination with age-appropriate measurement techniques, and the degree of hearing loss will be quantified. The next step is the development of an aural rehabilitation plan. The plan will vary depending upon the nature and degree of the hearing loss and whether it is prelingual or postlingual. Many plans entail a consideration of communication mode (e.g., oral language, American Sign Language, Total Communication), listening device (e.g., hearing aid, cochlear implant, FM system), and intervention program (e.g., a center-based program, a home-based program).

Throughout the course of this aural rehabilitation process, families and their children will need sensitive counseling and support from their speech and hearing professionals. This counseling includes both informational counseling and personal adjustment counseling. Informational counseling informs families about the nature and ramifications of the hearing loss and about intervention options. Personal adjustment counseling helps them adjust to the emotions associated with having a child with hearing loss and provides them with needed support.

Detection of a Hearing Loss

With rare exception, learning that a baby has not passed a screening test is a traumatic and unexpected experience for new parents. Not only are there the natural emotions of excitement and stress of becoming new parents, but there is the physical exhaustion and emotional upheaval of childbirth. The news that their baby may have hearing loss may prove to be overwhelming.

It is important that parents not be waylaid with professional jargon. If possible, the audiologist or person who performed the screening should avoid using the word *failed* in conveying the news. At this point, parents need to be reassured that a referral following a screening test does not necessarily mean that their baby has a hearing loss, but they must also be encouraged to pursue a follow-up examination. Every attempt must be made to schedule the comprehensive diagnostic evaluation as soon as possible. The fast scheduling will ensure that parents spend as little time as possible in that emotionally fraught haze of uncertainty and that their baby does not "slip through the cracks" of the medical system and fail to be identified as having hearing loss until much later in development. If the baby does have a hearing loss, then early identification can result in early intervention, which in turn will promote communication skills that are more comparable to children who have normal hearing (National Institutes of Health, 2006).

As is the case with newborn hearing screening, many referrals due to school screenings may occur in the presence of normal hearing. The speech and hearing professional will explain to the parents or guardians the nature of screening and encourage them to schedule an audiological evaluation.

Diagnosis of a Hearing Loss

If follow-up diagnostic testing reveals a true hearing loss, the information will likely be a shock to the family, and members will appreciate the audiologist's sensitivity and compassion in conveying the news and in providing informational and personal adjustment counseling. Table 9-5 suggests some general guidelines to follow when counseling parents following diagnosis. Ideally, the test results will be shared with both parents (and a parent support person if in attendance) in a private, comfortable location with comfortable seating and with the baby or child present. Telephones will be turned off. An audiologist may issue a "warning-shot" comment like, "I know you've been anxious about today" or "I'm afraid I have some difficult news," and then go on to describe the test results succinctly, using layperson's language and referring to the baby by first name. For instance, the audiologist might say, "I've completed testing Jason's hearing. My results indicate that he has almost no hearing in one ear and what we call a moderate hearing loss in the other ear. I'm very sorry." The results should not be minimized or presented with unnecessary qualifications that might create false hope. Eye contact, slowed or softened speaking, and attention to the parents' body language will serve to convey compassion and empathy. After sharing the test results, the audiologist will want to wait quietly and allow parents to absorb them, and will acknowledge their verbal and nonverbal reactions. Silence or tears may follow, and an audiologist may have to overcome an urge to relieve his own discomfort by offering reassurance or launching into a detailed description of the test procedures and results. During this visit, the audiologist will want to offer realistic hope and to explore what the diagnosis means to the family and to validate and encourage emotions (VandeKieft, 2001).

Some of the questions parents may ask upon diagnosis include the following (English, Naeve-Velguth, Rall, Uyehara-Isono, & Pittman, 2007, p. 687):

■ Are you sure?

■ Why did this happen? What is the cause?

■ Will my child talk?

■ What should I do now?

■ Shouldn't I get a second opinion?

■ How many children have you tested?

■ Can this be fixed? Is there a surgery or medicine to fix this problem?

■ Will my baby have to wear a hearing aid?

■ Might my other and/or future children have hearing loss too?

■ How will we communicate with him?

TABLE 9-5 General Guidelines to Follow When Counseling Children's Parents (or Guardians) Following a Diagnosis of Hearing Loss

• **Keep it simple.** Relate what you say to what parents already know. Avoid using excessive jargon.
• **Be sensitive.** This may be the first time parents are hearing the news that you give them, whether it be an initial diagnosis or a change in hearing. Ask the parents what they want to do next or what they are ready for.
• **Provide written information for the parents to take home.** It is likely that the parents will not remember much of what you tell them after the fact that the child has a hearing loss. Always allow them to take notes and be sure to send them home with written information even at follow-up visits or annual evaluations. Don't assume the parents understand everything you are telling them even if it is not their first visit to your clinic. Just because the parents have been told something before does not mean they remember it or that they understood it the first time. Even if the child has been wearing hearing aids for years, you may be surprised at how little the parents really understand about the child's hearing loss and they are just afraid to ask.
• **Explain what you are doing as you test and what you are looking for from the child.** Sometimes parents of very young children don't understand what is being done in terms of testing. If you explain what is happening, they can often be very helpful in identifying responses from the child. Always let them know what you are expecting from the child and from them. Never forget, they know their child better than you do.
• **Remember that parents will come to you at different stages of the grieving process over the years.** Remember that stages of grief and adjustment can be repeated at different points in a child's life. Try to understand where the parents are coming from and don't be afraid to ask what they are thinking or feeling. Don't assume how parents will react to the news you are delivering, whether it is the initial diagnosis or changes later. Even if you have seen the parents for appointments before, their emotional state may be different from visit to visit.
• **Let parents know it is okay to get a second opinion if they would like.** If you are the person bearing bad news, parents may want a second opinion or they may want to go to someone else for future service. This is not a personal affront to you as a professional and should not be taken as such.

Continues on next page

Continued from previous page

> • **Be patient.** Parents may need time to make decisions about intervention, technology, and other matters involving their child's hearing loss. Although clinics are usually busy and there may be limited time to spend with parents, take the time to give the information needed and provide them with opportunities to ask questions.
>
> • **Remember that the child's hearing loss may not be the only issue that the family is confronting.** There may be other health concerns with the child or other children, family issues, or any number of issues that may take priority for the family. As professionals, we need to respect this and avoid making judgments. Whether it is their choice in intervention, the speed with which they follow up with you, or their reaction to news you have given them, you cannot know all of the considerations factoring into their choices.

Source: Catherine Schroy, personal communication, March 1, 2010.

The family will likely not retain much of what is said after the diagnosis, so it is important to write down key information and provide diagrams if appropriate. More detail about hearing and the audiogram can be relayed at a later visit.

Emotional responses to a diagnosis of hearing loss may evolve over time and may range from shock, denial, and grief to guilt and anger and ultimately to acceptance. These stages are not necessarily sequential, and parents may revisit stages of emotional adjustment each time a child approaches a new milestone. For instance, when a child enters preschool with children who do not have hearing loss, a parent may realize that the child may never have the same speech production skills as other children, and this may cause a wave of sadness.

Development of an Aural Rehabilitation Plan

Following diagnosis, the next appointment is scheduled as soon as possible, so that intervention can begin quickly and also so that parents begin to feel like they have a positive and definitive course of action to pursue and not feel as if they are floundering. If there is a time lag between diagnosis and a follow-up appointment, the audiologist may provide parents with reading materials and informational videos so that they feel as if they have something tangible and positive to do while they are waiting.

Starting at the follow-up visit, an aural rehabilitation strategy will be formulated, one that will include early intervention. The goals of this intervention will be to enhance the child's development, minimize any developmental delay, and maximize the family's ability to accommodate the child's hearing loss. Typically, after diagnosis the family is put into contact with personnel from available early intervention services in the family's region. In cases in which the child is of school age, the diagnostic information will be conveyed to the child's school system, and appropriate intervention services will be initiated.

In the next months and years, many choices will have to be made and many interventions will be initiated. Families will be actively involved with their audiologist in making these decisions. The child will likely begin to use appropriate listening devices, which will entail the family learning how to handle the devices and how to ensure appropriate usage. The parents will learn about communication modes and will receive information and support in selecting the optimum one for their child and their family. For instance, some families may not be receptive to learning sign language, so an oral method will be selected. Parents will be encouraged to model effective communication behaviors and will receive information about various intervention services and early intervention programs. They will be encouraged to become actively involved with intervention choices and may be encouraged to seek support from extended family and parent support groups. A parent support group provides opportunities for parents to share their feelings related to having a child with hearing loss and allows them to discuss hearing-related issues with others who have experienced them firsthand.

As this litany of choices and actions suggests, this will be a busy and perhaps emotionally wrenching time for parents. Their speech and hearing professionals will need to show them kindness and empathy and express hope and confidence often, while being careful not to minimize the situation. The importance of parent–child bonding should never be overlooked, and occasionally some parents may need to be reminded to relax and enjoy their beautiful child. To establish healthy attachment, some audiologists provide parents with a notebook to record their baby's various behaviors and not just their auditory responses. For example, parents might consider such questions as, "What seems to soothe or delight your baby?" or "How does she tell you she is sleepy?" (English, Kooper, & Bratt, 2004). The goal is to promote a deep, enduring bonding between child and parent that is not defined by the child's hearing loss.

Formal Education

Children with hearing loss typically leave an early intervention program at about the age of 3 or 4 years and matriculate into a preschool. The next decade and a half of education will present both rewards and challenges, and a child's experiences will be influenced by the magnitude of the hearing loss, the family, and the educational and support systems available in the child's home community. By preschool, the child and family will have adopted a communication mode, and ideally the child will have been fitted with an appropriate listening device such as hearing aids or a cochlear implant. Changes in communication mode or listening device may subsequently occur, depending upon the child's progress. Children with significant hearing loss often demonstrate delay in their language and speech development, and often in their academic achievement. For instance, reading and writing may be adversely affected, in part due to deficits in vocabulary and syntax. Children may require special interventions, which may range from being placed in a self-contained classroom to being placed in a full-time mainstream classroom. Mainstream classroom placements often entail interactions with an itinerant teacher and optimized classroom acoustics, as with a soundfield FM system. Parents and family will need to be kept apprised of a child's progress and forewarned about potential academic difficulties.

As the child progresses through the school system, he or she may need special support, both academically and psychosocially, and continued family involvement should be encouraged. In instances in which the child enters the mainstream, the classroom teacher will need information about accommodating a child with hearing loss in the classroom. Fellow students may need to learn about hearing loss and its ramifications. A speech and hearing professional may provide an in-service to classroom teachers and classmates about hearing loss and accommodations in the classroom.

Psychosocial Adjustment

Children and teenagers with hearing loss are at greater risk for developing a poor self-concept and experiencing psychosocial problems than are children with normal hearing (Wallis, Musselman, & MacKay, 2004). Self-concept is the understanding of who we are and is the foundation of self-esteem as we grow into adulthood. Psychosocial problems may include social isolation, naiveté about peer interests and customs, difficulty in empathizing, limited understanding about internal states such as feelings, and feelings of frustration or intimidation during social interactions (see Tye-Murray, 2009, for a review). The severity of psychosocial problems tends to vary with degree of hearing loss. For example, a child with a borderline hearing loss "may be unaware of subtle conversational cues that could cause [him or her] to be viewed as inappropriate or awkward" whereas a child with a moderate loss may be "significantly affected, and socialization with peers with normal hearing [is] increasingly difficult" (Anderson & Matkin, 1991, pp. 17–18).

Assessment instruments for assessing psychosocial adjustment for school-age children include the following:

- *The Meadow Kendall Social Emotional Assessment Inventories for Deaf and Hearing-Impaired Students* (SEAI; Meadow-Orlans, 1983)
- *The Children's Peer Relationship Scale* (English, 2002)
- *The Self Assessment of Communication-Adolescent* (Elkayam & English, 2003)

For example, the SEAI includes 59 items that index social adjustment, self-image, and emotional adjustment. Norms are available for children ranging in age from 7 to 21 years. A classroom teacher who knows the student well rates the student's behaviors on a five-point scale, ranging from "Very true" to "Does not apply."

A few programs have been developed to enhance the development of social skills (e.g., Gfeller & Schum, 1994; Paul & Jackson, 1993; Schloss & Smith, 1990; Schum, 1991). For instance, Suarez (2000) developed a program that includes an interpersonal problem-solving training program and lessons of social skills. Students learn to identify emotions portrayed in drawings and photographs and to consider the causes of emotions. They also learn specific social abilities, such as how to apologize or negotiate with peers. Training activities include modeling, role playing, feedback, and homework. Other programs and recommendations are aimed at the classroom teacher. For instance, a classroom teacher might be provided with the following suggestions (Oticon, 2006, pp. 6–7):

- Develop a program that includes coping strategies.
- Enable the student to accept how hearing loss makes him or her different, while still enabling him or her to realize that hearing loss is not the student's primary descriptive characteristic.
- Identify attributes that describe the student as a valued individual.
- Help the student and classmates to understand the nature of hearing loss.
- Develop activities to foster inclusion.
- Create situations that encourage a student to take chances.

Deaf Culture

Some children with significant hearing loss may choose to associate with the Deaf Culture, if their parents have not already made that decision for them early in their growth. The Deaf Culture is comprised of individuals who lost their hearing early in life and who share a common language (e.g., American Sign Language), beliefs, customs, arts, history, and folklore. Membership in the Deaf Culture is determined by orientation and not degree of hearing loss. For many, membership is a source of pride, which may stave off some of the psychosocial adjustment issues experienced by many children with hearing loss. Members of the Deaf Culture can communicate with fellow signers, believe that their cultural differences are reason for celebration, and are free of some of the anxieties that arise when a person with hearing loss attempts to function in a hearing world.

CASE STUDY

Grandparents Are Involved, Too!

When 4-year-old Bobby Benton came in for his annual hearing evaluation, he was accompanied by his single-parent mother and his grandmother. After testing, the audiologist explained the results to the family. Bobby's hearing was stable, revealing a mild-to-moderate hearing loss, but Bobby did need new earmolds. Bobby's grandmother, who babysits him while her daughter works, quickly interjected that the expense of new earmolds was unnecessary because Bobby did not wear his hearing aids during the day. Instead, the grandmother made a point of speaking loudly and of turning up the television set volume. The use (or non-use) of the hearing aids was clearly a bone of contention between the boy's mother and grandmother. Bobby's mother said that both she and the boy's speech-language pathologist had tried to convince the grandmother of the importance of hearing-aid usage, especially as Bobby was demonstrating delays in his speech and language development. The audiologist tactfully questioned the grandmother about her reluctance. The grandmother admitted that she thought hearing aids would make Bobby stand out as being disabled and as a result people would treat him differently. The audiologist acknowledged the grandmother's sentiments and empathized with her feelings of wanting only the best for her grandson. He asked if she would be open to meeting other grandparents of children who have hearing loss so that they could talk and share their experiences and feelings. The audiologist then discussed the importance of hearing aid use for normal language acquisition. He provided her with written information and a video about hearing loss and speech and language development to take home. The grandmother agreed to have Bobby wear the hearing aids for the following week. When the family returned to pick up the new earmolds, the audiologist congratulated the grandmother on Bobby's hearing aid usage and encouraged her to keep a log of his use and to report back occasionally. The audiologist also placed her in contact with another woman who babysits her grandchild who has a hearing loss. By the following year, Bobby was a full-time hearing aid user. As Bobby's story demonstrates, enlisting the support of extended family is important as they may spend as much or more time with the child as the parents.

CONCLUDING COMMENTS

Hearing loss is one of the most prevalent health conditions in the United States. Over 30 million adults have hearing loss (Taylor & Hansen, 2002), and over 1.4 million children have what is termed *a significant loss* (National Institutes of Health, 2006). With this high incidence, it is likely that most speech and hearing professionals will interact with someone who has hearing loss at some point during the course of their career. In this chapter, we have considered the ramifications of hearing loss acquired in adulthood and the counseling that may be involved in addressing listening difficulties and ensuring appropriate use of listening devices. We have also considered the ramifications of hearing loss acquired in early childhood and the counseling skills needed for interacting with both the family and child as the child progresses from infancy through the school years.

Because the initial contact with an adult patient or with parents may entail delivering "bad news," the therapeutic relationship often begins on a somber note. The adult may be saddened by the loss of physical ability and the loss of easy communication and may be dismayed to learn that what was once only suspected—a hearing loss—is indeed fact. A young child's family may be grief-stricken as they cope with the loss of a hoped-for future for their child and as they separate from a significant lost dream (Kurtzer-White & Luterman, 2003). During the course of intervention, the therapeutic relationship will evolve and may become one of the many rewarding experiences in the life of a speech and hearing professional. Launching patients and families on a course of aural rehabilitation and seeing them through the process requires not only professional expertise, but empathy, sensitivity, and insight into human nature. Rewards are many and the opportunity for personal growth immense.

Discussion Questions

1. What skills do you have that will help you with psychosocial counseling of patients who have hearing loss? Do you have any life experiences that would help you better understand patients who have hearing loss?

2. What might you say to a patient who has isolated himself because of hearing-related communication difficulties?

3. Provide examples of a solution-based approach to aural rehabilitation.

4. What do you believe is the most important aspect of counseling adults with hearing difficulties?

5. What might you do if your ideas about what the patient needed were different from what the patient thought he needed? Give an example of such a situation.

6. When should you refer a patient who has a hearing loss to an outside counselor?

7. Do you think that being a parent yourself would be an advantage to counseling parents of children with hearing loss? Why or why not?

8. What type of information might you provide for a child's teacher about the child's hearing loss?

9. How much information should you give parents on their initial visit? How would you decide how much? What clues might you look for to indicate that you have said enough?

10. Discuss a patient-centered orientation. Describe how a patient-centered orientation might affect your counseling with a businesswoman versus a stay-at-home mother.

11. Discuss the difference between congenital and perilingual hearing loss. How might your counseling for parents vary as a function of each type of hearing loss?

12. List four questions that parents might ask you after finding out that their child has been diagnosed with a hearing loss. How might you answer these questions? Consider both your choice of words and the content that you would include.

Role Plays

1. Practice explaining an audiogram with a friend, making eye contact and using clearly articulated speech. Have the friend feign a hearing loss. When communication breakdowns occur, pay attention to how you attempt to repair them. Was your explanation effective? Were you able to convey your message even after an initial communication breakdown?

2. Practice using empathy and compassion when telling a mother and father that their child has a hearing loss. Pretend that the parents express initial denial of their child's hearing loss. Role play how you might respond and facilitate their gradual understanding and acceptance.

References

Anderson, K. L., & Matkin, N. D. (1991). Relationship of degree of long-term hearing loss to psychosocial impact and educational needs. *Educational Audiology Association Newsletter, 8,* 17–18.

Brooks, D. N. (1979). Counseling and its effect on hearing aid use. *Scandinavian Audiology, 8*(2), 101–107.

Demorest, M. E., & Erdman, S. A. (1987). Development of the Communication Profile for the Hearing-Impaired. *Journal of Speech and Hearing Disorders, 52*(2), 129–143.

Dillon, H., James, A., & Ginis, J. (1997). Client Oriented Scale of Improvement (COSI) and its relationship to several other measures of benefit and satisfaction provided by hearing aids. *Journal of the American Academy of Audiology, 8*(1), 27–43.

Elkayam, J., & English, K. (2003). Counseling adolescents with hearing loss with the use of self-assessment/significant other questionnaires. *Journal of the American Academy of Audiology, 14*(9), 485–499.

English, K. (2002). *Counseling children with hearing* loss. Boston: Pearson Education Company.

English, K., Kooper, R., & Bratt, G. (2004). Informing parents of their child's hearing loss: "Breaking bad news" guidelines for audiologists. *Audiology Today, 16*(2), 10–12.

English, K., Naeve-Velguth, S., Rall, E., Uyehara-Isono, J., & Pittman, A. (2007). Development of an instrument to evaluate audiologic counseling skills. *Journal of the American Academy of Audiology, 18*(8), 675–687.

Gagné, J. P., & Jennings, M. B. (2000). *Audiological rehabilitation intervention services for adults with acquired hearing impairment.* New York: Thieme.

Gatehouse, S. (1999). Glasgow hearing aid benefit profile: Derivation and validation of a client-centered outcome measure for hearing aid services. *Journal of the American Academy of Audiology, 10,* 80–103.

Gfeller, K., & Schum, R. (1994). *Requisites for conversation: Engendering world knowledge.* Washington, DC: Alexander Graham Bell Association for the Deaf.

Grice, H. P. (1975). Logic and conversation. In P. Cole & J. Morgan (Eds.), *Syntax and Semantics 3: Speech Acts* (pp. 41–58). New York: Academic Press.

Hétu, R., Getty, L., & Waridel, S. (1994). Attitudes towards co-workers affected by occupational hearing loss II: Focus group interviews. *British Journal of Audiology, 28(6),* 313–325.

Hogan, A. (2001). *Hearing rehabilitation for deafened adults: A psychosocial approach.* Philadelphia: Whurr.

Kochkin, S. (2005). MarkeTrak VII: Hearing loss population tops 31 million people. *The Hearing Journal,* 16–29.

Kurtzer-White, E., & Luterman, D. (2003). Families and children with hearing loss: Grief and coping. *Mental Retardation and Developmental Disabilities Research Reviews, 9*(4), 232–235.

Meadow-Orlans, K. P. (1983). *Meadow-Kendall Social/Emotional Assessment Inventory for Deaf Students.* Washington, D.C.: Gallaudet University.

National Council on Aging. (1999). *The consequences of untreated hearing loss in older persons.* Washington, D.C.: National Council on Aging.

National Institutes of Health. (2006). *Fact sheet: Newborn hearing screening.* Washington, D.C.: Author.

Oticon. (2006). *Teacher's guide.* Denmark: Oticon.

Paul, P. V., & Jackson, D. W. (1993). *Toward a psychology of deafness: Theoretical and empirical perspectives.* Needham Heights, MA: Allyn & Bacon.

Schloss, P. J., & Smith, M. A. (1990). *Teaching social skills to hearing-impaired students.* Washington, D.C.: Alexander Graham Bell Association for the Deaf.

Schum, R. L. (1991). Communication and social growth: A developmental model of social-behavior in deaf-children. *Ear and Hearing, 12*(5), 320–327.

Suarez, M. (2000). Promoting social competence in deaf students: The effect of an intervention program. *Journal of Deaf Studies and Deaf Education, 5*(4), 323–333.

Sweetow, R. W., & Barrager, D. (1980). Quality of comprehensive audiological care: A survey of parents of hearing-impaired children. *ASHA, 22*(10), 841–847.

Taylor, B., & Hansen, V. (2002). Change yourself, change the industry. *The Hearing Review, 9,* 28–56.

Taylor, K. S., & Jurma, W. E. (1999). Study suggests that group rehabilitation increases benefit of hearing aid fittings. *Hearing Journal, 52*(9), 48–54.

Tye-Murray, N. (2009). *Foundations of aural rehabilitation: Children, adults, and their family members* (3rd ed.). Clifton Park, NY: Delmar, Cengage Learning.

Tye-Murray, N., Mauzé, E., & Schroy, C. (2010). Receive readily, recognize genuinely: Small talk and cooperative behaviors. *Seminars in Hearing, 31(2),* 154–164.

Tye-Murray, N., Spry, J., & Mauzé, E. (2009). Professionals with hearing loss: Maintaining that competitive edge. *Ear and Hearing, 30 (4),* 475–484.

VandeKieft, G. K. (2001). Breaking bad news. *American Family Physician, 64*(12), 1975–1978.

Ventry, I. M., & Weinstein, B. E. (1982). The hearing handicap inventory for the elderly: A new tool. *Ear and Hearing, 3*(3), 128–134.

Wallis, D., Musselman, C., & MacKay, S. (2004). Hearing mothers and their deaf children: The relationship between early, ongoing mode match and subsequent mental health functioning in adolescence. *Journal of Deaf Studies and Deaf Education, 9*(1), 2–14.

PART

III

The Therapeutic Process with Challenging Situations and Behaviors

Part III of this text emphasizes challenging situations and behaviors that our clients and their families sometimes present. Our evaluations and therapy for children and adults, and our interactions with their family members, inevitably involve complex emotional reactions and needs. In pragmatic terms, clinicians work with hearing, speech, language, cognitive, and swallowing disorders of clients of all ages in a wide variety of settings; however, skills and strategies for interacting that lessen their anxiety can help the therapy process go more smoothly. Clinicians' sensitivity and understanding can do much to relieve anxiety and emotional distress. Understanding and communicating with people about sensitive issues can enhance therapy and ultimately help clinicians be more effective.

Some client or family behaviors may trigger strong emotional responses on the part of the clinician. This section of the text will help you better understand the people you are working with, how to respond with more empathy, and how to remain cool when surface client behaviors appear to be defensive, resistant, self-defeating, or counterproductive. Certain counseling issues and situations may occur more frequently depending on the setting you are working in and the stage of therapy. However, challenging interpersonal and emotional issues may surface at unexpected times and places. Challenging situations are not confined to certain work settings or particular stages of therapy, but may depend upon the client and family's personality styles (as well as the clinician's personality style) and clinician–client interactions. These challenging situations may reflect responses to certain situations such as receiving bad news and experiences of loss in combination with the coping styles and defenses that clients and their families bring to bear on these situations. By better understanding some of these phenomena and the counseling principles that are associated with them, clinicians are more likely to navigate these situations successfully.

CHAPTER 10

Defense Mechanisms Relevant to Speech-Language Pathologists and Audiologists

CHAPTER OUTLINE

- Introduction
- Defense Mechanisms
- Concluding Comments
- Discussion Questions
- Role Plays

INTRODUCTION

Defense mechanisms (or ego-defense mechanisms) are automatic, involuntary mental processes that people use as protective responses to stresses, threats, and anxiety (*Diagnostic and Statistical Manual of Mental Disorders-IV-TR*, 2000). The concept of defense mechanisms has its origins in Freud's psychoanalytic therapy (Freud, 1923) and was expanded by his daughter Anna Freud (1936), who listed additional defense mechanisms observed in individuals. It is a concept that continues to be used in theoretical discussions of personality development, psychopathology, and psychotherapy (Gabbard, 2005; Masterson & Lieberman, 2004; Maxmen & Ward, 1995). Individuals are often unaware of defense mechanisms, as they operate to provide a mental refuge from situations with which a person cannot currently cope. While we all use defense mechanisms, some defenses are central to certain personality styles (Horowitz et al., 2001; Johnson, 1994) and some defenses are characteristic of particular personality disorders (Gabbard, 2005; Lingiardi, Lonati, Delucchi, Fossati, Vanzulli, & Maffei, 1999; Masterson & Lieberman, 2004; Ryder, McBride, & Bagby, 2008; Zanarini, Weingeroff, & Frankenburg, 2009). There has been a plethora of research on defensive styles and their prevalence in certain populations; for example, defensive styles have been researched in child and adolescent populations (e.g., Dollinger & Cramer, 1990; Goodman, Quas, & Ogle, 2010; Noam & Recklitis, 1990; Sadock, Kaplan, & Sadock, 2007), elderly populations (e.g., Yu, Chamorro-Premuzic, & Honjo, 2008), and in patients with anxiety and depressive disorders (e.g., Knijnik, Salum, Blanco, et al., 2009; Olson, Presniak, & MacGregor, 2009). Some studies also have shown that defensive styles can change during the course of psychotherapy (Bond & Perry, 2004). Defense mechanisms protect a person from being overwhelmed by anxiety through adaptation to situations and through distortion or denial of events or facts. Defense mechanisms are essential for helping people cope with failure, stress, and loss while maintaining a positive self-image. They are used to combat the anxiety generated by everyday stresses as well as the overwhelming angst caused by significant losses. As Comer (2003) says, "The defense never rests."

Defense mechanisms serve a person's emotional and psychological survival (e.g., children with traumatic experiences often repress many of them; veterans who have seen combat often repress many of those memories). In other instances, however, defenses can interfere with personal growth, such as when a person's excessive rationalization interferes with taking responsibility for his own behavior. It is important to remember that everybody uses defense mechanisms; however, some are healthier than others. Defense mechanisms can be considered to exist along a continuum (Vaillant, 1994; Vaillant, Bond, & Vaillant, 1986) from those that are relatively healthy (i.e., they help the person cope without significant distortion of reality) to those that are unhealthy (i.e., they help the person cope but with significant distortion of reality). Although people may use a variety of defense mechanisms, they tend to have a preferred defensive style; that is, they may tend to use the same relatively healthy two or three defenses in most situations in which defenses are necessary to cope. However, under extremely stressful conditions, people may use less healthy defenses that are not characteristic of their normal, everyday coping styles. We need to consider that in much of our work, particularly with children and adults who have significant impairments, clients and family members are likely to view the situation as extremely stressful and, therefore, may temporarily use less healthy defenses than they otherwise might. It is important, then, to recognize and to respect our clients' needs for defenses to shield them from overwhelming experiences of threat, loss, and emotional or physical trauma.

As long as people employ relatively healthy defenses to assist them in coping with the stresses of hearing loss, communication delays, disorders, injury, illness, treatment, recovery, or death, their defensive styles often do not come to the attention of clinicians or interfere with therapy. For example, a person may use humor, laughing at the amusing aspects of her current medical condition or treatment to diffuse the anxiety she feels. Another person may use self-assertion, appropriately expressing the limits of tolerance for multiple appointments and demands in a single day. A third person may deal with stressors, such as receiving news about a poor prognosis by affiliation, appropriately turning to others to share feelings and to receive support to avoid intense feelings of anxiety.

In contrast, when clients use less healthy forms of defenses, they can impact interpersonal relationships and create obstacles to forming or maintaining a therapeutic relationship. In these situations, defenses may interfere with the professional's attempts to work on therapy goals (Gabbard, 2005; Masterson & Lieberman, 2004). This chapter provides illustrations of these situations and some clinician responses that may be used to keep the therapy on track.

There are a few general guidelines that should be considered when deciding whether or not to address a person's defenses. First, a clinician should not interfere with a person's defenses unless they persist in posing obstacles to therapy. Many times an individual's defenses occur briefly and help the person to register the challenging situation or crisis at his own pace. If, on the other hand, a person's defenses persist and interfere with therapy, our job is not to attempt to remove the defenses or to criticize them, but to respond in a respectful way that tries to reestablish the treatment process and empower the person. Clients' and families' defensive strategies, however, can put clinicians to the test. Because, on the surface, defenses often seem like illogical responses, some clinicians may grow impatient, frustrated, or angry. They also may take personally the client's defensive actions. It is easy to get "hooked" into these negative interactions with people (Benjamin, 1996). However, another rule of thumb is to maintain a calm, professional demeanor and to avoid the power struggles in which we may feel pulled.

Although the *DSM-IV-TR* (2000) discusses 27 different defense mechanisms (acting out, affiliation, altruism, anticipation, autistic fantasy, denial, devaluation, displacement, dissociation, help-rejecting complaining, humor, idealization, intellectualization, isolation of affect, omnipotence, passive aggression, projection, projective identification, rationalization, reaction formation, repression, self-assertion, self-observation, splitting, sublimation, suppression, and undoing), not all are typically relevant to the work of SLPs and Auds. Some of the defenses are more commonly associated with severe psychological problems. The following are discussions of defense mechanisms that our professions may likely encounter and therapeutic responses to them. The definitions we present are based on those provided in the *DSM-IV-TR* (2000).

DEFENSE MECHANISMS

Acting Out

When a child or adult is **acting out**, the individual is dealing with emotional conflicts or internal or external stressors by actions rather than reflections or feelings. In stressful or challenging situations, some individuals manage their anxiety and external demands by responding in inappropriate ways. For example, a child with a hearing impairment who is teased or taunted by classmates may act or strike out at his tormentors, or a child who has reading problems who must read in front of the class may act out by throwing her book to avoid reading, or an elderly patient having to eat pureed food he detests may push the tray off the table. It is important to note that not all forms of a child or adult's misbehavior can properly be considered acting out. Acting out pertains only to behavior that is prompted by emotional conflict or stress. Acting out refers to a person acting upon feelings rather than talking about them. Children, in particular, have difficulty understanding and talking about their anxieties, fears, and the demands placed on them at school and home. They may use acting out behaviors (e.g., cursing, slamming books down, yelling at an adult, or disrupting therapy) as ways to express their feelings.

It is important to determine if a child's behavior is typical age-related behavior (e.g., the result of boredom) or acting out, because that judgment will determine what response will be most therapeutic. If, for example, a child in group therapy begins disrupting the therapy by talking or playing, you may determine that the behavior is *not* the result of the child experiencing anxiety or stress, and manage the behavior using a behavioral approach such as rewarding more appropriate behavior. However, if you determine the child's disruptive behavior is the result of anxiety or stress that may be caused by his speech or language problems, then addressing his feelings (e.g., "It looks like you don't want to be here right now" or "It looks like some things are bothering you. Would you like to talk about them for a little while?") may be more helpful. When possible, spend a few minutes with the child alone to talk about any feelings the child may have that are contributing to the acting out behavior, for example, embarrassment and frustration. Putting words to the child's painful emotional feelings may diminish the need for acting out behaviors.

Adults also may use acting out behaviors when they feel stress or emotional conflict and feel unable to voice their true feelings. For example, a client may "fire" a therapist who has asked him about a sensitive topic rather than confronting the difficult subject. Another client may get drunk upon learning that he will have to care for a chronically ill child. Resisting the impulse to pass judgment is key for clinicians at these moments, as they may be able to be much more helpful and therapeutic by encouraging the client to speak about his painful or distressing feelings.

COUNSELING SKILLS IN ACTION

Acting Out—or Not?

The examples below contrast situations in which children are acting out versus situations in which they are not.

Acting Out: Sanjay is a moderately disfluent 12-year-old who is anxious about his upcoming oral book report. During recess he instigates a fight with another boy and gets sent to the principal's office for the afternoon, thereby missing his oral book report presentation.

Acting Out: Rochelle is extremely anxious about her parents' frequent arguments and fears her dad will leave home. At school she yells at her male speech therapist and calls him a jerk.

Not Acting Out: Leslie is participating in a speech group therapy session, but she continues to play with the board game pieces after the SLP has asked her to stop. She is not anxious, but is simply captivated by the novelty of the new game.

Not Acting Out: Joey is a bright, energetic boy who is bored by his teacher's lesson. He understands the teacher's lessons and has mastered the current academic material. He pesters the girl next to him and makes paper airplanes and throws them across the room.

The clinician needs to make distinctions between acting out and mischievous behavior or misbehavior which may represent boredom, inattention, or lack of understanding of social cues. When acting out behavior occurs, the clinician needs to address the feelings or the motivations behind the behavior rather than simply trying to eliminate (extinguish) it. However, when a clinician believes some of the child's acting out behavior, feelings, or motivations are beyond her scope of practice to address, a referral to a counselor or psychologist may be appropriate.

In medical settings we cannot always predict which patients will act out and when, and therefore it is best to take steps to try to prevent these episodes from occurring rather than simply dealing with the aftermath. Some individuals, particularly patients with TBIs at Levels 4 (Confused-Agitated) and 5 (Confused, Inappropriate, Non-Agitated) on the

Rancho Levels of Cognitive Functioning (Hagen, 1998), because of their neurologic impairments, exhibit disruptive behaviors. These patients have heightened states of activity, make purposeful attempts to remove restraints or tubes, may crawl out of bed, and may exhibit aggressive or flight behaviors. Patients with TBIs often are able to cope with minimal auditory, visual, and tactile stimuli (external stressors). These stimuli cause internal stress and may reach a level beyond what patients can tolerate, at which time they are likely to demonstrate acting out behaviors. These patients also are responding to internal stimuli such as pain or discomfort and a general sense of confusion about where they are, how they got there, and why they are in the hospital.

It is helpful to obtain information from family members about the patient's premorbid coping skills. Prior to a TBI, some patients may have had tendencies to be aggressive or abusive, and the TBI results in diminished capacity for self-control. In addition, some patients may view their clinicians as persecutors and punishers because of impairments in their cognitive functioning. It is important to keep in mind that patients are doing the best they can and that their acting out behaviors are not under their cognitive control at this time. Clinicians need to remember that no matter what Confused-Agitated patients say or do (including swearing, striking out, etc.), not to take it personally but to maintain an empathic stance with acceptance of the patient's emotional, cognitive, and physical conditions. Clinicians should treat patients with respect and dignity and give them personal space (Kriege, 1993).

Working with Acting Out Behaviors

While working in acute care hospitals I have seen many patients of all ages with TBIs demonstrate acting out behaviors such as cursing and even striking out at rehabilitation therapists (PTs, OTs, and STs) and nurses. The acting out behaviors typically occur when patients feel stresses from the demands of rehabilitation programs. SLPs can adjust the complexity, amount, rate, and/or duration (CARD) of therapy tasks and stimuli to accommodate each patient's levels of tolerance to decrease internal and external stresses. That is, SLPs may choose to simplify a complex task, decrease the amount of stimuli presented or number of repetitions of a task, slow the rate of presentation of the stimuli or requested rate of the patient's responses to the stimuli, and/or decrease the length of time the patient is performing a task or in a therapy session. (See Chapter 13 for further discussion.)

CLINICAL QUESTIONS

1. You notice one day that your 8-year-old client Jonathan is stealing pencils from your desk area. What questions might you ask Jonathan (and yourself) to determine whether this is acting out behavior?

2. Imagine that your hospitalized adult patient who is usually polite and cordial in her interactions with you begins to swear at you one day. What questions might you ask her (and yourself) to determine whether this is acting out behavior?

Speaking to patients in gentle, respectful, and nonthreatening tones may help to keep the therapy on an even keel. Initially, this may involve avoiding startling the patient by approaching the patient from the front, slowing down your pace, and maintaining a calm, self-controlled demeanor. Setting aside your agenda or therapy plan and simply being with the patient can be soothing. The payoff may be the prevention of time-consuming conflicts and explosions as well as possible physical injury to you. Also, keep in mind that patients who are prone to aggressive behaviors or acting out episodes may try to push you into a demanding or threatening posture that then serves as a trigger (or excuse) for them to blow up.

When other acting out episodes occur, polite but direct confrontation and limit-setting may be warranted in order to inform the patient of guidelines for appropriate behavior during therapy. It also may be important to give the patient specific examples of permissible behavior, keeping in mind the limited amount of information the patient can process. For example, you might say "Mr. D., please do not swear at me. You can tell me that you are angry and what you want, but do not swear at me." If you think a patient cannot process that much information, then simply saying "Swearing at me is not appropriate" may be the best method to set limits. Your tone of voice is important; it should be firm rather than harsh. It is better to emphasize and reinforce appropriate behavior rather than confront inappropriate behavior. For example, you might say, "Thank you for waiting patiently the last few minutes" or "I appreciate it when you speak softly."

We need to remember that acting out behavior means that the person, child or adult, is dealing with emotional conflicts and stressors that the person cannot manage in a more socially appropriate manner. If we can determine the conflicts or the stressors that are precipitating the acting out behaviors, we may be able to prevent or deter the behaviors. Determining the conflicts or stressors requires that the clinician listen to the patient for clues about anxieties and fears and try to behave in ways that help to calm the patient or de-escalate the situation.

Altruism

SLPs and Auds may occasionally recognize **altruism** in the behavior of family members. Normally, altruism is not a significant concern to clinicians; however, we need to be aware of altruism when it interferes with family functioning and negatively affects our work with a client. In many cases, altruistic behavior, in which the individual becomes focused on meeting the needs of others, is considered a healthy response to stressful situations. Family members are often anxious and fearful about the well-being and future of their loved one. In essence, individuals distract themselves from their own guilt or anxiety by performing helpful deeds for others. These deeds or acts may be gratifying in themselves or may elicit gratitude from others. In either case, internal anxiety is channeled into creating a positive interpersonal experience.

In some cases, family members may make healthy adjustments to a disability or illness situation by engaging in altruistic behavior. For example, a mother who took drugs during her pregnancy may take on a second or third job to pay for extra services her child needs to maximize the child's potential. A husband may take on a caregiver role when his mate develops multiple sclerosis. Another example may involve a young adult who has a TBI while living independently, and his parents may act altruistically by having the adult son move back into the family home in order for them to become his caregivers. Sometimes adult children bring their elderly parents into the home to live with them. This can create additional family stress and what is commonly known as the "sandwich generation" where a couple is raising their own children and at the same time caring for one or more of their own parents. (This latter situation also may have advantages because the grandparent may be able to help care for or monitor the grandchildren, and a strong grandparent–grandchild relationship may develop.) Unfortunately, an increasingly common example of altruism involves grandparents who take in and care for one or more grandchildren when neither of the parents can nor will care for their children (Fuller-Thomson & Minkler, 2001).

On a larger scale, some individuals take on a mission to help others who have experienced a similar loss or disability by becoming active in support organizations at the local, state, or even national levels such as C.H.A.D.D. (Children and Adults with Attention Deficit Disorders), M.A.D.D. (Mothers Against Drunk Driving), or S.H.H.H. (Self-Help for Hard of Hearing People). This kind of altruism is the foundation of many organizations that offer an educational perspective, a supportive network, and practical resources for individuals who have common experiences of loss.

In some cases, altruism may become problematic if it results in neglect of important areas of the person's life. A mother who focuses altruistically on her disabled child may neglect self-care, her other children's needs, or her marriage. This example illustrates that altruistic behavior towards one person may cause a disruption or damage to other family relationships. Despite this mother's positive intentions, she and her family may need brief counseling from a professional counselor to recognize imbalances in the family and reorganize family roles. In these examples it is important to note that the individuals who are behaving altruistically are not simply acting responsibly, but are using this strategy to channel their own anxiety into productive action.

In general, as clinicians our primary responses to an altruistic family member might be: (1) acknowledgement and validation in order to show empathy for the family member's focus on the person with the acute or chronic disorder; or (2) if the clinician feels the altruism is causing neglect of other important areas of the family member's life, a referral to a counselor or psychologist may be appropriate. The psychologist may proceed by inquiring about the neglected aspects of the family member's life, and by helping the person find solutions that respect the family member's need to behave in an altruistic manner.

Denial

In response to news or information that is overwhelming, some people respond with the basic defense known as denial. The *DSM-IV-TR* (2000) defines **denial** as an emotional conflict or internal or external stressors that the individual deals with by refusing to acknowledge some painful aspect of external reality or subjective experience that would be apparent to others. In some cases, denial is a coping strategy that reflects feelings of inadequacy that are triggered by significant losses, injury, or impairment. The person may admit that the problem exists, but is not engaged emotionally. Even well-adjusted people may initially employ denial to protect themselves from overwhelming anxiety (Gladding, 2009). Short-lived denial is a common response to receiving news of a diagnosis of

Working with Challenging and Difficult Emotional States

CHAPTER OUTLINE

INTRODUCTION

Speech-language pathologists and audiologists typically work with children and adults who present various challenging and difficult emotional states, some of which may be enigmas to us. It is important to remember that clients and patients are experiencing disabilities with one of the most important and fundamental human skills—the ability to communicate. Therefore it is natural that a considerable amount of emotion often surrounds these challenges and impairments. In addition to our clients' emotional responses, family members frequently experience strong emotional reactions to the challenges they are confronted with when a loved one has a significant communication impairment. Viewing our clients and their families holistically allows us to work with more than just the speech, language, cognitive, swallowing, or hearing problems they present. Holistic therapy involves focusing on the whole person (mind, body, and spirit), and the goal is the growth of the whole person (Bourne, 2005; France & Kramer, 2001; Gladding, 2009; Nystul, 2005; Shames, 2006).

As SLPs and Auds, our responsibility is not to "cure" or remove the negative emotional states or possible mental health conditions that exist in the individuals we are trying to help. Our responsibility is to work with each individual in such ways that his emotional states do not interfere or significantly hinder therapy progress. We can explore through various microskills (see Chapter 4) the negative feelings the client, patient, or family members are experiencing and attempt to understand them. In some cases, our understanding and therapeutic responses will lead to a reduction in the individual's negative emotional states or the development of better coping abilities to manage distressing emotional states.

We need to be careful not to function outside of our scope of practice when dealing with challenging emotions and behaviors and to make the appropriate referrals. Meanwhile, we also need to recognize the counseling skills that may be appropriately used to respond to emotionally distressed clients and their families. As discussed in Chapter 3, we need to avoid "pathologizing" clients and family members by labeling them as paranoid, depressed, neurotic, or compulsive. However, some aspects of what we observe may be relevant in our description of our clients. In such cases it is best to use descriptions of behaviors that reflect our observations rather than global pathologizing terms. We can describe situation-specific behaviors but not label or diagnose the individual's general emotional state or disorder. Even though a client has a certain set of behaviors that are observed in a particular situation, it does not mean these are typical of the person. As clinicians, we may consider whether behaviors, characteristics, or symptoms are understandable reactions to a particular experience, or whether the experience may be excessive and/or causing impairment in the client's emotional functioning. In general, we can describe emotional, behavioral, or psychological symptoms but we cannot diagnose an emotional or psychological disorder.

ANXIETY AND FEAR

Anxiety is an inevitable part of life. It is important to appreciate that there are many situations that occur in everyday life in which it is appropriate and reasonable to react with some anxiety. A lack of feeling of any anxiety in response to potential loss or failure would be abnormal. Anxiety is a distressing feeling of uneasiness, apprehension, or dread. The anxiety may be rational and based on actual events, or irrational and based on anticipated events that likely will not occur. Anxiety occurs in children and adolescents as well as adults. Children may have separation anxiety from their parents (we sometimes see this during initial evaluations of young children in clinical practicum) or anxiety about being abandoned or sent away from home. A main source of anxiety for both children and adults is the fear of being separated from other people who are felt to provide emotional security (Bowlby, 1969; Erdman & Cafferty, 2003). However, when an individual's anxiety is chronic and not traceable to any specific cause, or when it interferes with normal activity, the individual may need professional help (France & Kramer, 2001; Stewart, 2005). SLPs and Auds need to avoid pathologizing a person's emotional response to a situation by labeling it an anxiety disorder. *Anxiety Disorder* refers to a group of disorders that includes Acute Stress Disorder, Generalized Anxiety Disorder, Social Phobia, and others (*DSM-IV-TR*, 2000). Only appropriately trained mental health professionals can diagnose these disorders.

Anxiety and Communication Disorders

Anxiety is a common component of many communication disorders (Andrews & Summers, 2002; Bloodstein & Bernstein Ratner, 2008; Crowe, 1997; Holland, 2007; Luterman, 2008; Shames, 2006; Shipley & Roseberry-McKibbon, 2006; Tanner, 2008). SLPs and Auds work with individuals and families who are confronted with acute anxiety, social anxiety, and panic attacks. In some cases, clients' anxiety may interfere with their performance on some language and cognitive assessments. For example, a child who is anxious during an evaluation may respond with a shorter mean length of utterance during a language-sampling task than she would in a situation in which she feels more comfortable. Also, an anxious child may respond with incomplete answers to problem-solving assessments, which may lower her scores. Some sources of anxiety for children, adults, and their family members are reflected in the questions they ask. Figure 11-1 lists some of these types of questions.

While some anxiety is inhibiting, some anxiety serves an important function by providing a state of tension that motivates individuals to action. Anxiety can be viewed from a time perspective, that is, acute versus chronic (Clark & Beck, 2009; Rolland, 1994). Acute anxiety states have a sudden onset, occurring perhaps as a reaction to severe external stress, and tend to be relatively brief in nature (e.g., receiving a diagnosis of a CVA). Chronic anxiety, however, runs a prolonged course and may not be associated with particular stressful events. Individuals with chronic anxiety often worry excessively and tend to respond to many situations with undeserved anxiety and trepidation. Anxiety can appear at different levels of intensity, from mild feelings of uneasiness to panic attacks (Bourne, 2005; France & Kramer, 2001).

A different way of viewing anxiety is to analyze it in terms of its triggers and causes (Beck & Emery, 1985; Clark & Beck, 2009). Situational (situation-dependent) anxiety refers to anxiety that tends to occur in relatively limited situations and times, for example, just before an examination or just before a job interview. Situational anxiety is the most common form of anxiety that individuals with communication disorders experience (e.g., anxiety regarding being understood in front of the class, stuttering when speaking to a person of the opposite gender, or performing adequately at work following a stroke). One of the paradoxical features of anxiety is that clients often bring on the situation they fear the most (Beck & Emery, 1985). That is, the anxiety causes the very symptoms they fear and detest.

Anxiety frequently manifests itself as the result of opposing or conflicting wishes, desires (e.g., wanting to stay home and be with the children and also wanting to pursue a career), beliefs (e.g., believing that the work environment should always run smoothly but experiencing conflict between co-workers), life events (e.g., the serious illness of a loved one), or stress resulting from conflict between roles (e.g., being a parent and a professional). The more difficult the decision between two opposing drives or pressures, the more severe the anxiety. When people cannot deal with anxiety through appropriate rational methods, they often resort to ego-defense mechanisms (see Chapter 10). Defense mechanisms may operate until the person is better able to confront or manage the situation and stressors. This is a normal process that all people employ. Defense mechanisms do not extinguish anxiety; they try to bind or keep it from awareness (Stewart, 2005).

The distinction between anxiety and fear is not always clear. Lang and McTeague (2009) and Craighead and colleagues (1994) consider anxiety and fear as being on a continuum. However, anxiety may be distinguished from fear in several ways. When people experience anxiety they often cannot specify what it is they are anxious about. On the other hand, individuals often misidentify the cause of the anxiety, for example, being anxious about traffic on the freeway when the underlying anxiety is about being late for work again and a supervisor's job evaluation. The focus of anxiety is frequently more

Figure 11–1 Questions that reflect anxieties for counseling

"Will cochlear implants help my child?"

"Can my mouth be fixed so I don't sound like I'm talking through my nose?"

"Will my baby's cleft lip and palate affect the way he talks?"

"Do you think my child's frequent ear infections have affected his speech?"

"Do you think tubes (pressure-equalizing tubes) will help my child's hearing?"

"Can cytomegalovirus cause hearing problems in my baby?"

"My daughter had meningitis when she was three years old. Can that cause hearing problems?"

"Do you think that all the antibiotics my son was on for such a long time could have affected his hearing?"

"Will hearing aids help my daughter? How much will they cost?"

"How much do you think hearing aids will help me?"

"Will my child's Down's syndrome interfere with his language development and learning?"

"Will my son grow out of his stuttering?"

"Can I learn to talk without stuttering?"

"Will he ever learn to make his /s/ and /r/ right?"

"Can I someday make my /s/ and /r/ right?"

"Can I ever learn how to read?"

"Will his CAPD (or ADD) affect his school work? His social development?"

"How much will my son's head injury affect the way he talks? Will he be able to do well in school again?"

"Do you think I can do okay in school after I had the accident?"

"Will my voice get any better with therapy?"

"Do you think my husband will have another stroke?"

"Can I ever get back to work after my stroke?"

"Will my Meniere's disease get worse?

"Is presbycusis curable?"

"What are we going to do in therapy?"

"Will I ever be able to take care of myself?"

"Will I be a burden to my family?"

"Are you a really good audiologist/SLP?"

"How much will all this cost?"

internal than external and is a response to a vague, distant, or even unrecognized danger such as losing control, feeling that something bad is going to happen, or threats to self-esteem (Bourne, 2005). Certain individuals are anxious about their overall job performance, what others will think of them, or whether they will be rejected by a partner. The anxiety is diffuse and not particularly tied to a specific event. However, when people are experiencing fear, it is usually directed toward some concrete, external object or situation. Fear is an innate, primitive alarm response that is often accompanied by manifestations of fight or flight (Clark & Beck, 2009; Craighead et al., 1994; De Becker, 1997). The object or event that is feared is usually within the realm of possibility; for example, fearing a burglar when a person hears unfamiliar noises during the night, fearing an attack when a ferocious animal approaches, or fearing destruction of one's home upon hearing a tornado warning.

Psychological, Physiological, and Behavioral Effects of Anxiety and Fear

Anxiety and fear affect people simultaneously in three ways: psychologically, physiologically, and behaviorally. Psychologically, anxiety is a subjective state of apprehension and uneasiness. Other mental symptoms may include irritability, poor concentration, mental tension, fear of losing control, fear of impending disaster, and worrying. There may be a reduction in awareness of the environment and surroundings, with the person appearing disoriented to person, place, time, and purpose (i.e., disoriented × 4). However, some individuals may become hypervigilant regarding the source of apprehension or fear (i.e., becoming excessively watchful and alert to danger). Individuals may have a decrease in emotional responsiveness, often finding it difficult to experience pleasure in previously enjoyable activities. Depressive symptoms are common for people with chronic anxiety (Barlow & Campbell, 2000; Bear, Connors, & Paradiso, 2007; Bourne, 2005; *DSM-IV-TR*, 2000; France & Kramer, 2001; Morrison, 2008).

On a physiological level, anxiety and fear may cause tightness in the chest and throat; respiratory distress; shaky or tremulous voice; queasiness in the abdomen; dizziness or feelings of light-headedness; skin pallor; dry mouth; difficulty swallowing; increased pulse rate and urinary frequency; mild exertion producing undue increase in heart rate; muscle tension; headaches; sweating, flushing, or chills; and an exaggerated startle response. Sleep may be disturbed with difficulty falling or staying asleep, restlessness, or unpleasant dreams. Newly hospitalized patients may be given sedatives to help decrease their anxiety during the day and to allow them to sleep better at night. Behaviorally, the presence of anxiety may include a strained-looking face, furrowed brow, tense posture, clenched fists, restlessness, and pale skin (Bear et al. 2007; Clark & Beck, 2009; Craighead et al., 1994). Anxiety may cause people to speak rapidly and somewhat incoherently. Voice volume (often decreased or erratic), pitch (unusually high because of tense vocal folds), and quality (strained, hoarseness) may be affected by anxiety (Boone, McFarland, & Von Berg, 2009).

There may be several contributors to anxiety, including heredity, biological factors, family background and environment, recent stressors, self-talk and personal belief systems, ability to express feelings, and conditioning. A single-cause theory of anxiety overlooks the often-necessary combinations of contributors that may occur for any one person in any single circumstance (Barlow, 2000).

Heredity or biological sensitivity is a possible contributor in some individuals who are predisposed to excessive anxiety. Some individuals may inherit anxious, inhibited temperaments that predispose them to strong reactions to relatively mild-threatening stimuli. Childhood factors and social learning also may contribute to childhood, adolescent, and adult tendencies toward anxiety. For example, parents who communicate an overly cautious or fearful view of the world, or parents who are overly critical with excessively high standards, may contribute to children becoming excessively anxious or fearful. Children who experience neglect, rejection, abandonment through divorce or death, or emotional, physical, or sexual abuse may develop emotional insecurity and dependency that form a background for anxiety reactions to stresses in later life (Bourne, 2005; Canino & Spurlock, 2000).

In one puzzling syndrome that appears to have a strong anxiety component, children who develop selective mutism exhibit partial or complete withholding of vocal communication (Rubin, Sataloff, & Korovin, 2006). Although there are believed to be numerous possible causative factors, social anxiety is considered to be a key variable. In fact, Anstendig (1999) speculates whether selective mutism is a symptom of an anxiety disorder rather than a distinct psychological disorder. Some studies have shown that children with selective mutism have social phobia or avoidant anxiety (Black & Uhde, 1995; Dummit, Klein, Tancer, Asche, Martin, & Fairbanks, 1997). In fact, Johnson and Wintgens (2001) state that children with selective mutism "learn to avoid anxiety by not attempting to speak" (p. 17). Additional predisposing factors may be the child's wariness and hypersensitivity, as well as a family history of shyness, social isolation, or selective mutism. Evidence of trauma or abuse in the histories of children with selective mutism has not been consistent (Black & Uhde, 1995). Adults may develop long-term or permanent functional aphonia (elective mutism) after events of acute stress (Andrews, 2006; Boone, McFarlane, & Von Berg, 2009).

Stressors and Anxiety

Short-term stressors may precipitate or trigger anxiety, such as a significant personal loss (e.g., loss of a job or loss of a loved one). However, cumulative stress over time may be a significant contributor to anxiety (e.g., health impairments, marital problems, employment uncertainty, or long-term impairment of communication abilities secondary to a CVA). Anxiety produced by cumulative stress is more enduring and often less easily managed than that produced by short-term stress. In other cases, anxiety may be the result of the accumulation of several life events, that is, events that change the course of a person's life and that require adjustment and reordering of priorities. While one or two events each year are common and manageable for most people, a series of many life events over a one- to two-year period can lead to chronic stress. Holmes and Rahe (1967) developed the *Life Events Survey* (also known as *The Social Readjustment Scale*) to assess the number and severity of life events that occur in a two-year period, and this instrument may be used as a general measure of cumulative stress (Bourne, 2005). Over time, stress can affect the neuroendocrine regulatory systems of the brain, which are important in mood and anxiety

(Bear, Connors, & Paradiso, 2007). Biological causes of anxiety refer to physiological imbalances in the body or brain that are associated with anxiety, which may be the result of specific hereditary vulnerability and/or cumulative stress over time.

There are many possible factors that can contribute to an individual's level of anxiety: hereditary or temperamental factors, childhood history, cumulative stresses, or biological and medical factors. It is important to keep in mind that even positive events such as marriage, the birth of a child, a move to a new location, or a new job can be stressful. Therefore, avoiding being judgmental and focusing on an empathic approach to the person who is demonstrating anxiety will be beneficial to the therapeutic relationship.

Social Anxiety

Social anxiety involves fear of embarrassment or humiliation in situations in which a person is exposed to the scrutiny of others. The anxiety level may vary depending on a variety of factors such as to whom the person is talking, how many people are listening or watching, their ages, their social status, and so forth. The anxiety or fear may be strong enough to cause individuals to avoid situations. Severe levels of social anxiety may be diagnosed by a psychologist or psychiatrist as Social Phobia and treated by individuals in those professions. A diagnosis of Social Phobia includes avoidance that interferes with work, social activities, or important relationships (*DSM-IV-TR*, 2000).

Children and adults who stutter frequently experience high levels of social anxiety when talking in front of a classroom, at meetings, or in front of groups. Talking to individual people, particularly those who are perceived as having a higher status, can create significant anxiety and increase stuttering behaviors. For individuals who stutter, one of the highest levels of anxiety occurs when attempting to talk openly about their stuttering (Aten, 2008; Conture & Curlee, 2007; Gregory, 2003; Guitar, 2006; Ramig & Dodge, 2010; St. Louis, 2008; Zebrowski, 2002).

Fogle (2008) discusses the emotional and social effects of each of the major areas of communication disorders. Some children with moderate to severe articulation or phonological disorders may demonstrate symptoms of social anxiety in their avoidance of interacting with other children or talking to adults because of fear of not being understood and fear of embarrassment. Children with repaired cleft lips and/or hypernasality may avoid speaking to others and may be considered shy by other children or teachers. When coerced to speak in front of a group, for example, giving a required speech or oral book report, these children may have panic attacks that are related to being embarrassed or humiliated. Adults with neurological impairments resulting in moderate to severe apraxia, dysarthria, aphasia, or cognitive disorders may avoid social settings or work environments in which they had been very comfortable and successful for decades. These adults may choose to remain in their homes and minimize outings in order to avoid potential difficulty communicating in public and being embarrassed or humiliated. An adult with a neurogenic communication problem who chooses to avoid normal social contacts may cause stress within the family because of the limited activities he now enjoys. It is important for clinicians to appreciate that some of our patients may have had significant social anxiety prior to their neurological damage; the neurological impairment can exacerbate their social anxiety to the degree that it becomes a social phobia.

GENERAL APPROACHES TO ADDRESS SOCIAL ANXIETY

General approaches that may be helpful for clients and patients who are experiencing social anxiety related to their communication disorders include systematic desensitization, relaxation training, cognitive therapy, and group therapy (Andrews, 2006; Boone, McFarlane, & Von Berg, 2009; Bourne, 2005; Clark & Beck, 2009; Craighead et al., 1994; Gregory, 2003; Guitar, 2006). These approaches are discussed in the following sections.

SYSTEMATIC DESENSITIZATION   Many clients with voice disorders or fluency disorders benefit from systematic desensitization in which the person is asked to create a hierarchy or list various situations in her life that ordinarily produce some anxiety. The person is then asked to arrange those situations in a sequential order from the least to the most anxiety provoking. Wolpe (1987) developed this therapeutic approach in which a person is taught relaxed responses to anxiety-evoking situations. In a stepwise fashion the person learns to approach and master one anxiety-provoking situation after another, moving from the least anxiety-provoking situations to the most anxiety-provoking situations (Beck & Emery, 1985; Clark & Beck, 2009).

RELAXATION TRAINING   Many clients with voice disorders and fluency disorders benefit from relaxation training; however, most people with normal stresses in their lives also may benefit from this approach. Because people often cannot change their worlds, they need to learn to change their responses to them (Elliot, 1994). Regardless of who we are or what we do, good things, bad things, and tragedies are going to occur in our lives. Learning relaxation responses to stressful situations can help people maintain their emotional equilibrium so they can better maintain their ability to function satisfactorily in their work life, home life, and social life. Essentially, relaxation training helps people become more aware of their physiological state of tension and then provides ways to achieve a state of mental and physical calm.

COGNITIVE THERAPY   The process of change in cognitive therapy initially involves the use of behavioral strategies to increase activities, especially those that give the person a sense of mastery and pleasure. In addition to these behavioral strategies, the following cognitive procedures also are used: (1) identification of dysfunctional and distorted cognitions and realization that they produce negative feelings and maladaptive behaviors; (2) self-monitoring of negative thoughts or self-talk; (3) identification of the relationships of thoughts to underlying beliefs and feelings; (4) identification of alternative and more productive thinking patterns; and (5) hypothesis testing regarding the validity of the person's basic assumptions about himself, the world, and the future (Beck & Emery, 1985; Clark & Beck, 2009; Prochaska & Norcross, 2009). Overall, the intention of cognitive therapy is to help the person change the way she thinks about a situation, which in turn will help her change the way she feels about the situation. (See Chapter 2 for more details and applications of cognitive therapy.)

GROUP THERAPY   Group speech therapy is commonly used in public schools in order to manage large caseloads of children. However, group therapy also provides benefits for both children and adults who have anxiety about their communication problems.

Learning to speak openly in small groups can help them gain confidence and prepare them to speak in larger groups, such as in front of a class or a business meeting. Group therapy has long been used with individuals who stutter (Gregory, 2003; Guitar & Reville, 2006; Ramig & Dodge, 2010; Van Riper, 1982; Van Riper & Erickson, 1996; Zebrowski, 2006). Sheehan (1970) felt that stuttering was a social problem and, therefore, was best worked with in a social (i.e., group therapy) environment. Group therapy and support groups for individuals with neurological disorders or laryngectomies have been incorporated into hospital, rehabilitation center, and university programs for many years. Support groups have been very helpful for many parents of children who are deaf or hard of hearing, providing the opportunity for parents to meet and interact with others who are in a similar situation.

Acute Stress Response

Acute stress response (which may evolve into Acute Stress Disorder) involves development of anxiety and possible disabling symptoms after a traumatic event and may be considered a response to a crisis event (see Chapter 14). The initial trauma involves exposure to an event that carries the threat of death or serious injury. In an acute stress response the symptoms subside in less than one month; however, if the symptoms last beyond one month a psychologist may change the diagnosis from Acute Stress Disorder to Posttraumatic Stress Disorder (see Chapter 14). Causes of acute stress responses in individuals SLPs and Auds may include CVAs, TBIs, sudden loss of hearing, and other causes of rapid or abrupt onset of communication disorders. These individuals may have a subjective sense of emotional numbing (being out of touch with feelings), feelings of detachment or estrangement from others, absence of emotional responsiveness, loss of interest in activities that used to be pleasurable, reduction of awareness of surroundings and environment (i.e., not being oriented to person, place, time and purpose; being in a daze), or derealization (feeling the experience is not real). The symptoms cause significant distress and interfere with normal functioning (Bourne, 2005; *DSM-IV-TR*, 2000).

Individuals with acute stress responses also may have symptoms of despair and hopelessness that may be sufficiently severe and persistent to be diagnosed as a major depressive episode by a psychologist. Some patients may be the survivors of traumas in which other people were killed or injured (e.g., motor vehicle accidents, terrorist attacks, etc.) and the survivors may feel guilt about having remained alive or about not providing enough help to others who were injured or died. These individuals often perceive themselves to have greater responsibility for the consequences of the trauma than is warranted (Bourne, 2005; *DSM-IV-TR*, 2000).

PANIC ATTACKS (PANIC REACTIONS)

Panic is an extreme level of an alarm reaction that a person has in response to a perceived threat, whether physical or psychological. In some cases there may be no perceived threat and the panic attack may emerge without any noticeable provocation, out of context, and without apparent reason. Physiologically, during a panic attack the autonomic (involuntary) nervous system's sympathetic branch (sympathetic nervous system) mobilizes several different bodily reactions rapidly and intensely. The adrenal glands release a large amount of adrenaline, causing a sudden surge or jolt, often accompanied by a feeling of dread or terror. Within seconds the extra adrenaline causes several reactions: (1) significantly increased heart rate, (2) shallow and rapid respiration, (3) profuse sweating, (4) trembling and shaking, and (5) cold hands and feet. Muscles throughout the body contract, and in extreme cases a person may be too scared to move, exhibiting a "deer in the headlights" phenomenon. Muscles in the chest and throat contract, making it difficult to breathe or make any sound. An excess of stomach acid is released and there may be nausea; there is a release of red blood cells by the spleen and release of glucose by the liver. There is an increase in metabolic rate and dilation of the pupils (Bear, Connors, & Paradiso, 2007). Each physiological reaction during a panic attack is the result of the fight-or-flight response. Panic attacks tend to last approximately 30 minutes, during which time the kidneys and liver reabsorb the adrenaline that was released. Individuals who have recurrent panic attacks may have a panic disorder and should be evaluated by a psychologist or other mental health professional.

Some children who stutter may experience panic attacks when they are told they must speak in front of the class and may exhibit a flight response by not attending school that day or avoiding the experience any way they can. Children with other communication disorders such as hypernasality secondary to a cleft palate or significant articulation or phonological disorders may panic at the thought of speaking in front of the class. Avoidance of an anxiety-producing or feared situation is one of the most common defenses used by children and adults with communication disorders (Fogle, 2008). Avoidance may be accomplished by delaying the feared communication situation or refusing to perform or communicate. Avoidance provides relief from threats to self-esteem caused by fears of communicating inadequately. Whereas avoidance prevents the feared experience from occurring, escape provides immediate and effective relief from the feared situation at hand (Tanner, 2008).

Escape may be used when postponements or refusals (i.e., attempts at avoidance) are not successful. People with severe communication disorders, such as severe apraxia, dysarthria, or aphasia, may not be able to verbalize their anxiety and fears, but observations of their facial expressions and body language and attempts to understand their limited verbal communications can help us appreciate the intensity of their feelings. Some hospitalized patients leave the hospital by checking out against medical advice (AMA), that is, without the approval of their physicians. Patients may be escaping anxieties or fears of further invasive medical procedures, perceived isolation, or uncomfortable or painful rehabilitation procedures. This can have serious medical consequences, but it may provide patients with immediate (albeit temporary) relief from the feared situation.

ANXIETY RELATED TO PLACES AND SITUATIONS

Some individuals have significant anxiety or fear of being in places or situations from which escape might be difficult or in which help may not be available in the event of a panic reaction. The anxiety may lead to pervasive avoidance of a variety of situations such as being home alone or being alone outside the home, being in a crowd of people, or traveling in a car or airplane. Psychologists use the term *agoraphobia* for this disorder, with the essence of agoraphobia being fear of panic attacks. These individuals not only fear panic attacks, but what other people will think of them should they be seen having a panic attack (Bourne, 2005).

Although SLPs and Auds cannot diagnose or treat agoraphobia, we may see the problem in some individuals with whom we work. For example, individuals with cerebral palsy, CVAs, or TBIs may avoid going out in public for fear of being embarrassed by their handicaps or becoming lost if they go too far from home. It is as though they are under a self-imposed house arrest. Likewise, some patients in skilled nursing facilities may refuse assistance from OTs or CNAs to get out of bed and into their wheelchairs so they can spend time in the day room or dining room.

Working with a Patient with Agoraphobia

I worked with a patient with dysphagia in a skilled nursing facility. She had been an elementary school teacher for over 30 years before she retired. Her husband had died and her adult children lived in other states. The patient had made a comfortable "little nest" with her bed and side table. She had stacks of magazines, material for her needlework, a radio, and telephone. She was always happy to see me and did the necessary therapy tasks to improve her swallowing to be a safe, independent eater. However, she chose to have all her meals in bed and refused assistance from anyone to get out of either her bed or the room. I discussed this with the nursing staff, who said that she was probably afraid to leave her room and that she had become quite comfortable with her limited surroundings. Encouragement or coaxing did not help her get out of the room and expand her world. Sometimes all we can do is support and encourage a patient, but ultimately it is each person's choice regarding the best way to live one's life.

CLINICAL QUESTIONS

1. How might you communicate with this client about her limited world?

2. How might you convey both acceptance and yet question whether she has fears that inhibit her? At what point might you view this conversation as outside your scope of practice?

3. What information might lead you to refer this client to a mental health professional for an assessment of a possible anxiety disorder?

Co-occurrence of Anxiety Responses

Since the mid-1990s there has been increasing recognition that many people have more than one anxiety trigger, response, and/or disorder. For example, individuals with social phobias also may have panic attacks, and people with panic attacks also may have agoraphobia (Bourne, 2005; Clark & Beck, 2009). This is important for SLPs and Auds to appreciate because some of our clients and patients may have experienced some type of anxiety symptoms prior to their current health-related anxiety responses. Individuals who previously experienced social anxiety now may be experiencing an acute stress response because of a hearing loss or aphasia. The communication impairment may exacerbate their previous social anxiety.

Summary

Some level of anxiety is normal for most children and adults who have their hearing, speech, language, cognition, or swallowing evaluated. A client's anxiety also may be evident during the treatment phase. In many cases, we see individuals who are trying to cope with situational anxiety, which may not be reflective of their general manner of managing and coping with other areas of their lives. However, when an individual's anxiety interferes with the evaluation process we must consider whether the test results are valid or an underestimate of the client's abilities. Also, when anxiety interferes with therapy, the client may benefit from the incorporation of anxiety management techniques into the therapy. We are not attempting to manage an anxiety disorder (the purview of psychologists and counselors), but we may be helping individuals learn and develop ways of recognizing, managing, and coping with the anxiety that is preventing or interfering with their gains in using hearing aid devices or improving their speech, language, cognitive, or swallowing abilities.

DEPRESSION

Many people feel depressed during some point in their lives, but their symptoms may not warrant a clinical diagnosis of depression, particularly when grieving after a significant loss (see discussion of the stages of grief in this chapter). Other people may suffer from more severe symptoms that together constitute a clinically diagnosed disorder of depression. Because SLPs and Auds are not qualified to diagnose depression, we are primarily concerned with depressive symptoms and, in this text, refer to depressive symptoms as depression.

Depression is a common response to a significant loss of speech, language, cognition, swallowing, or hearing abilities (Holland, 2007; Schow & Nerbonne, 2006). Depression is the most common psychological reaction to stroke-related communication disorders, particularly aphasia (Tanner, 2003, 2008) (see Chapter 8). Young children with hearing loss or developmental communication delays or disorders may experience some depression if they sense disapproval or rejection from their peers or parents. The parents of these children may experience some level of depression (along with guilt) as a consequence of fears of possibly causing the delays or disorders (e.g., a mother's abuse of drugs or alcohol during pregnancy). Parents also may experience guilt and depression if they feel they did not recognize and have the hearing or communication problem evaluated earlier and follow the recommended course of therapy (Schow & Nerbonne, 2006; Tye-Murray, 2009).

Hospitalized patients and residents in skilled nursing facilities may show signs of depression for a variety of reasons: lack of stimulation, absence of family and friends, loss, loneliness, awareness that they may never see their home again, and being ill and weak. Some communication problems associated with depression are (Wallace, 2007):

- **Communicative withdrawal**   Depressed patients make little effort to interact with other people and may reject social contacts and attempts to get them involved in activities. They may refuse therapy.

- **Decrease in the quantity and complexity of communication**   When depressed individuals communicate, there is usually a paucity of words and the use of simple, direct sentences. When they are feeling a little more upbeat, they are more likely to participate and even enjoy therapy.

- **Reliance on body language and other nonverbal signals**   In the absence of verbal communication, some depressed patients rely on nonverbal communication (body language and facial expressions) to convey feelings and needs.

The *DSM-IV-TR* (2000) discusses symptoms of individuals with depression. These symptoms may include being sad, depressed, hopeless, discouraged, or angry; a loss of interest or pleasure in activities that were previously enjoyable (anhedonia); difficulty sleeping; and loss of appetite or possibly excessive sleeping and/or eating. Many individuals with symptoms of depression report impaired ability to think, concentrate, or make decisions. They may appear easily distracted or complain of memory difficulties. In children, a precipitous drop in grades may reflect poor concentration caused by depression. In adolescents, irritability or substance abuse may reflect a depressive condition (Birmaher, Arbelaez, & Brent, 2002; Zuckerbrot, Cheung, Jenson, & Stein, 2007). In elderly people, memory difficulties may be the chief complaint and may be mistaken for early signs of dementia (pseudodementia) (Kindermann & Brown, 1997). You may observe psychomotor behaviors including agitation (e.g., hand wringing, pacing, pulling or rubbing the skin) or psychomotor retardation (e.g., slowed speech, thinking, and body movements; low voice volume; little or absent voice inflection; or functional aphonia). Individuals often describe or demonstrate decreased energy, tiredness, and generalized fatigue, with even the smallest tasks requiring substantial effort. A sense of worthlessness or guilt may be associated with depression, with ruminations over minor past failings. Frequent thoughts of death or suicidal ideation may occur.

In general, depressed mood reveals itself as sadness; depressed cognition refers to a negative evaluation of one's self, the world, or the future or impoverished thought (i.e., minimal thought processes with decreased ability to provide elaboration); and depressed behavior may include lethargy, isolation, and disturbed eating and sleeping patterns (Beck, 1967; Lambert, 2008). Depressive symptoms can become intensified over time and may be debilitating. Our goal is to recognize the signs and symptoms of depression in order to make the appropriate referral to a professional who can manage the problem. However, whether or not a counselor, psychologist, or psychiatrist becomes involved with our clients and patients, SLPs and Auds must provide therapy only in our areas of expertise.

Some individuals may have experienced depression prior to acquiring a hearing or communication disorder, and their new communication disorder may exacerbate their depressive symptoms. Individuals with chronic, low-level symptoms of depression may be experiencing dysthymia (*DSM-IV-TR*, 2000) Also, family members may have chronic, low-level symptoms of depression prior to their loved one's communication impairment and may show difficulty finding the energy or motivation we might expect of them to help the patient. It is important to consider whether clients or family members are depressed or if they are unable to comply with the SLP or Aud's recommendations. If the client is suffering from depression, even a low-level depression such as dysthymia, the condition may need to be treated before he can become more amenable to therapy. Likewise, if the primary family caregiver has undiagnosed and untreated dysthymia, she may not have the emotional or physical energy to sufficiently care for the patient once he is brought home. The family caregiver may benefit from professional counseling and possible pharmacological intervention.

Interviewing

When interviewing clients or patients it is appropriate to ask about medications they are taking. In medical settings, information about psychotropic drugs is available in medical charts, which should be reviewed prior to first seeing patients. Psychotropic drugs affect the psychological function, behavior, and experiences of a person (Anderson, Keith, & Novak, 2007). Although we may ask clients in general terms about medications, we do not specifically ask if they are taking anti-anxiety or antidepression medications. Clients may not feel the need for the SLP or Aud to know that information and therefore may deny the use of medications or may report taking some medications but not others. If, during the interview and evaluation of the client, we see signs of depression or the person reports symptoms of depression, we may choose not to comment on it at that time, but to take note of our observations and be alert to them in future contacts with the person. Symptoms of depression may be secondary to a medical disorder (Morrison, 1997) and need to be evaluated by a mental health professional or physician. The challenge for SLPs and Auds is to work with individuals who have symptoms of depression that may interfere with therapy. A few approaches that are within our scope of practice may help improve the client's coping abilities and enhance the benefits of therapy.

General Approaches to Use with Symptoms of Depression

There are several approaches clinicians can take to help clients with symptoms of depression, including the cognitive-behavioral approach, the humanistic approach, and the interpersonal approach. The theoretical foundations of these approaches are discussed in more detail in Chapter 2.

COGNITIVE-BEHAVIORAL APPROACH

Cognitive-behavioral therapy (Beck, 1967, 1995; Craske, 2010; Farmer & Chapman, 2008; Hollon & Beck, 2004) attempts to help individuals identify coping strategies, such as listening to uplifting music and reading positive books or other material. Clients can be encouraged to call or visit family and friends who are supportive and whom they enjoy. Speaking to people who have survived or worked through similar communication problems can help clients recognize that their goals in therapy are not insurmountable. Positive self-talk and affirmations can help change clients' negative views of themselves and their rehabilitation potential. Clinicians may compliment the person when she is well dressed, neat, or looks nice. Reinforce smiles, jokes, and light-hearted conversation. The purpose of this is not to encourage the client to hide or mask her feelings, but to attempt to reinforce the person's more positive and upbeat behaviors, which may influence the person's mood. A client who is enjoying positive relationships and feedback is more likely to engage in and enjoy the tasks of therapy than a client who is focused on the negative side of life experiences.

HUMANISTIC APPROACH

Following the humanistic approach (Cain, 2010; Rogers 1951, 1957, 1961, 1980), the clinician will want to maintain genuineness, empathic understanding, unconditional positive regard, and acceptance of the client. Focus on "being with" the client rather than on what to say. Occasional reflections of feelings, such as "It looks like you are feeling a little low today," spoken in an accepting, empathic manner, can help the client feel that you recognize her mood and understand her. This interaction can be very important to a depressed client who feels invalidated or ignored by others. It is often helpful to mirror the nonverbal communication of the client (see Chapters 3 and 4) who has symptoms of depression (e.g., speaking softly to match the client's voice and moving slowly and gently in a manner that does not abruptly contrast with the client's). This mirroring can help the client feel that you are "in tune" with her, which may help her be more responsive to you and the therapy (Corey, 2008; Prochaska & Norcross, 2009).

INTERPERSONAL APPROACH

Clients with symptoms of depression sometimes express themselves in ways that elicit negative responses from others (e.g., whining, moaning, complaining) (Sullivan, 1953, 1972; Benjamin, 1996; Weissman & Klerman, 1991). If we feel ourselves becoming irritated, the client is probably having a similar effect on other people too, including family and friends. We need to avoid responding in ways that the client has learned are predictable of other people, such as with impatience, irritation, harshness, or anger. Responding in a predictably negative manner reinforces the vicious cycle that the client is already experiencing with others (Anchin & Kiesler, 1982; Klerman & Weissman, 1993; Weismann, Markowitz, & Klerman, 2007). We need to be supportive and encouraging, not demanding. Our tone of voice and body language are as important as the specific words we say.

Summary

Depression is a common response to a significant loss of hearing, speech, language, cognition, or swallowing abilities. SLPs and Auds need to be aware of the signs and symptoms of depression and make appropriate referrals to other mental health professionals when it appears that the symptoms are chronic and interfering with the person's life. We need to recognize when symptoms of depression are the likely result of the newly diagnosed or long-standing communication problem and consider the client's affect as a part of the total person and her capacity to engage in the treatment process. Although we cannot diagnose or treat depression, there are approaches we can incorporate into our therapy that may improve our clients' receptivity to treatment and coping abilities.

GRIEF

Loss is a natural consequence of living; similarly, grief and bereavement are human reactions to loss. Life-threatening illness or injury is not only a medical crisis; it precipitates a psychological, social, and spiritual crisis as well. Loss is a fundamental aspect of any disability, including those involving hearing, speech, language, cognition, and swallowing. The client or patient has lost some level of function, and family members have lost a loved one as the person they knew. Ultimately, the clinician's interaction with the grieving person can affect the overall prognosis for recovery of function (Hansson & Stroebe, 2007; Rolland, 1994).

Loss can have both real and symbolic meaning. Real loss involves loss of either a person (death or separation of a significant person), function (use of an arm), ability (hearing, speaking), or meaningful object (a prized possession). Symbolic loss includes a loss of either self-esteem, personal or professional standing, or the role a person plays in his family. A hearing loss or communication disorder can result in both real and symbolic losses (Tanner, 2003, 2008).

The expression or outer manifestations of the inner grief experience can be quite varied. How individuals grieve, particularly for the loss of a loved one (including the person as he had been prior to a significant impairment), is often influenced by their age, gender, and cultural background (Sanders, 1998; Stroebe, Hansson, Schut, & Stroebe, 2008). In addition, there are indications that early socialization has an effect on the way children respond to loss. The grieving behavior of a child is often similar to that of the surviving parent of the same gender. For example, after his mother's death, a son may try to be stoic and "strong," much as he sees his father trying to be. While family and friends may say in an admiring way, "What a little man you are being!" or, "He is acting so grown up!" these comments tend to discourage the boy's important emotional expression.

Understanding death involves comprehending the concepts of irreversibility, finality, and causality (Corr & Balk, 2010). Kenyon (2001) and Slaughter and Griffiths (2007) found that, in general, prior to age 3, children may recognize an absence among those in their immediate world and miss a familiar person who is gone, but they are unlikely to understand the difference between absence and death. Preschool children may talk about death but still expect the person to come back. By age 9 or 10, most children have developed an understanding of death as final, irreversible, and inescapable. Children in general may express their grief for the loss of a loved one in the following ways (Potter, 2006; Worden, 2008):

1. Prolonged withdrawal, apathy, sustained acting out of anger, denial, crying spells, and rejection of others

2. Depressed mood that fluctuates, irritability, low levels of energy, loss of attention to people and tasks, loss of interest in friends and previously enjoyable activities, escaping by watching excessive amounts of television or playing video games

3. Weight changes as a result of not eating or overeating

4. Insomnia because of worry or fear of bad dreams or hypersomnia—sleeping too much

5. Psychomotor changes with either a significant decrease in activity levels or an excess of activity

6. Feelings of guilt, worthlessness, and low self-esteem

7. Difficulty concentrating and a decline in school performance

8. Prolonged ruminations about death and possible talk of self-harm

9. Frequent somatic complaints such as headaches and stomach aches

10. The need for extra or constant attention and fear of the living parent, grandparent, or sibling leaving or dying

Men and women tend to express their grief differently. Women who are grieving tend to exhibit the following characteristics (Doka, 2007; Margo, 2006; Worden, 2008):

1. Express anguish in tears and laments

2. Show willingness to talk about their grief

3. Seek support from family, friends, and social networks

4. Reminisce about the loved one

5. Have difficulty expressing anger

6. Experience guilt feelings

7. Provide caregiving to friends and family

8. Maintain the family circle

9. Cope by engaging in destructive behaviors, such as excessive use of tobacco, alcohol, or drugs

Men who are grieving may exhibit the following behaviors and tendencies (Doka, 2007; Margo, 2006; Worden, 2008):

1. Feelings may be blunted, limited, or toned down

2. Self-control may be valued

3. Thinking precedes and often dominates feelings

4. The focus may be on problem solving rather than expression of feelings

5. The outward expression of feelings often involves anger and/or guilt

6. Intense feelings may only be expressed privately; there may be a general reluctance to discuss feelings with others

7. Intense grief is usually expressed immediately after the loss or at post-death rituals such as funeral services

8. Some may try to return to structured routines as soon as possible and immerse themselves in work or activity. Some may cope by engaging in destructive behaviors, such as excessive use of tobacco, alcohol, or drugs

Grieving reactions may be viewed along an affective-cognitive continuum (Sanders, 1998). Females tend to invest more energy toward the affective end of the continuum, while males tend to invest more energy in cognitive processes. Perhaps because many women express grief in an emotionally expressive manner, caregivers tend to overlook masculine (husband, father, son, grandfather, brother) reactions to grief and focus instead on the feminine (wife, mother, daughter, grandmother, sister) reactions to grief (Doka, 2007; Worden, 2008). Although there are masculine and feminine cultural traditions of grieving, many men and women have transcended these traditional patterns of grieving, and therefore these common characteristics may not predict a particular individual's processing of grief. Whatever the individual's response to grief entails, clinicians need to remember to be respectful and not try to short-circuit that process. For example, when clients or family members are expressing their grief through tears, we should not attempt to relieve our own discomfort by offering reassurance or launching into a detailed description of our assessment procedures to distract them from their grief.

Stages of Grief

Elisabeth Kubler-Ross (1969) discussed the grieving process in her book *On Death and Dying*. Our discussion of the grieving process expands Kubler-Ross' model to grieving the loss of hearing, speech, language, cognitive, and swallowing functions and, in a way, a loss of sense of self (Rolland, 1994; Tanner, 2003, 2008). Grief is not considered a single reaction, but a complex progression involving many emotions and attempts to adjust and cope with loss. Kubler-Ross presents five stages in the grieving process: denial, anger, bargaining, depression, and acceptance. Parents of infants and children who are diagnosed as deaf or hearing impaired frequently go through the grieving process. The child who seemed so normal now may have a profound handicap that will affect all aspects of communication and many aspects of life. The parents may begin to envision possible restrictions and difficulties in their child's education, friendships and relationships, and eventual employment. The parents also will likely consider the challenges they will be facing in their parental roles and how the child's hearing impairment might cause limitations in the family's future plans. For example, the added expenses for hearing evaluations, hearing aids, and possibly special schooling for the child with a hearing impairment may limit financial resources for other things the parents had hoped for and planned.

It is helpful to keep in mind that clients, patients, and families with communication problems may go through the stages more than once. For example, a child with a head injury and his parents may progress from denial to acceptance while in the hospital and rehabilitation settings, but when the child returns home and he and the family begin to recognize his severe limitations in that environment, they may have denial about new issues and eventually have to progress to acceptance again. Furthermore, when the child returns to school and is confronted with his severe losses by being moved to a lower grade level or into special education and adaptive physical education, and begins to see how his friends and teachers treat him differently, the child may again go through the stages of grief. For example, the child may experience denial ("I don't need to be in special ed! I'm still smart!"); anger ("I won't do this stupid work!"); bargaining ("If I do everything you want me to do, can I go back to my real classroom?"); depression ("I can't do this stuff like I used to. I'll never be smart again!"); and acceptance ("I have to stay in this class, I guess, even if I don't like it.").

DENIAL

Denial has been discussed in some detail (see Chapter 10), but a few concepts may be reviewed in the context of discussing loss. In response to news or information that is overwhelming, some people respond with the very basic defense of denial. A person's first reaction may be a temporary state of shock from which she recuperates gradually (Kubler-Ross, 1969). Even well-adjusted people may initially employ denial during times of overwhelming anxiety (Gladding, 2009). Short-lived denial is a common response to receiving news of a diagnosis of a disability or a serious illness or injury and is not considered an unhealthy response. The client, patient, or family member may protest, "No, I don't!" or "No, it can't be true!" This form of denial may be a relatively short-lived response when the person must make a radical adjustment to her self-image and expectations as this new information is processed. Denial is the barrier that many people temporarily erect as they try to adjust to a profound change in their lives. Denial becomes a concern when it persists for an extended period of time and interferes with sound judgment, logical problem solving, and investing in needed therapy.

Some clients may need confirmation of a diagnosis (e.g., APD or dysphagia) and request a second opinion, particularly if the client does not understand the nature of the problem or is uncertain of the clinician's expertise. In many cases, clients do not present a total denial of a diagnosis or the need for therapy, but a partial denial in which they acknowledge some part of what is explained, but are not ready to accept all of the diagnostic implications or commit to a therapy regimen. Later, when the client has progressed to the stage of acceptance, there may be times when the person reverts back to denial and again may need to work through the stages, although the progression is usually more rapid than the first time.

Parental denial of a child's hearing or communication problem can delay or even prevent the child from receiving much-needed help. In some cases, parents may admit a problem exists but not be sufficiently emotionally engaged to make the arrangements or carry out the needed management for the child (e.g., having the child's hearing tested by an audiologist, purchasing hearing aids, or enforcing the child's wearing of them). We need to keep in mind that denial is a plea for help and not a dereliction of duty on the parents' part (Friehe, Bloedow, & Hesse, 2003; Luterman, 2008).

When a person denies or minimizes a communication problem for which she needs an evaluation and therapy, it is helpful to gently but clearly state the problems you see and the need for intervention. A strong statement about the need for therapy may result in stronger denial and resistance. Letting the person know that there is some urgency about beginning therapy and the reasons for the urgency may help the person accept therapy before she truly accepts the loss.

ANGER

Anger is discussed in some detail in Chapter 13, but a brief review of a few concepts may be helpful as they relate to grief. When the first stage of grief cannot be maintained any longer, it is replaced by feelings of anger and possibly rage (Kubler-Ross, 1969; Rolland, 1994; Stroebe et al., 2008). The parents, child, or adult may ask aloud or to themselves, "Why me?" Although people do not wish hardships on others, they may be thinking, "Why couldn't it have happened to someone else?"

Anger in the grieving process can be very difficult to cope with because it may be displaced in many directions and projected onto the environment at unexpected times. Sometimes anger is projected onto people who have what the client has lost. For example, patients who must begin eating pureed meals with thickened liquids may become angry toward the therapist who ordered them, the individuals who deliver them, and even toward patients who have regular meals and thin liquids.

Clinicians need to remember that the client or patient's anger is not a personal reaction to the clinician or the therapy program. The clinician needs to understand the anger and its source, and not judge it or automatically react to it. This perspective can be shared with family members, who often have particular difficulty responding to a grieving person's anger. Family members may have a tendency to avoid or reject the patient for her angry behaviors. Helping the family understand the grieving process and the need for acceptance of the individual's moods and behaviors can help the grieving person feel accepted and loved.

Children and adults with severe communication problems often are not able to adequately express their feelings verbally, and may use angry behaviors to express the depth of pain they are experiencing. If reprimands are needed for physical displays of anger, they should be reserved for acts that are destructive or could harm the person or other individuals. Letting the patient know that the anger is understandable can go a long way towards giving the person permission to express the anger directly (i.e., through words) rather than indirectly or through destructive action.

BARGAINING

In the first stage of grief, the person is unable to accept the difficult facts of the diagnosis and the need for management, and in the second stage the person is angry with others, even God. In the third stage, the person attempts to enter into an agreement that may postpone or reduce the effects of the loss. The bargaining stage, like denial and anger, is normal and helpful in the process of eventually achieving acceptance of loss. The person may bargain with whomever he feels may have some power or control over the loss: God, physicians, nurses, clinicians, or family. Some individuals even bargain with themselves, saying, for example, "I will never take drugs again if I can just get my speech back." People often bargain for time or "one more chance"; however, when the bargained-for time has passed or one more chance has not occurred, they bargain for more time and more chances. During the bargaining stage patients often are motivated and enthusiastic in therapy, which may be the result of hope for a rapid improvement or recovery. Bargaining is about hope and trying to reverse the loss or change the outcome; however, when the hope for the ending or alleviation of the loss does not materialize through bargaining, the person will likely move to the fourth stage of grieving, depression.

DEPRESSION

Depression, discussed in some detail earlier, is discussed now in its relationship to the grieving process. When grieving people find that their denial does not make the problem go away, their anger does not frighten it away, and their bargaining does not gain them anything, they move into the fourth stage, depression. We need to keep in mind that people's loss of hearing and loss of communication abilities represent changes in their lives that can have profound effects. From these losses countless other losses may follow: loss of positive self-image, loss of self-esteem, loss of relationships as the person has known them, loss of employment with resulting loss of income and financial dependence, and many others.

As clinicians, we may only see the "tip of the iceberg" of a person's loss. Our focus is on the person's hearing, speech, language, and swallowing problems. Although we try to view our clients, patients, and their families holistically, we can never imagine the total magnitude of losses they may be experiencing or the depth of depression and despair they may be feeling. The cost of evaluations and therapy, hearing aids, and assistive devices can burden families so heavily that "little luxuries" may need to be dispensed with, and even household and family necessities reevaluated and possibly eliminated. Financial burdens can weigh heavily on the individual and family, adding to their depression.

Friends or family may attempt to cheer up the grieving person; however, this response may reflect a lack of sensitivity and an implicit devaluing of a person's losses and need to grieve. The grieving person may try to smile or laugh to please or appease the individuals who are trying to be cheerful, but the person will likely revert back to grief when those people are gone. Grieving individuals should not be told to find the silver lining or to look at the brighter side of life. Such admonitions are usually for the benefit of the family and friends who make them; they often reflect their inability to tolerate another's sadness for an extended period of time. Rather than cajoling or attempting to cheer the grieving person, family and friends can be most helpful by being quietly present and not placing demands or having expectations of their conversations or interactions with the grieving person.

Some people may remain in the depression stage for only a few days, but for others it may last for a few months or longer. How long a person remains in this stage depends on a variety of factors, such as what was lost and how much was lost; the cognitive capacity of the person (e.g., patients with severe brain injuries may not be aware of the extent of their losses); the preexisting personality; and the support of family and friends. Brief episodes of depression can even be triggered by photographs of the person or family members or other visual, auditory, or tactile sensations that remind the person of who or what the person was before the loss. Some people do not pass successfully through this stage but become stuck in the depression stage (Tanner, 2003, 2008).

People who are grieving and depressed often have difficulty attending and staying focused in therapy and may be generally unresponsive, lethargic, and pessimistic. There may be a significant change from the motivated and enthusiastic attitude the person had during the bargaining stage to an "It's no use" attitude during the depression stage. Individuals in this stage of grieving need to be monitored for signs of severe clinical depression, which may require mental health intervention. Our goal as SLPs and Auds is not to eliminate the depression, but to show empathy and facilitate the natural process so that the grieving person can advance to the stage of acceptance.

ACCEPTANCE

Acceptance is an admission and acknowledgement of the truth: the loss did occur, and denying it, being angry about it, bargaining over it, and being depressed about it will not change it. There is a resignation to the loss, and the person is no longer resistant to it.

The person may have consciously resolved to accept the way things are and to move on from there. In essence, the person has gone through each of the three ways people change: (1) *revolution* (a significant event in the person's life has changed the way she thinks and believes); (2) *evolution* (the person has progressed through the stages of grief); and (3) *resolution* (the person has accepted things as they are and that she must move forward from there).

The acceptance or integration (Luterman, 2008, p. 71) stage is characterized by getting the disorder into a life perspective. The changes caused by the disorder are integrated into a new lifestyle with different values. The client and family learn to live with the disorder and to spend time and energy on other matters. They realize that "beating" the disorder is not always a matter of reaching normalcy, but rather of learning to live life to the fullest in the face of the disorder (Luterman, 2008, p. 72).

Summary

Although there is general agreement that grieving involves a dynamic process in which individuals progress through multiple stages, a particular stage model (such as Kubler-Ross') may not apply to all individuals. The stages of grief are not clear-cut, and people may show signs of being in more than one stage at a time. Also, stages may recur: a person who appears to have advanced to the acceptance stage may suddenly appear to have returned to the bargaining or depression stage. Nevertheless, knowledge of this model may help to provide a framework for understanding patients who experience loss and whose reactions may not always appear logical or helpful.

Most of us have had a significant loss in our lives and know how it feels, although we may not have known or recognized various stages of our own grieving. In general, people tend to remember the last two stages, depression and acceptance, because they are often more long-lasting than the denial, anger, and bargaining stages. However, we may not see clients, patients, or family members progress through all the stages, particularly in acute-care medical settings where patients are discharged after a few days or weeks. While in therapy in outpatient clinics and rehabilitation centers, clinicians may see patients and families work through the latter stages and arrive at some level of acceptance. In university clinics it is common for clients and families who have been living with their losses for some time to have reached the acceptance stage and to appreciate the continued therapy available to them.

GUILT AND SHAME

Guilt and shame are both negative emotions that often occur in the context of illness or injury. Although guilt and shame are distinct and different emotional experiences, they may coexist (George & Cristiani, 1995; Stroebe et al., 2008). Guilt is a feeling that frequently occurs when people believe that they may have in some way contributed to the cause of a loved one's problem (e.g., a mother and child are in a motor vehicle accident and the child is seriously injured), or that they have caused their own problem (e.g., not taking blood pressure medication and having a CVA). Parents often feel some guilt for a child who has a congenital condition. Parents of children with hearing impairments often state that if bad news is communicated poorly, our clients and their families may never forgive us; however, if bad news is communicated well, they may never forget us.

Presenting bad news is a particular communication challenge that may be especially trying and possibly go poorly without sufficient understanding of several basic principles. Although SLPs and Auds do not present the initial news to clients, patients, and family members about life-and-death issues or serious physical illnesses (e.g., cancer of the larynx or a brain tumor), the difficult information we must convey may be perceived by the receiver as more serious, profound, or life-changing than we might expect. How we share bad news can make an important difference as to how it is received and accepted. In addition, if a person has received bad news from several other professionals in a short amount of time (e.g., a serious medical diagnosis from a physician, nursing concerns, and physical therapy and occupational therapy diagnoses), our bad news may be "the straw that breaks the camel's back," and the person may become emotionally distraught as a result of the accumulation of negative news. This can occur in educational settings as well, for example, when parents attending an Individualized Educational Plan (IEP) meeting are presented discouraging information about their child by the school psychologist, the classroom teacher, the resource specialist, the audiologist, the SLP, and others (Lawrence-Lightfoot, 2003).

Greenberg (1999) describes a training program to help SLPs and educators increase their sensitivity about sharing bad news with parents. In the initial training she had participants recall an occasion when they received bad news about their own children, another family member, or themselves. Responses typically were sadness, shock, anger, disbelief, fear, anxiety, guilt, or despair. The memories of these occasions also were vivid in how the participants were told the bad news, and typically the memories were not positive. The same group was then asked to recall a time when they had to share bad news and how they felt. The participants described a variety of fears associated with giving the news, including fear of causing pain, being blamed, feeling they had failed, and losing control of their own emotions. This exercise may be helpful for other SLPs and Auds to increase their understanding and empathy when sharing disappointing or bad news with clients, patients, and their families. The following is a discussion of six principles from Buckman and Kason (1992) and Hallenbeck (2003) that are helpful when giving bad news, particularly as it relates to medical environments.

The Physical Environment and Presentation of Yourself

Walk into the room at a normal or slightly slower pace. Avoid a fast pace that may give the impression that you are in a hurry. Shake each person's hand, the patient's hand first, then those of other family members or individuals invited by the family. Shaking the patient's hand first demonstrates that the patient comes first and is the focus of the time together. Buckman and Kason (1992) and Hallenbeck (2003) recommend that the patient be touched at least once during the meeting to reduce perceived emotional separation between you and the patient and that the initial handshake may be the best time for an initial touch. A handshake at the end of the meeting or a brief touch of the arm may confirm to the patient or relative the respect and empathy we hope they felt throughout the meeting.

If possible, take the patient or family members to a quiet room, which may require "the long walk." You may want to give an explanation such as, "I know that it's a bit of a walk, but it will be much easier to talk if we are in a quiet area" or "You'll find it easier to ask questions if we find somewhere quiet and private." If you will be talking to an inpatient in a hospital, draw the curtains (which gives a modicum of privacy and makes neighboring patients or visitors aware that they should not be listening). Before patients and families hear what you will share they are often sensitive to your body language, such as haste or composure, tension or comfort.

The worse the news is, the more private the environment should be. A relatively small, quiet room feels more intimate and confidential than a large, open, noisy room. There should be few or no distracting noises such as telephones ringing or fax machines whirring. There should not be potential for intruders who could walk in at the moment you are disclosing the bad news, during the time the patient or family is trying to process the information, or during the time of emotional reaction to the news. The only people who should be present are the ones who are directly involved with the situation. There should not be any curious bystanders within hearing distance. If appropriate, introduce yourself again and your professional title because the person may have heard numerous names and titles already that day. All people should be sitting down because the reaction of the person receiving the information may cause a loss of strength in the legs or a loss of balance. The worse the news that must be presented, the more time should be devoted to the person for processing and reacting to it. Some people, however, may have very strong emotional reactions to information you may feel is not particularly serious. Everybody's stress tolerance and ability to manage stressful situations is different. Plan ahead so that you can avoid giving the bad news and then rushing off to another appointment. Even though you may not do or say very much after you have shared the information, your presence will likely be appreciated. Ideally, a desk or table should not be positioned between you and the receiver of the bad news. However, sitting at a corner of a table or desk facing one another can facilitate a sense of openness as well as connectedness. Sitting within arms' reach of the person also gives a feeling of caring and warmth and allows the person to take your hand or allows you to touch the person's hand if you feel it is appropriate and helpful. The desk or table should have an area cleared of clutter so the person receiving the information has some place to rest hands and arms, and possibly even the head if weeping occurs. Cups or glasses of water on the table for each person present, including yourself, are a thoughtful gesture. An emotional situation can cause people to have a dry mouth, which can make talking more difficult. A box of tissues should be within easy reach of both you and the other person. The physical environment can convey support and acceptance of people's emotional responses, and therefore it is wise to prepare the room before bringing the patient and family into it.

Your body posture is also important. You should sit in a relaxed posture (a rigid posture increases both your tension and the family's), but not appear excessively casual either because that degrades the importance of what you are saying. Use open body language (legs uncrossed, arms uncrossed, hands open) and lean forward slightly. Your facial expressions should convey concern and empathy, rather than strain or stress. Make eye contact with each person as best you can without appearing as though you are staring, allowing them time to react to what you are saying. Give the majority of your attention to the patient if she is present. If the patient is not present, give the majority of your attention to the spouse or closest relative present in the meeting.

Use a gentle but not faltering tone of voice with moderate loudness so that each person can hear you and will not have to ask you to repeat yourself. If the person asks you to repeat the information because of difficulty registering or believing what was just heard, repeat the same information in as close to the same words and tone as you just said it. This allows the person to confirm that she heard you correctly without having to compare new words or word order. Speak slowly and pause after each important statement to allow each person to process the information and to ask questions. Use as few technical words as possible. Speak in layman's terms. Professional and medical jargon ("medicalese") distances you from the person and makes it more difficult for the person to process the information you are trying to convey. The therapeutic goal is to assist the person in processing what will likely be unsettling information.

What Does the Person Already Know?

If appropriate, ask the patient or family what they know about the problem. For example, "Mr. Farris, I'd like to know what you understand about your hearing problem," "Mrs. Adams, what do you understand about your husband's stroke?" or "What did the doctor tell you about . . . ?" This gives you the opportunity to assess the accuracy of the person's understanding and the level of sophistication of communication the individual has, which allows you to adjust your level of communication so you are not speaking either above or below the person's language ability. If the person says that no information has been given, consider that the person may have received the information and may be confused about it or cannot recall what, if anything, had been said.

Communicating the News

Reinforce the accurate information the patient or family relates about the patient's problems, using the person's own words if possible. This helps give the individuals confidence that what they understand is correct. Educate the patient or family further about the communication problems of the patient, which may involve the presentation of some new information or correction of information that was previously misunderstood.

It is helpful to alert the person that something serious is coming using a statement such as "Some of what I need to tell you may be new information and it will require the use of some special strategies." For example, "Mrs. Childers, there are some problems with your swallowing that affect the diet that will be safe for you to eat" or "Mr. and Mrs. Mehta, the evaluation results on Jenna indicate that she is having problems in several areas." Then tell the patient or family the news straightforwardly and objectively. It is helpful to imagine yourself in the person's situation and consider how you would want to receive such information. Avoid being judgmental or accusatory with your tone of voice, facial expressions, and choice of words. Be careful not to suggest any innuendo that implies the person could have prevented this difficulty or in some way caused it. The person already may have a strong sense of guilt, and any negative insinuation you convey may unnecessarily intensify the person's psychological burden (e.g., a mother who was taking illegal drugs during her pregnancy and now has a child with a serious handicap).

Disclosing the bad news may only take a moment, or there may be a number of areas that must be covered, for example, the person's hearing ability, speech systems (respiratory, phonatory, resonatory, and articulatory), speech intelligibility, receptive language, expressive language, cognition, and swallowing. It is possible that the person has significant impairments in each of these areas; therefore, some information may not seem particularly disturbing, while other information may be very upsetting. There also may be a cumulative effect in which the first information presented may not elicit a strong emotional response but the accumulation of information may be very disturbing to the client. If there are a few areas with serious impairments, it may help the person process the information if you have a momentary pause after you present portions of information to allow the person to consider what you said and to ask questions for clarification. Asking yes-no questions may help you recognize whether the person is understanding you well, for example, "Was the last part clear?" or "Am I going too fast?" Such questions allow the person time to process the information, encourage the person to ask questions, help the person feel an element of control over the meeting, and validate the thoughts and feelings of the person by inviting her to join in the discussion.

It is best not to assume that the person will feel the same way you would if you received that particular information. The person may process the information in a different way than you. The person may have anticipated the news and have mentally and emotionally prepared for it. However, based upon your previous interactions with the person, you may anticipate how the person will likely respond to the information and then fashion your presentation accordingly. After you have shared the news, an empathic response is appropriate when a person is trying to process disturbing information, for example, "This must be very upsetting for you." It is best not to say, "I know how upsetting this is to you," because you do not really know. You also may want to say, "This is a lot of difficult information to receive at one time" or "You have heard a lot of people talking about your child's problems today. It can be overwhelming to hear so much all at once."

If the news or explanation is complex or contains multiple components, you may wish to provide recall aids (Back & Curtis, 2002). For example, you may give the patient a handout with a brief summary of your findings, diagnosis, and core treatment recommendations. Some patients are more visually oriented, and having a sheet of paper that summarizes the main points can both help to orient their attention visually and give them a permanent document of the findings to refer back to or to show other family members. Sometimes patients are so upset that they "forget" what they were told or only recall portions of the important feedback (Luterman, 2008). For example, a patient may hear a dreaded diagnosis and then fail to process any information thereafter. One Stanford University website (Kincer, Zipper, Crenshaw, & Solley, Retrieved February 6, 2010) that instructs physicians and other health care workers on how to give bad news emphasizes that "patients retain only 10% of what they hear." This is a good reason to provide patients and their families with a written summary.

Finally, in giving bad news, it is critical to promote hope or optimism (Groopman, 2004; Sweeny & Shepperd, 2007). This can often be accomplished by focusing on the potential for beneficial treatment and the possibilities for an improved quality of life. Be careful not to exaggerate the likely positive treatment outcomes, however, as this can cause later disappointment and can impair the trust the patient and family have in the clinician.

Overall, during this difficult time of communication we need to be able to manage our own feelings so they do not interfere with the patient and family managing theirs. We need to remain professional and poised in all interactions with clients, patients, and family members. We can reflect on our own experiences with our colleagues and our own families, but should not allow our feelings to cloud our ability to focus on our patients when we are with them.

Reactions to Bad News

Reactions to the bad news may range from stoicism to a wide range of emotions and behaviors. Tears and crying are perhaps one of the more difficult responses we must be ready to see. Crying is not an emotion; it is a symptom. It can be a symptom of several emotions: fear, pain, frustration, anger, rage, despair, depression, and even joy, love, humor (laughing so hard you cry), and others. Some people are moved to tears easily and cry when almost any emotion reaches a moderate level of intensity, while other people do not cry even when passionately moved.

Many people (including SLPs and Auds) are not comfortable when others become tearful and distraught. As clinicians, we are often uncertain how or whether to give comfort. Buckman and Kason (1992) and Hallenbeck (2003) suggest practical steps for professionals to use when a person cries.

MOVE CLOSER TO THE PERSON

Most people feel very vulnerable when crying and feel even worse if they perceive disapproval or rejection for crying. Depending on what you feel is the person's comfort level, you may lean forward in your chair toward the person or move a little closer, but at least do not move away. Maintain eye contact with the person, which helps convey interest and empathy for the person's suffering. In contrast, looking away when a person cries may convey discomfort, criticism, or disapproval.

OFFER A TISSUE

Make certain there are tissues available in the room where you are meeting with the patient or family. If none are available and the person begins to cry, go get several or, ideally, a box of tissues. Providing tissues does several things: it gives the person permission to cry; it gives the person a means to restore her appearance (it is difficult to talk normally if your nose is running and your eyes are wet with tears); it brings you into closer proximity with the person; and offering the person a tissue gives you something to do that is supportive and helpful.

TOUCH THE PERSON

If you feel that both you and the person crying will be comfortable with physical contact, a light and brief touch of the person's hand or arm may show comforting support. The clinician needs to be alert to the person's response to this gesture and be prepared to withdraw the hand and refrain from further touch. Do not encourage a person to cry on your shoulder because this can easily be misconstrued by patients, family members, and colleagues.

TRY TO IDENTIFY THE STRONG EMOTION AND THE CAUSES

The cause of the person's tears may be obvious, in which case you can use an empathic response (e.g., "It's understandable that you would be very upset with this news [new information]"). If the cause is not obvious, a question may help you understand the source of the tears (e.g., "Can you tell me what is upsetting you at the moment?"). Sometimes it is an aspect of the news that we do not anticipate that sparks an intense emotional reaction in patients. We do not know everything about the family's history, and so we cannot always predict what part of the news will be easiest to digest and what part of the news will be most disturbing and upsetting.

REMAIN PRESENT UNTIL THE PERSON REGAINS COMPOSURE

By planning ahead you may have the time to be present during the acute reaction to the bad news. If you cannot remain with the person, try to find someone else who can be with the person for a while (e.g., the patient's family member or a close friend). If the person asks to be left alone for a while, honor the request. Crying as an acute reaction to bad news is normal; however, prolonged, uncontrollable, and unstoppable crying is rarer and more serious (Buckman & Kasson, 1992; Hallenbeck, 2003). If the person frequently cries during other meetings or sessions with you, ask her what she is feeling. You also may get a sense of how upset she is by asking her to rate her distress on a scale of 1 to 10. Some people are very emotionally expressive, and their tears may not upset them as much as they do you.

Planning and Follow Through

Patients and families typically feel very alone and isolated immediately after receiving discomforting news. If the professional who presents the bad news does not have any follow-through plan, then the patient or family may feel even more isolated and discouraged. It is important for the bearer of bad news also to be the bearer of directions for support. By having a plan for help, you are therapeutically responding to the isolation the patient or family might be experiencing by emphasizing that support is available to them (recall the discussions in Chapter 2 on existential uncertainty, meaninglessness, and isolation). Many patients may look to the clinician to guide them as they may feel disorganized or "lost" right after receiving bad news. In these situations, the clinician may be helpful in providing some initial direction, such as indicating, "Mrs. Smith, the first strategy we need to work on is. . . . After that, we can discuss the next steps for you to improve. . . ." Here, the clinician provides some initial organization and direction until the patient can get "back on her feet" emotionally and feel ready to contribute to the decision-making process.

It is important to try to get a sense of the patient's or family's priorities and mesh the treatment planning with their priorities. If what you feel is important is not quite what the patient or family feels is important, the family may not comply with the recommended interventions or strategies. In order to get a sense of their priorities you may want to ask them what is important to them at this time. This helps the patient or family feel somewhat in control of the situation, which is a perception that is therapeutic when there is an overall feeling of loss of control of one's life.

The clinician also can identify the patient's and family's coping strategies and sources of support and attempt to work with them. Most people have some kind of support network, such as family, close friends, church members, or co-workers. These will be the pillars on which people lean during difficult times. This is a time most people feel a pressing need for relationships. You might want to say to the person something like, "You have had to deal with some very difficult times in your life. What or who has helped you get through those times?" This kind of statement and question shows recognition of the strength the person has shown in past difficult circumstances and shows that you are trying to identify sources of support for them to possibly reach out to again. However, many people, particularly the elderly, have few if any people they can call upon and expect support. Most of their family may be at a great distance or deceased, and friends may be too frail or have their own burdens that prevent them from providing the support they would like to give. There are no easy solutions for situations in which a person does not have family, friends, or community support; however, contacting social services agencies in the hospital or medical facility may be helpful.

Usually when SLPs and Auds are presenting evaluation results, something positive can be pointed out to the patient or family. It may not outweigh the unsettling information, but it may help provide them some hope. Providing the more positive information after the disturbing information may help the patient and family recognize that the patient is doing well, or at least better in some areas. Sometimes SLPs and Auds feel a need to cheer people up even when it may be inappropriate. This is not a time to introduce levity or cheeriness to help decrease your own discomfort and anxiety. Maintaining an earnest manner provides respect for the significant changes that are likely to occur in the patient's and family's lives and the adjustments they will need to make.

After the information has been shared and the client and family have processed it, at some point everyone must depart. Maintaining an attitude of sensitivity, compassion, and professionalism can help the client and family leave with the sense that you are someone they can rely on to be a part of their support system. If they do not already have your business card or professional telephone number, provide it with encouragement to call you if they have any questions. Often after individuals have processed disturbing news they begin to have numerous questions they could not pose at the time they first learned it.

Communicating Bad News to Children

Whatever difficulties exist in breaking bad news to adults, they are compounded when dealing with children. Audiologists and SLPs frequently have to give potentially upsetting information to children about their hearing, speech, language, and sometimes their swallowing. Even when a child is thought too young to be told, some facts may be impossible to withhold as the child grows older. If children find out unexpectedly about their impairments and have not been gradually introduced to them, they can feel angry and cheated. It is wise to judge carefully how much information should be given, at what stage of development, and by whom. Buckman and Kason (1992) and Lloyd and Bor (2004) provide guidelines for communicating bad news to children.

HAVE A CLOSE ADULT RELATIVE PRESENT IF AT ALL POSSIBLE

If at all possible, talk to the parent or caregiver first and agree on when, where, and how the information will be shared with the child. The adult may want to participate (which you should welcome) and may have valuable insights into what will be the most difficult areas for the child. If the adult has no particular suggestions, describe how you will share the bad news with the child and ask the adult for her impressions.

CHECK YOUR COMMUNICATION LEVEL FREQUENTLY

With children of all ages it is difficult to be certain of their developmental level of understanding. Check your communication level frequently to determine if the information you are providing aligns with the understanding of the child. Answer the child's questions with the words and language level he will likely understand. Remember that even though a child may be a certain age, his comprehension may be considerably younger than his actual years, particularly if he is ill, injured, or under emotional stress. Emphasize what the child will be able to do, thereby giving realistic hope.

BE READY TO REPEAT WHAT YOU HAVE SAID

Children often require repetition of information, usually to be reassured that they have understood correctly. Be patient if the child asks the same questions several times or in different ways. This may be the child's way of assuring herself that you really mean what you say.

UNDERSTAND MAGICAL THINKING

Magical thinking refers to children's (and adults') beliefs that their bad thoughts or actions can magically cause negative events to happen in their world (Wachtel, 1994). Magical thinking attributes unrealistic power to a child's thoughts and ascribes a cause-and-effect relationship to unrelated thoughts and actions. The young sister of an ill or injured boy may feel guilty and believe that her angry wish that her brother was dead caused her brother's illness or accident. The injured child also may engage in magical thinking and imagine that his illness or accident is punishment for "bad thoughts" about a sibling or parent. Although children are not likely to express their magical thinking directly, it is important to make clear to children that the illness or injury is nobody's fault ("Your mother's illness [stroke] is not her fault, or your daddy's fault, or your brother's fault, and definitely is not *your* fault").

MAKE A REFERRAL IF YOU FEEL THE CHILD WOULD BENEFIT

Children who are seriously ill or injured often have difficulty communicating their thoughts and feelings to their families, and families often do not know what to say to their children. In addition to the ill or injured child, siblings also may be struggling emotionally as they try to understand the illness or injury and its causes (Corr & Balk, 2010). Pediatric psychologists may help these children communicate their thoughts and feelings and help the parents as well as the other professionals better understand how these children are processing the bad news.

Summary

Sharing bad news is a part of our professional responsibility no matter what setting we work in. It is never easy telling parents about serious hearing, speech, language, cognitive, or swallowing problems of their children, and often it is not any easier when sharing such information with their family members. Sharing bad news with children may be some of the most sensitive and challenging work we do. We sometimes work with the tragedies of life: TBIs in children, unusual and severe medical syndromes, CVAs and other neurological impairments in adults of all ages, laryngeal cancer that requires a laryngectomy. Our professional role requires us to maintain our poise and to be as sensitive, insightful, and empathic as possible when sharing discomforting news with clients, patients, and their families.

HIDDEN AGENDAS

Hidden agendas are undeclared or covert intentions of a person that may become evident during an interview or therapy session (Menahem, 1987; Wagner, Lentz, & Heslop, 2002). Clients and family members usually have explicit concerns or goals that are shared with the clinician during an evaluation or family conference. Meanwhile, they also may have concerns or goals that remain implicit or concealed. When hidden agendas occur, there is usually some potential gain for the person that differs from the stated intentions or goals. When a clinician suspects a client or family member has a hidden agenda, she may view the person as being indirect or manipulative and may experience countertransference reactions or become irritated with the person. These clinician responses are not helpful; however, there may be much to gain by understanding the source of the person's hidden agenda. For example, clients and family members may be reluctant to communicate directly about certain desires or goals because of emotions such as anxiety, embarrassment, and shame. It is important to recognize their discomfort with expressing certain feelings, thoughts, or information and maintain an empathic view toward clients and families so that these issues can be explored in a nonjudgmental manner.

When we recognize that a person has a hidden agenda during an evaluation, therapy session, or family conference, probing questions such as, "What other concerns do you have? or "Is there something you would like to talk about that we haven't discussed yet?" or "You seem to have something else on your mind. Would you like to talk about it?" can help the person more openly discuss a hidden agenda. Once the clinician recognizes the presence of a hidden agenda, she should explore what it is about and then help the client or family member problem-solve the issues around the theme. Hidden agendas may include a family member's reluctance to admit her personal needs and to assume certain responsibilities for a patient. Often, family members may become more able to express their needs directly if the clinician shows an accepting and nonjudgmental attitude, for example, by conveying that it is *understandable* that a family member is not able to take on such a large amount of responsibilities.

We may need to deal with the hidden agenda as *the* issue, that is, the primary issue, regardless of what was anticipated to be the focus of the session. If the hidden agenda is not recognized and sufficiently managed, the issue may become a recurrent theme and may interfere with the therapy process. Unresolved hidden agendas sometimes become apparent when clients are noncompliant. If this happens, maintain a professional stance of curiosity and encourage the client to share what is standing in the way.

RECURRENT THEMES

Recurrent themes represent issues and problems that arise more than once that need to be addressed. As mentioned above, occasionally the recurrent theme may begin as a hidden agenda. Recurrent themes may involve most any issue, including the client's concerns about a clinician's qualifications, the direction of therapy, or the cost of therapy. When recurrent themes emerge, it is usually a signal that the client harbors some level of anxiety about the issue, and until the issue is addressed, anxiety may increase. The client may have difficulty focusing on therapy tasks until the recurrent theme is recognized and sufficiently discussed. If the issues are not addressed, a second issue emerges. The first anxiety-provoking issue is the recurrent theme, and the second anxiety-provoking issue becomes the client's negative feelings about the clinician for failing to recognize the initial issue.

It is important to address the recurrent theme directly and to show nonjudgmental curiosity. Clinicians can explore the recurrent theme using the open-ended reporters' questions (what, when, who, and how) to gain general and specific information to help understand the client's concerns. For example, clinicians can acknowledge what has happened repeatedly (e.g., the client comes late to sessions or the client omits certain homework tasks while following other recommendations) and ask the client what he thinks may be going on. Once the client responds, requests for clarification (e.g., asking the client if you understood him correctly or summarizing the conversation in order to clarify or confirm what was said) can help the clinician discern the accuracy of understanding.

VERBOSE BEHAVIOR

Some clients and family members are overly talkative and do not give the clinician time to provide the information or deal with the issues that need to be addressed. New clinicians (and some experienced clinicians) may have considerable difficulty trying to "get a word in edgewise" with clients who are very talkative (Mosak & Maniacci, 1998). The clinician may begin an interview or discussion using normal verbal encouragers (head nods, "um hums"), and then find that no encouragement is needed for the person to continue talking. These individuals often talk rapidly and with somewhat of a monotone so that the listener does not get a cue as to the ending of a statement (i.e., a time to "jump in" to the conversation). They often use numerous "ands" as though each statement or topic is intimately related to the previous one. Their conversations may be rambling and convoluted, leaving the listener in a quandary about the main topic or point of the conversation. These individuals may not be aware of or may simply ignore turn-taking pragmatics. Individuals with neurological disorders (particularly right-hemisphere damage) may have "press of speech" and may not be aware of verbal or nonverbal cues from the listener that the listener wants to speak (Worrall & Frattali, 2000).

When the clinician becomes aware of the client's overly talkative manner or pressured speech, the first strategy may be to attempt to redirect and refocus the discussion. In order to do this, the clinician may need to intentionally interrupt the person using vocal, non-verbal, or verbal interrupters. These are used to signal to the person that it is the clinician's turn to talk or that some redirection is desired. Examples of vocal, nonverbal, and verbal interrupters include clearing the throat, interjecting a short "ah," checking a clock or watch, raising a finger to indicate "stop for a moment," getting a calendar to indicate you are scheduling another appointment, touching the client's hand or arm to get the client's attention, or saying, "Let me interrupt (stop, interject something, add something, etc.) for a moment." The clinician may need to use an assertive statement such as "I will discuss your concern as soon as I finish what I need to say." In some cases such a statement may need to be made using the broken record technique. Another technique to inhibit overly verbose behavior is to use primarily closed questions to try to elicit brief responses.

If the client's pressured and overly talkative speech occurs repetitively, then the clinician may wish to set some ground rules (Mosak & Maniacci, 1998). For instance, the clinician can let the client know that he (the clinician) needs to review five points during their therapy session, and he may need to interrupt the client in order to keep the session moving along. Then, once the client becomes talkative, the clinician can remind her of the ground rules, for example, that they have three more issues to discuss in today's therapy session and the clinician wishes to get back "on track." This can be a polite and effective way to maintain the structure of the session and to avoid getting caught up in the client's whirlwind of ideas.

However, in some cases, the client's loquacious speech is the result of excessive anxiety or stress. In these situations, the client may need to know that she is "being heard" before she can move on to the next topic. Reassuring or supportive comments about the client's fears and anxieties may reduce the tendency to talk too much. For example, the clinician may acknowledge, "I know you are having a tough time getting along with your mother and that is weighing on your mind. Do you think we can stop and take a deep breath and then get back to our speech exercises?" This acknowledges that you understand the client's source of stress, and sometimes clients will stop their repetitive activity once they get this acknowledgement. The second part of the example (asking the client to take a deep breath) helps to demarcate the goal-directed portion of the session from the free-flowing thoughts and ideas.

MANIPULATIVE BEHAVIOR

Manipulation refers to behavior that covertly elicits desired responses from others and implies an element of inauthenticity or deceit (Feltham & Dryden, 2005). However, perceptions of manipulation are in the eye of the beholder and may reflect how secure (or insecure) we are feeling with an individual. When clinicians feel tricked, fooled, or frustrated by a person, they sometimes describe that person as manipulative. Clinicians do not like to think of themselves as gullible and easily manipulated, and sometimes clinicians deal with those feelings by blaming the client. However, when we are comfortable with our clinical skills and have an understanding of our client's motivations and typical interpersonal patterns, we are much less likely to pathologize the person's behavior and apply this derogatory term. A child or adult who may be viewed as manipulative is probably trying to gain some measure of control and self-esteem in a situation where the person feels vulnerable and does not currently possess better coping or interpersonal skills.

Children may use indirect means to avoid working on therapy tasks. They may try to distract the clinician with playful and charming antics and conversation. These children may be attempting to avoid or postpone doing tasks that are difficult for them and threatening to their self-esteem. Therefore, the problematic behavior is not so much directed towards "tricking" the clinician but is primarily intended to distract the clinician from the child's speech and language problems that may be embarrassing or shameful to the child. In response to a child who is using such tactics, the SLP may respond with, "I know these exercises are difficult for you, but by doing them your speech will get better, and I'm sure you will be happy about that." This response acknowledges the child's difficulty with the tasks (but does not focus on his embarrassment or shame) and provides an opportunity for a nonthreatening discussion about the therapy.

In some situations, manipulative behavior occurs when a person has a sense that his goal is not socially acceptable. The classic example of manipulation in adults is the malingering patient. **Malingering** involves intentional simulation of an illness or disorder with a conscious motivation of external incentives or gains, such as financial compensation from insurance, or avoiding expectations of others, such as returning to gainful employment (Johnson & Jacobson, 2006). SLPs may see patients who are malingering who have neurological damage but feign symptoms of more severe impairments than evaluation results indicate in order to gain financial compensation. Auds may see malingering in individuals who consciously pretend to have a hearing loss or be deaf to avoid some responsibility or seek concessions or compensation.

If a clinician experiences a client's behavior as manipulative, consider first the motivations and feelings of the client. Is the client fearful or uncertain about what is being asked in therapy? The clinician can use a reflection of feeling to help identify and understand what the client may be feeling. Confrontations are seldom effective or useful in these situations; they only cause the person to retreat or assume a defensive posture. In response to the patient who is suspected of malingering, the clinician may respond with, "I wonder if you are feeling uncertain or even a little fearful about your future and the possibility of returning to work." These reflections acknowledge the patient's struggles and convey an empathic, respectful tone which may help the client to feel more comfortable in expressing his anxieties or avoidant behaviors.

Mr. D.

Mr. D., a patient in an acute-care hospital where I worked, was receiving physical, occupational, and speech therapy following a mild stroke. After a few sessions with each of the rehabilitation team members we began to suspect the patient was malingering. Upon my initial evaluation, I noted specific receptive and expressive language problems; however, as Mr. D. had opportunities to observe other patients in

Continues on next page

Continued from previous page

their rehabilitation programs who had strokes, he began to take on some of their impairments. I noticed inconsistent signs of dysarthria and apraxia, and his receptive and expressive language problems varied from day to day. He also began to have more difficulty walking and using his right arm. Further brain imaging techniques conducted by the radiologist revealed no additional cerebral hemorrhages or other complications. I discussed with Mr. D. the possibility that he may have concerns about returning to his former job and not performing at the level that was expected of him. I asked him if he was willing to meet with the social worker to discuss his concerns. He agreed and the referral was made. Mr. D. began making more rapid improvements in all areas of rehabilitation and did not show new signs of impairments. He eventually returned to his work, albeit at a lower level of expectations and performance.

CLINICAL QUESTIONS

1. What are some other ways that you might question a patient whom you suspect of malingering?
2. How might your hypotheses about malingering affect your treatment plan?

When we have not fully explained our therapy strategies and goals or clients do not fully understand them, they may view our therapeutic interventions as sophisticated forms of manipulation and may understandably respond with resistance. Clients want to maintain control of their own lives, perhaps saying to themselves, "No one is going to get me to do something I don't want to do." If the clinician thinks this type of resistance may be occurring, she may need to review the rationale for the therapy goals and strategies with the client and encourage a collaborative process. We want our clients to feel that they have respectful, open relationships with us and receive straightforward explanations from us so that they do not feel manipulated in any way.

EMOTIONAL LABILITY

Emotional lability, or affective dysregulation, refers to uncontrolled and often rapidly changing expressions of emotions or mood swings (Feltham & Dryden, 2005; Gabbard, 2005). While emotional lability or affective dysregulation are most commonly seen in psychiatric settings in which patients have Mood Disorders (such as Bipolar Disorder) and Borderline Personality Disorder (Gabbard, 2005), SLPs may be most familiar with this phenomena when it is secondary to neurological impairment (Brookshire, 2007; Palmieri, Abrahams, Soraru, et al., 2009). Patients in whom emotional lability is more common are those with CVAs or TBIs, which may cause a loss of inhibitory control, along with the patient's intense emotional responses to loss of former abilities and competencies. The most common sign that the patient is emotionally labile is that the patient cries easily or appears overreactive to neutral situations or conversational topics. The patient's overreactions may include other emotional expressions, such as inappropriate laughter in situations that are not humorous or excessive laughter in response to mildly amusing stimuli. Emotional lability also may be manifested as unexpected anger or rage. In some instances the lability may be a reflection of an emotionally significant thought, feeling, or event (e.g., feeling overly controlled by one's family), but in other instances the emotional lability may not have an apparent emotional context (e.g., a strong reaction to being served scrambled eggs at breakfast). Some contexts or topics may understandably precipitate emotional reactions, but in other cases labile behaviors may reflect the neurological impairment more directly.

Helping the Person Who Is Expressing Emotional Lability

Rollin (2000) makes several suggestions about helping patients who are emotionally labile. He suggests not bringing attention to the behavior if it is only a momentary lapse of emotional control and continuing on with the planned therapy. Normalizing the behavior also may be helpful; for example, "What you are experiencing now is natural considering what you've been through," "Because of your stroke, it's hard to control your feelings all the time," or "As you improve physically, you'll have better control of your crying" (p. 51). In some cases, the clinician may choose to reflect the patient's feelings of sadness, uncertainty, or anxiety and provide empathy about the feelings and reactions. Gently acknowledging the patient's behavior and asking a probing question may help the clinician better understand what the patient is thinking and feeling; for example, "You are crying. Is there something we are talking about or doing that has upset you?" If the clinician feels a therapy task has precipitated the labile response, changing the task may help the patient regain his composure. Having tissues on the table or nearby can help the person manage tears. We need to remember that patients are often embarrassed about their crying and to reassure them that it is quite all right and understandable.

REPAIRING COUNSELING ERRORS

We can assume that if we are working with people who have complex communication and emotional issues that affect their lives, we occasionally are going to make mistakes in what we say, how we say it, and what we do (Kottler & Blau, 1989). Our education and training provide the foundational skills for being SLPs or Auds, but our advanced skills come mainly from on-the-job-training. This is true not only for our professions, but all professions. Clinicians have sometimes said, "Physicians bury their mistakes, but our mistakes live on to talk about us." The adage is still true; however, mistakes with dysphagia patients can be life threatening. Most of our counseling errors, however, have less serious ramifications and involve not communicating with our clients, patients, and their families in the most sensitive manner or not being sufficiently aware of nonverbal messages our body language may be projecting. Clients, patients, and family members may recognize our counseling errors more easily than we can. They know when we have said something in an insensitive manner, and they may read our body language better than we can read our own.

During undergraduate and graduate clinical training, clients and their families are usually very tolerant of student mistakes. Clients may be bewildered and families may see humor in the errors student clinicians make. Ultimately, in the university setting the faculty supervisor must take responsibility for what is said and done by the student clinician. However, once students graduate, the professional responsibility is on their shoulders.

Most clinicians would likely agree that with each person they try to help, they make some error(s) in what they say and do. In *The Imperfect Therapist: Learning from Failure in Therapeutic Practice* (1989), Kottler and Blau reveal and discuss errors they and other highly regarded psychotherapists have made. Regardless of the attention and empathy we give to our clients and their families, we are still going to make errors. How we repair our errors depends first on whether we are even aware of them. If we notice the client or family wincing from something we have said, we should quickly reflect whether our verbal and nonverbal messages were received in the way we had intended. Were we clear and accurate in what we said? Were we congruent? Were we sensitive and empathic? Did we say too much or too little? Did our statements sound critical or blaming? Was the information presented prematurely or in a harsh manner? It is important to ask these questions and, based upon our self-evaluation, determine what needs to be said or done to repair the error. Even when a person responds to us with a stoic expression, we need to be asking ourselves these questions. Individuals who have a stoic presentation and give little visual or verbal feedback can be more difficult to work with than those who give us considerable feedback. We tend to misread or read into expressionless faces. Negative feedback is easier to work with than no feedback. We need to keep in mind that some of our neurologically impaired patients may have expressionless faces but may still have strong feelings in response to what we communicate to them through our words, tone of voice, and actions.

Pipes and Davenport (1998) and Morrison (2008) emphasize that the possibility of a clinician error needs to be consistently acknowledged and that the clinician must be willing to listen to client feedback and change behavior or expectations to increase the clinician's credibility and enhance the therapeutic alliance. When we realize that we have made an error, we have some options regarding how to manage it. The first possibility, of course, is an apology followed by a correction. Most people accept such apologies and recognize that everyone (including clinicians) makes mistakes, and that everyone has good days and bad days. Appropriate and timely apologies can enhance the client–clinician relationship. For example, if a clinician makes an error with the client's name, a rapid apology and saying the correct name is all that is needed. However, it is not necessary to provide personal reasons for the error, such as, "I'm sorry. I'm very tired. I didn't sleep well last night." Sometimes an apology may seem like an overstatement, and a brief revision or correction of what we said is sufficient. If the error is not corrected, the person may harbor some ill feelings about us and we may never really understand what caused the change in the person's attitude toward us. As clinicians, we tend to be sensitive to other people and recognize subtle changes in their behaviors toward us. If we feel that something is wrong, we may try to talk to the person about it, but we may not get open, honest responses. What is left unsaid by the client or by us may haunt us for a long time. At best, sometimes all we can do is learn from our mistakes and try to do better the next time. We will always remain imperfect clinicians.

CONCLUDING COMMENTS

The nature of our work is that we must give bad news to children, clients, patients, and families about evaluation results and lack of progress in therapy. Although we try to sandwich the bad news between good news about a child's hearing, speech, language, or general behavior or about the preserved abilities of an adult, usually some negative information needs to be presented. The setting, timing, and manner in which the information is presented can have important effects on how well it is received and accepted. Skills in presenting bad news in an honest and yet sensitive manner are essential for our professions.

In our clinical work, some clients and family members may have hidden agendas that become evident during an interview or therapy session. Recognizing and appreciating the person's discomfort with expressing certain feelings, thoughts, or information helps us to respond in a therapeutic manner rather than allowing ourselves to feel the person is being manipulative and become irritated. Sometimes hidden agendas become recurrent themes if they are not recognized and openly discussed by the clinician. Recurrent themes often signal areas of client anxiety and concern, and until the issue is recognized and sufficiently resolved, the anxiety will likely continue and possibly escalate.

There are other common client behaviors that can interfere with the process and progress in therapy. Verbose behavior is a challenge for many clinicians. Although we should be good listeners, some clients' verbalizations become excessive, repetitive, or tangential. At these times, we may feel the session is out of our control and our professional time is being wasted. Learning how to politely interrupt and redirect an overly talkative client can facilitate therapeutic progress and help the client make gains more quickly. Emotional lability is fairly common in patients with neurological impairments and may become evident when patients cry easily and display overreactions to minor events. The clinician's empathic manner of responding to the lability can help patients accept and better manage their uncontrolled emotions.

Whether we are new or experienced clinicians, we make mistakes in what we say, how we say it, and what we do. The more complex and the more sensitive the issues, the greater the likelihood that something we say or do will not be received well by someone. We first need to engage in self-evaluation to recognize an error and then consider options for ways to manage it. Appropriate and timely apologies can enhance the client–clinician relationship and can increase the client's trust in the clinician.

Discussion Questions

1. Remember a time when you were given some bad news, perhaps medical news regarding yourself or a family member. What positive strategies did the professional use who gave the bad news? How could the delivery of bad news be better communicated?

2. Recall a time when you had to give a client, a loved one, or a friend some bad news. What do you think you did well? What do you wish you had done differently?

3. Recall a situation in which you discovered that the client had a hidden agenda. Empathically describe what motivated the client's hidden agenda. How did you manage the situation after you recognized the hidden agenda? How might you help the client more directly express her needs now?

4. Recall a time when you recognized a client's recurrent theme. How did you respond to it once you recognized that it was important to the client? How might you respond differently now?

5. If you have had a client or family member who demonstrated verbose behavior, how did you manage the situation? In retrospect, what additional strategies might you have employed to better manage the conversation?

6. If a colleague comes to you and complains that he feels manipulated by a client, what might you say to help the colleague analyze and resolve the situation?

7. Have you had a client with emotionally labile behaviors? How did you manage the situation? What might you do differently now?

8. Recall a time when you made an error when counseling with a client or family member. Discuss the situation and how you handled it to try to repair the therapy relationship. How might you handle it differently or better now?

Role Plays

1. Divide the class into client–clinician pairs. Ask the "clinicians" to practice giving bad news to an adult client or the parents of a child client. Ask the "clients" to respond emotionally and have the clinicians use their best therapeutic skills to respond to their reactions. Afterwards, ask the clients how well the clinicians did and what strategies were used to provide the bad news in a sensitive manner.

2. Again, divide the class into client–clinician pairs. Ask the "clients" to play the role of individuals with indirect communication and difficult behaviors (e.g., verbose behavior, emotionally lability, or hidden agendas) but with well-meaning underlying motives. Ask the "clinicians" to respond in a sensitive and therapeutic manner and to try to discern the underlying concerns of their clients.

Working with Resistance and Anger

CHAPTER OUTLINE

- Introduction
- Resistant and Noncompliant Attitudes and Behaviors
- Angry or Hostile Attitudes and Behaviors
- Communicating and Responding to Angry Behavior
- Concluding Comments
- Discussion Questions
- Role Plays

INTRODUCTION

This chapter presents situations and behaviors that are often difficult for clinicians to manage. The focus of this chapter is on providing tools for better understanding and managing resistant, angry, or hostile attitudes and behaviors in the clinical setting. Although these situations may not arise often, they can be particularly challenging to handle in a safe and therapeutic manner. In all cases, the clinician's safety as well as the client's is the first concern. However, by recognizing potentially escalating behaviors, the speech-language pathologist or audiologist can often avert potentially threatening situations and respond in a way that preserves the working alliance.

RESISTANT AND NONCOMPLIANT ATTITUDES AND BEHAVIORS

When clients present themselves for assessments and therapeutic assistance, it can often be frustrating and puzzling to clinicians when their clients do not adhere to their professional recommendations. Freud (1912/1958, 1917) first described these opposing forces in clients: the apparent desire to change and the desire to maintain the status quo. Clients tend to safeguard against unpleasant feelings, and the resulting behaviors that may gain the clinician's attention may include being late for appointments, forgetting to pay the bill, forgetting the clinician's advice or recommendations, and focusing on unimportant information during the sessions (Gabbard, 2005). These behaviors, which interfere with the progress of therapy, are often referred to as resistance. *Resistance* and *noncompliance* are terms that are frequently used to label behaviors of a client or family member who makes the clinician feel inadequate (Morrison, 2008; Pipes & Davenport, 1998; Teyber, 2005).

Although resistance and noncompliance are not synonyms, they are often used interchangeably by SLPs, Auds, and other rehabilitation specialists. *Resistance*, however, suggests an unconscious ambivalence about doing what is asked or recommended in therapy, while *noncompliance* refers to conscious, intentional failure to comply or follow through with what is asked or recommended, as well as unconscious attempts to thwart the therapy process. However, the clinician can never know all of the client's thoughts and feelings and rarely knows whether ambivalence or refusal is at the heart of the matter. In view of the overlap in the behaviors that are often considered examples of both resistance and noncompliance, we use the term *resistance* to include noncompliant behaviors.

Resistance is a natural occurrence when people fear change, are uncertain about a new situation, or perceive the danger of being overwhelmed (Freud, 1914). The paradox is that many people who seek therapy become resistant to it (e.g., consider the client who states a strong desire to stop stuttering but resists the therapy). People in general are likely to show resistance when they feel frightened or threatened (Arkowitz, 2002; Safran & Muran, 2000). Resistance does not mean that people are being irresponsible or obstinate in order to make our work difficult. Resistance may reflect long-standing defensive patterns of coping with anxiety-provoking feelings (Gabbard, 2005). Their resistance serves to protect them from giving up familiar patterns of behaviors (e.g., disfluent speech and social avoidance). Resistance also can serve to protect people from facing a change in identity; that is, engaging in therapy means accepting that something has changed (e.g., the loss of ability to communicate because of a CVA) or needs to change (e.g., wearing hearing aids). Because resistance is frequently the result of a fear of change, clinicians can seek to understand the meaning of resistance for each client instead of simply viewing it as an obstruction to progress in therapy. People change in essentially three ways:

1. *Revolution* occurs when a significant event in a person's life dramatically and abruptly changes the way she thinks, believes, or behaves (e.g., marriage, parenthood, a stroke).

2. *Evolution* occurs when a person slowly, sometimes almost imperceptibly, changes over time (e.g., normal maturation and growth, education, rehabilitation).

3. *Resolution* occurs when a person decides that it is now time to change (e.g., going back to school, stopping alcohol or drug abuse, taking responsibility for improvement in therapy).

SLPs and Auds work with clients and families who are changing or have changed in each of these ways. A negative *revolutionary* event for a person may be, for example, a CVA, TBI, sudden hearing loss, or parents receiving a diagnosis of autism for their child. A sudden loss of communication or hearing abilities, or a diagnosis of a significant problem in a family member, may result in apparent initial resistance (denial) to accepting the loss or diagnosis and the need for management because there was little or no adjustment time to register the significant changes in the patient's or family's life.

Change through *evolution* is perhaps the easiest and least painful way people change in both positive and negative ways, and often only after a significant amount of time do individuals retrospectively realize that much change has occurred. Education and skill development on the job are examples of positive evolutionary changes. A gradually progressive hearing loss or growth of a brain tumor are examples of negative evolutionary changes.

However, as clinicians, we know that both habilitation and rehabilitation are slow, evolutionary processes, and typically clients and families are anxious for the process to be completed and for the client to be "normal."

Resolution is an important step in therapy for clients and families; that is, clients need resolve to cooperate with the therapist, attend sessions on a consistent basis, and do the tasks that are designed to be helpful. Families need resolve to be supportive of therapy and follow the clinician's recommendations. Clients who do not have this resolve may demonstrate resistance by not attending therapy consistently, refusing to do therapy tasks, or doing them in a perfunctory manner. Families who do not have this resolve may demonstrate resistance by not supporting therapy or by refusing to follow the clinician's recommendations. If we can view client or family resistance as a signal of fear that deserves our empathy and support rather than as an annoying obstacle, it becomes easier for us to maintain the therapeutic alliance and encourage the person to work toward change. Our ability to offer the best of ourselves rather than withdrawing or becoming adversarial when we sense resistance is what inspires clients to persevere even when they are fearful.

In therapy we are likely to see resistance expressed by a variety of behaviors such as passive-aggressive behaviors ("Oops! I forgot my appointment again!"), denial ("I don't think my son's speech problem is that bad"), shifting the focus of the conversation ("Have you ever had somebody in your family have a stroke?"), being late for therapy, canceling therapy, subtle or overt forms of inattention, disagreement with something we say, tense silence, wanting to end therapy sessions early, or not doing assignments or exercises. In medical settings, a patient who takes pride in his independence and self-sufficiency may appear resistant because his medical condition has deprived him of a former sense of self-control and has created a sense of shame about depending upon others for self-care, including meals. The patient may be resisting being a patient. Coming to therapy may constitute a continual reminder that he has disabilities. Similarly, attending school-based speech therapy may stimulate a child's painful emotional feelings about being different from other children or fears of rejection by peers. In contrast, and paradoxically, some patients may fear the consequences of regaining certain abilities because it could mean losing emotional or financial support; therefore, forgetting appointments or failing to do therapy homework may reflect resistance to recovery (compare this to the concept of malingering, discussed in Chapter 12 under "Manipulative Behavior").

Reluctance

Before considering therapeutic responses to client resistance and noncompliance, it is necessary to discuss a related process that is often mistaken for resistance; that is, *reluctance*. Reluctance, in contrast to resistance, has an interpersonal basis (Pipes & Davenport, 1998; Teyber, 2005). Reluctance arises out of interactions with the clinician, while resistance arises primarily out of ambivalence within the client. Reluctance may be the result of fear or mistrust of the clinician or failure of the clinician to achieve an agreement about the goals and tasks of therapy, while resistance represents the client's own personal fear of change and growth. In both cases, the client hesitates or refuses to attend therapy or do certain therapeutic tasks, but the reasons behind the hesitation or refusal differ. The classic example of reluctance is a child's initial reluctance to come to the first therapy session;

however, the reluctance is easily resolved once the child discovers the clinician is non-threatening and friendly.

Clients may be reluctant (either temporarily or permanently) to perform recommended tasks or to continue therapy because the therapeutic alliance was insufficiently established or has deteriorated. Clients who feel unsupported or offended may show considerable reluctance to follow a clinician's goals or recommended exercises, at least with *that clinician*. The client is conveying that something about the clinician or something the clinician has said or done is not acceptable or tolerable. It is the client's perception that matters, and until the client feels sufficiently reassured and supported, maximum gains in therapy cannot be accomplished.

The relationships we form with clients and family members are often the basis of therapeutic cooperation and change. Many clients and family members agree to therapy or to do difficult assignments because they like, respect, and want to please their clinician. However, clients who feel slighted, discounted, unappreciated, or treated disrespectfully by a clinician are likely to be reluctant to fully engage with the clinician or to comply with the clinician's recommendations. Clients have both hopes and fears: hopes that they can be helped by their clinician and fears that they may not be helped. From the client's perspective, the clinician is the unknown quantity at the outset of the therapy. The client may know something about his communication problem, but initially knows little or nothing about the clinician. How the clinician treats the client can minimize or prevent the development of the client's reluctance to engage in therapy.

Clients sometimes are reluctant to share their problems with an SLP or Aud out of concern that the clinician may develop some control over their lives. This is not altogether unreasonable. A child who stutters may be reluctant to attend therapy for fear that his therapist will ask him to do things that might embarrass him, or that the therapist and his parents will encourage him to make difficult changes. A patient with dysphagia may be reluctant to be evaluated by an SLP because she knows that a roommate received a swallowing evaluation and was placed on pureed foods and thickened liquids. We cannot assume that all of our clients will immediately like and trust us and be willing to do the things we believe will help them.

Another reason clients or family members may be reluctant to participate in therapy or do particular tasks is their lack of understanding of the therapy goals and rationales and the connection between the therapy tasks and the goals. If a client's behavior is contrary to the tasks and goals of therapy, we need to first be certain that the client clearly understands what we are recommending and why. Second, we should not expect that one persuasive five-minute explanation will be sufficient for the client to understand and follow through with all of our therapy suggestions and recommendations. Reluctance often can be successfully resolved by adequately answering the client's questions and reassuring the client. As we respond sensitively, the client's growing confidence in the clinician often causes the initial reluctance to dissipate.

Poor Motivation Versus Resistance

As explained at the beginning of this chapter, resistance involves an internal conflict in which the client simultaneously wants to improve but has some reasons for fearing change. In this case, the client's ambivalence or contradictory motivations should be examined.

Poor motivation, however, does not necessarily involve internal conflict; that is, the client does not have the incentive or enthusiasm to improve and, therefore, chooses to only minimally or perfunctorily participate or to discontinue therapy altogether. Some clients come to therapy because of external pressure, motivation, or encouragement; for example, family members may want therapy for their child, or an employer may tell an employee that if her speech (e.g., fluency or voice) does not improve significantly, the employee's job may be in jeopardy. In such cases, the client may agree to enter or continue therapy to please or meet the demands of another person. External motivation alone is not conducive to improvement in therapy. Once in therapy, the externally motivated client is likely to exert minimal effort in complying with tasks or making changes. Internal motivation, however, refers to the client's personal desire to be in therapy and to put forth the effort to create desired changes. Clients with strong internal motivation usually have the best chance for achieving their maximum potential in therapy. Often, however, there is a mixture of external and internal motivation in a particular client, and the proportion of each may change over time. If a client's internal motivation wanes over time, the external motivators (parents, teachers, friends, colleagues, employers, etc.) may be sufficiently powerful for the client to continue progressing in therapy.

Poor motivation to engage in the tasks of therapy also may occur when the clinician is not able to sufficiently address the client's initial reluctance or does not recognize differences in the client's and clinician's goals. Trying to understand the client's goals and helping the client to understand ours may help increase the client's motivation. In addition, the effects of illness, injury, or medication can significantly affect a patient's motivation. Patients who are very ill, in pain, or sedated may not be sufficiently motivated or able to attend therapy and do therapy exercises. Patients with neurological disorders, particularly TBIs or CVAs with frontal lobe damage, may have significant cognitive impairments that affect their personality and character. Individuals who, prior to the neurological insult, were typically industrious, highly motivated people now may be apathetic and lethargic and not have the incentive to be in therapy or do therapeutic tasks (Andrewes, 2001; Tanner, 2003). This can be particularly frustrating to the patient's family and friends who knew the person as a hard worker and willing to do what it takes. In therapy we must do all that we can to stimulate, encourage, and reinforce the patient's participation. We should persevere, exercise tolerance, and move at a pace that benefits the patient. These patients may not be able to comprehend long-term goals, so more immediate goals should be identified and emphasized. However, regretfully, SLPs sometimes must discharge such patients from therapy because of lack of participation or frequent cancellations of therapy.

Responding to Resistance

Morrison (2008) and Teyber (2005) emphasize that the crucial ingredient for responding to resistance is to refuse to adopt an adversarial stance and instead to "join" with the client, thereby providing client support, lessening the client's fear, and encouraging discussion about what might be causing the resistance. This can be viewed as a three-part process. First, draw the client's attention to the resistant behaviors in as nonthreatening a manner as possible. For example, you might say in a noncritical tone, "You seem to be rather quiet today," "These exercises seem to be more difficult for you than usual," or

"For a while you were always on time for our appointments, but lately I notice that you've been five to ten minutes late for each session." If you can show genuine interest in what the client is thinking and feeling rather than annoyance, the client will have an easier time beginning to explore some of the reasons for the resistance. However, empathizing with the client's feelings does not mean that you support the resistance.

The second step, which may be combined with the first step, is to identify the specific context in which the resistant behavior occurs. For example, you may note, "Just when we begin talking about how your stuttering is affecting your job, you change the subject," "You seem reluctant to talk about how your voice sounds when talking to your father," or "The last time we met you looked rather angry, and then you cancelled the next appointment." The more sensitive, threatening, or fearful the issue is to the client, the more resistant or defensive he likely will be. Being quietly supportive rather than accusatory will help the client feel more comfortable sharing his thoughts and feelings.

The final step is to invite the client to explore what is going on for him. Approaching the exploration with genuine curiosity and interest can be helpful in conveying an open, noncritical attitude. Clinician congruence is essential during this process; that is, the clinician's thoughts, feelings, and emotional tone should match her behavior. Steps one and two are intended to prepare the client for the third step, and all three steps may be taken in a single brief interaction. Probing questions can help obtain information from the client to understand his thoughts and feelings. You may merge the three steps in a series of brief statements such as, "You seem to be rather quiet today. The last time we met you appeared a little angry, and then you cancelled the next appointment. How have you been feeling about the therapy and our work together?" (or, "What are your feelings about what I have just said?"). Other examples are, "You are generally very open when talking about your stuttering and how it affects different parts of your life, but now, just when you begin to tell me about how your stuttering is affecting your job, you change the subject. I'm wondering if this subject is especially difficult to talk about. Would you tell me about what's going on?" or "These exercises seem to be more difficult for you than usual and you are having some trouble getting them done. What do you think makes these exercises more difficult than the ones you have done in the past?" or "You seem to be in a rush when we are meeting and not focusing on your voice when we're together. Your speech sounds more pressured than in the past. Can you help me understand what might be going on for you?"

Clients are not always immediately able to respond to these questions in a meaningful way. However, these questions may trigger the client's reflections and introspection and open the door for further exploration at a later date. Essentially, these questions give the client permission to discuss difficult and negative feelings with the clinician so that the resistance can be overcome.

When the clinician invites such exploration she needs to be willing to hear anything the client says, even if it reflects the client's negative or hostile feelings toward the clinician and the therapeutic relationship. The invitation to explore is done supportively, unapologetically, and nondefensively. If, in fact, the clinician erred in some way, she needs to be willing to acknowledge the error nondefensively. This can strengthen the therapeutic alliance by legitimizing the client's feelings and by showing respect. The clinician's apology also provides a good model for the client that being human and making mistakes does not have to destroy one's self-respect or a relationship (Morrison, 2008; Pipes & Davenport, 1998).

Summary

When dealing with resistance and poor motivation, SLPs and Auds need to avoid slipping into a defensive or adversarial mode that can jeopardize the therapeutic relationship and sabotage future progress in therapy. If clinicians can reframe the client's resistance as a normal and expected component of therapy, they will find it easier to remain empathic while simultaneously encouraging the client to explore what she is thinking and feeling and the fears she may have about change.

ANGRY OR HOSTILE ATTITUDES AND BEHAVIORS

We have all experienced being angry or having someone's anger directed toward us. Anger is a normal human emotion. Whatever a person is angry about, that person likely feels strongly about. Ordinarily, people do not get angry about things they do not care about. When handled appropriately and expressed assertively (i.e., directly and without violating the rights of others or hurting oneself), anger can be a positive, creative communication that may lead to problem solving and productive change. However, when channeled inappropriately and expressed as verbal aggression (verbal attacks on others) or physical aggression, it can be a destructive and potentially life-threatening force (Keltner, Schwecke, & Bostrom, 2007).

Broadly speaking, anger is an affective response to frustration or perceived injustice and can encompass behavioral acts of hostility, self-defense, or protection of others and reactions against threats to our physical or emotional well-being (Feltham & Dryden, 2005). Hostility suggests a feeling of unfriendliness, animosity, or antagonism towards others. Anger and animosity towards others may be expressed in many ways. Anger can range in intensity from mild annoyance to rage and fury. Angry behavior spans a continuum from mild irritation and arguing to verbal or physical abuse, to uncontrolled rage and violence (see Table 13-1).

Anger can be released in more controlled ways, such as cynical or sarcastic humor, or it can be released in verbally or physically explosive behavior. The problem is not usually the anger itself but the way in which a person manages his anger. In some cultures and in some families, expressing anger is not acceptable and so people do not learn how to manage their anger effectively and constructively (Dahlen & Deffenbacher, 2001). Many people occasionally get angry and channel their feelings appropriately when they do. Other people may be chronically irritable and angry and behave as though they have a constant "chip on their shoulder." Others may be rarely angry, but when they do get angry it is as though a volcano erupts. They have stored anger for a long time until finally something triggers its release.

There are complex psychological bases for expressions of anger, including a person's temperament, general ability to regulate emotional states, historical factors such as history

TABLE 13-1 Expressions of Anger

Feelings that may Accompany Anger	Behaviors Towards Others	Behaviors Toward Self
Disappointment	Irritation	Crying
Inferiority	Sarcasm or cynicism	Ruminating
Sense of guilt	Arguing	Self-doubt
Sense of failure	Blaming	Self-criticism
Envy	Contempt	Self-condemnation
Feelings of injustice	Hostile behavior	Self-loathing
Low self-esteem	Insulting	Limit options
Feeling violated	Defensiveness	Restrict self
Integrity compromised	Yelling/Screaming	Self-negation
Mistrust	Intimidation	Erratic behavior
Demoralization	Defiance	Self-sacrifice
Cheated	Rage	Grieving
Depression	Withdrawal	Emotional numbing
Alienation	Non-disclosing behavior/ Passivity	Self-neglect (e.g., poor hygiene and nutrition)
Desperation	Protesting	Risk-taking behaviors (e.g., reckless driving)
Somatic symptoms (e.g., head-aches or stomachaches)	Punishing	Substance abuse (alcohol or drugs)
Powerlessness	Vengeful behavior	Self-destructive behavior
Helplessness	Verbal abuse	Self-mutilation (e.g., cutting behavior)
Hopelessness	Aggressive behavior/Assault	Suicidal behavior

Delmar/Cengage Learning

of trauma or mistreatment, and current factors such as stress levels. Poorly controlled or frequent expressions of anger can be detrimental to self-esteem and can damage relationships. Counseling approaches to anger help individuals learn how to manage anger rather than to eliminate it (Dahlen & Deffenbacher, 2001; Deffenbacher, 2006). The clinician's understanding of anger, its causes and expressions, and constructive responses can help clinicians to feel less threatened by a client's anger (Matsakis, 1998).

The Neurochemical and Neurophysiologic Basis of Anger

Anger and hostility, like all emotions, have a neurochemical and neurophysiological basis. An important trigger for anger is a feeling of frustration that accompanies the belief that obstacles have been imposed by others and the fear of not achieving one's objectives. Another common trigger is the perception of being threatened or endangered either physically or emotionally (e.g., our self-esteem or self-image), which creates fear. Goleman

(1995) and Bear, Conners, and Paradiso (2007) describe the neurophysiology of fear. Perceptions of threat or danger act as triggers for the hypothalamus and cause a surge in the limbic system. One part of the surge is a release of catecholamines (the neurotransmitters dopamine, norepinephrine, and epinephrine), which generate a burst of energy that lasts for a few to several minutes, which is sufficient time for the fight-or-flight response. Meanwhile, an amygdala-driven response through the adrenocortical branch of the nervous system creates a general background of action-readiness that lasts longer than the catecholamine energy surge. The generalized adrenocortical excitation can last for hours to days, keeping the emotions in readiness for arousal, and becoming a foundation on which subsequent reactions can rapidly build. This adrenocortical arousal process helps explain why people are more prone to anger if they have already been provoked or irritated by something else. Stress of all kinds creates adrenocortical arousal, lowering the threshold for what provokes anger.

We usually visually identify people who are angry before we hear their angry remarks. There are unique patterns of facial muscular contractions that are associated with primary emotions, including anger, and an angry face can be recognized by people around the world (Burgoon et al., 2002; Tian, Kanade, & Cohn, 2005). Tense facial muscles are often the first indication that a person is angry. The muscles of the brow move inward and downward, creating a frown and a foreboding appearance about the eyes, which seem to be fixed in a hard stare toward the object of anger. The nostrils dilate and the nares of the nose flare out. The lips may be tightly pursed and the chin tightened, or the lips may be open and drawn back in a rectangle-like shape, revealing clenched teeth. Often the face flushes red because of a rapid increase in blood supply. The observer will likely get a clear message that the person is frustrated and is either holding back an angry response or about to have a display of anger. The angry facial features allow the listener (observer) to make some adjustments in what she is saying or doing to manage or quell the anger and therefore avoid a verbal or physical attack. However, individuals who "telegraph" few or no visual signs of anger but simply lash out at a person are particularly dangerous because the listener has little or no time to adjust the communication or assuage the anger.

The Assault Cycle

Stuart (2008) discusses Smith's stress model (1981), which includes the assault cycle with five phases of a predictable pattern or chain of aggressive responses to emotional or physical stress (see Figure 13-1). Assault is legally defined as any behavior that physically or verbally presents an immediate threat of physical injury to another individual (Garner, 2009). SLPs and Auds are rarely confronted with assault (except perhaps with patients with TBIs at Level IV of the Rancho Scales—Confused-Agitated); however, the assault cycle model can help us understand an anger cycle.

The five-phase cycle adapted from Smith (1981) and described by Stuart (2008) includes the following:

1. *Triggering phase*. The stress-producing event occurs, initiating the stress responses (e.g., in an IEP meeting a parent hears difficult information about her son from the classroom teacher, resource specialist, and SLP, or a patient in rehabilitation is

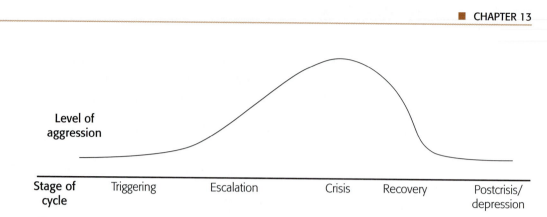

Figure 13–1 The assault cycle (Adapted from Smith, 1981).

in physical pain and the SLP asks him to work on tasks which he either feels are of questionable value or does not understand). Observable behaviors may include muscle tension, changes in voice quality, tapping of fingers, pacing, repeating statements with increasing intensity, restlessness, irritability, anxiety, perspiration, glaring, or changes in breathing.

2. *Escalation phase.* Responses represent escalating behaviors that indicate a movement toward the loss of control (e.g., the parent begins displaying defensive strategies such as denial and devaluing, or a patient starts refusing to do therapy tasks). Behaviors that may be observed include pale or flushed face, loud voice, swearing, agitation, threats, demands, loss of reasoning ability, or clenched fists.

3. *Crisis phase.* A period of emotional and physical crisis involving loss of control occurs (e.g., a parent begins yelling, screaming, and cursing at the staff, or the patient begins to verbally and/or physically attack a hospital staff member). Observable behaviors may include loss of control, swearing, fighting, hitting, kicking, scratching, and throwing objects.

4. *Recovery phase.* A period of "cooling down" occurs, in which the person slows down and returns to normal responses (e.g., the parent stops yelling and cursing the staff and sits with arms folded, or the patient lowers his voice and sits back in the chair with a defiant expression). Observable behaviors may include decreased body tension, lowered voice volume, and change in conversational content to include more rational problem solving.

5. *Post-crisis depression phase.* A period in which the person feels remorseful or contrite and attempts reconciliation with others (e.g., the parent feels embarrassed and apologizes for her outburst and asks forgiveness, or the patient rationalizes his explosive behavior and then asks to continue therapy). Observable behaviors may include apologies, crying, and reconciliatory interactions.

Clients may become angry when they feel that they have been threatened or treated unjustly, their rights have been restricted or violated, they feel criticized or devalued, or they feel abandoned. Anger often involves cognitive characteristics such as distortions and catastrophizing (Martin & Dahlen, 2005). For example, a client may respond to an unfortunate event with exaggerated and dramatic thoughts such as, "Everything bad happens to me. I always get 'the short end of the stick.'" Not every client will have the same anger triggers and so clinicians cannot always predict when clients will become angry. When people get angry, they are attempting to influence someone (e.g., to obtain a desired intervention or to avoid a dreaded intervention), while in other cases anger simply communicates a painful emotion.

Clinicians tend to have a much harder time responding empathically to client anger than to softer client emotions such as sadness, anxiety, and depression (Hess, Knox, & Hill, 2006; Matsakis, 1998). While client anger can be a scary emotion for the clinician to experience, especially when the client directs these feelings towards her, it is important to try to help the client de-escalate the situation as well as to discover what the client is trying to communicate. Further, it is important for the clinician to try to keep calm while attempting to help the client return to a more rational way of expressing his thoughts and feelings.

A key element in preventing and managing angry client behavior is to understand the triggering phase, that is, the stress-producing event or events that initiate the stress response that lead to the angry behavior. Almost anyone experiencing significant or catastrophic change will experience some anger. Moreover, even though the person may not be aware of the anger or may be unable to express it, the anger is present nonetheless (Luterman, 2008; Rollin, 2000; Tanner, 2008). The person's anger may emerge or become apparent at a later date or unexpected time. Immediate and appropriate angry reactions are often considered healthy expressions and verbal signals to others. Expressions of anger may be viewed as behavior-toward-others or behavior-toward-self (Fein, 1993; Stuart, 2008). Some people tend toward more internalizing styles, and their anger is expressed predominantly in behaviors toward themselves. Other individuals tend toward more externalizing styles, and their predominant ways of expressing anger are in behaviors toward others. In some people, however, anger is expressed both toward self and others (see Table 13-1).

Clients may become angry when they receive a diagnosis of a severe hearing or communication disorder or when they receive bad news in an insensitive manner (see Chapter 12). Sometimes client or family anger is displaced onto the professional, and the professional can easily become the "lightning rod" for negative feelings. People sometimes "slay the messenger" when they do not like the message. When disability in a family is present, life options are narrowed and people may become angry at these restrictions (Luterman, 2008). Clients may become angry when they realize that they cannot be "cured" or the result of therapy was a less favorable outcome than they had hoped for. Family members feel angry when someone (e.g., a drunk driver) physically injures a loved one. Parents feel angry when their child is permanently injured because of a tragic accident. Sometimes family members even become angry with a spouse or parent who is seriously injured, disabled, or killed. The spouse or child may feel that the person has abandoned them and may say to themselves, "But you promised me you would always be there for me. Where are you now when I need you most?"

Once again, anger is a normal feeling and reaction to many disturbing situations; however, it is the manner in which the anger is expressed that becomes the challenge to clinicians. Anger from clients and family members can provoke strong emotional responses in clinicians (including anger, anxiety, and fear) and can test our patience and tolerance. We may not feel we are being treated with proper respect. We need to keep in mind that anger is likely the surface behavior that hides emotional or physical pain, anxiety, frustration, fear, and a sense of helplessness or hopelessness.

Despite the natural tendency to respond defensively when someone demonstrates anger toward us, it is important to reflect on our possible contributions to the person's feelings. For example, clients and family members may become angry with us if we are not communicating with them sufficiently to keep them abreast of progress, if we are late for appointments, if we are explaining information at too technical a level, or if we do not truly understand what they are telling us because of lack of careful listening (Wachtel, 1993; Shipley & Roseberry-McKibbon, 2006). By considering what we may have said or done to engender anger toward us, we can decide if an apology or making amends is needed and thereby decrease or eliminate some or all of the frustration contributing to the person's anger.

The first goal as a clinician is to try to understand the source of the person's anger and the feelings that are being masked or overshadowed by the anger. Knowing the client's case history may help us understand whether the communication problems may be perceived by the client and family as an acute threat to their emotional well-being. Also, it is helpful to understand whether the person is experiencing chronic frustration because expected improvements have not been achieved or feeling a sense of helplessness, that little or nothing may ever change. By considering the feelings that underlie the anger, we are able to more easily respond in an empathic and therapeutic manner. We need to respond consciously and carefully to the client's angry behavior to maintain the therapeutic relationship. The first step in responding is to try to hear the client's concerns while not becoming emotionally intimidated or retaliatory. It is important that our response helps the client feel greater trust in us rather than damages that trust.

Some clients have difficulty expressing their anger appropriately and may benefit from learning more appropriate cognitive, communication, coping, and relaxation skills (Deffenbacher, 1999, 2006; Deffenbacher, Oetting, & DiGiuseppe, 2002). The SLP may teach these skills to some children and adults (particularly those with neurological impairments) who have problems with pragmatic language, especially when they are angry or upset. Learning how to express their anger can help clients maintain amiable and respectful relationships with other people.

Mosak and Maniacci (1998), Gordon (2000), and Bippus and Young (2005) distinguish between "You-messages" and "I-messages" and how they can be effective as a teaching device for clients. Clients frequently experience difficulty expressing anger and other emotions, particularly when they are upset, and teaching them how to use "I-messages" can help improve their communication skills. "I-messages" place the responsibility of the person's feeling on herself, not the other person. Three-part sentence stems are used: "When you . . . I feel . . . because . . ." For example, clients who are having difficulty communicating their anger can be taught to say, "*When you* don't understand what I'm saying, *I feel* angry *because* I don't think you are paying attention to me." The first part of the stem ("When you") describes the behavior that is producing the emotion; the second part ("I feel") names the emotion; and the last part ("because") helps the client express the reason for feeling that way. Through role playing, clients can practice these skills and learn to use them both within and outside the therapy environment.

As clinicians we can use the same technique to communicate our feelings toward a client or family members. "I feel" statements allow us to help people understand how we are feeling about something they have said or done without sounding accusatory. Instead of saying "You did this . . ." or "You make me feel . . . ," we are simply stating how we feel, for example, "When you talk to me in a loud voice, I feel uneasy because your words and tone of voice sound rough and hostile."

If you are working in a medical setting where you see many patients with TBIs, it may be helpful to develop a behavioral management team where each team member agrees on specific management approaches to use with individuals displaying hostile, angry, or aggressive behavior. A 1-to-10 scale may be used to measure an individual's anger or aggression, with 1 indicating very mild anger and 10 indicating rage. Some patients can quickly escalate from 1 or 2 to 8, 9, or 10. The goal is to teach the patient to identify his anger before it escalates and to employ coping skills to prevent the anger or aggression from escalating. Reflections and probing questions may help reveal the source of the frustration, hostility, irritation, anger, or fear; for example,

- "You seem a little annoyed with . . ."
- "You seemed to have had a difficult experience with . . ."
- "I sense that you're irritated about . . ."
- "You seem angry right now. Can you tell me what you are thinking about?"
- "You seem a little more tense than when I saw you last time. Would you like to tell me what's going on?"
- "You seem a little more tense today. I'm wondering if I have paced the exercises a little too fast. What do you think?"
- "Therapy can be a little frightening because it is difficult to predict how much improvement will be made. Do you feel concerned about that sometimes?"
- "Besides what we have been talking about, what other concerns do you have?"

Reflections and probes allow the person an opportunity to ventilate and express his thoughts and feelings and communicate to the person that his feelings are respected. The anger and aggression scale and therapeutic communication techniques should be taught to all staff working with patients who are neurologically impaired so the staff have consistent and predictable strategies to deal with problem behaviors.

COMMUNICATING AND RESPONDING TO ANGRY BEHAVIOR

The following are a number of principles and strategies for dealing with angry behavior:

1. Respond with unconditional positive regard.
2. Maintain your poise.
3. Be aware of the person's defense mechanisms.
4. Maintain good eye contact and listen without interrupting.

5. Give the person time to blow off steam.

6. Pause briefly before responding.

7. Offer empathic statements or reflections of feelings.

8. Give the person the opportunity to respond more appropriately.

9. Provide opportunity for the person to save face.

10. Help the person feel validated and important.

Respond with Unconditional Positive Regard

The general approach is to respond to the person with unconditional positive regard (Rogers, 1951), that is, acceptance of the person without reservation, rather than trying to control or manage the person's anger. Consistently nonjudgmental responses can allow the person to feel accepted and, therefore, more relaxed. While it is important to accept the person, we do not necessarily have to accept all of the person's behaviors. When people feel accepted, they feel less tense and more calm, which can defuse some of the angry feelings and diminish angry behaviors.

Maintain Your Poise

When you do not get angry in return, the person does not have anything to "push against" and it destabilizes him, which allows him to try a different tactic or behavior other than anger. In other words, some clients may be looking for a fight; do not give them one. Maintaining your poise is the most important strategy you can use to reduce a person's anger.

Be Aware of the Person's Defense Mechanisms

Remember that the person is probably feeling overwhelming anxiety. He may be using defense mechanisms such as denial, displacement, passive-aggressive behavior, or devaluing to protect himself from anxiety or frustration (see Chapter 10 for more information on defense mechanisms). It is important that you not become defensive yourself. You need to be aware of your own defensive tendencies, how you deal with your own anger, and how you can channel it into constructive, productive actions. You cannot defuse a person's anger or aggression when you are in a similar emotional state, and any retaliatory anger on your part will likely intensify or escalate the person's anger.

Maintain Good Eye Contact and Listen Without Interrupting

If you must interrupt, do it politely. Listen intently but not tensely; that is, try to stay calm, relaxed, and in control of yourself so the person does not think he is getting to you. In a calm voice, call the person by his last name to show respect, for example, "Mr. Adams, I want to explain something." Being courteous and respectful may be surprising to the person and help defuse the anger.

Give the Person Time to Blow Off Steam

Once a client is very angry, it may take some time before he is able to regain his composure. If you feel it is in the best interest of the therapeutic relationship, you may choose to hear the person out. However, if you feel that the person's anger is escalating and that he may not be able to control himself, it is quite justifiable to tell the person that you will be happy to talk again when he is less angry and can talk in a more appropriate manner, and then discontinue or postpone the rest of the session. Discontinuing an interaction when a person is very angry may help to protect a relationship, as things are often said "in the heat of the moment" that may later be regretted.

Pause Briefly Before Responding

Your willingness to listen to the person, and a brief pause before you speak, lets the person know that you are in control of yourself. Speak calmly and slowly, and use a low-volume voice. A rapid or loud verbal response can escalate a feeling of threat to the person, and his anger may intensify. Maintain good eye contact when you speak, which can help the person feel that you are confident about what you are saying.

Offer Empathic Statements or Reflections of Feelings

A statement such as, "Mr. Adams, you are understandably upset" reflects empathy and being nonjudgmental. Do not tell the person, "I understand how upset you are" because you probably do not really understand the intensity of his feelings. Other empathic statements may be, "Mr. Adams, this must be hard for you" or "Mr. Adams, I know this situation is quite upsetting." A collaborative statement might be, "Mr. Adams, let's try to figure this out together."

Give the Person the Opportunity to Respond More Appropriately

Some people calm down spontaneously after a brief moment of anger. In other cases, you may feel the need to facilitate this transition. After offering empathic statements such as, "It's understandable that this situation is very upsetting," you may try to join with the person by asking if he would like to take some slow, deep breaths with you. For example, you might offer, "Let's sit back in our chairs for a moment and take a few deep breaths. Sometimes that helps in gaining some distance and perspective."

Provide an Opportunity for the Person to Save Face

Many times people are embarrassed after they have displayed excessive anger. If the person wants to apologize for his angry outburst, allow it. However, it is good to avoid the social response "That's all right" because that may give the false impression that the angry behavior is acceptable. An empathic response such as, "Your anger is understandable" validates his feelings but not his behavior. Saying "Thank you" after an apology acknowledges that you have accepted it. Sometimes just nodding your head once slowly with a concerned facial expression is sufficient to acknowledge the acceptance of the apology. If the person does not spontaneously offer an apology, do not ask for one. This could set up more resistance and intensify the person's feelings of shame and anger.

Help the Person Feel Validated and Important

If you can return to therapy tasks, the tasks need to help the client feel some measure of success. Provide reinforcement for any behavior that is appropriate, but avoid sounding patronizing or condescending with your choice of words or tone of voice.

Various Therapeutic Approaches to Angry Behavior

In addition to the general principles for responding to client anger described above, the following illustrations provide some different approaches to dealing with angry behavior, including the behavioral approach, culture-sensitive approach, humanistic approach, and interpersonal approach. For further information regarding theoretically-based counseling approaches, refer to Chapter 2.

BEHAVIORAL APPROACH

If the person's anger is mildly inappropriate but transient (e.g., swearing at you), you may simply ignore the behavior and appear more attentive and engaged when the person expresses himself in a more rational and appropriate manner. You may attempt to "shape" appropriate behavior and extinguish inappropriate behavior. You do not want to reinforce inappropriate, angry behavior.

CULTURE-SENSITIVE APPROACH

Some cultures are socialized to express their emotions in an open, demonstrative, even dramatic way. Be careful not to inaccurately label or overestimate the person's emotional reaction to the situation. Instead of interpreting the person's feelings (e.g., "Mr. Jones, you certainly seem angry"), it is better to inquire about his feelings (e.g., "That information got a strong response from you, Mr. Jones. How are you feeling about things right now?"). In other cultures, individuals are discouraged from expressing anger directly and so they may develop a habit of suppressing the feeling and/or expressing it indirectly. You may encourage healthy modes of expressing feelings by "normalizing" the feeling and letting the person know that it is understandable to feel anger in a situation like this. This provides the person with permission to express a previously taboo feeling.

HUMANISTIC APPROACH

You can express empathy and acceptance of the person's angry feelings while encouraging the person to explore the feelings that may underlie the surface emotion (e.g., frustration, anxiety, fear, sense of helplessness). A therapeutic response might be, "It is understandable that you are upset (empathy). Would you like to say more about how you are feeling now (exploration)?" In this way, you can convey unconditional positive regard for the person despite the negative feelings that have been expressed.

INTERPERSONAL APPROACH

Avoid getting "hooked" by the person's anger. The person may have a history of eliciting defensive, angry, or retaliatory responses from others, and is demonstrating the same tactic with you. Resist the urge to respond with counter-hostility and, instead, provide a response that reflects the person's feelings toward you at the moment, for example, "I can see that you're upset that I don't have all the answers." This provides the person with a different interpersonal response than the one he is accustomed to eliciting. By interrupting an ingrained interpersonal pattern, you are helping the person to reflect on his behavior rather than simply acting it out. Over time, the individual can learn new interpersonal patterns for expressing anger in more constructive ways.

Rage or Potential Physical Abuse (Catastrophic Reactions)

Although SLPs are unlikely to be confronted with a person's rage or potential physical abuse, it has occurred, particularly in acute medical and rehabilitation settings with patients with TBIs at Level IV (Confused-Agitated) on the Rancho Scales. However, patients with CVAs, especially in the posterior left frontal lobe area, are susceptible to catastrophic reactions (Tanner, 2008). We need to keep in mind that when such patients have catastrophic reactions it is secondary to the nature of the neurological damage and that the patients' behaviors are not completely under their cognitive control. As a result, SLPs working with these patients need to take a significant amount of responsibility for managing the potentially dangerous behaviors until patients can manage their own anger and angry behaviors.

Catastrophic reactions may be seen as explosive outbursts by patients with potentially uncontrolled rage (Brookshire, 2007; Tanner, 2008). The causes of the reaction may be the same or similar to the anger or rage response, that is, frustration and fear. Some clinicians have been physically injured by patients, resulting in worker's compensation claims and loss of work time needed for recovery. However, if a clinician injures a patient during an attempt to protect herself, legal entanglement may occur.

In therapy rooms within medical settings, where you are likely to work with patients who have had CVAs and TBIs, it is prudent to arrange your therapy table so that the patient and you both have the door to your sides rather than having the door behind you or in front of you. Having the door to your sides without any hindrance for either you or the patient may help both of you feel unimpeded if there is a need to quickly leave the room. If, for example, the table is arranged so that the patient is behind the table with his back to the far wall and he becomes agitated and wants to leave the room immediately, you may be blocking the exit (Figure 13-2A). On the other hand, if you are behind the table with your back to the far wall and the patient becomes agitated and possibly threatening, you may be trapped (Figure 13-2B). Your exit or the patient's can be expedited with the table arranged so that either you or the patient can simply turn and walk out of the room (Figure 13-2C).

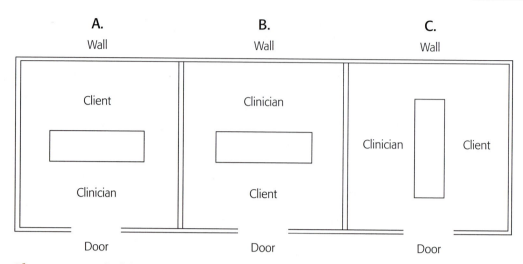

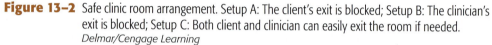

Figure 13–2 Safe clinic room arrangement. Setup A: The client's exit is blocked; Setup B: The clinician's exit is blocked; Setup C: Both client and clinician can easily exit the room if needed.
Delmar/Cengage Learning

Fein (1993) discusses methods for clinicians to manage client rage and potential physical abuse. He emphasizes that the clinician's safety is essential. The first priority for dealing with problem anger must be avoiding injury to yourself and others, and, secondarily, to the angry person. The best way to protect against problematic anger is to anticipate it. If frustration is what triggers a person's anger, if at all possible remove the cause of the frustration. Fein describes several ways this can be done.

REMOVE THE INDIVIDUAL FROM THE SOURCE OF ANXIETY

It is prudent for clinicians to be aware of an expedient method to move a patient from one environment to another. This can prevent the patient from harming other staff or patients and can prevent an altercation between patients. Patients do not only strike out at staff but may attack other patients who cannot escape or defend themselves.

Removing a Patient from an Anxiety-Producing Environment

I was working in a skilled nursing facility during the summer. The social service director had arranged for an entertainer to come into the facility for an afternoon and the residents were encouraged to attend. Many of the staff, including myself, assisted residents into the large room, and many of them were in wheelchairs. The room became crowded, and personal space for some of the residents was violated. One man in a wheelchair who was surrounded by other residents became agitated. Before any of the staff could reach him, he began cursing at another resident and hit him with his fists. A CNA who had earlier cared for the agitated resident quickly told

Continues on next page

Continued from previous page

the staff that she knew him well and could take care of the situation. She rushed to the resident and knelt down beside his wheelchair and in a soothing way tried to calm him; however, the resident struck out at her with his fist and hit her in the face. I reached the CNA and resident in an instant, helped the CNA off the floor, started moving other residents to clear a path for the agitated man, and quickly wheeled him out a side door and into an open courtyard to get him away from what precipitated his agitation—the violation of his personal space. Fortunately, the CNA was unhurt and realized the error she had made by placing her face within arm's reach of the resident.

CLINICAL QUESTIONS

1. Describe how you might have tried to intervene with this agitated patient.

2. What are the preventive steps you would take if you were working with this patient and another special event was announced?

MOVE THE SOURCE OF ANXIETY

For some patients, a particular staff person may not be tolerated well and, for whatever reason, may trigger or escalate a patient's uncontrolled anger. If a staff member recognizes that his presence is frustrating or agitating a patient, it is wise for that staff member to remain out of view and voice range of the patient as much as possible.

DISTRACT THE ANGRY PERSON FROM THE SOURCE OF ANXIETY

Directing the patient's attention and gaze to something more tolerable to the patient may briefly take his focus away from the offending person or situation. Distractions and diversions provide a more agreeable stimulus that is incompatible with anxiety and anger. Having the patient focus on some interesting visual stimulus or initiating some casual and enjoyable conversation may be sufficient to divert the patient's attention away from the anger-producing person or situation.

INTERCEDE BETWEEN THE ANGRY PERSON AND THE SOURCE OF ANGER

When the angry person cannot physically reach the source of frustration or anxiety, a physical and psychological barrier allows the person to cool down. The time may allow the person to regroup and calm himself sufficiently to begin to manage the angry behaviors. This time also allows the clinician an opportunity to assess the situation and consider another more permanent strategy to manage the person's aggressive anger. The clinician should keep in mind that it is not prudent to place herself between the angry person and the source of frustration without being at least a leg's distance from the person.

Calming Techniques

The eventual goal is for the patient to be able to calm himself and control his anger, which, from a language perspective, may be considered a pragmatic skill (i.e., the ability to communicate anger appropriately through both verbal and nonverbal channels). From a cognitive perspective, anger reduction serves a therapeutic purpose as anger often impairs cognitive processes. To be able to calm himself and control his own anger, the patient must recognize what triggers his anger and the signs that he is getting angry. The clinician may introduce calming techniques that may later become a part of the patient's behavioral repertoire for self-management. These coping strategies can help the person feel some control over stressful situations. Calming techniques may be implemented by the angry person himself or by those nearby. When the person can implement them, he is in a better position to develop and maintain positive social interactions. Calming techniques include the use of safe places, safe persons, and safe activities (Fein, 1993). The following calming techniques may be incorporated within a typical therapy session that works on other areas of language or cognitive therapy:

SAFE PLACES

The purpose of a safe place is to remove an agitated or enraged person from a frustrating environment that may escalate the anger. Most people tend to calm down once they are no longer provoked. The person or situation causing the frustration is removed, or the angry person is moved to a more neutral location. The patient's antagonist is asked to leave the room, or the patient may choose to leave. This reduces the patient's stress, frustration, or fear. If the SLP has learned who or what may provoke a patient, that person or situation should be kept away from the patient. Most clinicians attempt to create a warm and inviting therapy environment; however, in a busy hospital noise levels and visual distractions are often difficult to control and make safe places a premium.

SAFE PERSONS

Patients typically relate better to some staff than others, and the SLP may be the least threatening or anger-provoking person in the patient's environment. Physical and occupational therapists, nurses, and physicians may place demands on patients or touch or prod them in ways that are irritating. Patients with TBIs may have catastrophic reactions when their threshold of tolerance is exceeded and more is asked of them than they can comfortably do. The SLP may be the professional who is particularly sensitive to subtle signs of frustration, anxiety, or irritability. The SLP also may be the person whom other staff members recognize as having a good or excellent rapport with a patient and the range of abilities to communicate in a nonthreatening manner. Therefore, it is quite possible that for a particular patient with uncontrolled anger, the SLP may be the safe person, the person who can most easily calm and soothe the patient.

To calm or soothe a patient, our voices should be reassuring and our demeanor nonthreatening. Our language should be easily understood with words of support and encouragement. Similarly, our body language should convey openness and comfort, with no obvious indication of being prepared to defend ourselves or to escape (although we must be ready to do either). The message safe people want to convey is that they are not angry, frightened, or demanding and, therefore, have no reason to be frustrating or threatening to the patient. Successful calming depends upon trust, which the clinician must earn from the patient. The angry person can only be calmed if he feels safe with the person trying to calm him. The clinician needs to convey that she is on the side of the patient and must behave in a nonconfrontational and nondemanding manner. When talking to an aggressively angry patient, the clinician must be sincere and avoid coercive behaviors and patronizing or condescending language. This may take considerable self-restraint on the part of the clinician. The SLP must recognize when she does not feel that she has the resources (emotional strength, physical health, patience, or sensitivity) to take on such a challenging task and defer the task to someone who can manage the situation better at that time.

SAFE ACTIVITIES

Frustration usually arises from not attaining what is urgently desired. Patients need a feeling of accomplishment and respect. They also may need a quiet, nonthreatening environment, people they enjoy, relief from pain, being able to stop an activity they cannot tolerate, or having the foods or food textures they like. If we can discern what the patient wants or needs and if possible provide it, the anger may rapidly subside. However, if the desired activity or item cannot reasonably be provided, then a diversionary activity may help calm the person.

When an angry patient shifts focus to another task, he also may shift immediate priorities. What the person no longer is focused on loses its importance and, therefore, its frustrating effects (e.g., an intensely angry person can be encouraged to take a walk with you). Physical activity requires concentration that can be drawn away from the frustrating person or situation. Physical activity also uses energy that can be dissipated toward healthier and safer pursuits. Fatigue produces a sense of tranquility. If, however, because of physical limitations the patient can do little or no physical activity that may be sufficiently distracting and/or fatiguing, the patient may be asked to do nothing at all, that is, to sit quietly for a few moments. The person may be left alone (if you feel the person or your office will be safe) or may be placed in a quiet room with few distractions, not as a punishment but as an opportunity to try to settle himself. He may find this time peaceful and welcoming. He also can learn this as a strategy for managing himself when he is feeling intense anger in the future.

Cue Training

Cue training is a technique aimed at helping people induce self-control, based on the assumption that few people willingly lose self-control; that is, their anger gets out of hand and they cannot restrain it. Once they become enraged, they cannot think clearly and are less likely to get their wants, needs, thoughts, and feelings understood and met. Cue training involves helping the patient become aware of escalating anger and the triggers for it. Increased self-awareness of escalating anger may involve reflection on one's moods, physiological responses (tense jaw, clenched fists, perspiration, etc.), and interpersonal behavior (raised voice, hostile language, impatience, etc.). In this way, the patient can recognize his own anger in an early stage and, hopefully, prevent it from intensifying. Being more aware of these cues can help the patient better manage himself by using such techniques as moving himself away from the frustrating or anxiety-provoking person or situation, calmly asking the person to leave, finding a quiet, peaceful place to be alone for awhile, and so forth. The goal is to help the patient learn to manage his intense feelings as well as aggressive angry behavior. This allows the patient to become more self-confident in hospital or rehabilitation settings as well as social situations.

Summary

Angry or hostile attitudes and behaviors from clients, patients, or family members may be some of the most difficult challenges clinicians are confronted with, and such challenges may occur in any setting. It is important for us to appreciate that anger is a normal feeling and reaction to many disturbing situations. It is important to discover the source of the client's anger and whether it is a reaction to life circumstances (such as illness or loss) or whether it is a reaction to something you have said or done (e.g., the client feeling criticized, ignored, or humiliated). Behind angry or hostile behaviors there are usually feelings of frustration, threat, or fear. If clinicians can recognize the feelings behind the anger, they can better communicate with the patient who is angry and be instrumental in helping to diminish the patient's anger. Clinicians must also be aware of their own tendencies to become defensive or angry in response to another person's anger. There are numerous principles for communicating with a person who is angry and techniques for managing catastrophic reactions.

CONCLUDING COMMENTS

Resistance is a natural occurrence when people fear change or are uncertain about a situation. Some people who seek therapy also are resistant to it, particularly if they feel frightened or threatened by the challenges and tasks put before them. A sudden loss of hearing or communication abilities may result in resistance to accepting the loss. Viewing an individual's resistance as a signal of fear that deserves our empathy and support can help us avoid responding in a defensive manner, and provide a better opportunity to maintain the client–clinician relationship.

Anger is an affective response to frustration or perceived injustice that can be recognized behaviorally in a variety of ways. Clinicians may become "lightning rods" for intense emotional reactions when clients or families feel threatened by a diagnosis of a communication disorder or therapy has not progressed as fast or as far as hoped. We need to manage our natural tendency toward defensiveness and counterproductive emotional responses in order to respond in a therapeutic manner toward our clients.

Discussion Questions

1. Discuss clinical examples of reluctance and resistance and productive strategies for responding to those client experiences and behaviors.

2. Think of a time when you had low motivation or felt reluctant to do something that was asked of you. What was your resulting behavior? How did you communicate your reluctance or low motivation?

3. Recall a situation in which you felt a client or family member might have been reluctant to do what you asked. What do you think was the source of that reluctance? How did you help the person go beyond the reluctance to do what you felt was therapeutic?

4. What are examples of noncompliance that may not be appropriately classified as resistance?

5. Describe your educational career and progress, using the concepts of revolution, evolution, and resolution and how you have developed and changed.

6. Discuss a client with whom you worked and how change occurred through revolution, evolution, and resolution.

7. What are some of the manifestations of resistance you have experienced with clients and their family members? How did you handle the resistance therapeutically, or how would you handle it if you had another chance?

8. Describe some situations in which clients became angry. How did they express their anger? What do you think was the source of their anger?

9. How well have you handled client anger in the past? What strategies for handling client anger will you be likely to use in the future?

10. Recall Smith's assault cycle as it relates to your own anger. What triggers an angry response in you? What escalates it? What do you do when you have an angry outburst? How do you cool down? How do you feel afterwards?

11. Remember an incident when you observed someone have an angry outburst. What do you think triggered it? What escalated it? What did the person do during the outburst? What helped him cool down? How do you think he felt afterwards?

12. What are some reflections and probing questions you might ask a client that may help you understand his frustration, irritation, fear, or anger? What are some supportive verbal or nonverbal messages you might communicate when a client is angry?

13. Have you ever intervened to calm a very angry or enraged person? What did you do that helped calm the person? What did not help?

of life apart from the crisis, for example, family life or employment; and (5) limited duration, that is, the experience is temporary, not chronic (George & Cristiani, 1995; Nystul, 2005).

Crises overload a person or family's coping abilities, making their usual problem-solving strategies unworkable and ineffective. A crisis, by definition, is an emotionally hazardous situation in which a person experiences a significant sense of threat; however, it also may represent an opportunity. A crisis creates a time of turmoil and transition that may bring about important changes in a person or family system by forcing individuals to adopt new perspectives or allow role changes as a means of adapting to changing conditions (Dattilio & Freeman, 2007; Flannery & Everly, 2000; Goldenberg & Goldenberg, 2007).

It is important to keep in mind that the defining characteristic of a crisis is not the apparent gravity of the instigating event, but rather the person's difficulty in coping with the situation (Roberts, 2005; Zaro, Barach, Nedelman, & Dreiblatt, 2000). Although a crisis usually is the result of a catastrophic situation such as the death of a family member, SLPs and Auds are more likely to see patients or families in crisis following the survival of a catastrophic event, such as a stroke or traumatic brain injury. However, SLPs and Auds also may see families in apparent crisis following a diagnosis, a school's decision during an IEP meeting, or a family's challenging decision making regarding caregiving roles.

Common physiological responses to the perception of a crisis include tense muscles, racing pulse, pounding heart, dry mouth, queasy stomach, and sweating. Some general reactions to a crisis range from being noticeably anxious to being extremely upset or in a state of panic. The person may be visibly agitated, moving quickly and aimlessly. The person's speech may be rapid and pressured. The person is likely somewhat confused and shows impaired judgment, with difficulty making even very simple decisions, and therefore wants and needs considerable direction from others. Some individuals may become hypersensitive to the environment and other people, or withdrawn and noncommunicative (Roberts, 2005).

In contrast, some individuals are able to rise to the occasion, muster their resources, and perform even better under very stressful conditions. In crisis situations, some people seem to be able to exercise an extraordinary degree of energy and focus to accomplish the task at hand. After such experiences, there is often a sense of accomplishment and self-discovery of personal resources they did not know they had.

There are many kinds of crises that occur in people's lives, and one crisis may lead to another. For example, a motor vehicle accident resulting in a child having a TBI creates a crisis around the child's neurological damage and the initial concern about his survival. Crises can have a cascading effect in which the effects of one crisis compound the effects of the next one. Additional crises that may occur following the scenario described above are the parents' loss of time from work, expenses that are incurred that insurance will not cover, attempts to care for the other children at home, and countless other "little crises" that arise, all of which can be magnified by the parents' loss of sleep. As SLPs and Auds we can reasonably assume that a previously normally functioning individual who now has a moderate to severe communicative or cognitive problem is in crisis, and so is the family. Even seemingly mild problems can throw some people into a crisis. Although we are not crisis counselors, we must work with clients, patients, and families who are in crisis. Understanding general principles of crisis management can help our patients and their families maximize the benefits they receive from therapy during the acute stage. Crisis management should be a team approach in which all the professionals working with a patient or family are following similar strategies to help them cope with the crisis as best they can.

Turning Personal Crisis into an Opportunity for Professional Growth

Several years ago a graduate student's father died while she was in the middle of a semester. She, of course, flew home to attend the funeral. When she returned a few days later to resume her classes and clinical work, I felt that she was still in crisis and talked to her about possibly cancelling therapy that week with her adult voice client. She assured me that she wanted to go ahead and see the client and that she would be all right. I observed her carefully during the next two sessions and noticed that her therapy was the best I had ever seen. She was tuned in to every nuance and emotion of the client. This actually was the beginning of significant clinical growth for the student. In some cases a crisis may interfere with a student or professional's work; in other cases a crisis may enhance the clinician's performance and mark the beginning of significant personal growth.

CLINICAL QUESTIONS

1. Reflect on a time when you experienced a crisis in your personal life. Did you need time right away to process the loss or threat, or were you able to invest your attention in educational or work matters?

2. Think of a challenging situation that was experienced as stressful for your family and discuss who (i.e., which family member) experienced it as a crisis. Why might it have affected that person more intensely?

Crisis situations can create intense feelings of frustration, inadequacy, and incompetence in clinicians. To some extent the clinician may experience many of the feelings of the person in crisis, for example, anxiety, uncertainty, and confusion. These reactions are natural and understandable, but the clinician must be in control of them when talking to the person in crisis. The clinician should convey an attitude of concern, but not alarm, and model a rational problem-solving approach to the situation. It is through education, training, and experience that SLPs and Auds will be able to manage crisis situations with some degree of confidence. Maintaining a calm composure creates a safe environment that allows the person to process the crisis and then to develop practical strategies to address the problems at hand.

Three-Stage Crisis Intervention Model

A number of authors (Burnard, 2005; Flannery & Everly, 2000; George & Cristiani, 1995) outline a crisis intervention model and crisis management principles that are applicable to a wide range of crisis situations. The model presented below can be used whether the SLP or Aud is working independently or as part of a crisis management team.

FIRST STAGE

During the first stage of this model (Burnard, 2005; George & Cristiani, 1995) the clinician attempts to establish an understanding of what the individuals in crisis are going through—the fears, feelings, and confusion. This helps the clinician establish an alliance with the individuals and allows the patient to recount the crisis situation. At this stage, the clinician can gather the facts, encourage the patient's expression of difficult emotions, and inquire about the impact that the crisis has on this family. For example, the parents of a child newly diagnosed with a hearing loss, APD, or cerebral palsy may be in crisis due to fears that the child has significant problems that may affect schooling, social interactions, and family life. In addition, through exploration of the family's life and routines *before* the crisis, the clinician may get a sense of the family's pre-crisis level of functioning. As the clinician works with the family through the period of crisis, one goal will be to help the family learn to function as independently and successfully as possible. However, the emotional toll that crises take on families can temporarily impair that capacity.

Another example of a clinician working with a family in crisis concerns a young father with a TBI. Depending on what level he is in on the Rancho Scales (Hagen, 1998), he may have little or no awareness of his deficits. However, each family member is likely to experience a sense of crisis: the wife, the children, the man's parents, his siblings, and possibly others. As the patient progresses through the Rancho Levels and develops increasing recognition of his impairments, he may begin to go through the crisis stages. In some medical settings the SLP may be chosen to be a member of a behavioral or crisis management team. This is not surprising given the areas of expertise of SLPs (e.g., neuropathologies) as well as the communication skills for managing challenging situations.

The two important processes of the first stage of crisis management are establishing rapport and assessing the situation. To establish rapport, the clinician creates an environment that allows each person to discuss the crisis. The clinician's emphasis should be on communicating genuine warmth and empathic understanding. The manner in which a clinician talks with each person in crisis may either help de-escalate the sense of crisis or escalate it. Using a slower-than-normal rate of speech and calm tone of voice may help moderate the intensity of speech of the person in crisis. The clinician also needs to make an assessment of the crisis situation, which involves getting a sense of how the individuals understand what has happened and their accompanying fears and problems.

SECOND STAGE

The second stage of crisis management involves facilitating the patient's understanding of the crisis event or the patient or family's knowledge of the communication disorders. This information should be tailored to the patient's and family's level of knowledge and understanding. For example, during the interview of parents whose child is newly diagnosed with APD or ADHD, the clinician should learn what they already know and understand about these problems. Only after evaluating the child's auditory processing, speech, language, and cognition can the clinician provide clarification about the areas that need attention from an SLP and/or Aud. In a medical setting, the clinician may or may not meet with the family before she does her evaluation of the patient with a TBI. If she does meet with the family briefly before the evaluation, she may follow the processes of the first stage, that is, establish rapport and assess the situation. After the evaluation of the patient, the clinician can provide feedback about the patient's speech, language, cognition, and swallowing to the patient and family. During this time, the clinician can observe the reactions of family members to determine whether they are perceiving a crisis situation. Encouraging recognition and understanding of the problems helps family members accept the realities of the symptoms, illness, or injury. The clinician should avoid false reassurance and resist the temptation to prematurely assure the patient or family in crisis that everything will be all right because the situation may *never* be all right, only tolerated or accepted.

The transition from the second stage to the third stage of crisis management can be made most smoothly if the clinician summarizes and reviews her evaluation and perceptions with the patient and family. This serves two functions: (1) it reassures the patient and family that the clinician has a good understanding of the patient's problems and the crisis as they may perceive it, and (2) it helps the clinician recognize whether the patient and family understand the need for therapy and its goals. Once the clinician, patient, and family agree on the need and direction of therapy, they are ready for the third stage of the process, in which a plan of action is determined.

THIRD STAGE

The purpose of the third stage of crisis management is to determine what problem-solving strategies, treatment goals, and procedures are warranted. Although this may not appear different from the normal process we would follow of establishing rapport, assessing the situation, evaluating the patient, and then determining appropriate therapy goals and procedures, there are a few additional factors that need to be considered when the patient or family is in crisis. Most people can deal with serious problems more easily if they are not overwhelmed by the magnitude of the situation; therefore, breaking up the crisis into manageable parts can be very helpful. Considering and approaching manageable parts of a crisis helps people feel less overburdened and frustrated. If one small part of a crisis can be managed, then another small part also may be managed. Encouraging the individuals in crisis to help themselves by actively seeking help from family or friends can lessen their dependence on the clinician and allows more independent decision making on their part. Once the immediate crisis has passed and individuals are more open and capable of learning new skills, the SLP or Aud may want to teach a few strategies or coping skills to help them manage future stresses or crises. The following sections describe examples of coping skills SLPs and Auds may teach clients, patients, and family members.

Monitoring Self-Talk

Oftentimes family members experiencing emotional distress make themselves feel worse as a consequence of the negative statements they make to themselves (e.g., "My daughter will never do well in school because of her language and learning problems," "I will never be able to work again because I can't talk normally after my stroke"). These negative statements also contribute to a sense of helplessness or hopelessness about a situation. Self-statements are often automatic, and individuals do not realize they are contributing to their distress. They may say them aloud to loved ones or only silently to themselves. Clinicians can have individuals in crisis monitor their self-statements or self-talk and change negative statements to positive statements, such as changing "I can't cope with losing my hearing" to "I *can* cope with losing my hearing"; "I don't know if I can make it through this time" to "I'm *going* to get through this time"; "My speech is getting worse" to "My speech is getting *easier* and more fluent"; or "I can't cope with all of this" to "I *can* cope with this." The process of replacing negative appraisals of life events with more positive ones is sometimes referred to as **cognitive restructuring** and is a common technique used by cognitive-behavioral therapists (Baron et al., 2008; Dattilio & Freeman, 2007; Zebrowski, 2002; also see Chapter 2). This technique is based on the understanding that negative thoughts can lead to negative or distressed feelings while positive thoughts can contribute to positive feelings and actions.

Affirmations

An affirmation is a conscious, positive thought that helps change a particular image or belief a person has about herself. Affirmations allow people to believe in themselves and to put their thoughts into action. Affirmations begin with the first person ("I") and are in the present tense, positive form (e.g., saying "I am not sad" is not as helpful as saying "I am coping well during this difficult time" or "I am very patient with my kids during this crisis"). Affirmations may be helpful in times of crisis as well as times of relative calm. The purpose of affirmations is to focus on what is wanted, not what is unwanted. A metaphor may be helpful to understand the notion of focusing on what is wanted. When a horse that a person is riding begins to head in the wrong direction or toward a hazard (e.g., a cliff), the rider does not keep looking in the wrong direction; the rider looks in the direction he wants the horse to go. The rider's body then automatically uses its muscles to move the horse in the right or safe direction. Affirmations help the mind stay focused on what the person wants, which allows it to begin finding ways to achieve its goals. By saying affirmations using the first person, present tense, and positive form it is as though what is desired is already acquired, as if it is spoken into existence. Examples of affirmations include, "I am speaking more fluently now," "I am using my esophageal speech easily," and "I am using the chin-tuck position with every bite." Affirmations are powerful tools that many highly successful athletes and various types of performers use before and during competition.

Visual Imagery (Visualizations)

Visual imagery is the deliberate exercise of imagining scenes designed to have helpful or therapeutic value (e.g., speaking confidently in front of a classroom or visualizing using safe-swallow techniques). Often relaxation strategies are taught first so that the person is calm when they imagine their desired outcome. By using visual imagery techniques, the clinician can help the client in crisis "see" successful completion of activities and tasks that meet the client's goals. Visualizing desired goals also may help the person to feel hopeful about the future.

Relaxation Techniques

Relaxation techniques such as progressive muscle relaxation can be an effective tool to increase coping abilities (Craske, 2010; Wolpe, 1958, 1987). To use this technique, the person begins by alternately flexing and relaxing groups of muscles (e.g., the hands) to appreciate the difference between relaxed and tense muscles. The person can then move to other muscle groups such as the arms, shoulders, back, and so forth. Controlled breathing also is helpful, with slow, deep, relaxed breathing being most helpful. Various progressive relaxation CDs are available commercially. A relaxed person can think and problem-solve more clearly than a very anxious one.

Problem-Solving Skills

Clinicians can teach problem-solving skills that may be helpful in managing the communication problem, for example, teaching patients to observe people's faces as they are talking, asking people to get the patient's attention before they begin to speak, writing down information to reduce the need to rely on auditory memory, having an electrolarynx by the bedroom telephone for a laryngectomee, or wearing a MedicAlert™ bracelet.

Other factors that may need to be explored in the third stage of crisis management are the resources and support immediately available to the client and family. For example, the child with APD or ADHD may have a teacher or reading specialist who is very supportive of him, or the patient with a TBI may have family and friends who can take care of the well siblings while the patient is in the hospital and the spouse is visiting. Note that there may be an overlap in the information the SLP and social service staff in the hospital obtain; however, this can help patient care conferences go more smoothly because there is a better general understanding of the family's support system. The client and family may benefit from information about support groups (e.g., ADHD or stroke support groups) so they can network with other people who have had similar experiences and crises and understand the problems the client and family may encounter in the future.

CASE STUDY

Limitations

Many people, particularly those in convalescent hospitals, do not have family or friends available for support. Many elderly people have outlived the rest of their family and are essentially alone in life. Regrettably, the hospital staff usually are a poor substitute for close family and friends during a time of crisis. During a summer when I was working in a convalescent hospital I had an elderly patient who had a stroke that resulted in aphasia, cognitive impairments, and dysphagia. Both the patient and his wife were in the hospital and were roommates. The hospital staff had arranged the room so that it resembled a small apartment, and the couple was happy to be together. The wife was relatively healthy and able to watch over and take care of her husband in various ways. The couple had been together in this environment for many months when one of them died—the wife. The man was very confused and did not understand what happened to his wife, although it was explained to him many times by hospital staff. He wandered around the hospital in his wheelchair, often searching for her. All the staff and rehabilitation team, as well as a psychologist who evaluated the patient, felt helpless in this situation. This vignette illustrates our limitations in helping some patients who may experience acute emotional distress.

CLINICAL QUESTIONS

1. How might you talk to or provide support for this patient?

2. What strategies might you try to suggest in order to help the patient through this crisis?

The three crisis management stages may move along very quickly or they may take several meetings or sessions to work through; however, during this time you probably will have initiated therapy for the patient. As discussed above, one crisis may precipitate a cascade of other crises. Some crises may fall out of our scope of expertise, and therefore patients and their family members may not discuss all of these matters with us. If a patient or family appears to be advancing in coping skills and then experiences a sudden change in therapeutic progress or motivation, it may reflect that a new crisis has occurred that has not been shared with the clinician. In this case the clinician may empathically question the patient and family about the changes noticed. If the changes in therapy progress reflect issues that are within the clinician's expertise, they may be addressed; otherwise the clinician may wish to refer the patient or family to a counselor, psychologist, or social worker who can address these new crises. However, although the clinician may make such a referral, an appointment may never be made by the patient or family, and the clinician may be left to do the best she can with individuals who may be moving in and out of various crises.

Summary

Clinicians in all settings, who are working with clients or patients of all ages and their families, encounter crisis situations. The defining characteristic of a crisis is not the instigating event, but rather the person's difficulty coping with the situation. Some crisis situations may cause cascading effects that make the initial crisis more difficult to manage. We can reasonably assume that a person who functioned normally all his life but now has a moderate to severe communication problem is in crisis, and so is the family. Understanding general principles of crisis management can help clients and their families better cope with the crisis situation. A three-stage model for crisis management was presented; the first stage involves the clinician establishing an alliance with the client or family that helps them develop confidence in the clinician. The second stage involves clarifying the problems based on the clinician's assessment of the client. The third stage is to determine the treatment goals and possible procedures. Although these stages may appear routine to the clinician, additional factors may be involved to help the individuals in crisis manage their thoughts and feelings in productive ways to allow maximum gains from therapy.

THREAT OF SUICIDE OR SELF-HARM

Over 30,000 recorded suicides occur annually in the United States, ranking it as the 11th leading cause of death in this country among adults and the third leading cause of death among young people between the ages of 15 and 24 (Holmes & Holmes, 2005).

Suicide is the second leading cause of death among college students, and their suicide rate is 50 percent higher than that of the general population (Gladding, 2009). In addition, approximately 10,000 people over age 60 kill themselves each year (Hooyman & Kiyak, 2001; Shiner, Scourfield, Fincham, & Langer, 2009).

Suicide at any age is tragic, and it is even more so with children. School-based and other clinicians need to be alert to any indications of depression or warning signs that a child may be thinking of harming himself and make referrals to the school counselor or other mental health professionals, as well as informing the parents. For many of these children, the speech and language problems that are central to the SLP's interventions are also symptoms that interfere with the child's ability to communicate his thoughts, feelings, and experiences to the counselor.

There are various terms associated with suicide and suicidal behavior. *Suicidal ideation* refers to thoughts of wanting to die, but do not necessarily signify suicidal intentions. *Parasuicide* indicates an action that results in self-harm but is not intended to cause death (e.g., when a person overdoses on medication and then calls someone for help). In this case, the parasuicidal behavior is a "cry for help." A *suicide gesture* refers to an act that results in minor self-harm, such as taking a half-dozen aspirin tablets or scratching but not cutting the wrists. The problem with suicidal gestures and parasuicidal behavior is that sometimes an individual miscalculates the level of harm caused by a particular act and suicide results. *Attempted suicide* signifies that an act that may have led to death has been prevented. Regardless of the severity of suicide ideation or an attempt that is made, all self-harm thoughts and actions should be taken seriously, and immediate action should be taken to determine the seriousness of the suicidal behavior and to prevent a tragedy.

A "Code 3" Call

During my years as an ambulance driver and attendant (EMT) in Southern California, I had many emergency ("Code 3") calls when people had attempted or accomplished suicide. Some people were very creative in their choices of ways to die. I had learned and later experienced that women often choose overdosing on medications or other "quiet" means for suicide, while men tend to choose more dramatic forms such as shooting themselves with a pistol or shotgun.

One evening my driver and I received a Code 3 call to a residence. When I entered the home two young boys, ages about five and eight, pointed to the garage and said "Mommy's in there!" When I opened the door from the house into the garage I saw an automobile running and a woman behind the steering wheel slumped over. I immediately opened the garage door to get fresh air inside and the carbon monoxide outside. I then shut off the engine of the car, pulled the woman out, put an oxygen mask over her face, and began pumping oxygen into her. On the way to the hospital the boys rode in front of the ambulance with the driver while I continued pumping oxygen into their mother in the back of the ambulance. She survived, although I have often wondered how much brain damage she may

Continues on next page

Continued from previous page

have sustained and whether she ever needed speech therapy. As SLPs in acute-care hospitals and rehabilitation centers, we see patients a significant amount of time after they have been brought to the hospital's emergency room. Often the life-saving and "brain-saving" work has been done days before we see them as our patients.

CLINICAL QUESTIONS

1. Why might it be helpful to read the emergency room physician's report as well as the patient's current attending physician's report in a medical chart before you begin your evaluation?

2. Why might it be helpful to read the Social Service report in a medical chart before you begin your evaluation of a patient?

Important Points About Suicide

Sommers-Flanagan and Sommers-Flanagan (1999) present several important points about suicide.

■ Twenty-five to 50 percent of people who commit suicide have previously attempted to do so. Previous suicide attempts are one of the better predictors of future attempts.

■ People who eventually commit suicide often have tried to communicate their despair to others in a variety of ways. They also usually give clues or warnings, either verbally or through their behavior, that they are contemplating suicide; however, older people (60 years and above) tend to communicate their suicidal intentions less often than younger people.

■ Medical patients are often at risk for suicide if they are depressed and/or in extreme pain.

■ People who attempt suicide are more likely than other psychiatric patients to use disinhibiting substances (including alcohol) in the 24-hour period before the attempt. The disinhibiting substances can help people get up the nerve to follow through on thoughts of killing themselves.

■ Men are about three times more likely to complete suicide than women, while women are about three times more likely to attempt suicide than men (men's completion of suicide may be partly the result of their more drastic and violent means).

■ Almost all people in the presuicidal state experience ambivalent feelings. They want to die and also to be saved. They want to escape from an intolerable situation and they also wish that the intolerable situation could be changed so that they could continue living.

Myths About Suicide

Numerous myths are associated with suicide (Nystul, 2005), including the following:

■ *Myth: Suicide is only committed by people with severe psychological problems.* Reality: Most individuals who commit suicide have not been diagnosed as having a psychological disorder.

■ *Myth: Suicide usually occurs without warning.* Reality: Most suicides are preceded by warning signs such as a sudden change of behavior, verbal threats of suicide, talk of hopelessness, and depression.

■ *Myth: Discussing suicide may cause the person to carry out the act.* Reality: The opposite is true; talking with a caring person can often prevent suicide.

■ *Myth: When a person has attempted suicide and pulls back from it, the danger is over.* Reality: Another period of danger may be during the upswing period, when the person becomes re-energized following a severe depression and has the energy to commit suicide.

■ *Myth: People who are suicidal will always be prone to suicide.* Reality: Most people who become suicidal do not remain in that state through the rest of their lives. They may be struggling through a temporary personal crisis, and once they work through the crisis they may never be suicidal again.

Risk Factors

There are certain risk factors for suicide that clinicians should be aware of, although none can predict suicidal behavior in a particular individual. SLPs and Auds should never attempt to predict which clients or patients may be at risk for suicidal ideation. The relationship between depression and potential suicide is well documented, with about 80 percent of suicide attempts being made by people of all ages who are depressed (Gladding 2009; Morrison & Anders, 2001; Sommers-Flanagan & Sommers-Flanagan, 1999). A strong sense of hopelessness is an important predictor of suicide. The risk of suicide escalates as the person's suicidal ideation intensifies and becomes more frequent. Almost everyone has had fleeting suicidal thoughts, but only some individuals ruminate about it. It is more dangerous if the person has a plan, particularly a detailed plan.

In general, some of the major risk factors for suicide are a history of suicide attempts, severe hopelessness, a family history of suicide, acute overuse of alcohol, and loss or separations (Mattas-Curry, 2000). Interpersonal causes of suicides can include feeling no sense of belonging to a valued group or relationship or perceiving that one is a burden to loved ones (Joiner, Van Orden, Witte, & Rudd, 2009). In fact, a study by Shiner, Scourfield, Fincham, and Langer (2009) found that relationship problems or breakdowns were the main trigger for suicide in over one-half of the suicide cases. In suicide cases of individuals under the age of 25 years, damaged family attachments were a major triggering factor and included negative childhood experiences such as physical and sexual abuse, neglect, and separation. However, knowing these risk factors only reveals the statistical risk of suicide; these factors cannot tell a clinician what the risk is for a particular child or adult.

The Speech-Language Pathologist's and Audiologist's Role

SLPs and Auds may have long careers without having a child or adult verbalize suicidal ideation or intention. During informal surveys conducted by the author (P. F.) in cities around the country with SLPs, Auds, PTs, and OTs (primarily those working in medical settings) who attended seminars on counseling skills, many indicated that they have had patients who either attempted or completed suicide. The possibility is of increasing concern, and we need to know how to respond to it. Recognition of suicidal tendencies and appropriate preventive interventions by professionals and family members may save a person's life.

It is the mental health professionals' responsibility to conduct a systematic and thorough suicide evaluation. The SLP or Aud, however, can provide critical information to these professionals that may facilitate their determination of the level of suicide risk for a particular person. In order to gather this critical information, the primary task of the clinician is to listen carefully and perhaps to ask the client to elaborate on his suicidal thoughts. In some cases, the clinician may discern that the person has no intention of carrying out the suicidal thoughts. In other cases, the clinician may learn that the person has a general or specific plan for suicide. The clinician may ask general questions such as, "Tell me more about your thoughts about hurting yourself (committing suicide, taking your life)." Depending on what the person discloses, the clinician may ask specific questions (described in the following sections) about suicidal history, lethality, and specificity. However, it is important to remember at all times that the clinician should not attempt to conduct a full suicide evaluation. This means that all disclosures of suicidal ideation must be reported immediately to a mental health professional, regardless of the clinician's impressions of the level of suicidal risk. SLPs and Auds are *mandated reporters*, and it is up to the mental health professional to determine the level of risk.

In most situations, if you plan to break confidentiality in order to ensure the patient's safety, it is advisable to inform the patient of your intention. This action may help preserve a trusting relationship between yourself and the patient. For example, in response to a patient who voices self-destructive or suicidal thoughts, the clinician may say, "Mrs. S., in order to ensure your safety, I feel it is necessary to share this information with the nurse and your doctor (psychologist, etc.). They will be able to take the appropriate steps to make sure you do not harm yourself." If the patient protests your disclosure of this confidential information, you can apologize for opposing the client on this matter while maintaining that your primary concern and responsibility at this time is for the patient's safety.

Obtaining Information from a Patient Threatening Suicide

I was working in a convalescent hospital during the summer and had a patient with cognitive impairments whom I was seeing on a daily basis. One day I wheeled him into the therapy room, and after we worked for a few minutes, he told me he was going to kill himself. I talked to him about it at length because I felt we had a good working relationship and that he would share information with me that he

Continues on next page

Continued from previous page

might not easily share with others. As an SLP, I cannot do a suicide assessment but I can obtain as much information as possible to share with the other professional staff. At the end of our therapy session I did not take him back to his room as I normally did, but wheeled him to the nurses' station where there were several people to oversee him. I then told the charge nurse, in private, about the patient's suicidal ideation and followed up by informing the director of nursing, the social service director, and the administrator. Appropriate measures were taken and the patient was put on "suicide watch," which meant a staff member was with him 24 hours a day, observing him eat, sleep, and use the bathroom. A review of his medical chart revealed that he had attempted suicide previously by setting himself on fire. A psychologist was called in for a suicide assessment; he interviewed and evaluated the patient extensively and decided the patient was not a risk to himself at this time. After approximately seven days, the patient was taken off suicide watch.

CLINICAL QUESTIONS

1. What are some additional steps you might have taken in this situation?

2. What steps are most critical to take in a situation like this one?

Be prepared to write a detailed report on what the patient says and does. Careful documentation is essential and must be immediate. Document what the patient said verbatim as much as possible, being concrete and without drawing inferences or interpretations (these are left to the mental health professionals). Record what steps you took to alert other professionals to the patient's suicidal thoughts. Report relevant details in the sequence or order they occurred so appropriate professionals can evaluate them and draw conclusions. It is also useful to report on any questions the patient refused to answer, for example, "After declaring she wanted to end her life, the patient refused to elaborate on whether she has a plan to do this."

The following sections describe signs and symptoms that SLPs and Auds will want to be alert for when talking with individuals who express thoughts of self-harm. The information is summarized from several sources, including Burnard (2005), Gladding (2009), Meir and Davis (2000), and Morrison (2008).

LISTENING FOR SIGNS OF DEPRESSION

It is difficult to know how best to talk with a person who is expressing suicidal or self-destructive thoughts; however, there are guidelines that can be helpful. Listen closely to the person's thoughts and feelings. Throughout the conversation or interview, your tone of voice, facial expressions, and body language should convey warmth, caring, concern, and empathy. You may be the first person to whom the individual has ever voiced these thoughts and feelings. The person needs to feel that you hear accurately how miserable and desperate she is. Avoid expressions of shock or surprise when a person begins to talk about suicide. Responding to the person in a calm, concerned manner suggests that you have dealt with such issues before and, therefore, that you are competent to listen and respond appropriately. Many of the suicidal individuals SLPs are likely to work with have some neurological damage from CVAs or TBIs. Therefore, their speech, language, and cognitive functioning may be significantly impaired with resulting difficulty expressing their thoughts and feelings. These physical limitations may contribute to their frustration and rationale for wanting to end their lives. In addition, some individuals may experience an impaired capacity for self-control, which may put them at higher risk for suicide.

Depression is implicated in many of the risk factors for suicide, and therefore one of the first questions you may reflect on is how the person is feeling. Sad? Depressed? Helpless? Hopeless? From the person's perspective, helplessness may indicate a feeling or belief that she is unable to make any changes necessary to feel better on her own. The person's feelings of helplessness may represent an indirect request for help from the clinician. She may believe that while she is unable to effect change in her own life, someone else might be able to do so for her. If the person feels hopeless regarding the possibility of positive changes and believes no one can help, she may make statements such as, "I don't see how things will ever be any different," or "I've felt like this for a long time and I'll probably always feel like this."

A common sign of depression is withdrawal from friends, family, and usual activities. Listen for indications that the person has lost some interest in activities she used to enjoy and people she used to enjoy being with. Depression is often accompanied by somatic changes such as loss of sleep or sleeping much more than usual, loss of appetite, or an unusual amount of eating (particularly comfort foods). People who show signs of depression may have **psychomotor retardation** with slowed movements and speech as well as cognitive changes such as slowed thinking, difficulty remembering, inability to concentrate, and difficulty making decisions and solving problems. The opposite may also occur; the person may appear agitated and anxious, speak rapidly, pull on her hair or clothing, rub her hands together, or pace back and forth. The agitation may indicate the person has the energy to commit suicide or, in some cases, may suggest a Bipolar Disorder, in which the person suffers from both depression and mania.

LISTENING FOR SUICIDAL IDEATION

When individuals make vague references to suicide (e.g., "I'm going to end it all," "Soon it will be over," or "It doesn't matter anymore"), an SLP or Aud may ask, "I'm wondering what you are thinking about doing (what your intentions or plans are)." In general, asking a person about self-harm does not cause this behavior, but to be on the safe side, the SLP or Aud should only ask general questions rather than be the first to bring up the topic of suicide. Use open-ended questions so that your questions cannot be interpreted as a suggestion.

If the person answers "yes" to any questions about suicidal ideation or intent, open-ended follow-up questions may help get more specific information, for example, "Could you tell me more about your thoughts?" Most suicidal people will admit self-destructive thoughts when asked about them.

LISTENING FOR SUICIDE PLANS (SLAP-I)

The acronym SLAP-I refers to various areas that require careful listening by a clinician; that is, Specificity, Lethality, Availability, Proximity, and Intent. These areas can provide a framework for listening to or teasing out important information embedded in the sometimes rambling or disjointed information a cognitively impaired or depressed client may provide. The clinician can then report essential information to the mental health professional in an organized manner. SLPs and Auds do not need to try to make judgments about the client's level of suicide risk, but simply be responsible for reporting the information as quickly and accurately as possible.

SPECIFICITY Specificity refers to the details the person has thought through about how he would carry out suicide; the more specific the plan, the higher the risk. You may ask about the person's plan, for example, "Do you have a plan about how you would kill yourself?" At this point the person may assure you that he really does not have a plan and does not intend to kill himself even though he has thought about it. The person may give reasons why he would not carry it out, such as religious beliefs, children, or other family members. If the person assures you that he will not commit suicide and provides the reasons that would prevent such action, do not continue pursuing questions about a plan. However, if the person describes a plan to carry out the suicide, you may question him further.

LETHALITY Lethality refers to how quickly or effectively the person's method of attempt could cause death. The greater the lethality, the higher the suicide risk; for example, firearms, overdose of medications, or driving a car off a bridge have different levels of lethality. If the person has already indicated he has a specific plan to commit suicide, you may ask a "how" question in order to gauge the level of lethality, for example, "How might you carry out your plan?" A patient may report a plan to take an overdose of aspirin, which may not be as lethal as an overdose of sleeping pills, or may describe a plan to drive off a low bridge into a shallow stream, which may not be as lethal as driving off a high bridge into a rocky ravine. Sometimes children or individuals with cognitive impairment who are genuinely distressed and report self-injurious ideation do not have very realistic or lethal ideas about how to hurt themselves.

AVAILABILITY Availability refers to how quickly a person could potentially carry out the suicide plan. Does the person actually have the means to implement the plan? An elderly person in a convalescent hospital may talk about driving a car off a bridge, but if he is unable to ambulate or drive and there is no bridge in the vicinity, the plan is unlikely to be carried out. However, this does not mean the person is any less serious about a suicide attempt, but it may indicate that he does not have the cognitive capacity to have a workable plan. Many people have sufficient medications in their home medicine cabinets to achieve a lethal overdose. The immediacy of the availability is also important; for example, there is a difference between a person who says, "I'm going to go out and buy a gun," and the person who says, "I have a loaded gun in my car." Therefore, the clinician who hears that the patient wants to shoot himself may want to ask, "Do you have a gun?" In most cases, considering the availability of a suicide method is a key variable in determining suicide risk and whether or not immediate intervention (e.g., hospitalization and suicide watch or protective custody) is needed.

PROXIMITY   Proximity refers to how close helping resources are to the person who is planning to attempt suicide, that is, other individuals who could intervene and rescue the person if an attempt is made. Does the person live alone or with family or friends? Are there neighbors nearby who know and look after the person? Never let a potentially suicidal person leave a therapy session alone. Call a relative or friend of the person to drive the person home and do what you can to have someone with the person at all times or to check in on the person frequently. Nighttime is usually the worst (i.e., the most vulnerable) time for someone who is considering suicide, and some of these individuals have been discovered by family or friends the next morning.

INTENT   Intent refers to how determined the person is to carry out the suicide. Some people are resolute in seeking self-destruction and, short of hospitalization or being placed in protective custody, it may be nearly impossible to prevent them from killing themselves. Asking the person to rate herself on a 1-to-10 scale, with 1 being no intent and 10 being total intent, may provide an indication of the person's determination. A rating scale that provides the terms absent (1—no intent), low (2–3), moderate (4–6), and high (7–10) provides terms that reflect the numbers of the scale.

SUICIDE-PREVENTION CONTRACTS

Suicide-prevention contracts may be either verbal or written, and are sealed with a handshake. Many suicidal people will honor such a contract, which also buys time for you to contact other professionals and family members. A contract may be as simple as having the person agree not to hurt herself until you can get mental health professionals or family members involved in providing a safety plan. Because it may be too easy for the person to say, "Sure, I won't do anything until I see you again," it may be better to give the person the option of declining the contract offer by saying, "I only want you to agree to this contract if you really believe you can follow through with it." Suicide-prevention contracts also help assess a person's self-control and intent. If a person is willing to agree to a suicide prevention contract, the person is probably in some control and may have only low to moderate intent. However, a person with low self-control or high intent usually will not agree to a suicide prevention contract.

It is best not to give a person who has reported suicidal thoughts your cell phone or home phone number; rather provide the telephone number of the local suicide hotline. This service can provide a lifeline that the person can use 24 hours a day to speak with people who are well-trained and experienced in dealing with such a life-threatening crisis. Above all, you should recognize that if you are engaged in such a discussion with a patient, you need to document the discussion, make a referral to a mental health professional immediately, and do not leave the patient alone.

A TEAM APPROACH

A mental health professional must become involved in the care and management of a patient who is contemplating suicide. However, even though such a professional may quickly establish a therapeutic alliance, the professional will likely recognize and appreciate the relationship you have already established with the patient (which is probably the reason the suicidal ideation was disclosed to you). Therefore, the mental health professional may encourage you to continue seeing the patient using a team approach to help manage the suicidal risk. Careful documentation of each session is essential, and discussing each session with the mental health professional can help you and the team of professionals work for the best interest and welfare of the patient.

Summary

A person's threat of suicide can be a very unsettling experience for SLPs and Auds, and when it occurs it *cannot* be ignored. We are mandated reporters, and therefore the concern for breaking professional confidentiality is secondary to the responsibility of preventing self-harm. SLPs or Auds may be the professionals to whom clients or patients first voice their suicidal ideation because of the close therapeutic alliance we have established, with our emphasis on helping people communicate their wants, needs, thoughts, and feelings. We are often the only professionals whom clients or patients see who give them undivided attention for half an hour to an hour each day. The consistency of seeing patients on a regular basis for several days, weeks, or sometimes months, and the close working relationships we develop may encourage them to share thoughts and feelings with us that they have not disclosed to others. Our initial and primary goal is to help ensure the patient's safety. By understanding risk factors for suicide and our professional role within the suicide prevention team, we may make an important difference in averting a tragic situation.

CLIENTS WITH POSTTRAUMATIC STRESS DISORDER

The concept of Posttraumatic Stress Disorder (PTSD) has existed since World War I when soldiers were observed to suffer chronic anxiety, nightmares, and flashbacks for weeks, months, or even years following combat (Briere, 2004). At that time the condition was known as "shell shock." Since then it has been recognized that all wars and combat experiences can result in PTSD for the men and women involved.

Beyond war experiences, PTSD can occur in anyone following a severe trauma outside the normal range of human experience. These are traumas that would produce intense fear, terror, and feelings of helplessness in anyone, and include natural disasters and catastrophes such as earthquakes or tornadoes, motor vehicle accidents, plane crashes, rape, assault, or other violent crimes against oneself or loved ones (Bourne, 2005), and more recently, terrorist attacks (Pyszczynski, Solomon, & Greenberg, 2003). The frequency of PTSD may be increasing in children and adolescents, especially those who live in the inner city, where stressors such as violent crime and domestic violence are common. Juvenile PTSD may be among the most underrecognized of mental health disorders (Morrison & Anders, 2001; Mueser, Rosenberg, & Rosenberg, 2009).

The *DSM-IV-TR* (2000) lists the symptoms of acute stress, including a subjective sense of numbness; detachment or absence of emotional responsiveness; a reduction in awareness of surroundings; derealization (a subjective sense of the world being unreal); depersonalization (a loss of the sense of being the person one usually is; a feeling of being outside oneself in the role of an onlooker); and dissociative amnesia (an inability to recall important personal information that is too extensive to be explained by the normal forgetfulness usually related to a traumatic or stressful experience). Following the trauma, the event is persistently re-experienced, and the person has a marked avoidance of stimuli that may arouse recollections of the event. For example, a person who was injured in a motor vehicle accident may become fearful of driving. The symptoms typically last for at least two days but do not persist beyond four weeks after the traumatic event. When symptoms last beyond four weeks, PTSD is considered.

Beyond the above symptoms, the *DSM-IV-TR* (2000) uses the following diagnostic criteria for PTSD: the person has been exposed to a traumatic event in which both of the following were present: (1) the person experienced, witnessed, or was confronted with an event or events that involved actual or threatened death or serious injury, or a threat of physical harm to self or others, and (2) the person's response involved intense fear, helplessness, or horror. The traumatic event is persistently experienced in one or more of the following ways: (1) recurrent and intrusive distressing recollections of the event, including images, thoughts, or perceptions; (2) recurrent distressing dreams of the event; (3) acting or feeling as if the traumatic event were recurring, including a sense of reliving the experience, illusions, and dissociative flashback episodes; (4) intense psychological distress at exposure to internal or external cues that symbolize or resemble an aspect of the traumatic event; and (5) physiological reactions (e.g., shaking or a "chill") on exposure to internal or external cues that symbolize or resemble an aspect of the traumatic event. Other symptoms of PTSD may include difficulty falling asleep or staying asleep, irritability or outbursts of anger, difficulty concentrating, hypervigilance, and exaggerated startle response.

Acute PTSD is considered to last less than three months, and chronic PTSD has a duration of more than three months. Delayed onset of symptoms is considered when symptoms begin to emerge at least six months (and in some cases, many years) after the traumatic event. Awareness of the phenomenon of delayed onset of symptoms began in the mid-1970s with Vietnam veterans who began experiencing signs and symptoms of the disorder approximately 10 years after being in that war. We need to be aware that even though an individual may appear to be coping well with a traumatic event, it may take several months or longer before symptoms begin to emerge, at which time the clinician may have difficulty recognizing the original source of the symptoms.

It is important to note that not all people who experience severe trauma develop PTSD. There are a number of factors that may operate as either protective or risk factors in a particular individual (Morrison & Anders, 2001; Meuser et al., 2009), including the following:

- Duration and severity of the stress and the duration of the evoked terror
- Proximity to the traumatic event
- The emotional stability of the child, adolescent, or adult
- Reactions shown by parents and other family members
- The community's social network
- Cultural and political factors (e.g., national tragedies)

SLPs and Auds typically do not have information about a client's prior trauma history, which may exacerbate the impact of the current trauma. It is important for clinicians to be aware of the symptoms of PTSD in order to make referrals for counseling when these symptoms are recognized. Likewise, adults may have experienced emotional and/or physical traumas that have long-term effects on their cognitive and emotional responses to their environment. The following are symptoms of Posttraumatic Stress Disorder described in the *DSM-IV-TR* (2000).

Symptoms of Posttraumatic Stress Disorder

- Repetitive, distressing thoughts about the event
- Nightmares related to the event
- Flashbacks so intense that the person feels or acts as though the trauma were occurring all over again
- An attempt to avoid thoughts or feelings associated with the trauma
- An attempt to avoid activities or situations associated with the trauma
- Avoidance of social settings or situations related to or reminiscent of the trauma
- Emotional numbness—being out of touch with feelings
- Restricted range of affect
- Inability to recall important aspects of the trauma
- Feelings of detachment or estrangement from others
- Reduced interest in activities that used to give pleasure
- Persistent symptoms of increased anxiety, such as falling asleep, difficulty concentrating, startling easily, or irritability and outbursts of anger
- Symptoms of depression
- Symptoms of guilt
- Fear of being hurt (again) or of dying soon

In addition to these symptoms, children with PTSD may exhibit separation anxiety, regressive behavior, clinging behavior, reluctance to return to school, behavior disturbances, problems with concentration, and re-enactment of the traumatic event (La Greca, Silverman, Vernberg, & Roberts, 2002; Mueser et al., 2009). Our role as SLPs and Auds is not to diagnose Posttraumatic Stress Disorder, but to recognize its symptoms in our clients and patients and to make the appropriate referrals to mental health professionals.

WORKING WITH ACTIVE DUTY MILITARY AND COMBAT VETERANS

In 2003 I was invited by the Chief of the Army Audiology and Speech Center at Walter Reed Army Medical Center (WRAMC) in Washington, D.C. to present an in-service training to the speech-language pathologists at the center. I was invited to present because of my background in counseling and because I could speak to the clinicians from the experience of being an Army combat veteran (medic, Vietnam, 1969) (Fogle, 2009b). The clinicians, most of whom were in their 20s and 30s, had been working extensively with wounded active duty military (ADM) from Iraq and Afghanistan, and a few were having some difficulty (as would be expected) working with young men and women who were age peers with such devastating TBIs and severe wounds to all areas of their bodies. The clinicians also needed to provide feedback and SLP counseling with the families of the wounded warriors. This is not easy for anyone, and it is not uncommon to become emotionally engaged in the tragedies that patients and their families are trying to cope with and will likely have to manage for the rest of their lives. I emphasized to the clinicians that they, like the men and women who they were helping, would never forget the experiences they were having—that some memories would be with them every day for the rest of their lives.

The most common psychological disturbance during battle is *combat stress reaction* (CSR)—a psychological breakdown on the battlefield. However, CSR may, in many cases, crystallize after the war experience for both ADM and combat veterans into Posttraumatic Stress Disorder (Corso, Bryan, Morrow, Appolonio, Kanzler, & Dodendorf, 2009; Roth, Mashima, & Cornis-Pop, 2010). (It should be noted that even though soldiers may be experiencing CSR, they are usually able to carry out their missions effectively, which is an indication of their ability to suppress severe mental stresses in order to perform their duties as soldiers). The general symptoms of PTSD as related to ADM and combat veterans include severe interpersonal problems, depression, anxiety, anger or rage, paranoid ideation (e.g., mistrust of people and the safety of the surroundings), hypervigilance, intrusive combat-related thoughts and images, nightmares, avoidance of stimuli reminiscent of the traumatic stressors, and withdrawal (Cantrell & Dean, 2005; Roth, Mashima, & Cornis-Pop, 2010).

In Iraq and Afghanistan, closed head injuries (CHIs) and mild to moderate TBIs from explosions (e.g., bombs and artillery) and blasts (e.g., improvised explosive devices [IEDs] and rocket-propelled grenades [RPGs]) are more common than penetrating head injuries from bullets and shrapnel (Veterans Health Administration, 2008). Overall, nearly two-thirds of the soldiers in Iraq who arrive at Walter Reed Army Medical Center have some kind of TBI (explosions and blasts can produce unique patterns of injury seldom seen outside of combat, including severe burns). In an explosion there are *primary* injuries from the blast air wall that can result in traumatic amputations of limbs, *secondary* injuries from shrapnel striking the head, neck, and other exposed body parts, and *tertiary* injuries from being thrown to the ground or against something solid causing blunt traumas such as fractures and crush injuries. *Quaternary* effects of blast injuries refer to all explosion-related injuries, illnesses, or diseases such as burns, angina, hypertension, and respiratory problems, which are often the result of inhalation of smoke or toxic fumes (Gaylord, Cooper, Mercado, Kennedy, Yoder, & Holcomb, 2008; Samson, 2004; Wallace, 2006).

As a result of major advances in body armor technology (e.g., Kevlar helmets and vests) and battlefield medicine, many military personnel are surviving injuries that would have been fatal in previous wars (Lew, Poole, Alvarez, & Moore, 2005). There has been a reduction in penetrating brain and thoracic injuries, although many soldiers receive concussions (i.e., CHI and TBI) from explosions and blasts. Shrapnel and burns cause facial and body disfigurements, and limbs may be traumatically amputated. Soldiers with such wounds are diagnosed as *polytrauma* patients, that is, as suffering concurrent injury to the brain (TBI) and several body areas or organ systems that result in physical, cognitive, and psychosocial impairments (multiorgan/multisystem injury) (Veterans Health Administration, 2005).

Because of exposure to extremely traumatic events, the loss of health and independence, and body disfigurement, these ADM and combat veterans are at risk for a host of psychiatric disorders, including PTSD, which is currently the primary mental health diagnosis being treated at VA hospitals. Many PTSD symptoms overlap with symptoms of mild traumatic brain injury, such as headaches, dizziness, irritability, decreased concentration, memory problems, fatigue, visual disturbances, sensitivity to light and noise, judgment problems, anxiety, and depression (Cantrell & Dean, 2005; Hoge, Castro, Messer, McGurk, Cotting, & Koffman, 2004; Mora, Ritenour, Wade, Holcomb, Blackbourne, & Gaylord, 2009; Rogers & Read, 2007). Similarities in the behavioral characteristics of patients with TBI, postconcussion syndrome, and PTSD can complicate the rehabilitation team's diagnostic and treatment efforts (Cornis-Pop, 2006; Wallace, 2006; Warden, 2006).

Lew and colleagues (2007) state that the following elements are essential to the sequential assessment and treatment of postconcussion syndromes: (1) a complete description of altered consciousness and history of functioning from immediately after injury to the present; (2) counseling that targets postconcussion syndromes as early as possible by instilling coping and adaptive strategies; (3) medical treatment and cognitive therapy to address any conditions that affect cognitive functioning; and (4) a comprehensive neuropsychological evaluation to guide further rehabilitation if cognitive difficulties persist.

Soldiers who suffer polytrauma often need to have an extensive interdisciplinary team involved to keep them alive, stabilized, and rehabilitated. The medical treatment team may include a physiatrist (i.e., a rehabilitation physician) or other physician as the team leader; specialists in surgery, neurosurgery, and internal medicine; advance nurse practitioners; infectious disease specialists; wound care nurses; respiratory therapists; physical therapists; occupational therapists; speech-language pathologists; kinesiotherapists; prosthetics specialists; orthotics; physical therapy amputee case managers; rehabilitation counselors; psychiatrists; neuropsychologists; recreational therapists; blind occupational therapists; audiologists (Helfer, Jordan, and Lee [2005] reported that deployed military to Iraq were 50 times more likely to have noise-induced hearing loss than military who were not deployed); social work case managers; education specialists; veteran benefits specialists; military liaisons; and chaplains. Each of these medical, health care, and rehabilitation specialists has specialized expertise in caring for the polytrauma patient and family and is essential to help ensure comprehensive and optimal outcomes. Speech-language pathologists are part of the core team for polytrauma patients.

Micaela Cornis-Pop (2006), a speech-language pathologist and rehabilitation planning specialist headquartered in the VA Medical Center in Richmond, Virginia, described a typical polytrauma patient. Sgt. S. was transferred from WRAMC to the Richmond VAMC. He arrived by ambulance accompanied by his parents and fiancé. At 26 he had survived an Iraq car bombing that caused a terrible combination of injuries, including moderate-to-severe TBI, traumatic right arm amputation above the elbow, complex bone fractures in the right leg, and a significant visual field defect. He had a tracheostomy tube, feeding was by PEG tube, and the initial evaluation showed severe-to-profound cognitive and communication impairments. Rehabilitation challenges were related to the complexity of injuries sustained that affected multiple organs and body parts with consequences for communication and cognition, including brain damage, vision and hearing problems, facial trauma and disfigurement, and emotional and behavioral problems (e.g., agitation and aggression).

A full range of psychological reactions may be seen in newly returning soldiers who may have multiple symptoms and comorbid disorders such as PTSD, depression, anxiety, personality disorders, and substance abuse problems. Speech-language pathologists and audiologists must fully understand their patients' psychological histories and diagnoses and the psychologists' priorities for treatment. Patients, their families, and significant others need to receive appropriate education, training, and counseling to increase their knowledge of the patients' injuries, disabilities, and treatment needs and learn the skills and behaviors that promote recovery and maximize function (Cantrell & Dean, 2005; Sayer, Cifu, McNamee, et al., 2009).

The Counseling Roles of Speech-Language Pathologists and Audiologists

What are the counseling roles of speech-language pathologists and audiologists when working with active duty military and combat veterans and their families? As always, we need to appreciate that we cannot clearly separate our discipline-specific therapy role from our counseling role: from moment to moment they may blend. It is also important to understand that it is not only SLPs and Auds working in VA hospitals who care for wounded soldiers; many of these soldiers are eventually released from VA hospitals and sent to local civilian community hospitals for further rehabilitation. Although SLPs and Auds are treating the cognitive-linguistic, speech, hearing, and swallowing disorders of these casualties, these clinicians are treating a different type of patient than they see with more typical civilian traumas, and a new paradigm of rehabilitation and counseling care is needed to address the complexities of the wounded combat veterans and their families (Cornis-Pop, 2006; Fogle, 2009b; Roth, Mashima, & Cornis-Pop, 2010).

The most likely mental health diagnosis that SLPs and Auds will be confronted with for ADM and combat veterans is PTSD. Although we are not mental health professionals, we need to be willing to listen to the "stories" and experiences that these men and women are willing to share. During this process, we are developing rapport, earning trust, and learning about their speech, language, memory, and cognitive problems. During our listening and observation of these patients we also need to be alert to any hint of suicide or self-harm ideation. The information provided in this chapter in the section on the speech-language pathologist's and audiologist's role in dealing with threats of suicide or self-harm is particularly applicable when working with active duty military and combat veterans.

Families are a vital part of the initial and ongoing rehabilitation process (Cantrell & Dean, 2005). Part of the SLP's and Aud's outreach is educating families how to stimulate and work with patients. Getting family members involved helps them feel they are doing something meaningful. However, families are often processing their own emotional reactions to their loved one's injuries. SLPs and Auds can provide support as well as education to help them understand the patient's injuries, impairments, and limitations. Many ADM and combat veterans have severe relationship problems with their families and difficulty maintaining employment. However, being married and having a supportive relationship with one's spouse considerably reduces the negative impact of combat experiences and greatly aids in the recovery and healing process. On the other hand, the emotional well-being of spouses of veterans can be negatively impacted too. Studies of wives of ADM and combat veterans with PTSD indicate that these women tend to perceive negative emotions and lowered intimacy with their wounded spouse and also experience greater severity of psychiatric and somatic symptoms of their own (Manguno-Mire, Sautter, Lyons, et al., 2007).

Family members of injured ADM and combat veterans have questions that they commonly ask, often of more than one medical or rehabilitation team member. It is helpful if the various team members provide similar answers to decrease confusion among family members. Although each team member may view patients from their own professional perspective, there can be commonalities in their responses to family members' questions (Cantrell & Dean, 2005; Sayer, Cifu, McNamee, et al., 2009). The following are two frequent questions with possible responses to family members.

1. Why is he or she so tired all of the time after the TBI? Frequent (chronic) fatigue is very common after a TBI of any kind. Many of the cognitive functions that are automatic and reflexive for people without cognitive impairments take two or three times more conscious mental effort for people with TBIs. The following are some strategies families may use when communicating with their wounded veteran:
   - Use everyday language, not "medicalese" or "VA language," for instance, "Anyone who has gone through what you have would need the stress level reduced" rather than "You have PTSD."
   - Patients respond better to closed-ended questions and choices, such as, "Are you feeling good or bad today?" rather than "How are you feeling?"
   - If he needs to be involved in important decisions, try to get him involved when he has the greatest amount of energy, which is usually in the morning.
   - Make as many activities as possible into a routine to minimize choice and to save mental energy.
   - Use of an organizer of some kind is essential for him to plan and understand his daily activities and to decrease the amount of mental energy it takes to make it through a day.

2. Why is he angry all of the time? The anger expressed by ADM and combat veterans may be a reaction to several cognitive and emotional factors. A wounded soldier's cognitive deficits, such as slowed ability to process information, reduced attention span, difficulty managing more than one thing at a time (i.e., multitasking), memory problems, visual-spatial impairments that affect the way he perceives his environment, and other cognitive problems make the world a difficult place for him to comprehend and cope with. Sometimes he might get extremely upset (a catastrophic reaction) with what would seem like a minor annoyance to other people.

When family members recognize that anger is present or escalating or that a catastrophic reaction of any kind is brewing, they can try to reduce unnecessary demands or stressors. Family members may suggest to their wounded loved one that perhaps there is too much for him to deal with right now, and then offer to reduce the amount of tasks he has to think about or complete at the moment. Speaking to him quietly and with numerous pauses can help him "catch up" with what is being said. (For additional information that may be helpful to family members dealing with angry behavior, see Chapter 13.) Some additional points to consider when talking to ADM and combat veterans include:

- Always speak with a respectful tone of voice and choice of words.

- Listen intently to what the patient is willing to tell you about his combat experiences, but do not probe for details.

- Appreciate that the ADM or combat veteran may cry occasionally or even frequently, particularly during the early days and weeks after returning to the United States.

- If they ask you to do something that is within your power (and appropriate), do what you can to carry out their request.

- Sleep, appetite, energy level, and concentration can be impaired in the postdeployment phase as a result of traumatizing experiences, regardless of physical wounds.

- Appreciate that two of the greatest concerns ADM and combat veterans have is how their family will accept them and how they will return to and function at school or their previous employment. Many of the Iraq and Afghanistan War military are in the National Guard or Army Reserve and were activated and deployed, forcing them to leave schools, jobs, and families where they may have been the primary financial providers.

Family members, because of their love and concern for their wounded warrior, may feel that he is not receiving good enough medical care and may complain or express anger. We need to understand and appreciate that some families may have a tendency to displace their feelings onto the institutions or professionals who are trying to help. Often a family's anger does not appear during the acute phase, in which coping with disaster is paramount. However, suppressed feelings of anxiety, fear, frustration, uncertainty, helplessness, and others may emerge when the loved one is in the outpatient setting and engaged in the long-term process of rehabilitation. The family may feel that it is now safe to express how overwhelmed they feel.

Appropriate responses to family members who are exhibiting angry behaviors may help to solidify or maintain the therapeutic relationships with the family and the veteran. To help the family understand their loved one's rehabilitation, provide information in both verbal and written form, and patiently repeat the information as often as the family seems to need it. Family members often want (and may demand) predictions and prognoses when there are no clear answers. Acknowledge that not having definite answers is hard, but you have given them all that you know at this time. Referring the family to a local support group can help them find a sense of meaning among families who are experiencing similar tragedies and challenges. It is not uncommon for families to first experience a "honeymoon" phase of reconnection marked by euphoria, excitement, and relief that their loved one is home. However, a period of discomfort, role confusion, and renegotiation of relationships and roles can follow this initial phase. (For additional information about working through these challenging situations, see Chapters 6 and 13).

Clinicians who may have an opportunity to work with active duty military or combat veterans would be wise to keep the following sources and phone numbers nearby:

- National Suicide Prevention Hotline: 1-800-273-TALK (8255); press "1" for Veterans.

- Hearts Toward Home International provides excellent support and educational material for ADM, veterans, and their families: (360) 714-1525 (inquire@ heartstowardhome.com).

- It is also helpful to learn some basic military terminology. You can Google "established military terms" for such a listing.

Finally, and in contrast to the challenging scenarios described above, it is important to keep in mind the fundamentals of developing a rapport with our wounded patients. First, recognize that most men and women who have served their country experience immense pride in serving, fulfilling their missions, and surviving. They appreciate being acknowledged for their efforts and sacrifices. Few men and women who have seen combat boast about their war experiences and many typically will only talk about their experiences when asked, and then often only briefly. Returning warriors are usually very respectful and may address the clinician as "ma'am" or "sir." If their cognitive abilities permit, they may approach each therapy session and task wholeheartedly, as though it is a "mission." They may work on tasks as if their lives or someone else's life depends on it. Most combat veterans have a strong sense of duty and are willing to work hard without complaining. They take little for granted, including cold water and warm food. They see beyond the trivialities and stay focused on the big picture—their mission. Veterans are often a joy to work with and are very appreciative of all the care and assistance they receive. One of the most important things you can do for a veteran is to simply say, "Thank you for your service." This brief acknowledgement can help veterans feel appreciated and can be very meaningful (Fogle, 2009b).

CONCLUDING COMMENTS

Crisis situations may occur in any setting at any time; however, what defines a crisis is the combination of an unusually threatening or dangerous situation and a person's difficulty coping with that situation. Some crises may cause cascading effects that make the initial crisis more difficult to manage. People in crisis may have intense feelings of frustration, inadequacy, and incompetence. Helping clients cope with a crisis and find their inner resources can help them develop problem-solving skills and self-confidence, and allow them to maximize gains from therapy.

A threat of suicide or self-harm is one of the most difficult experiences a clinician may be confronted with, and every threat must be taken seriously. Many people who threaten or attempt suicide have signs and symptoms of depression. Although SLPs and Auds are not able to perform suicide assessments, the fact that a client or patient has disclosed self-destructive thoughts or intentions to us indicates some level of trust. Clinicians can listen for both direct and indirect suicidal references and share those with the appropriate administrative and mental health professionals. A team approach with a mental health professional may be used, in which the clinician continues working with the patient and meanwhile monitors the patient's thoughts and feelings about suicide.

Posttraumatic Stress Disorder is a common outcome for individuals who have experienced domestic violence, shootings in schools and workplaces, national crises such as terrorist attacks, natural disasters, and wartime injuries. While not everyone who experiences a traumatic event develops PTSD, it is important to recognize the symptoms that may indicate the presence of this disorder and to make a referral to a mental health professional.

Working with active duty military and combat veterans and their families is both an honor and a challenge. There are numerous unique rehabilitation and psychosocial concerns and problems that must be managed that are significantly different from traumas seen in civilian life. Clinicians who have the opportunity to work with these men and women need to develop many additional skills beyond their education, training, and civilian work experience.

Discussion Questions

1. What coping skills have you used to manage crises in your life?

2. Discuss a child or adult client who shared a crisis experience with you? How did the crisis affect your client? How did it affect your therapy? What did you do or say that you felt was helpful? What did you do or say that may not have been helpful?

3. Considering the client situation discussed in question 2, how were you helpful to the client's family members? How could you have used counseling skills to be even more helpful to the family?

4. What do you feel is the role of the speech-language pathologist or audiologist with children or adults who threaten self-harm or suicide?

5. How might you respond to an adult client who says she is so depressed and miserable with her life that she might as well "put an end to it all"?

6. Have you had an adult client who suffered from posttraumatic stress symptoms? What was the client's experience? What were the symptoms? How did the symptoms affect the client's communication or cognitive problems?

7. What are some things you might tell the wife of an injured veteran when she asks, "How can I cope with all of these changes in my husband?"

Role Plays

1. Role play an initial interview in which you discover that your adolescent client does not feel "life is worth living." How would you respond? What steps would you take next?

2. Have the class divide into clinician–patient pairs and instruct the clinician to interview the "adult combat veteran patient" who has some cognitive impairment and gets angry over minor issues. Have the clinician practice a variety of supportive and therapeutic responses. After the role play, ask the patient which responses felt most respectful and validating and which ones were not helpful.

Taking Care of Ourselves

CHAPTER OUTLINE

- Introduction
- Therapeutic Failures
- On Death of Patients
- Symptoms of Posttraumatic Stress Disorder in Clinicians
- Peer Counseling
- Professional Counseling for the Clinician
- Professional Burnout
- Concluding Comments
- Discussion Questions
- Role Plays

INTRODUCTION

Speech-language pathologists and audiologists must learn how to take care of themselves emotionally, physically, socially, recreationally, and spiritually in order to best help others. One source of professional stress and emotional fatigue may come from our ongoing emotional involvement with our clients, patients, and their families and the challenges they present. Another source of professional stress can come from our own appraisals of our work, including our perceived shortcomings and imperfections. Strong negative emotions can influence our clinical perceptions, decisions, and treatment approaches. When we feel burdened by our errors and failures, are disappointed by third-party reimbursement policies and decisions, feel grief for our patients who suffer or die, or experience professional burnout, we cannot provide the best care that our clients, patients, and their families deserve. Taking care of ourselves, which may include seeking professional help, reflects our personal responsibility and commitment to ourselves, the people with whom we work, and our profession. In this chapter, we discuss some of the sources of professional stress and some ways that clinicians may take care of themselves. Ultimately, if we do not take care of ourselves, symptoms of stress and professional burnout may be the result (Fogle, 2006).

Most clinicians are reluctant to discuss their insecurities and therapeutic failures. Even experienced clinicians may still wonder with each new client or patient, "Will the client like me? What if he has a problem I don't know very much about? Will this be the client who discovers my weaknesses? What if I fail and the client tells her family or friends that I am incompetent, or worse, tells my colleagues?" With every client we are putting ourselves "on the line," bringing all our knowledge and skills to bear. We take risks with every person we try to help: will we be the right clinician at the right time with the right approach for this client? Although we may perceive the failure as ours, in reality, the client is the one who has the most to lose. The client's improvement may be delayed or, even worse, the client may not have the chance for therapeutic success again. Many children and adults who stutter have worked with only one SLP in their lives, and if that therapist was not able to successfully manage their stuttering, no other SLP was given the opportunity to try.

THERAPEUTIC FAILURES

Chapter 12 discusses repairing counseling errors and the fact that it is inevitable that we are going to make errors in our interactions with clients and their families. Beyond making specific errors, we also may experience therapeutic failures in which a child or adult does not make the improvements in hearing, speech, language, cognition, or swallowing that they and we would like. Clinical failures may be the result of making a variety of errors and, in some cases, perhaps only a single fateful error (e.g., with dysphagia patients). Failures also can be the result of factors outside of our control, such as when clients or patients have physical or emotional illnesses that prevent them from receiving maximum benefit from therapy, or when they move or terminate therapy early. Errors and failures are not synonymous, and we need to recognize that we can make a variety of errors and still have a successful outcome.

There are countless client and family variables that interact to determine the outcome of therapy, such as the age and motivation of the client, the nature and severity of the problem, multiple communication problems, support of the family and other professionals, medical complications (e.g., syndromes or diabetes mellitus), and intellectual and cognitive impairments of the client. Clinician variables also play a part in the success of therapy, such as the clinician's education and training, professional experience, therapeutic skills, up-to-date information on disorders and management approaches, and availability to provide consistent and ongoing therapy.

Historically, therapeutic failures seldom have been discussed in either the SLP, Aud, or psychology literature. However, increasing attention is being given to the potentially harmful effects in some psychotherapy cases (Barlow, 2010; Castonguay, Boswell, Constantino, Goldfried, & Hill, 2010; Dimidjian & Hollon, 2010). Many clinicians may feel uncomfortable about admitting or making public their failures. Frequently, professors and supervisors prefer to discuss their successes and may not mention their therapeutic errors and failures to their students. Our failures can become private experiences that haunt us and contribute to professional stress and burnout, but this experience can be turned around. Castonguay and colleagues (2010) urge supervisors and trainees to be alert for the factors that can sometimes contribute to harmful therapeutic effects such as a weak alliance, poor collaboration, and negative interpersonal behavior (e.g., the therapist's belittling and blaming). While negative effects may be even less common in the work that SLPs and Auds do, the emerging literature in the psychotherapy field is an important source of information about the kinds of factors that can be helpful versus harmful.

Therapeutic challenges, and even failures, are often our best learning experiences (Orlinsky, Botermans, & Ronnestad, 2001; Stahl, Hill, Jacobs, Kleinman, Isenberg, & Stern, 2009) because we need to evaluate and reevaluate what we did that worked and did not work. We tend to remember our failures more clearly than our successes, and sometimes dwell on them to the detriment of our self-confidence. When we have a failure, we are sometimes reluctant to take on a similar case because we may not be certain that we, or the client, will do better than the last time. Kottler and Blau (1989) point out that psychologists and counselors teach their clients to forgive themselves (and others), to accept themselves as they are, to view their weaknesses as aspects of their uniqueness, and to welcome their failures as opportunities for learning. However, psychotherapists (as well as SLPs and Auds) do not easily apply this valuable wisdom to themselves.

Sometimes an initial error can lead to a cascade of errors and result in therapeutic failure. For example, if a child or adult is misdiagnosed and the therapy is focused on the presumed impairment, then little if any success will result. There are consequences for diagnoses that represent either false positives or false negatives. For example, if a client is diagnosed with a problem that he does not have (a false positive) and therapy is designed to remediate a problem that in fact does not exist, therapeutic failure is likely (e.g., a misdiagnosis of a phonological disorder when the real problem is childhood apraxia of speech). Likewise, if a diagnosis is overlooked (a false negative), then therapy may not be made available (e.g., when a cognitive impairment or swallowing disorder is missed).

Judging whether or not treatment has been successful can depend upon the goals or criteria the SLP or Aud and client have established. We tend to think in terms of improvement, while clients and patients often think in terms of cure. *Cure*, however, is not a word we typically use in our professional vocabulary. It tends to be reserved and more appropriate for the medical profession. Some illnesses and diseases can be cured. The cause or causes of communication problems may include anatomical, physiological, cognitive, affective, social, and behavioral factors; therefore a single cause may never be identified or eliminated (Shames, 2006). Our clients and patients may "improve," "make significant gains," "reach their therapy goals," or "reach their rehabilitation potential." We write functional goals that identify a practical outcome. We write measurable goals so that we can quantify the degree of success—or lack of success. In order to be considered a good or at least competent clinician, we need to have successful outcomes far more often than unsuccessful outcomes and we need to be able to develop the positive relationships with clients that facilitate clear communication and goal-directed therapeutic work.

Benefits of Therapeutic Failures

Although no one wishes or intends to have therapeutic failures, there are lessons that can be learned from these experiences. Kottler and Blau (1989) discuss the benefits of therapeutic failures in psychotherapy. Many of these points are applicable to SLPs and Auds as well.

Failure is a signal that something has not worked in the way it was intended. It is part of a feedback loop that provides information on the effects of our therapy, which allows us to reflect and then make adjustments in our behavior so that we have better (or at least different) results the next time. If we can appreciate failure as much as we appreciate success, it becomes a valuable source of information for us to improve our skills.

Failure teaches us to be persistent. If we fail once, it does not mean we will be successful the next time; however we persist in learning and trying new techniques and approaches until we have successful results with our clients. Every client is a single-subject research design for which the final conclusion in the discussion is "Further research is needed." Even though we may have a successful outcome with a client, could we have had the same outcome with a different approach? Could our therapy have been more efficient with more expeditious success? Which aspects of the therapy were problematic?

Failure is a stimulus. Because we do not have all the answers for any of the disorders we work with (the data are *never* all in), our clinical failures stimulate research and experimentation with new or better techniques.

Failure makes us introspective. More self-reflection likely takes place after a failure than after a success. After a success we quickly move on to the next client, but after a failure we ruminate and consider what went wrong. We learn our limits from our failures. If we have success after success, we may begin to see ourselves as omnipotent—"Who could have done a better job with that client?" "I am such a good clinician!" When an inevitable failure occurs, it shakes us enough to keep our egos in check and have more appreciation of other clinicians who also experience failures.

In time, we learn to tolerate some failures; that is, to fail, accept them, learn from them, and move on to the next challenge. We have the choice to pat ourselves on the back for what we have learned or to beat ourselves up for what we failed to do well. We need to avoid making excuses for our failures and instead ask ourselves what we can learn from them. In short, a healthy stance for clinicians is to be nondefensive about the errors we have made and failures we have experienced and be willing to reflect on them. Our errors and failures can teach us lessons about ourselves, our clients, our knowledge, human nature, the therapy relationship, and the limitations of doing therapy (Stahl et al., 2009). In contrast, clinicians who have not learned from their errors tend to externalize blame; that is, they tend to blame others for what has not gone well. We will always be imperfect clinicians.

In addition to the factors that clinicians *may be able* to control, there are other factors that clinicians *cannot* control that can contribute to clinician stress and fatigue.

ON DEATH OF PATIENTS

Over the years of supervising graduate students during their internships at various hospitals throughout California, several students have had patients who died (fortunately, not during therapy sessions). I (P. F.) asked some of these students to write detailed narratives of their reactions to their patients' deaths. They also wrote about how they were informed of the deaths, what support (if any) was provided for the students by onsite hospital supervisors, and what the students felt was most helpful to them to cope with the loss. The information obtained may be helpful for student interns and supervisors in hospitals who are processing the death of a patient. One graduate student, Carla, wrote, "My experience of the loss of a patient was quite remarkable. I don't think I will ever forget that day." Carla remembered talking to her patient about five minutes before he passed away. She had left the room for a few minutes to allow a physical therapist to fit the patient's prosthesis and was about to return to finish her therapy when over the hospital's intercom system she heard "STAT, STAT" and the room number of her patient. When she arrived at her patient's room, the door was closed and the person fitting the prosthesis was standing outside. He told Carla that the patient was not doing well. At the nurses' station, Carla overheard a nurse calling the patient's wife, telling her that her husband had another stroke and for her to come to the hospital. Carla's SLP supervisor was with her by this time and was the one who told Carla that her patient was "gone." "It was almost a surreal experience. I said 'What?' in disbelief and with the attitude of, 'That couldn't have happened. I just talked with him.' The next moment it hit me that it was the truth, the patient had died. My eyes immediately filled with tears. I couldn't hold back my emotions. My supervisor comforted me, and then told the other staff who were around, 'Oh, it's her first one.'" Carla's supervisors were very caring and allowed time for her to "gather" herself. She chose to stay at the hospital the rest of the day and found it helpful to talk with other SLPs about similar experiences they had and how they coped with the loss. Later that day, Carla saw the wife of her patient crying, and "again the tears filled my eyes and my heart went out to her." Carla felt fortunate that she was surrounded that day by other supportive staff.

Another student's experience also is enlightening. Jenna had begun an evaluation of an 81-year-old male patient who had dysphagia and was nonverbal secondary to a CVA. After completing a portion of her evaluation, a nurse told Jenna that the patient needed his shower. Jenna finished what she was working on and as she was about to leave the room the patient "grabbed my hand and squeezed it. I patted him on the shoulder and I can't remember my last words to him, however, I was thinking 'you are a sweet man.'" Later she heard over the hospital's intercom "Code Blue East 5, Code Blue East 5." Jenna distinctly remembers her knees getting weak, feeling that the code was for her patient. Her stomach started to "feel funny, and a million thoughts were running through my head: Did I accidentally unplug his oxygen when I was moving the table or lowering the bed? No! I had to reassure myself that he wasn't receiving any oxygen. Did I do something wrong? I continued to reassure myself that I didn't do anything wrong, but I wasn't convinced."

As soon as she was able, she went to the patient's room where she saw numerous hospital staff standing inside and outside her patient's room. "My stomach sank. I went to the nurses' station where I saw my supervisor, who said, 'Mr. P. coded.'" Jenna watched the code team working on him. "I couldn't see his face, just his body, and I was drawn in. From what I could tell, they got him back." Jenna asked her supervisor if the patient had his shower, "partially because I wanted to know what happened and mostly I wanted to know if I was the last person to see him. I really needed some reassurance that I didn't do something to cause all this." Jenna thought about the patient all night, and when she got to the hospital the next day her supervisor told her that Mr. P. had died. "I was told by my supervisor and the head of the department that people on rehab don't often code and the last one was probably 10 years ago. I really needed to hear that this was not my fault but I didn't in so many words from any of the people I work with. I just don't think it occurred to them that I needed reassurance even though I felt I was hinting at it."

A week later Jenna was talking to a friend of hers, a medical student at the University of California, San Francisco, explaining the experience to her, when "in the middle of my story she stopped me and said, 'Jenna, his death was not your fault.' I kind of laughed but felt sort of relieved and said, 'I know.' She said something along the lines of 'I just felt that I had to say that to reassure you because sometimes it is just good to hear it.' Instantly I felt better and it is amazing how good that feels."

Some Lessons for Students

There are some lessons to be learned from these students' experiences:

■ Do not be afraid to show your emotions, although it is more appropriate to restrain them until you are away from the patient's family. Other staff may have strong reactions as well, depending upon how closely they worked with that patient.

■ Seek support from other staff members immediately after the incident. Staying at the hospital to be around co-workers may be better than leaving for the day and returning to an empty apartment or house.

■ If reassurance that the death was not your fault is not explicitly provided by your supervisor or other rehabilitation or nursing staff members, specifically ask for that information or reassurance.

■ Discuss the experience with your university supervisor if you feel that would be helpful to you.

■ Seek help from the hospital psychologist, counseling, or chaplain service if you feel the need.

Lessons for Supervisors and Staff

Lessons from these students' experiences for hospital supervisors and staff include:

■ Try to respond empathically. Even if you respond less emotionally, consider that the student or young professional is reacting in a normal, expected manner to loss.

■ Provide immediate reassurance in explicit language that the student was not the cause of the death—that she was not at fault. The student may need to hear that reassurance more than once. If the student brings up the incident hours, days, or even weeks later, consider it an indication that she again may need reassurance or someone to help her process the series of events and her role in them.

■ Encourage the student to remain at the hospital for the rest of the day so that she can be around other supportive people who understand and can help the student process the experience.

■ Spend time with the student over a cup of coffee or lunch to allow the student to process the experience in a comfortable environment.

■ Avoid explaining to other staff the student's reaction to the death by saying, "Oh, it's her first one." This can sound demeaning and patronizing.

■ If the student insists on leaving the hospital for the day, ask if there will be someone at home when she gets there. It will likely be better for the student not to be alone for a while.

■ Realize that the death of the patient may cause the student to reflect on the death of a friend or family member. The student's reaction may be compounded by other experiences with loss.

■ Consider that the student may process the experience by moving through stages of grief, perhaps not going through each stage, but possibly a few of them such as denial, depression, and acceptance. Again, the ability to move through these stages may be complicated by the student's previous personal experiences with loss.

Over time, many hospital-based clinicians develop self-protective strategies so that they can continue to function effectively in spite of the death of patients. However, for clinicians as well as other health care workers, the loss of patients near their own age, and especially children, may cause strong emotional reactions and long-term (sometimes lifelong) memories of the experience regardless of their professional maturity. A registered nurse (my wife) shared with me an experience that she had when she worked in emergency rooms. After a two-year-old girl died, the child's mother held her daughter and said, "Talk to me! Talk to me!" The experience occurred over 35 years ago and it still brought tears to the nurse's eyes. Sometimes it may not be the death of a patient that touches us, but the reactions and grief of family members that we remember most.

When clinicians experience a series of therapeutic disappointments and failures, or the loss of patients, they may become susceptible to conditions such as Posttraumatic Stress Disorder or burnout. Fortunately, there are a number of steps that clinicians can take to avoid or mitigate these outcomes.

SYMPTOMS OF POSTTRAUMATIC STRESS DISORDER IN CLINICIANS

Posttraumatic Stress Disorder and how it can affect children and adults is discussed in Chapter 14. SLPs and Auds also may experience PTSD. They may be exposed to tragic situations directly, or they may empathically experience a client's or family's pain and tragedy. SLPs in public schools where tragedies (e.g., shootings) have occurred most likely spent many hours trying to assist children, parents, and school personnel in any way possible to cope with their physical and emotional traumas. How much and what kind of professional help the SLPs received to manage their own stress has not been documented. In addition to being on the site of a school tragedy, many people (including clinicians) may experience trauma symptoms at various levels of intensity as a result of other local and national tragedies, such as terrorist attacks or natural disasters. Clinicians who have worked with children or adult clients who were injured or killed in such disasters may respond with anxiety and other strong feelings. Psychologists have recognized that professionals who absorb their clients' emotional pain may suffer from "compassion fatigue" as they empathically experience their clients' emotional roller coasters themselves (Boscarino, Figley, & Adams, 2004; Figley, 2002). In a similar vein, psychologists have identified the problem of "vicarious traumatization" (McCann & Pearlman, 1990; Harrison & Westwood, 2009), which occurs when therapists experience the cumulative effects of working with clients who have lived through horrific events and losses. This experience is believed to be due to the deleterious effects of the clinician's empathic involvement over time.

After a direct experience with loss or trauma (i.e., being injured or physically present during a traumatic experience) or indirect experience (learning about a traumatic event but not being physically injured or present at the scene), clinicians may initially react with acute stress from anxiety and fear. Unless mental health professionals evaluate clinicians, a diagnosis of Acute Stress Disorder cannot be made, although it may exist. It is important to recognize that while many clinicians may not have the breadth and severity of symptoms necessary to be diagnosed with either PTSD or Acute Stress Disorder, they may suffer some of the symptoms. Boscarino, Figley, and Adams (2004) note that compassionate therapists (i.e., those vulnerable to compassion fatigue) should be alert for signs of stress, such as:

- Withdrawal from family or friends
- Emotional numbing or hyperalertness
- Anhedonia (a loss of interest in everyday pleasures and activities)
- A preoccupation with clients' problems
- Physical symptoms such as headaches and muscle tension
- Insomnia

All clinicians should become aware of their responses to stress, regularly assess themselves, and take steps to rebalance their lives when necessary.

Treatment for Posttraumatic Stress Disorder

Psychological treatment for Posttraumatic Stress Disorder is complex and multifaceted (Bourne, 2005). Many of the strategies used for other anxiety disorders are helpful (e.g., hierarchy analysis, relaxation training, and cognitive-behavioral therapy), but additional techniques may be used as well. *Exposure therapy* involves helping the individual confront fearful situations. In some cases, the work is begun with imagination exposure in which the person working with a mental health professional repeatedly reviews fearful memories of events, objects, or persons associated with the original trauma. With real-life (in vivo) exposure, the person returns to the actual situation in which the trauma occurred. Repeated exposure helps the person realize that the fearful situation is no longer present. *Support groups* help individuals understand that they are not alone and that other people are having similar reactions to the traumatic experience. *Family therapy* may be needed to help educate family members about how to understand and support the person who is experiencing Posttraumatic Stress Disorder. *Medication* that helps to reduce the physiological aspects of anxiety may be helpful, especially when the symptoms are severe and long-lasting.

PEER COUNSELING

Fortunately, most SLPs and Auds have co-workers and friends in their profession. It often takes someone in the same profession to understand and appreciate the trials and tribulations of our work. We can be the first line of comfort and support for one another by relating and empathizing with another clinician's experiences and feelings. We can recognize when clinicians become frustrated with clients or family members. We also can recognize when clinicians become frustrated with supervisors, administrators, or "the system." We can often detect interpersonal difficulties among co-workers (and sometimes we may be the ones having or causing the difficulties). We can frequently recognize that external pressures are affecting our own or a co-worker's performance.

With a trusted co-worker, you may be able to share some of your challenges (insecurities, errors, failures, frustrations, etc.). In turn, co-workers may place confidence in you when they share their experiences and feelings. We need to be careful not to break that confidence or use it perniciously. In many cases, just listening to a co-worker relate an experience or feeling is sufficient, and there may be no need to try to help the person work through it. When a problem is severe or chronic, mentioning the value of additional (professional) guidance may be appropriate.

PROFESSIONAL COUNSELING FOR THE CLINICIAN

As students you may experience many of the same emotions as your clients and their families. It is normal to feel anxiety and even some fear when seeing a client for the first time or working with a disorder with which you have no experience and little or no course work. Report writing can be both mentally and emotionally draining. No matter how much education and training you have, you may feel anxious, fearful, and insecure during a clinical internship at a hospital, during your clinical fellowship year, and on your first job when you are expected to know what you are doing. There are three guarantees for all clinicians: (1) you are going to make mistakes, (2) you are going to get tired, and (3) you are never going to know everything.

As a professional, you may feel guilty that you did not try to learn more in your classes or attend a workshop or seminar that could have helped you learn how to better manage a particular client or patient. You may feel vulnerable that a client or family will too easily recognize your weaknesses and insecurities. You may feel resentment that you have to work late when you would really rather be at home. You may occasionally feel resentment or anger that you have to spend your time dealing with other people's problems when you have your own "crisis" at home that needs your attention. You may be fearful that your report writing and documentation may not be adequate for your supervisors, Medicare, insurance companies, or HMOs. You may feel vulnerable that the kinds of tragedies that befall your clients or patients could happen just as easily to you or someone you love, and say to yourself, "There, but for the grace of God, go I."

We need to find ways to take care of our own stresses and negative emotions. The information and strategies for helping our clients, patients, and family members with their challenging and difficult emotions also can be strategies we can use to help ourselves. The principle for helping others—"First, do no harm"—applies to ourselves as well. We need to take care of ourselves emotionally, physically, socially, recreationally, and spiritually to be balanced enough and strong enough to help others and still have reserve to enjoy the other aspects of our lives.

Counseling and therapy are very personal experiences that not only change the client but also change the clinician. SLPs and Auds tend to present a professional façade, appearing rather stoic about their own emotional struggles, and may not recognize or acknowledge when they need professional help. We can appear very secure and emotionally stable most of the time and then experience an emotional crisis or shock that puts us in a tailspin. We are all vulnerable to such reactions. We need to recognize whether we have enough personal resources to get us through a crisis or whether we need professional help. Do not think that it is a personal or professional stigma or failure to seek professional help. It may be the best thing we can do to help ourselves. Most health care and mental health professionals would benefit from professional help at some time in their lives. A basic principle of survival is: Take care of yourself so you can take care of others.

PROFESSIONAL BURNOUT

Professional burnout is a serious concern for people in the helping professions (Baker, 2003; Maslach, 2003; Maslach & Leiter, 1997; Rogers, 1987; Scott & Hawk, 1986; Zur, 1993) including speech-language pathology and audiology (Blood, Thomas, Ridenour, Qualls, & Hammer, 2002; Harris, Prater, Dyches, & Heath, 2009; Lubinski, Golper, & Frattali, 2007; Luterman, 2008; McLaughlin, Lincoln, & Adamson, 2008). Burnout is usually attributed to chronic stress. Over time clinicians are worn down (or out) by the chronic emotional strain of working closely with other people who are troubled or who have problems. Very seasoned professionals as well as novice professionals are susceptible to professional burnout. Burnout can become evident when a professional becomes exhausted, drained, depleted, or even apathetic about her clinical work. The burned-out professional may experience "emotional overload," feel low energy, and even become detached and callous about her work. For some professionals, burnout may be linked to unhealthy coping behaviors such as substance abuse and emotional conditions such as depression and anxiety (Zur, 1993). Even though job satisfaction tends to be high for the professions of speech-language pathology and audiology, chronic stress can take its toll on our feelings about our work and job performance. Burnout may occur even with the strongest personalities when stresses are prolonged, intense, or unresolved (Lubinski et al., 2007). Burnout is insidious and may take years to be recognized by a clinician, and by that time the clinician may not have the motivation, energy, or resources to reverse the process. However, despite the hazards of working closely with clients and their problems, there are strategies for preventing burnout. First, let us examine more specifically the sources of burnout, and then we will discuss what clinicians can do to balance their lives and prevent this unfortunate outcome.

Sources of Burnout

A multitude of factors can contribute to burnout, but there are three primary factors: client factors, professional situation factors, and personal factors (Baker, 2003; Lubinski et al., 2007; Skovholt, 2001). For any one clinician it is likely that a combination of several of these factors contributes to burnout.

CLIENT FACTORS

Client factors, such as age of clients, type of communication disorder and severity, and medical complications, can vary depending on the settings in which clinicians work. Because therapy is performance driven, clinicians must demonstrate (often in a relatively short amount of time) clinical success. When client or patient improvement is slow or is less than hoped for, increasing demands are often placed on clinicians. Even when there are good results, client or family appreciation may be modest. Client factors that may exacerbate the experience of chronic stress in clinicians may include chronic or life-threatening illnesses, client survivors of traumatic life events, and uncooperative, demanding, or unappreciative clients. Professionals cannot help but be affected by their clients' experiences and traumas, and no matter how much we try, we inevitably are impacted when our clients suffer, do not improve significantly, or blame us for their failure.

PROFESSIONAL SITUATION FACTORS

Professional situation factors that contribute to burnout for SLPs and Auds are numerous in all work settings. Blood and colleagues (2002) and Harris and colleagues (2009) discuss several factors that contribute to stress and burnout for public school clinicians, including the rise in technology assistance for children with communication disorders, new legal mandates requiring additional paperwork and meetings, new competencies in literacy, larger caseloads, instructional limitations, uncertainty in role identification and expectations, and salary. In some environments job security is relatively high, while in others, such as medical settings, there are many fewer salaried positions and more contracted and hourly arrangements, which results in clinicians being sent home if their caseload is down; consequently monthly income may not be consistent. There is always someone, some institution, or some organization or agency that oversees our work. We are never totally autonomous, even in private practice. Salaries may be inadequate, with little potential for significant increases, that create financial stresses on clinicians and feelings of being underappreciated, undervalued, and undercompensated for their education, training, and quality of work.

Documentation is a burden both in time and energy in all work settings. Most clinicians feel they could provide more and better therapy if they did not have to spend so many hours completing out forms, documenting results, and writing reports. However, the paperwork is needed for the "bottom line" of our employers, that is, financing our time and work and the institution's services. Even where the overall physical work environment is adequate or good, the space, equipment, and materials for SLPs and Auds may be grossly inadequate. There are still clinicians in the public schools who are working out of converted custodian closets and even restrooms. In many hospitals, there is not an office or room dedicated to speech therapy or audiology, which leaves the SLP or Aud to share counter space with other rehabilitation team members. Treatment rooms may have physical and/or occupational therapy tables and equipment filling the space.

Although we recognize the importance of our work, administrators, teachers, and other school personnel may not fully appreciate it (Blood et al., 2002; Harris et al., 2009). In medical settings, physicians and nurses commonly understand the goals of physical and occupational therapists more easily than they understand our goals to improve patients' speech, language, cognition, and sometimes even hearing. Swallowing disorders may be in the forefront of physician and nursing referrals partly because those professionals recognize the physical consequences of dysphagia more easily than they recognize the impairments of mild to moderate hearing loss, apraxia, dysarthria, aphasia, and cognitive impairments.

If clinicians work in private practice, a sense of emotional isolation can develop as clinicians must keep their client issues confidential (Zur, 1993). They may not have anyone to consult with on a regular basis to allay their professional worries or to help reduce the stress they feel about working with particularly difficult clients. Thus, clinicians are limited in what they are able to reveal about their professional lives, and this can create a sense of interpersonal distance from others. Some clinicians in private practice try to prevent this isolation by developing a consultation group of private-practice practitioners.

PERSONAL FACTORS

Personal factors of individual SLPs and Auds can be a source of burnout. Although many SLPs and Auds appear to be generally well-adjusted individuals, they often have perfectionistic tendencies that create self-imposed stress. We care deeply about the individuals we try to help and frequently go "above and beyond the call of duty" to provide the best therapy we can. When we feel children or clients have not improved to our (or their) levels of expectation, we often place the culpability on ourselves, feeling that we have failed them *and* ourselves.

Many clinicians tend to have high energy levels and are quick to please others, which means that additional tasks and responsibilities may be added to our daily workload. Because of good people skills and communication abilities, clinicians are often asked to be on time-consuming committees. Clinicians often have difficulty saying "no," which may reflect the need for approval from others rather than a genuine desire to accept more responsibilities. Accepting more tasks results in clinicians having more to do with less time and energy, which may cause the quality of their therapy to suffer, creating guilt for not doing their best at what they most enjoy. SLPs and Auds tend to be remarkably patient and tolerant people with everyone *except* themselves. We tolerate weaknesses and foibles in others that we do not tolerate in ourselves. We strive to be better clinicians and people, and never quite live up to our own expectations. Like other professionals, we also have family pressures and competing demands for our time. We feel the need to give 100 percent on the job and 100 percent at home. We sometimes behave as if we have joined the army, trying to "Be all we can be!" We have learned how to take care of others, but not sufficiently how to take care of ourselves.

Stages of Burnout

As clinicians, we need to be aware of the stages of burnout so that we can recognize the early signs in ourselves and our colleagues and begin to better care for ourselves and be supportive of our colleagues. The process of burnout may take one, two, or more decades; however, for some clinicians it may begin just a few years after beginning professional employment. Most new professionals in speech-language pathology and audiology have strong commitments to their chosen professions. On the other hand, some individuals may not have a particularly strong commitment and their initial enthusiasm for the day-to-day work of a clinician may quickly wane. They may become disenchanted with their work and burn out in a relatively short amount of time. Cherniss (1980) and Lubinski and colleagues (2007) describe a three-stage process of burnout for people in helping professions, while Baron and colleagues (1998) describe a four-stage process. The following is an integration of the two models.

STAGE ONE

In stage one there is an imbalance between the demands and resources to deal with job stress, with too few personal or institutional resources to equalize the increasing demands. New therapists often feel overwhelmed on their first job for the first several months. They realize that in many instances the "buck" stops with them. They must make the final decisions about diagnoses and treatment strategies. As they become increasingly proficient in their work and well-known in their work setting, additional demands are placed on them. At the same time, marriage and/or children may increasingly complicate their personal lives. Home and job demands and stresses collide.

STAGE TWO

Clinicians (as well as other professionals) react to stress and strain with feelings of anxiety, tension, cynicism, and negative views of others and their own work. They find it increasingly difficult to enjoy their co-workers and their own work. They begin to see their therapy as less pleasurable and more of a burden. They become impatient with others and wonder why the children or adults they are trying to help do not improve more rapidly. The negative attitudes may carry over into the home, causing family discord.

STAGE THREE

Emotional exhaustion develops and defensive mechanisms may emerge such as displacement (showing anger at home rather than on the job), help-rejecting complaining (complaining about stresses but rejecting co-workers' and family and friends' helpful suggestions), and passive-aggressive behavior (dealing with emotional conflict, stressors, or demands by indirectly and unassertively expressing aggression toward others). Clinicians may become emotionally detached from co-workers and withdraw, spending less time in their company and possibly spending it alone, brooding.

STAGE FOUR

Clinicians become physically exhausted and increasingly fatigued from a day of work. More sick days are taken, some because of increasing amounts of illness and others as a "take-care-of-myself" day. They have less energy for family activities in the evenings, often just wanting to rest. Marital conflict and family disharmony may be reflections of clinicians' dissatisfaction with their job or work environment. Getting up in the mornings and getting to work on time becomes more difficult. Weekends and vacations do not replenish and renew the energy and spirit needed to perform well on the job.

Preventing Burnout

Various authors discuss strategies for engaging in the self-care necessary to prevent professional burnout (Blood et al., 2002; Corey, 2001; Harris et al., 2009; Lubinski et al. 2007; Norcross & Guy, 2007; Shapiro & Carlson, 2009). Norcross and Guy (2007, p. 14) note that "self-care is not a narcissistic luxury to be fulfilled as time permits; it is a human requisite, a clinical necessity and an ethical imperative." They, and many other recent authors, emphasize the self-care that is critical to cultivate. The strategies that are recommended include changes in a clinician's professional conduct as well as ways to balance one's overall life. The emphasis is on clinician self-awareness and retaining or regaining control of one's life. The following is an integration of the strategies recommended by these authors.

KNOW YOUR STRENGTHS AND WEAKNESSES

As clinicians, we know the importance of working with clients' strengths in order to improve areas of weakness. Self-reflection helps us identify our own strengths, and we need to play to those. For example, if your strength and preference is working with children, then working in a setting where you see primarily children may be more satisfying than working in a setting (e.g., a hospital) where you may see relatively few children. Conversely, if you prefer to work with adults, the public schools may not be the best job setting for you even if the salary and vacation time is somewhat better in the school setting. If, after you have had some experience with dysphagia patients, you find that swallowing disorders are not an area you enjoy, find a setting where you can work with the age population you prefer and where dysphagia is not a significant part of your therapy duties. We are likely to be more resilient, even during trying times, if we are engaged in professional work that is meaningful to us.

Other strengths that are helpful for us to be aware of are our emotional strengths (e.g., being patient), character strengths (e.g., honesty and forgiveness), intellectual abilities, family support, friends and social connections, and spirituality (Plante, 2009). No one is equally strong and balanced in all areas of their lives, but recognizing what internal and external resources we can draw upon helps us feel self-confident and feel that we do not have to manage all our work challenges and life's vicissitudes alone. Having a professional mentor or joining a professional consultation group can help us to be more resilient practitioners (Skovholt, 2001). Our social community and professional networks can represent external resources that increase our coping abilities, while reflection on our internal strengths also can help us to be more resilient.

BE IN CONTROL OF YOUR OWN LIFE

When people feel that someone or something (particularly an impersonal institution or agency) is in control of their lives, they feel threatened, weakened, and impotent. Emotional and physical tension are often associated with feeling a lack of control, with fear that someone with power over us may say or do something that might harm us professionally or personally. Recognizing that we, as individuals, are responsible for the quality of our own lives places the burden of our happiness and success on our own shoulders. Reflecting on what *we can do* to change or influence a situation may help to shift our thinking from a helpless position to an empowered one.

An important principle of preventing burnout is to avoid managing other people's lives. Some people have a tendency to meddle and act as though they have all the answers for what other people need to do to improve their lives, but have difficulty effectively managing their own lives. By our nature we are helpers, but we need to avoid being "rescuers" in both our professional and personal lives. While taking responsibility for our lives, we cannot always change what others choose or do. Letting go of feeling overly responsible for others may help to free up some of our positive and constructive energy. Thus, maintaining clear boundaries can help clinicians to remain empathically engaged while honoring the limits of their sphere of influence (Harrison & Westwood, 2009).

FIND OTHER INTERESTS BESIDES YOUR WORK

Although we may enjoy our work and be happy to spend many hours involved in it, if the majority of our off-duty hours are consumed with thoughts of work, our minds do not have an opportunity to be renewed with other (perhaps more pleasant) diversions. We need to consider our motivations for being totally absorbed in our work. What do we want that we are not getting from a relatively normal amount of work involvement? Whom are we trying to please (or appease)? What rewards are we looking for? We may need to answer these questions before we can let go of our work and develop other interests and other areas of ourselves. We need to focus on developing ourselves as well-balanced individuals who have interests and passions besides our professional work. We should find and invest in relationships and activities that can bring joy and levity to our lives. Outside interests can help us to refuel mentally and physically and give us a richer perspective from which to draw when we are at work.

THINK OF WAYS TO BRING VARIETY INTO YOUR WORK

Boredom is an important cause of dissatisfaction with our work and a strong contributor to burnout. Doing essentially the same therapy year after year, where the only real changes are in the faces and names of the children and adults with whom we work, means we have lost our creativity and intellectual stimulation. Challenging ourselves to learn new therapy approaches or working to develop a new area of expertise can be professionally invigorating and help us stay on the "cutting edge" in our field. This can help us to feel empowered in our profession rather than stale or bored by a repetitive work routine.

We are fortunate in our professions to have a wide variety of work settings in which to practice and age ranges of individuals in which to specialize. For example, we can work in hospitals and for agencies with birth–three programs; preschool programs; public schools with kindergarten through high school levels; special programs in community colleges; a variety of hospital settings, including acute, subacute, and long-term care and inpatient or outpatient services; residential health care facilities; physicians' offices such as those of otolaryngologists; industrial settings for audiologists to administer hearing conservation programs; various clinics such as Easter Seals; home health agencies; private practice; and universities as instructors, professors, and clinical supervisors (Fogle, 2008).

With these diverse areas of employment opportunities, SLPs and Auds have options that perhaps few other professionals have. If a clinician begins to burn out working in one setting, she may have opportunities to work in others without having to relocate to another town or city. Clinicians also have the option of leaving the profession for a number of years (e.g., for an extended maternity leave) and returning later. Leaving the profession permanently is not the only solution to burnout (Fogle, 2006).

MONITOR YOUR PHYSICAL AND MENTAL HEALTH

Like most professions, speech-language pathology and audiology are stress producing. Having your blood pressure checked annually can forewarn you of your body's reaction to stress. Essential hypertension may be hereditary and/or stress related (Keltner et al., 2007). Illness caused by stress increases the difficulty of managing the stress. Most people know the importance of healthy diets and lifestyles, but for many professionals it becomes increasingly difficult to eat regular, healthy meals, exercise a few times a week, and get seven to eight hours of sleep a night. These self-care routines however can go a long way toward insulating individuals from feeling emotionally overloaded.

Another method for enhancing physical and mental well-being that has gained empirical support during the past few years is stress-reduction training, which can include relaxation methods and mindfulness meditation (Kabat-Zinn, 2003; Shapiro & Carlson, 2009; Siegel, 2007). While mindfulness training originates in Buddhist philosophy, it has been embraced by many Westerners who find that this way of thinking helps them to endure stressful situations as it encourages the individual to develop a detached way of noticing situations without trying to influence them (Plante, 2009; Shapiro & Walsh, 2007). Siegel (2007), who is a psychiatrist at the University of California, Los Angeles, conducts professional workshops to help train therapists as well as to teach therapists self-care skills. He summarizes the art of mindfulness in this way:

> Mindfulness heightens the capacity to become filled by the senses of the moment and attuned to our own state of being. As we also become aware of our awareness, we can sharpen our focus on the present, enabling us to feel our feet as we travel the path of our lives. We engage with ourselves and with others, making an authentic connection, with more reflection and consideration. Life becomes more enriched as we are aware of the extraordinary experience of being, of being alive, of living in this moment (pp. 14–15).

Siegel points out that mindfulness is not self-indulgent but actually enhances our ability to have caring relationships with others. Mindfulness practice also enables us to stay calm and grounded and to better tolerate ambiguity in life as well as to find hope in the face of suffering (Harrison & Westwood, 2009).

Clinicians approaching middle age need to be particularly aware of their physical health. It is during this time that some of the greatest demands are placed on us personally and professionally. Professionally, many middle-aged clinicians have advanced to administrative positions or have additional work-related demands on their time. Personally, they may have added domestic stressors, such as adolescent children. They also may be in the "sandwich generation" (Hooyman & Kiyak, 2008), meaning they are still raising their children and, in addition, are the primary caregiver for one or both elderly parents. In these situations, professional burnout may reflect an accumulation of both personal and professional stresses.

WORK SMARTER, NOT JUST HARDER

Clinicians often feel that if they work harder and put more time and energy into their work, they will be more successful and please more people. Working smarter includes working more efficiently, knowing what is expected of you on the job, and knowing what is not expected. Knowing who will be evaluating you and the criteria for evaluations can help you anticipate and prioritize which jobs and/or tasks are most important. On any new job, seek out a mentor to help you "learn the ropes" and "navigate the landmines." Procedures that you have learned in your academic training will not likely be the same ones that are used in any particular job setting. Also, on every job there are certain situations and/or people that tend to be challenging to work with—or around. Blood and colleagues (2002) and Harris and colleagues (2009) found that one of the more effective strategies for managing stress is obtaining social support from family, friends, co-workers, and supervisors. For a more detailed discussion of professional burnout see Lubinski and colleagues (2007).

Summary

SLPs and Auds need to be aware of the possibilities of experiencing professional stress and burnout beginning with their earliest years of professional work. Successful students have found ways to cope with professional stresses and prevent educational burnout in order to complete their graduate studies. Some of the strategies they have used as students may help them during their professional careers. Being aware of the numerous sources of professional burnout, the stages of burnout, and ways to prevent burnout can help lead to longer and more enjoyable and productive careers in the satisfying professions of speech-language pathology and audiology.

Maintaining Enthusiasm for Your Profession

At the beginning of each academic year, I tell the graduate students in my Neuropathologies of Adults course the following story.

In the ancient Olympics in Greece there was a race in which every runner had to carry a lighted torch. The winner was not the person who was the fastest, but the person who finished the race first with his torch still lit. The challenge for students is to finish their graduate work with their torch still lit with enthusiasm for learning and the profession.

CONCLUDING COMMENTS

Helpers and caregivers (including SLPs and Auds, mental health professionals, medical professionals, and others) sometimes are more conscientious about the care they provide for those who need their interventions than the care they provide for themselves. If we do not take adequate care of ourselves, we will have less mental and physical energy to help our clients and patients who depend on us. Our inevitable therapy errors and failures deserve self-reflection so that we can learn from them and provide better therapy to others. We need to forgive ourselves for our errors and failures as well as forgive our clients who we may feel have failed us in some way. Following personal or professional traumas, we need to reflect on our symptoms of stress, self-care strategies, and the possible need for professional help. The death of clients and patients can affect us deeply, and we need to have tools and resources in order to maintain our emotional stamina or regain our emotional equilibrium. Professional burnout is a very real problem, and attending state and national professional conventions may help to keep SLPs and Auds mentally fresh and connected to other professionals so that burnout is less likely. If we are aware of the professional and personal factors that could contribute to our burnout, we can take steps to prevent them, and in doing so, enrich our lives and the lives of others.

Discussion Questions

1. Discuss a case in which a client did not make the improvements in hearing, speech, language, cognition, or swallowing that either the client or you would have liked. What were some of the therapeutic errors or other contributing factors that may have resulted in less than an optimal outcome? How did you explain the lack of progress to the client? How did you feel about the experience? How did you "talk to yourself" about it? What did you learn from the experience?

2. Have you ever experienced symptoms of Posttraumatic Stress Disorder? What were your symptoms? How long did the symptoms last? What helped you resolve them? Have you experienced any residual symptoms, such as continuing to avoid certain situations?

3. Have you had a relative or friend who died? How were you told about the death? How do you wish you had been told? What support did you have immediately after you learned of the death? What support do you wish you had received?

4. Have you had a client or patient in your training who died? How were you told about the death? How do you wish you had been told? What support did you have immediately after you learned of the death? What support do you wish you had?

5. What clinical challenges do you share with your supervisor? How much do you share with your supervisor the personal and emotional impact that clients have on you? What forum (e.g., speaking with classmates or colleagues) have you found helps you the most to process challenging clinical situations and the emotional impact they have on you?

6. You have survived as a student through the rigors of undergraduate and much of graduate school. What strategies have you used to help prevent educational burnout?

7. If a student just beginning graduate studies asked you what you would suggest to prevent educational and clinical burnout, what would you tell the student?

Role Plays

1. Divide the class into small groups of 4–6 students each and discuss (1) the most stressful aspects of being a student and/or clinical work, (2) the signals of becoming overly stressed, and (3) the self-care strategies the students are using to manage the stress in their daily lives.

2. Ask the class to discuss how they would respond to a friend or colleague who appeared to be experiencing "compassion fatigue" or approaching professional burnout.

APPENDIX

Internet Resources

The following is a list of general and specific online and website resources that may be helpful to clinicians, clients, and families.

Note: At the time of publication, the Internet sites listed here were available. Given the nature of the medium, however, there is no guarantee that these sites continue to be available or at the same addresses.

www.aboutfaceusa.org
An organization whose aim is to connect individuals with similar experiences of living with facial differences.

www.aphasia.org
National Aphasia Association website that includes general and specific explanations of aphasia, apraxia, dysarthria, and dementia for professionals and the public. Includes how to communicate with patients and families about aphasia and the effects of aphasia on the family, with first-hand stories. Also includes information for families on how to find a speech-language pathologist, recommendations for books and articles, and links to other sites for more information about neurogenic disorders and rehabilitation.

www.apraxia-kids.org
Childhood Apraxia of Speech National Association (CASNA) website that provides general and specific information about CAS and whose mission is to strengthen the support systems in the lives of children with apraxia so that these children have their best opportunity to develop speech.

www.asha.org
ASHA's website for readings on all speech, language, cognitive, swallowing, and hearing disorders, including multicultural issues.

www.asha.org/public/speech/disorders/stuttering.htm
ASHA's website for stuttering.

www.ata.org
American Tinnitus Association website that provides information for professionals and the public about tinnitus and links to other websites for tinnitus.

www.audiology.org
American Academy of Audiology's website.

www.biausa.org

Brain Injury Association of America website that provides information for professionals and the public about the different severity levels and types of brain injuries, such as strokes, traumatic brain injury, diffuse axonal injury, concussion, shaken baby syndrome, and coma. It discusses the rehabilitation team for individuals with brain injuries and provides safety advice for preventing TBI in daily life as well as personal stories of those who made good recoveries from TBIs.

www.british-voice-association.com

British organization that provides information to international professionals and the public related to education and research about normal and abnormal voices and prevention of voice problems.

www.cleftadvocate.org

Website of the Cleft Palate Advocate, an organization whose mission is to educate and inspire families and to provide support networks.

www.cleftline.org

Website of the Cleft Palate Foundation that operates a toll-free hotline and produces free publications to professionals and the public that provide information about clefts and other craniofacial anomalies.

www.dysphonia.org

National Spasmodic Dysphonia Association website that provides information for professionals and support for individuals affected by spasmodic dysphonia.

www.facesofchildren.org

Website of Foundation for Faces of Children that provides a parent support network for awareness and education, particularly for parents just learning that their child has a craniofacial anomaly. English and Spanish versions are available.

www.friendswhostutter.org

National Association of Young People Who Stutter website that provides networking for children and teenagers who stutter.

www.healthlaw.org

National Health Law Program website that provides extensive information on health care law affecting families with children who have special health needs.

www.hospicecare.com

International Association for Hospice and Palliative Care website that provides information on hospice and palliative care centers around the world, as well as numerous links to help patients and families.

www.inspire.com

A website that connects children and adults, families, friends, and caregivers of individuals with communication disorders for support and inspiration.

www.listentoyourbuds.org

ASHA website designed to teach children how to use personal audio technology safely. It features an interactive game for children ages 6 to 12, information for parents, and resources for educators.

www.mayoclinic.org/voice-disorders.html

Mayo Clinic in Rochester, Minnesota website with information on voice disorders that is helpful to professionals and the public.

www.nad.org

National Association of the Deaf website that provides information on law and advocacy and whose mission is to promote, protect, and preserve the rights and quality of life for individuals who are deaf or hard of hearing.

www.netnet.net/mums/

Website of MUMS, a national parent-to-parent organization for parents and care providers of children with any disability, disorder, chromosomal abnormality, or health condition. The organization helps connect parents and care providers in their local area whose children have similar disorders or disabilities.

www.neuropsychologycentral.com

Brown University Medical School website that discusses behavioral and psychological aspects of TBI rehabilitation and the effects on a person's home life and social activities. It includes a search engine of links to hundreds of related sites.

www.speechdisorder.co.uk/Speech-and-Self-Esteem.html

A website developed for parents of children with communication disorders that provides information about articulation and other speech disorders as well as parent support groups.

www.stuttering.org

An umbrella association for national self-help associations for people who stutter.

www.stutteringhelp.org

Stuttering Foundation of America's online resources for services and support for those who stutter and their families.

www.tartamudez.org

Stuttering Foundation of America's Spanish version of the www.stutteringhelp.org website.

www.tinnitus.org.uk

British Tinnitus Association website that provides information for professionals and the public about tinnitus and links to other websites for tinnitus.

www.widesmiles.org

Wide Smiles website that includes information parents want to know about clefts, including stories, photographs, networking, and an active Internet discussion group.

GLOSSARY

acculturation The process of learning, incorporating, and adopting values, customs, and beliefs of a dominant culture.

acting out A defense mechanism in which the person deals with emotional conflicts by acting in inappropriate ways rather than by reflecting or talking about feelings.

action language Language that describes the client's specific behaviors and does not make inferences, pathologize, or label the client.

altruism A defense mechanism in which the person deals with emotional conflicts (e.g., those involving guilt and anger) by performing helpful deeds for others.

anosognosia A denial of or decreased awareness of deficits or disabilities that is often seen in patients with right-hemisphere damage; an impairment of an individual's ability to relate to parts of one's body.

anxiety A psychological and physiological state of emotional distress in which there are feelings of uneasiness, fear, or worry.

authoritarian parenting style A parenting style characterized by high expectations of conformity and compliance to parental rules and directions, while being less encouraging of open dialogue between parent and child.

authoritative parenting style A parenting style characterized by high expectations of maturity while placing limits and controls on child actions. Authoritative parents set clear standards while also being attentive to child needs and concerns.

autonomy Respect for the patient's right to determine his or her own choices in health care decision making.

beneficence The duty to act in the best interest of the patient or to promote the patient's best interest.

bicultural adjustment A positive state of psychosocial adjustment in which an individual feels comfortable in both the dominant and one's ethnic culture and has friends and interests in both cultures.

bioethics The attempt to understand and resolve ethical issues and problems in the health care setting.

boundaries The demarcation or differentiation between family members or family subsystems. Healthy boundaries enable appropriate levels of privacy (e.g., between parents and children), identity, and role differentiation.

case formulation A clinical tool that provides a comprehensive and integrated understanding of a client by relating all of the presenting complaints to one another and explaining why the difficulties have developed. A case formulation is a summarizing statement that captures the essence of a particular client's history, chief symptoms, and prognosis.

catastrophizing Faulty thinking that involves an exaggerated, negative view of the future (i.e., thinking that a catastrophe will occur).

circular questioning A therapeutic tool developed by family therapists to gain more comprehensive information about a family's interactional patterns. Circular questioning is done during the interview process and involves asking one family member what the other one does, as a way of getting the family to think about the motives, actions, and perspectives of the other family member.

classical conditioning A learning process in which a neutral stimulus (e.g., a nurse's presence) is repeatedly combined with another stimulus that elicits a physiological reaction (e.g., a painful injection). Over time, the person develops a physiological reaction to the neutral stimulus, in this case, growing fearful or anxious every time a particular nurse appears. The behaviorist Joseph Wolpe used this model to show how anxiety to any (previously neutral) stimulus can be learned.

clinical psychologist A professional with a Ph.D. or Psy.D. who specializes in assessment and treatment of individuals with psychological disorders and their symptoms.

cognitive distortions From a cognitive therapy viewpoint, these are various types of erroneous or faulty thinking that contribute to a person's fears, pessimism, and maladaptive behaviors. These include catastrophizing, "I should" statements, and dichotomous thinking.

cognitive restructuring The process of replacing negative appraisals of life events with more positive ones. In cognitive behavioral therapy, clinicians encourage clients to analyze and then restructure problematic (negative) aspects of their internal conversation. Thus, a client may be encouraged to change his typical self-talk from, "I always fail" to "I can do this if I try."

common factors approach The notion in counseling and psychotherapy that certain factors which are common to all forms of effective counseling such as a warm relationship and trust in the therapist are more potent factors than the techniques which are specific to particular theoretically-based approaches.

complex interpersonal message Communications that carry two often contradictory messages. On one level, the communication may sound benign or simply express a factual request (e.g., "When did you get your degree?"). On the second level, there is often a negative interpersonal message, for example, communicating doubt that the therapist has enough experience to help the client. Dysfunctional families are sometimes characterized by communicating frequent complex interpersonal messages to each other.

congruence The consistency between one's feelings and one's behaviors. According to humanistic therapists, healthy personality development occurs when children repeatedly receive the clear message (congruence) that they will be accepted even when they express their true feelings and experiences. Likewise, clinicians must demonstrate congruence in order to gain their clients' trust and confidence.

conversion reaction The concept that emotional pain can be expressed through physical mechanisms or symptoms. The specific physical symptoms that occur are considered symbolic of underlying emotional issues, and may reflect unresolved emotional feelings or wishes.

counseling Providing guidance, direction, or advice about personal matters. Psychological counseling is an applied social science that focuses on helping individuals to overcome adjustment problems or psychological problems that prevent them from dealing effectively with life situations. Applied to SLPs and Auds, counseling involves a helping relationship in which the clinician's intentions are to assist a person or family member to understand a hearing, communication, or swallowing disorder, its impact on their lives, and ways of preventing, managing, adjusting to, or coping with these disorders.

counseling psychologist A professional with a Ph.D. or Psy.D. who usually treats day-to-day adjustment problems in counseling settings, such as university or mental health clinics.

countertransference The therapist's perceptions, beliefs, wishes, and responses to a client, which are influenced both by the client's characteristics and behaviors and by the therapist's past experiences.

culture Any group of people who associate with one another on the basis of a common purpose, need, or background. The group often has shared beliefs, traditions, and values.

defense mechanisms Automatic mental processes that people use to protect themselves from intolerable levels of anxiety and internal conflict.

denial A defense mechanism in which a person deals with emotional conflicts by refusing to acknowledge some painful aspect of reality (e.g., the presence of a disorder or the severity of impairment) or a subjective experience (e.g., sadness and lethargy) that is apparent to others.

devaluation A defense mechanism in which a person deals with emotional conflict or stressors by attributing extreme, negative qualities to another person or object (e.g., the treatment). Devaluation may occur in the context of another defense mechanism, splitting, and may represent the "all bad" portion of the person's split perceptions.

dichotomous thinking Faulty thinking that tends to inaccurately divide all situations and people into "good" and "bad" categories rather than perceiving more subtle nuances or "shades of gray."

disengagement A family interaction pattern in which a family has minimal contact, structure, order, or authority. Family members feel disconnected and may experience little emotional support from one another.

displacement A defense mechanism in which a person transfers feelings about one person, object, or event onto someone else who is perceived as less threatening and/or less powerful.

diunital reasoning The ability to accept and understand world views that are divergent and at odds. This understanding may result in a change in one's own views when one ultimately places value on the practices of other cultures.

empathy An attitude of entering a client's world as if it were our own, allowing ourselves to feel what the client is feeling and communicating this to the client. Empathy is a key element in developing a positive therapeutic relationship with clients.

enmeshment A family interaction pattern in which there are weak boundaries and insufficient differentiation of roles and identity among the members. To others, the family members may appear "too close" and unable to tolerate healthy levels of autonomy among themselves.

ethics The philosophical discipline that is concerned with human conduct and moral decisions.

ethnography A common strategy in the social sciences to study human societies and cultures through observation of that culture. Research data is collected through interviews, questionnaires, and observation while the investigator is immersed in the culture.

existential isolation Our ultimate aloneness in the world—as we can never totally understand each other and our growth may lead others to reject us. This is a condition of life that produces anxiety, according to existentialist writer James Bugental.

existential meaninglessness The lack of an inherent meaning in life. The questions we ask about the significance of our existence highlight how tenuous our meanings are and how easily they can be changed or obliterated.

existential nonbeing The existential conditions of life such as uncertainty, meaninglessness, and isolation. In healthy personality functioning, the person grasps, admits, and grapples with these aspects of life.

existential uncertainty The uncertainty that we experience in our lives even as we take reasonable steps to shape, control, and predict it. This inescapable uncertainty is a source of anxiety in our lives, according to existential writers.

family myth A family's unspoken but entrenched notion about itself, which is prized and resistant to change but at odds with reality. Examples of family myths may be, "we all get along wonderfully," "we are all strong, honorable people," or "we don't have any problems." Families who subscribe to these seemingly positive myths may be intolerant of a family member who does not buy into the family's self-image or who speaks out against the family's self-image. A family member who opposes such a myth may find herself "divorced" or cast out from the family.

generalize The process of expanding newly learned skills from one environment to another.

gerontology The study of chronological, biological, psychological, and sociological age on elderly people.

help-rejecting complaining A defense mechanism in which a person expresses repetitive complaints or pleas for assistance but then systematically rejects all suggestions and recommendations that are offered. In this way, the client "defeats" the professional who is trying to help him.

hierarchy According to family systems theorists, a hierarchical organization is considered to be central to healthy family functioning. Functioning as the authority at the top of the hierarchy is usually the marital subsystem (i.e., the parents), which takes charge of the child or sibling subsystem. Families that do not function well often have vague or ill-defined hierarchies.

holistic A philosophical concept in which an entity (e.g., a person) is seen as more than the sum of its parts;

a prominent approach in psychology, biology, nursing, medicine, and other scientific, sociological, and educational fields of study and practice.

homeostasis The balance of roles and functions that is maintained in a family. A family's homeostatic functioning may be deemed as either healthy or unhealthy.

"I should" statements Faulty thinking that involves a moralistic or perfectionistic self-statement and an intolerance of personal flaws. Examples include, "I should always think of others first," "I should be able to control myself," and "I should always be organized."

informational counseling Counseling that focuses on providing education to clients and family members about a disorder, associated symptoms, and the rationale for specific treatment interventions.

informed consent The ethical and legal requirement to disclose all relevant risks and benefits associated with a given intervention, treatment, or procedure.

intellectualization A defense mechanism in which a person uses detached, logical, or abstract thinking in order to avoid an internal conflict or painful emotional feelings.

intermittent reinforcement schedule A pattern of providing a reward on only some of the occasions when the desired behavior occurs.

interpersonal style Recurrent patterns of relating to others; a learned style of communication and interaction. Examples of interpersonal styles can include friendly-dependent, hostile-suspicious, or controlling-devaluing.

licensed case social worker Usually a professional with a Master's degree who works with individuals and families and mobilizes community support systems.

malingering Feigning illness, impairment, or other incapacity (such as hearing loss, aphasia, or dysarthria) in order to avoid work or other responsibilities or to obtain benefits.

marriage and family therapist Usually a professional with a Master's degree who attempts to change the structure and interaction processes of a client's family in order to enhance their functioning.

medical family therapy A specialty discipline within the family therapy domain in which family therapists work collaboratively with physicians and other health professionals. In medical family therapy, therapists draw upon the literature in biopsychosocial health care to consider the psychosocial repercussions of biomedical events.

mental status examination (MSE) An important part of the clinical assessment process in psychological and psychiatric practice. The purpose of the MSE is to gain a comprehensive description of a client's mental state. Standard components of an MSE include the client's state of mind (e.g., rational or delusional), appearance, attitude, behavior, mood and affect, thought content, speech, cognition, insight, and judgment.

metacommunication In interpersonal psychology, metacommunication refers to dialogue that focuses on the immediate interpersonal process occurring between the clinician and client. For example, the client may choose to talk about topics unrelated to the therapy. The clinician may metacommunicate by asking the client whether she is having difficulty or experiencing anxiety about discussing her hearing impairment.

microskills Specific communication skills that enhance therapists interactions with clients and family members. Microskills include open-ended questions, nonverbal encouragers, paraphrasing, and reflections.

negative reinforcement The removal of an unpleasant or aversive stimulus that increases the frequency of a certain behavior. For example, a patient's cries or screams that halt an important but painful medical procedure may be negatively reinforcing to the patient.

neuropsychologist A specialty profession that focuses on brain functioning and the impact on brain functioning of various medical and psychological conditions. Neuropsychologists are licensed psychologists (typically with a Ph.D. or a Psy.D.) with special training in the links between behaviors and brain structures and systems. They can help to pinpoint the specific nature of cognitive alterations in a particular individual (e.g., one who has suffered a stroke or TBI) and thus assist in recommendations for rehabilitation.

nondirective therapy The style of therapy advocated by humanistic therapists in which clients are encouraged to direct the flow of conversation in sessions rather than having the therapist organize the agenda and direct session topics.

nonmaleficence The duty to do no harm in health care and rehabilitation interventions.

observational learning A process of learning through others who provide a model for certain behaviors (e.g., correct speech articulation).

operant conditioning Learning that occurs as a function of its consequences (e.g., rewards or punishments). Behavioral therapists have developed the notion of using operant techniques to modify a person's problematic behaviors.

overgeneralizations Faulty thinking that involves making incorrect inferences or "leaps in logic" from one situation to other situations that may not be related.

parentified role A form of role reversal in which a child is inappropriately given the role of meeting the emotional or physical needs of the parents or siblings. Parentified children may be expected to sacrifice play, friendships with peers, academic work, or their own age-appropriate emotional needs for nurturing and care in order to provide caregiving functions for other family members.

passive aggression A defense mechanism in which a person presents a façade of friendliness, compliance, or agreement while indirectly and unassertively expressing aggression or hostility. "Forgetting" and procrastination are classic examples of passive-aggressive behavior.

permissive parenting style A parenting style characterized by being indulgent, nondirective, or lenient and having few behavioral expectations for the child.

positive reinforcement Desirable consequences of a behavior that increase the frequency of that behavior. For example, a child who receives privileges (positive reinforcement) for attending and making an effort in his speech rehabilitation therapy sessions will learn to produce these behaviors more readily.

psychiatric social worker A professional with a Master's degree and specialized training in treating people in home, hospital and community settings who have mental health conditions.

psychiatrist A physician (M.D.) with postgraduate training in abnormal behavior, psychotherapy, and psychopharmacology who can prescribe medications as part of treatment for mental disorders.

psychoanalyst Either a psychiatrist or a psychologist who specializes in psychoanalysis, the treatment approach first developed by Sigmund Freud. In psychoanalysis, the therapist focuses on the patient's unconscious conflict, instinctual drives, and defense mechanisms that prevent the individual from functioning in an optimal, mature manner in daily life.

psychobiological disinhibition The brain's inability to inhibit unwanted or abnormal responses to stimuli and situations that may be caused by neurological damage, particularly in the frontal lobes.

psychoeducational approach An approach taken by psychologists that focuses on therapy as a learning process and teaches clients, patients, and their family members about relevant behavioral, developmental, or symptom patterns, as well as skills to improve or optimize functioning.

psychomotor retardation A slowing down of physical movements and thought processes, often occurring when a person is clinically depressed. This symptom may be present in other circumstances as well, such as in Parkinson's disease or as a side effect of psychotropic medication (i.e., medications prescribed for mental health disorders).

rationalization A defense mechanism in which the person uses self-serving and incorrect logic to explain his maladaptive behavior.

reinforcement contingencies The system of consequences associated with a person's behavior. Behavioral treatment plans typically develop a new system of reward contingencies to modify a person's behavior.

reinforcement schedule The frequency or consistency of applying a particular reward or reinforcement after a certain behavior has occurred. Reinforcement schedules can be altered to increase the likelihood of desired behaviors.

scapegoat A concept used by family systems therapists that refers to a person who is blamed for the family's unhappiness. Often this is a child whose misbehavior becomes the family's focus so that other problems or conflicts (e.g., marital conflict or a parent's substance abuse) can be avoided.

school psychologist/counselor A professional with a Master's degree in school psychology or educational psychology who works in school settings with children and parents and focuses on academic performance and behaviors or mental health conditions that interfere with academic success.

secondary reinforcers Consequences of a behavior that did not serve as the initial reinforcement, but help to maintain a desired behavior. Often they are not as powerful as the original rewards or else they acquire their value over time by being associated with a primary reinforcer. For example, following a period of formal rewards such as stickers or candy, a teacher's smiles and nods may become secondary reinforcers to a child. In a second example, a person who dislikes her job may find that her disability payments become secondary reinforcers for maintaining the illness behavior.

self-actualization A concept central to humanistic therapy that refers to the inherent human tendency to strive towards positive growth and emotional development.

self-concept The composite of ideas, feelings, and attitudes that a person has about his own identity, worth, capabilities, and limitations.

self-image The total concept, idea, or mental image that a person has of herself and her role in society.

self-esteem The degree of worth and competence a person attributes to oneself; personal judgment of self-worth.

social learning theory A perspective adopted by many behaviorists such as Bandura, which posits that most of human learning occurs through a process of observing and imitating others.

solution-focused therapy A form of psychotherapy that focuses on the present and what the client wants to change rather than on the past and underlying sources of the client's problems. This form of therapy focuses on the use of a collaborative relationship with the client so that practical solutions can be identified to help the client achieve her desired goals.

splitting A defense mechanism in which a person perceives others or situations in "black and white" or "good and bad" terms. By engaging in this dichotomous thinking, the person eliminates the challenge of confronting ambiguity and complexity in himself and others.

stimulus-response chain A pattern of behaviors and consequences that occurs with some predictability and consistency. For example, a child's stuttering behavior and the parent's subsequent taking over the conversation for her may develop into a predictable stimulus-response chain in which the child learns to let her parent speak for her.

stressor An environmental event or condition that causes stress to the individual. Stressors can be short-lived (e.g., an argument with a friend, losing one's keys, being late for a meeting) or long-lasting (e.g., poverty, fear of job loss, or dealing with a child's chronic illness). Some people may interpret certain situations as stressors while others may view the same situations as mere challenges or inconveniences.

structural family therapy A school of family therapy developed by Salvador Minuchin in the 1960s and 1970s. This therapy focuses on understanding and changing the unhealthy family structure and organization that maintains psychological symptoms in a family member.

successive approximations Client behaviors that gradually approach (i.e., approximate) the desired behavior. From a behaviorist viewpoint, it is generally advisable to provide reinforcement for the client's successive approximations so that he will continue to make progress toward a goal.

systematic desensitization A behavioral approach for treating learned anxiety responses and phobias that was developed by Joseph Wolpe. In this treatment method, a person learns to gradually approach a frightening situation (e.g., a dog or a medical procedure) while practicing a relaxation response. In this way, an anxiety response or phobia is unlearned.

technical eclecticism The practice of borrowing therapy techniques that appear to work from various theoretical perspectives, without necessarily embracing the theories in which the techniques are embedded.

temperament Those aspects of an individual's personality that are regarded as innate rather than learned. For example, some individuals may be considered to have a nervous temperament, while others may be considered to have an easygoing disposition or temperament.

theoretical integration The development of a cohesive conceptual or theoretical framework that blends ideas from two or more theoretical approaches.

therapeutic alliance The positive, interactive process between the clinician and the client, which includes: (1) a mutual understanding regarding the goals of therapy, (2) a shared commitment to the necessary treatment tasks, and (3) a sufficient emotional bond to withstand the strains that inevitably arise during the course of treatment. Core elements of the therapeutic alliance include the client's trust in the clinician, motivation to overcome her symptoms or disorder, and willingness to follow the clinician's instructions.

therapeutic communication Techniques for speaking with clients which promote trust-building, self-disclosure, increasing self-awareness and change. This concept highlights the interpersonal aspects of counseling and the communication of empathy to clients.

therapeutic distance This concept suggests that there is an ideal or optimal distance to maintain in the therapeutic relationship with the client. Optimal therapeutic distance suggests that we are optimally attuned and responsive to our clients. The optimal or ideal therapeutic distance may depend upon the type of client, stage of therapy and other factors. Maintaining a desirable therapeutic distance involves empathy and attention to the client's needs, with neither detachment nor overinvolvement in the client's life.

therapeutic error An intervention that either violates appropriate therapeutic boundaries or is the result of misattunement with a client's current needs and emotional states.

transference The client's perceptions of the clinician, which are influenced by past relationship experiences and certain unconscious elements as well as by the clinician's real qualities.

triangulation A process in which two family members recruit a third family member into an unhealthy alliance, often to avoid conflict with one another. Often, in unhealthy family functioning, children are triangulated into family interactions to avoid marital conflict. Triangulation can also involve situations in which a client or family member tries to develop an alliance with a clinician and to pit themselves against, reject, or blame other family members. Thus, clinicians must be aware of efforts by some clients to involve them in a web of problematic family relationships.

unconditional positive regard A key characteristic of therapists that was first described by the humanistic psychologist Carl Rogers. According to Rogers, therapists must show unconditional caring for their clients and positive regard for their inherent worth. Only by receiving this consistent and unwavering positive regard can clients feel free to reveal themselves in therapy and to accept themselves.

world view An individual's assumptions and perceptions of the world from a moral, social, ethical, and philosophical perspective.

REFERENCES

Achenbach, T. (2009). *Manual for the Child Behavior Checklist*. Burlington: University of Vermont Department of Psychiatry.

Ackerman, N. (2002). A theory of family systems. In I. Goldenberg & H. Goldenberg (Eds.), *Family therapy, an overview* (4th ed.). Pacific Grove, CA: Brooks-Cole.

Adams, P. (1993). *Gesundheit!: Bringing good health to you, the medical system, and society through physician service, complementary therapies, humor, and joy*. Rochester, VT: Healing Arts Press.

Adler, A. (1956). *The individual psychology of Alfred Adler*. H. L. Ansbacher & R. R. Ansbacher (Eds.). New York: Harper & Row.

Aiken, T. D. (2008). *Legal and ethical issues in health occupations* (2nd ed). Philadelphia: Saunders.

Ainsworth, S. (1945). Integrating theories of stuttering. *Journal of Speech Disorders, 10*, 205–210.

Alarcon, N., & Rogers, M. (2007). Supported communication intervention for aphasia. ASHA Self-Study CEU Program. Retrieved June 4, 2010, from http://www.asha.org/web/OLSDynamicPage.aspx?Webcode=olsdetail&title=Supported+Communication+Intervention+for+Aphasia

American Academy of Pediatrics. (2002). Policy statement: The medical home. *Pediatrics, 110,* 184–186.

American Counseling Association. (2005). *ACA code of ethics*. Alexandria, VA: Author.

American Psychiatric Association. (2000). *Diagnostic and statistical manual of mental disorders, TR* (4th ed., Rev.). Washington, DC: Author.

American Psychological Association. (2005, August). *Policy statement on evidence-based practice in psychology*. Washington, DC: Author.

American Speech-Language-Hearing Association. (2003). *National outcomes measurement system (NOMS): Adult speech-language pathology training manual*. Bethesda, MD: Author.

American Speech-Language-Hearing Association. (2007). Scope of practice in speech-language pathology. Rockville, MD: Author.

Anchin, J., & Kiesler, D. (1982). *Handbook of interpersonal psychotherapy*. Elmsford, NY: Pergamon Press.

Anderson, D., Keith, J., & Novak, P. (2009). *Mosby's Medical, Nursing & Allied Health Dictionary* (8th ed.). St. Louis: Mosby, Harcourt Health Sciences Company.

Anderson, J. D., Pellowski, M. W., Conture, E. G., & Kelly, E. M. (2003). Tempermental characteristics of young children who stutter. *Journal of Speech, Language, and Hearing Research, 46*, 1221–1233.

Andrewes, D. (2001). *Neuropsychology: From theory to practice*. New York: Psychology Press.

Andrews, M. (1986). Application of family therapy techniques to the treatment of language disorders. *Seminar in Speech and Language, 7*, 347–358.

Andrews, M. L. (2006). *Manual of voice treatment: Pediatrics through geriatrics* (3rd ed.). Clifton Park, NY: Thomson Delmar Learning.

Andrews, J., & Andrews, M. (1990). *Family based treatment in communicative disorders: A systematic approach*. Sandwich, IL: Janelle Publications.

Andrews, M., & Summers, A. (2002). *Voice therapy for adolescents*. Boston: College-Hill Publication.

Anstendig, K. D. (1999). Is selective mutism an anxiety disorder: Rethinking its DSM-IV classification. *Journal of Anxiety Disorders, 13*, 417–434.

Apatira, L., Boyd, E. A., Malvar, G., Evans, L. R., Luce, J. M., Lo, B., & White, D. B. (2008). Hope, truth, and preparing for death: Perspectives of surrogate decision makers. *Annals of Internal Medicine, 149*(12), 861–868.

Aram, D. M., Ekelman, B., & Nation, J. (1984). Preschoolers with language disorders: 10 years later. *Journal of Speech and Hearing Research, 27*, 232–244.

Aram, D. M., & Hall, N. E. (1989). Longitudinal follow-up of children with preschool communication disorders: Treatment implications. *School Psychology Review, 18,* 487–501.

Arkowitz, H. (1997). Integrative theories of therapy. In P. Wachtel & S. Messer (Eds.), *Theories of psychotherapy: Origins and evolution* (pp. 227–288). Washington, DC: American Psychological Association.

Arkowitz, H. (2002). Toward an integrative perspective on resistance to change. *Psychotherapy in Practice, 58,* 219–227.

Aronson, A. E. (1990). *Clinical voice disorders* (3rd ed.). New York: Thieme.

Arpin, K., Fitch, M., Browne, G. B., & Corey, P. (1990). Prevalence and correlates of family dysfunction and poor adjustment to chronic illness in specialty clinics. *Journal of Clinical Epidemiology, 43*(4), 373–383.

Aten, J. D., & Leach, M. M. (2009). *Spirituality and the therapeutic process: A comprehensive resource from intake to termination.* Washington, DC: American Psychological Association.

Aten, J. L. (2008). Overcoming fear and tension in stuttering. In *Advice to those who stutter* (2nd ed.). Memphis, TN: Stuttering Foundation of America.

Avent, J. (2004). Group treatment for aphasia using cooperative learning principles. *Topics in Language Disorders, 24*(2), 118–124.

Avent, J., Glista, S., Wallace, S., Jackson, J., Nishioka, J., & Yip, W. (2005). Family information needs about aphasia. *Aphasiology, 19,* 365–375.

Back, A. L., & Curtis, A. R. (2002). Communicating bad news. *Western Journal of Medicine, 176,* 177–180.

Baile, W. F., & Beale, E. A. (2001). Giving bad news to cancer patients: Matching process and content. *Journal of Clinical Oncology, 19*(9), 2575–2577.

Bailey, A., Channon, S., & Beaumont, J. G. (2007). The relationship between subjective fatigue and cognitive fatigue in advanced multiple sclerosis. *Multiple Sclerosis, 13*(1), 73–80.

Bailey, C. E. (2005). Assessment of parenting styles and behavior. In M. Cierpka, V. Thomas, & D. Sprenkle (Eds.), *Family assessment: Integrating multiple perspectives* (pp. 193–210). Ashland, OH: Hogrefe & Huber.

Bailey, D. B., McWilliam, P., & Winton, P. J. (1992). Building family-centered practices in early intervention: A team-based model for change. *Infants and Young Children, 5*(1), 73–82.

Baker, E. K. (2003). *Caring for ourselves: A therapist's guide to personal and professional well-being.* Washington, DC: American Psychological Association.

Baker, J. (1998). Psychogenic dysphonia: Peeling back the layers. *Journal of Voice, 12,* 527–535.

Baker, L., & Cantwell, D. (1982). Psychiatric disorders in children with different types of communication disorders. *Journal of Communication Disorders, 15,* 113–126.

Bandura, A. (1968). A social learning interpretation of psychological dysfunctions. In P. London & D. Rosenhan (Eds.), *Foundations of abnormal psychology.* New York: Holt, Rinehart & Winston.

Bandura, A. (1969). *Principles of behavior modification.* New York: Holt, Rinehart & Winston.

Barker, K. D., & Wilson, F. B. (1967). *Comparative study of vocal utilization of children with hoarseness and normal voice.* Paper presented at the convention of the American Speech and Hearing Association, Chicago, IL.

Barkley, R. (2005) *Attention-deficit hyperactive disorder: A handbook for diagnosis and treatment* (3rd ed.). New York: Guilford Press.

Barlow, D. H. (2000). *Anxiety and its disorders: The nature and treatment of anxiety and panic.* New York: Guilford Press.

Barlow, D. H. (2010). Negative effects from psychological treatments: A perspective. *American Psychologist, 65*(1), 13–20.

Barlow, D. H., & Campbell, L. A. (2000). Mixed anxiety-depression and its implications for models of mood and anxiety disorders. *Comprehensive Psychiatry, 41*(2, Suppl. 1), 55.

Barnett, D., Clements, M., & Kaplan-Estrin, M. (2003). Building new dreams: Supporting parents' adaptation to their child with special needs. *Infants and Young Children, 16*(3), 184–200.

Baron, R. A., Kalsher, M., & Henry, R. (2008). *Psychology: From science to practice* (2nd ed.). Boston: Allyn and Bacon.

Bateson, G., Jackson, D. D., Haley, J., & Weakland, J. (1956). Toward a theory of schizophrenia. *Behavioral Science, 1,* 251–264.

Battle, D. (2002). *Communication disorders in multicultural populations* (3rd ed.). Boston: Butterworth-Heinemann.

Baumrind, D. (1967). Child care practices anteceding three patterns of preschool behavior. *Genetic Psychology Monographs, 75*(1), 43–88.

Bayles, K. A., & Tomoeda, C. K. (2007). *Cognitive-communication disorders of dementia*. San Diego, CA: Plural.

Bear, M., Connors, B., & Paradiso, M. (2007). *Neuroscience: Exploring the brain* (3rd ed.). Baltimore: Lippincott Williams & Wilkins.

Beauchamp, T. L., & Childress, J. F. (2008). *Principles of biomedical ethics* (6th ed.). Oxford, UK: Oxford University Press.

Beck, A. T. (1967). *Depression: Causes and treatment*. Philadelphia: University of Pennsylvania Press.

Beck, A. T., & Emery, G. (1985). *Anxiety disorders and phobias: A cognitive perspective*. New York: Basic Books.

Beck, A. T., Rush, A., Shaw, B., & Emery, G. (1979). *Cognitive therapy of depression: A treatment manual*. New York: Guilford Press.

Beck, J. S. (1995). *Cognitive therapy: Basics and beyond*. New York: Guilford Press.

Becvar, D. S. (2007). *Families that flourish*. New York: W.W. Norton & Company.

Becvar, D. S., & Becvar, R. J. (2009). *Family therapy: A systemic integration* (7th ed.). Boston: Allyn & Bacon.

Beitchman, J., Wilson, B., Brownlie, E., Walters, H., Inglis, A., & Lancee, W. (1996). Long-term consistency in speech/language profiles: II. Behavioral, emotional, and social outcomes. *Journal of the American Academy of Child and Adolescent Psychiatry, 35*, 815–825.

Beichman, J., Wilson, B., Johnson, C., Atkinson, L., Young, A., & Adlaf, E. (2001). Fourteen year follow-up of speech/language-impaired and control children: Psychiatric outcome. *Journal of the American Academy of Child and Adolescent Psychiatry, 40*, 75–82.

Bellack, A. S., Hersen, M., & Kazdin, A. E. (Eds.). (1982). *International handbook of behavior modification and therapy*. New York: Plenum.

Bellis, T. J. (2003). *Assessment and management of central auditory processing disorders in the educational setting* (2nd ed.). Clifton Park, NY: Thomson Delmar Learning.

Benjamin, L. S. (1996). *Interpersonal diagnosis and treatment of personality disorders*. New York: Guilford Press.

Bennett, J. W., & Steele, C. M. (2006). Food for thought: The impact of dysphagia on quality of life. *Psychological issues related to dysphagia*. Rockville, MD: ASHA.

Berk, N. W., Cooper, M. E., Liu, Y., & Marazita, M. L. (2001). Social anxiety in Chinese adults with oral-facial clefts. *The Cleft Palate-Craniofacial Journal, 38*(2), 126–133.

Bernstein-Ellis, E., & Elman, R. (2007). Group communication treatment for individuals with aphasia: The Aphasia Center of California approach. In R. Elman (Ed.), *Group treatment for neurogenic communication disorders: The expert clinician's approach* (2nd ed.) (pp. 71–94). San Diego, CA: Plural.

Betan, E., Heim, A. K., Conklin, C. Z., & Westen, D. (2005). Countertransference phenomena and personality pathology in clinical practice: An empirical investigation. *American Journal of Psychiatry, 162*, 890–898.

Bippus, A. M., & Young, S. L. (2005). Owning your emotions: Reactions to expressions of self- versus other-attributed positive and negative emotions. *Journal of Applied Communication Research, 33*(1), 26–45.

Birmaher, B., Arbelaez, C., & Brent, D. (2002). Course and outcome of child and adolescent major depressive disorder. *Child and adolescent psychiatry clinics of North America, 11*(3), 619–637.

Bishop, A., & Scudder, J. (1990). *The practical, moral, and personal sense of nursing*. New York: University of New York Press.

Black, B., & Uhde, T. W. (1995). Psychiatric characteristics of children with selective mutism. *Journal of the American Academy of Child and Adolescent Psychiatry, 34*, 847–856.

Blood, G. W., Thomas, E. A., Ridenour, J. S., Qualls, C. D., & Hammer, C. S. (2002). Job stress in speech-language pathology working in rural, suburban, and urban schools: Social support and frequency of interactions. *Contemporary Issues in Communication Sciences and Disorders, 29*, 132–140.

Bloodstein, O. & Bernstein Ratner, N. (2008). *A handbook on stuttering* (6th ed.). Clifton Park, NJ: Delmar Cengage Learning.

Boles, L. (2002, November 23). *Counseling elders with communication disorders, their families and related professionals: Multicultural populations*. Institute Course,

American Speech-Language Hearing Association Convention, Atlanta, GA.

Boles, L. (2006). Counseling the elderly. In K. Shipley & C. Roseberry McKibbons (Eds.), *Interviewing and counseling in communicative disorders: Principles and procedures* (3rd ed.) (pp. 275–290). Austin, TX: Pro-Ed.

Boles, L. & Lewis, M. (2003). Working with couples: Solution focused aphasia therapy. *Asia Pacific Journal of Speech, Language and Hearing, 8,* 153–159.

Bond, M., & Perry, J.C. (2004). Long-term changes in defense styles with psychodynamic psychotherapy for depressive, anxiety, and personality disorders. *American Journal of Psychiatry, 161,* 1665–1671.

Boone, D. R. (1997). *Is your voice telling on you?* (2nd ed.). San Diego, CA: Singular.

Boone, D. R., McFarlane, S. C., & Von Berg, S. L. (2009). *The voice and voice therapy* (8th ed.). Boston: Allyn and Bacon.

Boone, H., & Crais, E. (1999). Strategies for achieving family-driven assessment and intervention planning. *Young Exceptional Children, 3*(1), 2–12.

Bordin, E. S. (1979). The generalizability of the psychoanalytic concept of the working alliance. *Psychotherapy: Theory, Research and Practice, 16,* 252–260.

Boscarino, J. A., Figley, C. R., & Adams, R. E. (2004). Compassion fatigue following the September 11 terrorist attacks: A study of secondary trauma among New York City social workers. *International Journal of Emergency Mental Health, 6*(2), 1–9.

Boscolo, L., Cecchin, G., Hoffman, L., & Penn, P. (1987). *Milan systemic family therapy: Conversations in theory and practice.* New York: Basic Books.

Boss, M. (1963). *Daseinanalysis and psychoanalysis.* New York: Basic Books.

Boss, P. (1993). The reconstruction of family life with Alzheimer's disease: Generating theory to lower family stress from ambiguous loss. In P. Boss, W. J. Doherty, R. LaRossa, W. R. Schumm, & S. K. Steinmetz (Eds.), *Sourcebook of family theories and methods: A contextual approach.* New York: Plenum Press.

Bourne, E. J. (2005). *The anxiety and phobia workbook* (4th ed.). Oakland, CA: New Harbinger Publications, Inc.

Bowen, M. (1978). *Family therapy in clinical practice.* New York: Jason Aronson.

Bowlby, J. (1969). *Attachment and loss: Vol. 1. Attachment.* New York: Basic Books.

Bradbury, E., & Hewison, J. (1994). Early parental adjustment to visible congenital disfigurement. *Child Care Health and Development, 20*(4), 251–266.

Brady, N., Skinner, D., Roberts, J., & Hennon, E. (2006). Communication in young children with fragile X syndrome: A qualitative study of mothers' perspectives. *American Journal of Speech-Language Pathology, 15,* 353–364.

Brammer, L. M. & MacDonald, G. (2002). *The helping relationship, process and skills* (8th ed.). Boston: Allyn and Bacon.

Brantley, H. T., & Clifford, E. (1979). Maternal and child locus of control and field dependence in cleft palate children. *Cleft Palate Journal, 16,* 183–187.

Breitenfeldt, D. H. (2008). Managing your stuttering versus your stuttering managing you. In *Advice to those who stutter* (2nd ed.). Memphis, TN: Stuttering Foundation of America.

Bressman, T., Sader, R., Ravens-Sieberg, U., Zeilhofer, H., & Horch, H. (1999). Quality of life research in patients with cleft lip and palate: First results. *German Journal of Mouth and Jaw Facial Surgery, 3,* 134–139.

Briere, J. (2004). *Psychological assessment of adult posttraumatic states: Phenomenology, diagnosis, and measurement* (2nd ed.). Washington, DC: American Psychological Association.

Brock, G., & Barnard, C. (1992). *Procedures in marriage and family therapy* (2nd ed.). Boston: Allyn and Bacon.

Broder, H. L. (2001). Using psychological assessment and therapeutic strategies to enhance well-being. *The Cleft Palate-Craniofacial Journal, 38*(3), 248–254.

Broder, H. L., Smith, F., & Strauss, R. (1994). Effects of visible and invisible orofacial defects on self-perception and adjustment across developmental eras and gender. *Cleft Palate-Craniofacial Journal, 31,* 429–436.

Broder, H. L., & Strauss, R. (1989). Self-concept of early primary school children with visible or invisible defects. *Cleft Palate Journal, 26*(2), 114–117.

Brodley, B. T. (2001). Observations of empathic understanding in a client-centered practice. In S. Haugh & T. Merry (Eds.), *Empathy* (pp. 16–37). Llangarron, UK: PCCS Books.

Broida, H. (1979). *Coping with stroke.* San Diego, CA: College Hill Press.

Brookshire, R. (2007). *Introduction to neurogenic communication disorders* (7th ed.). St. Louis, MO: Mosby.

Brown, J. E., & Handelsman, J. A. (2007). Professional autonomy and collaboration. In R. Lubinski, L. A. Golper, & C. M. Frattali (Eds.), *Professional issues in speech-language pathology and audiology* (3rd ed.) pp. 186–198). Clifton Park, NY: Delmar Thomson.

Brown, M. R., & Sourkes, B. (2010). Psychotherapeutic approaches for children with life-threatening illnesses. In C.A. Corr and D.E. Balk (Eds.), *Children's encounters with death, bereavement, and coping* (pp. 435–454). New York: Springer.

Brownlie, E. B., Beitchman, J. H., Escobar, M., Young, A., Atkinson, L., et al. (2004). Early language impairment and young adult delinquent and aggressive behavior. *Journal of Abnormal Child Psychology, 32*(4), 453–467.

Bruni, C., Mosconi, P., Boeri, P., Gangeri, L., Pizzetti, P., Cerrai, F., et al. (2000). Evaluation of quality of life in patients with malignant dysphagia. *Tumori, 86*(2), 134–138.

Bryan, K. (2004). A preliminary study of the prevalence of speech and language difficulties in young offenders. *International Journal of Language and Communication Disorders, 39*(3), 391–400.

Bryan, T., Donahue, M., & Pearl, R. (1981). Learning disabled children's peer interactions during a small-group problem-solving task. *Learning Disability Quarterly, 4*, 13–22.

Buckman, R., & Kason, Y. (1992). *How to break bad news: A guide for health care professionals.* Baltimore: Johns Hopkins University Press.

Bugenthal, J. F. T. (1965). *The search for authenticity: An existential-analytic approach to psychotherapy.* New York: Holt, Rinehart & Winston.

Burack-Weiss, A. (2006). *The caregiver's tale: Loss and renewal in memoirs of family life.* New York: Columbia University Press.

Burgoon, J., Buller, D., & Woodall, W. (2002). *Nonverbal communication, the unspoken dialogue* (3rd ed.). New York: McGraw-Hill.

Burnard, P. (2005). *Counseling skills for health professionals* (4th ed.). New York: Chapman and Hall.

Burns, G. W. (2001). *101 healing stories: Using metaphors in therapy.* New York: Wiley.

Butler, S. F., Flasher, L. V., & Strupp. H. H. (1993). Countertransference and qualities of the psychotherapist. In N. E. Miller, L. Luborsky, J. P. Barber, & J. P. Docherty (Eds.), *Psychodynamic treatment research* (pp. 342–360). New York: Basic Books.

Byrnes, A. L., Berk, N. W., Cooper, M. E., & Marazita, M. L. (2003). Parental evaluation of informing interviews for cleft lip and/or palate. *Pediatrics, 112*(2), 308–313.

Cade, B. & O'Hanlon, W. H. (1993). *A brief guide to brief therapy.* New York: Norton.

Cadman, D., Boyle, M., & Offord, D. (1988). The Ontario Child Health Study: Social adjustment and mental health of siblings of children with chronic health problems. *Journal of Developmental and Behavioral Pediatrics, 9*, 117–121.

Cain, D. J. (2010). *Person-centered psychotherapies.* Washington, DC: American Psychological Association.

Camarata, S., Hughes, C., & Ruhl, K. (1988). Mild/moderate behaviorally disordered students: A population at-risk for language problems. *Language, Speech, and Hearing Services in the Schools, 19*, 191–200.

Canadian Stroke Network. (2006). *Canadian best practice recommendations for stroke care: 2006.* Ottawa, Canada: Heart & Stroke Foundation of Canada.

Canino, I. & Spurlock, J. (2000). *Culturally diverse children and adolescence: Assessment, diagnosis, and treatment.* New York: Guilford Press.

Cantrell, B., & Dean, C. (2005). *Down range to Iraq and back.* Wake Forest, NC: Lash & Associates.

Cantwell, D. P., & Baker, L. (1991). Association between attention deficit-hyperactivity disorder and learning disorders. *Journal of Learning Disabilities, 24*(2), 88–95.

Caporael, L. R. (1981). The paralanguage of caregiving: Baby talk to the institutionalized aged. *Journal of Personality and Social Psychology, 40*, 876–884.

Capuzzi, D., & Gross, D. R. (2003). *Counseling and psychotherapy theories and interventions.* Englewood Cliffs, NJ: Prentice Hall.

Carrigan, N., Rodger, S., & Copley, J. (2001). Parent satisfaction with a pediatric occupational therapy service: A pilot investigation. *Physical and Occupational Therapy in Pediatrics, 21*(1), 51–76.

Carter, B., & McGoldrick, M. (1999). *The expanded family life cycle: Individual, family and social perspectives.* Boston: Allyn & Bacon.

Case, J. L. (2002). *Clinical management of voice disorders*. Austin, TX: Pro-Ed.

Cassell, E. (1996). *Talking with patients*. Cambridge, MA: The MIT Press.

Castonguay, L. G., Boswell, J. F., Constantino, M. J., Goldfried, M. R., & Hill, C. E. (2010). Training implications of harmful effects of psychological treatments. *American Psychologist, 65*(1), 34–49.

Castrogiovanni, A. (2002). *Special populations: Prison populations*. Rockville, MD: ASHA.

Cautela, J. R. (1977). *Behavioral analysis forms for clinical intervention*. Champaign, IL: Research Press.

Cecchin, G. (1987). Hypothesizing, circularity, and neutrality revisited: An invitation to curiosity. *Family Process, 26*, 405–413.

Centers for Disease Control and Prevention. (1995). *CDC quality of life as a new public health measure: Behavioral risk factor surveillance system*. Atlanta, GA: U.S. Department of Health and Human Services.

Chapey, R. (Ed.). (2008). *Language intervention strategies in aphasia and related neurogenic communication disorders* (5th ed.). Philadelphia: Lippincott Williams & Wilkins.

Chaudhuri, A., & Behan, P. (2004). Fatigue in neurological disorders. *The Lancet, 363*(9413), 978–988.

Chen, A., Frankowski, R., Bishop-Leone, J., Hebert, T., Leyk, S., Lewin, J., Goepfert, H. (2001). The development and validation of a dysphagia-specific quality-of-life questionnaire for patients with head and neck cancer. *Archives of Otolaryngology: Head and Neck Surgery, 127*, 870–876.

Cherniss, C. (1980). *Staff burnout: Job stress in the human services*. Beverly Hills, CA: Sage Publications.

Chmela, K. A., & Reardon, N. (2005). *The school-age child who stutters: Working effectively with attitudes and emotions, a workbook*. Memphis, TN: The Stuttering Foundation of America.

Christner, R. W., Stewart-Allen, J., & Freeman, A. (Eds.). (2007). *Handbook of cognitive-behavior group therapy with children and adolescents*. New York: Routledge.

Ciccia, A. E., Step, M., & Turkstra, L. (2003, December). Show me what you mean. *The ASHA Leader*.

Ciminero, A. R., Calhoun, K. S., & Adams, H. E. (Eds.). (1977). *Handbook of behavioral assessment*. New York: Wiley.

Clark, D. A., & Beck, A. T. (2009). *Cognitive therapy of anxiety disorders: Science and practice*. New York: Guilford.

Clarke, P., Marshall, V., Black, S. E., and Colantonio, A. (2002). Well-being after stroke in Canadian seniors. *Stroke, 33*, 1016–1021.

Clifford, E. (1969). Parental ratings of cleft palate infants. *Cleft Palate Journal, 6*, 235–244.

Clifford, E. (1987). *The cleft palate experience: New perspectives on management*. Springfield, IL: Charles C. Thomas.

Code, C., Hemsley, G., & Herman, M. (1999). The emotional impact of aphasia. *Seminars in Speech and Language, 20*, 19–28.

Cohan, S. L., Price, J. M., & Stein, M. B. (2006). Suffering in silence: Why a developmental psychopathology perspective on selective mutism is needed. *Developmental and Behavioral Pediatrics, 27*, 341–355.

Cohen, G. & Faulkner, D. (1986). Does "elderspeak" work? The effect of intonation and stress on comprehension and recall of spoken discourse in old age. *Language and Communication, 6*, 91–98.

Cohen, M. (2002, March). *Communicate, advocate and negotiate*. Paper presented at the California Speech-Language Pathology and Audiology Annual Convention, Los Angeles.

Cohen, M. S. (1999). Families coping with childhood chronic illness: A research review. *Families, Systems and Health, 17*, 149–164.

Collett, B. R., & Speltz, M. L. (2006). Social-emotional development of infants and young children with orofacial clefts. *Infants and Young Children, 19*(4), 262–291.

Colton, J. K., Casper, J. K., & Leonard, R. (2006). *Understanding voice problems: A physiological perspective for diagnosis and treatment*. Philadelphia: Lippincott Williams & Wilkins.

Colwell, H., Mathias, S., Pasta, D., Henning, J., & Hunt, R. (1999). Questionnaire for individuals with gastroesophageal reflux disease (a validation study). *Digestive Diseases and Sciences, 44*(7), 1376–1383.

Comer, R. (2003). *Fundamentals of abnormal psychology*. New York: Freeman.

Conti-Ramsden, G., & Botting, N. (2004). Social difficulties and victimization in children with SLI at 11 years of age. *Journal of Speech, Language, and Hearing Research, 47*, 145–161.

Conti-Ramsden, G., & Dykins, J. (1991). Mother-child interactions with language impaired children and their siblings. *British Journal of Disorders of Communication, 26,* 337–354.

Conti-Ramsden, G., & Friel-Pattie, S. (1984). Mother-child dialogues: A comparison of normal and language impaired children. *Journal of Communication Disorders, 17,* 19–35.

Contour, E. (2001). *Stuttering: Its nature, diagnosis, and treatment.* Boston: Allyn & Bacon.

Conture, E. G., & Curlee, R. F. (2007). *Stuttering, its nature, diagnosis, and treatment* (3rd ed.). New York: Thieme.

Cooper, E. B. (1997). Fluency disorders. In T. A. Crowe (Ed.), *Applications of counseling in speech-language pathology and audiology* (pp. 145–166). Baltimore, MD: Williams & Wilkins.

Corey, G. (2008). *Theory and practice of counseling and psychotherapy* (8th ed.). Clifton Park, NY: Cengage Learning.

Cornis-Pop, M. (2006). A new paradigm of rehabilitation for a new generation of veterans. *The ASHA Leader, 11*(9), 6–7, 28.

Corr, C., & Balk, D. (2010). *Children's encounters with death, bereavement, and coping.* New York: Springer.

Corsini, R. J., & Wedding, D. (Eds.). (2008). *Current psychotherapies* (8th ed.). Belmont, CA: Thomson Brooks/Cole.

Corso, K. A., Bryan, C. J., Morrow, C. E., Appolonio, K. K., Kanzler, K., & Dodendorf, D. M. (2009). Managing posttraumatic stress disorder symptoms in active-duty military personnel in primary care settings. *Journal of Mental Health Counseling, 31*(2), 119–123.

Cox, D., Fitzpatrick, R., Fletcher, A., Gore, S., Spiegelhalter, D., & Jones, D. (1992). Quality-of-life assessment: Can we keep it simple? *Journal of the Royal Statistical Society, Series A., 155*(3), 353–393.

Coy, K., Speltz, M. L., & Jones, K. (2002). Facial appearance and attachment in infants with orofacial clefts: A replication. *The Cleft Palate-Craniofacial Journal, 39,* 66–72.

Craighead, L., Craighead, W., Kazdin, A., & Mahoney, M. (1994). *Cognitive behavioral interventions: An empirical approach to mental health problems.* Boston: Allyn & Bacon.

Crais, E. R. (1991). Moving from "parent involvement" to family-centered services. *American Journal of Speech Language Pathology, 1,* 5–8.

Crais, E. R. (2009). Working with families of young children with communication and language impairments: Identification and assessment. In N. Watts Pappas & S. McLeod (Eds.), *Working with families in speech-language pathology* (pp. 111–130). San Diego, CA: Plural.

Crais, E. R., & Belardi, C. (1999). Family participation in child assessment: Perceptions of families and professionals. *Infant-Toddler Intervention: The Transdisciplinary Journal, 9,* 209–238.

Crais, E. R., Roy, V. P., & Free, K. (2006). Parents' and professionals' perceptions of the implementation of family-centered practices in child assessments. *American Journal of Speech Language Pathology, 15,* 365–377.

Craske, M. (2010). *Cognitive behavioral therapy: Theories of psychotherapy.* Washington, DC: American Psychological Association.

Crisp, J., & Taylor, C. (2008). *Potter and Perry's fundamentals of nursing.* Elsevier, Australia: Chatswood.

Crits-Christoph, P., Gibbons, M. B. C., & Hearon, B. (2006). Does the alliance cause good outcome? Recommendations for future research on the alliance. *Psychotherapy: Theory, Research, Practice, Training, 43*(3), 280–285.

Crowe, T. (Ed.). (1997). *Applications of counseling in speech-language pathology and audiology.* Baltimore: Williams and Wilkins.

Crowe, T. A., Walton, J. H., & Burnett, W. J. (1990). Voice disorders in a state penitentiary. *Corrective and Social Psychiatry and Journal of Behavior Technology, 36,* 8–12.

Culpepper, B., Mendell, L, & McCarthy, P. (1994). Counseling experience and training offered by ESB-accredited programs. *ASHA, 36,* 55–57.

Curlee, R. F. (2008). Why me? In *Do you stutter: A guide for teens.* Memphis, TN: Stuttering Foundation of America.

Dahlen, E. R., & Deffenbacher, J. L. (2001). Anger management. In W. J. Lyddon & J. V. Jones, Jr. (Eds.), *Empirically supported cognitive therapies: Current and future applications* (pp. 163–181). New York: Springer.

Damboise, C. & Cardin, S. (2003). Family centered critical care: How one unit implemented a plan. *American Journal of Nursing, 103*(6), 56AA–56EE.

Daniels, S., Schroeder, M., DeGeorge, P., Corey, D., Foundas, A., & Rosenbek, J. (2009). Defining and measuring dysphagia following stroke. *American Journal of Speech-Language Pathology, 18*, 74–81.

Darley, F. L. (1955). The relationship of parental attitudes and adjustments to the development of stuttering. In W. Johnson & R. Leutinegger (Eds.), *Stuttering in children and adults*. Minneapolis: University of Minneapolis.

Dattilio, F. M., & Freeman, A. (Eds.). (2007). *Cognitive-behavioral strategies in crisis intervention* (3rd ed.). New York: Guilford.

Davalbhakta, A., & Hall, P. (2000). Impact of antenatal diagnosis in the timing and effectiveness of counseling for cleft lip and palate. *British Journal of Plastic Surgery, 53*, 298–301.

Davidson, J., & Zhang, W. (2008). Treatment of post-stroke depression with antidepressants. *The Journal of Alternative and Complementary Medicine, 14*(7), 795–796.

De Becker, G. (1997). *The gift of fear: Survival signals that protect us from violence*. New York: Little, Brown and Co.

de Shazer, S. (1988). *Clues: Investigating solutions in brief therapy*. New York: Norton.

de Shazer, S., & Dolan, Y. (2007). *More than miracles: The state of the art of solution- focused brief therapy*. Binghamton, NY: Haworth Press.

Debout, L., & Bradford, A. (1992). Cross-cultural attitudes toward speech disorders. *Journal of Speech and Hearing Research, 35*(1), 45–52.

Deffenbacher, J. L. (1999). Cognitive-behavioral conceptualization and treatment of anger. *Journal of Clinical Psychology, 55*, 295–309.

Deffenbacher, J. L. (2006). Evidence of effective treatment of anger-related disorders. In E. L. Fiendler (Ed.), *Anger-related disorders: A practitioner's guide to comparative treatments* (pp. 43–69). New York: Springer.

Deffenbacher, J. L., Oetting, E. R., & DiGiuseppe, R. A. (2002). Principles of empirically supported interventions applied to anger management. *Counseling Psychologist, 30*, 262–280.

DeJong, P., & Berg, I. (2008). *Interviewing for solutions* (3rd ed.). Pacific Grove, CA: Brooks/Cole.

Dell, C. (2002). *Treating the school-age child who stutters: A guide for clinicians*. Memphis, TN: Stuttering Foundation of America.

Dimeff, L. A., Koerner, K., & Linehan, M. M. (Eds.). (2007). *Dialectical therapy in clinical practice: Applications across disorders and settings*. New York: Guilford Press.

Dimidjian, S., & Hollon, S. D. (2010). How would we know if psychotherapy were harmful? *American Psychologist, 65*(1), 21–33.

Dindia, K., & Canary, D. J. (2006). *Sex differences and similarities in communication*. London: Routledge.

Doherty, W. J., & McDaniel, S. H. (2010). *Family therapy*. Washington, DC: American Psychological Association.

Doka, K. J. (2007). *Living with grief: Before and after the death*. Washington, DC: Hospice Foundation of America.

Dolger-Hafner, M., Bartsch, A., Trimbach, G., Zobel, I., & Witt, E. (1997). Parental reactions following the birth of a cleft child. *Journal of Orofacial Orthopedics, 58*(2), 124–133.

Dollard, J., & Miller, N. E. (1950). *Personality and psychotherapy*. New York: McGraw-Hill.

Dollinger, S. J., & Cramer, P. (1990). Children's defensive responses and emotional upset following a disaster: A projective assessment. *Journal of Personality Assessment, 54*, 116–127.

Drotar, D. (2001). Promoting comprehensive care for children with chronic health conditions and their families: Introduction to the special issue. *Children's Services: Social Policy, Research, and Practice. 4*, 157–163.

Drotar, D., Baskiewicz, A., Irwin, N., Kennel, J., & Klans, M. (1975). The adaptation of parents to the birth of an infant with a congenital malformation: A hypothetical model. *Pediatrics, 56*, 710–717.

Druss, R. G. (1995). *The psychology of illness: In sickness and in health*. Washington, DC: American Psychiatric Press.

Dummit, E. S., Klein, R. G., Tancer, N. K., Asche, B., Martin, J., & Fairbanks (1997). Systematic assessment of 50 children with selective mutism. *Journal of American Academy of Child and Adolescent Psychiatry, 36*, 653–660.

Duncan, B. L. (2010). *On becoming a better therapist*. Washington, DC: American Psychological Association.

Dundas, J. (2006). An evaluation of use of the HADS scale to screen for post-stroke depression. *British Journal of Neuroscience Nursing, 2*(8), 399–403.

Dunst, C. (2002). Family-centered practices: Birth through high school. *Journal of Special Education, 36*, 139–147.

Dunst, C., Trivette, C., & Deal, A. (1988). *Enabling and empowering families*. Cambridge, MA: Brookline Books.

Ebert, K. A., & Prelock, P. A. (1994). Teachers' perceptions of their students with communication disorders. *Language, Speech, and Hearing Services in Schools, 25*, 211–214.

Eggenberger, S. K., & Nelms, T. P. (2007). Being family: The family experience when an adult member is hospitalized with a critical illness. *Journal of Clinical Nursing, 16*, 1618–1628.

Ehren, B. J., & Lenz, B. K. (1989). Adolescents with language disorders: Special considerations in providing academically relevant language intervention. *Seminars in Speech and Language, 10*, 192–203.

Ekberg, O., Hamdy, S., Woisard, V., Wuttge-Hannig, A., & Ortega, P. (2002). Social and psychological burden of dysphagia: Its impact on diagnosis and treatment. *Dysphagia, 17*(2), 139–146.

Elder, R. A. (1995). Individual differences in young children's self-concepts: Implications for children with cleft lip and palate. In R. A. Elder (Ed.), *Developmental perspectives on craniofacial problems*. New York: Springer-Verlag.

Eliopoulos, C. (2005). *Gerontological nursing* (6th ed.). Philadelphia: Lippincott.

Elliot, R. (1994). *From stress to strength: How to lighten your load*. New York: Chelsea House.

Ellis, A., & Grieger, R. (Eds.). (1986). *Handbook of rational-emotive theory* (Vols. 1–2). New York: Springer.

Elman, R. J. (2005). Social and life participation approaches to aphasia intervention. In L. LaPointe (Ed.), *Aphasia and related neurogenic language disorders* (3rd ed.). New York: Thieme Medical.

Elman, R. J. (Ed.). (2007). *Group therapy treatment of neurogenic communication disorders: The expert clinician's approach*. San Diego, CA: Plural.

Emmons, P. G., & Anderson, L. M. (2005). *Understanding sensory dysfunction*. Philadelphia: Jessica Kingsley.

English, K. (2002a). *Counseling children with hearing impairment and their families*. Boston: Allyn & Bacon.

English, K. (2002b). Psychosocial aspects of hearing impairment. In R. Schow and M. Nerbonne (Eds.), *Introduction to audiologic rehabilitation* (4th ed., pp. 225–246). Boston: Allyn and Bacon.

Erdman, P., & Cafferty, T. (Eds.). (2003). *Attachment and family systems*. New York: Brunner-Routledge.

Evens, D., Hearn, M., Uhlemann, M., & Ivey, A. (2008). *Essential interviewing: A programmed approach to effective communication*. Pacific Grove, CA: Brooks/Cole.

Faber, A., & Mazlish, E. (1995). *How to talk so kids will listen & listen so kids will talk*. New York: Avon Books.

Faber, A., & Mazlish, E. (2005). *How to talk so teens will listen & listen so teens will talk*. New York: Avon Books.

Fallowfield, L., & Jenkins, V. (2004). Communicating sad, bad, and difficult news in medicine. *Lancet, 363*(9405), 312–319.

Farmer, J. E., Marien, W. E., Clark, M. J., Sherman, A., & Selva, T. J. (2004). Primary care supports for children with chronic health conditions: Identifying and predicting unmet family needs. *Journal of Pediatric Psychology, 29*(5), 355–367.

Farmer, R. F., & Chapman, A. L. (2008). *Behavioral interventions in cognitive behavior therapy: Practical guidance for putting theory into action*. Washington, DC: American Psychological Association.

Fava, G., & Sonino, N. (2000). Psychosomatic medicine: Emerging trends and perspectives. *Psychotherapy and Psychosomatics, 69*(4), 184–197.

Fein, M. (1993). *Integrated anger management: A common sense guide to coping with anger*. Westport, CT: Praeger.

Feldman, R. (2005). *Essentials of understanding psychology* (6th ed.). New York: McGraw-Hill.

Feltham, C. & Dryden, W. (2005). *Dictionary of counseling*. London: Whurr Publishers Ltd.

Figley, C. (2002). *Treating compassion fatigue*. New York: Brunner-Routledge.

Fisher, R., & Ury, W. (1991). *Getting to yes*. New York: Penguin Books.

Fisher, R., Ury, W., & Patton, B. (2008). *Getting to yes: Negotiating agreement without giving in*. London: Penguin.

Flannery, R. B., & Everly, G. S. (2000). Crisis intervention: A review. *International Journal of Emergency Mental Health, 2*(2), 119–125.

Fogle, P. T. (1978, November). *A study of perceptions of parental attitudes and behaviors compared with how the parents believe their children perceive them*. Paper presented at the ASHA Convention, San Francisco.

Fogle, P. T. (1998, November). Preparing a feast for the senses. *Advance for Speech-Language Pathologists and Audiologists*. King of Prussia, PA: Merion.

Fogle, P. T. (2000, April). Forensic speech-language pathology: Testifying as an expert witness. *Advance for Speech-Language Pathologists and Audiologists*. King of Prussia, PA: Merion.

Fogle, P. T. (2001, February). Professors in private practice: Rediscovering the joy of therapy. *Advance for Speech-Language Pathologists and Audiologists*. King of Prussia, PA: Merion.

Fogle, P. T. (2003, December). A practical guide for the expert witness. *Benchmark Medical Consultants Newsletter*.

Fogle, P. T. (2004). *Safety issues of neurogenic patients in the hospital and home*. Paper presented at the ASHA Convention, Philadelphia.

Fogle, P. T. (2006). *Counseling skills for speech-language pathologists and audiologists: Taking care of ourselves*. Paper presented at the New Zealand Speech Therapy Association Convention, Christchurch, NZ.

Fogle, P. T. (2008). *Foundations of communication sciences and disorders*. Clifton Park, NY: Thomson Delmar Learning.

Fogle, P. T. (2009a). *Counseling skills: Recognizing and interpreting nonverbal communication (body language, gestures, and facial expressions)*. Gaylord, MI: Northern Speech Services/National Rehabilitation Services.

Fogle, P. T. (2009b, March). Being a veteran and speech-language pathologist. *Advance for Speech-Language Pathologists and Audiologists*. King of Prussia, PA. Merion.

Fogle, P. T. (2009c). *Cognitive rehabilitation: Collaborative brain injury intervention*. Paper presented at the Asia Pacific Society for Speech, Language, and Hearing Conference, Honolulu, HI.

Fogle, P. T., Reece, R. J., & White, J. E. (2008). *The source for safety: Cognitive retraining for independent living*. East Moline, IL: LinguiSystems.

Folkman, S., & Moskowitz, J. T. (2000). Positive affect and the other side of coping. *American Psychologist, 55*(6), 647–654.

Fouad, N., & Arredondo, P. (2007). *Becoming culturally oriented: Practical advice for psychologists and educators*. Washington, DC: American Psychological Association.

Framo, J. L. (1992). *Family-of-origin-therapy: An intergenerational approach*. New York: Brunner/Mazel.

France, J., & Kramer, S. (2001). *Communication and mental illness: Theoretical and practical approaches*. Philadelphia: Jessica Kingsley.

Franck, L. S., & Callery, P. (2004). Re-thinking family-centered care across the continuum of children's healthcare. *Child: Care, Health and Development, 30*(3), 265–277.

Frank, A. (2002). *At the will of the body: Reflections on illness*. Boston: Houghton Mifflin Company.

Frank, J. (1982). Therapeutic components shared by all psychotherapies. In J. H. Harvy & M. M. Parks (Eds.), *Psychotherapy research and behavior change*. Washington, DC: American Psychological Association.

Frankl, V. (1959). *Man's search for meaning*. Boston: Allyn and Bacon.

Freeman, J., Epston, D., & Lobovits. (1997). *Playful approaches to serious problems: Narrative therapy with children and their families*. New York: Norton.

Freud, A. (1936). *The ego and the mechanisms of defense*. In *The writings of Anna Freud* (Vol. 2). New York: International Universities Press.

Freud, S. (1910). The future prospects of psychoanalytic therapy. In J. Strachey (Ed. and Trans.), *Standard edition of the complete psychological works of Sigmund Freud* (Vol. 11, pp. 139–151). London: Hogarth Press.

Freud, S. (1912/1958). The dynamics of transference. In J. Strachey (Ed. and Trans.), *The standard edition of the complete psychological works of Sigmund Freud* (Vol. 12). London: Hogarth Press.

Freud, S. (1914). Remembering, repeating and working through. In. J. Strachey (Ed. and Trans.), *The standard edition of the complete psychological works of Sigmund Freud* (Vol. 12, pp. 145–156). London: Hogarth Press.

Freud, S. (1917). Resistance and repression. In J. Strachey (Ed. and Trans.), *The standard edition of the complete psychological works of Sigmund Freud* (Vol. 12, pp. 286–301). London: Hogarth Press.

Freud, S. (1923). The ego and the id. In J. Strachey (Ed. and Trans.), *The standard edition of the complete psychological works of Sigmund Freud* (Vol. 19, pp. 1–66). London: Hogarth Press.

Friedman, J. H., & Friedman, H. (2001). Fatigue in Parkinson's disease: A nine-year follow-up. *Movement Disorders, 16*(6), 1120–1122.

Friehe, M. J., Bloedow, A., & Hesse, S. (2003). Counseling families of children with communication disorders. *Communicative Disorders Quarterly, 24*(3), 137–142.

Fromm, E. (1941). *Escape from freedom.* New York: Holt, Rinehart & Winston.

Fromm, E. (1956). *The art of loving.* New York: Bantam Books.

Fuller-Thomson, E., & Minkler, M. (2001). American grandparents providing extensive child care to their grandchildren: Prevalence and profile. *Gerontologist, 41*(2), 201–209.

Gabbard, G. O. (2005). *Psychodynamic psychiatry in clinical practice* (4th ed.). Washington, DC: American Psychiatric Press.

Gabbard, G. O., & Wilkinson, S. M. (1994). *Management of countertransference with borderline patients.* Washington, DC: American Psychiatric Press.

Gallagher-Thompson, D., & Coon, D. W. (2007). Evidence-based psychological treatments for distress in family caregivers of older adults. *Psychology and Aging, 22*(1), 37–51.

Gardner, H. (2006). *Multiple intelligences.* New York: Basic Books.

Garner, B. (Ed.). (2009). *Black's law dictionary* (9th ed.). New York: West Group.

Gaylord, M. K., Cooper, D. B., Mercado, J. M., Kennedy, J. E., Yoder, L. H., & Holcomb, J. B. (2008). Incidence of posttraumatic stress disorder and mild traumatic brain injury in burned service members: Preliminary report. *Journal of Trauma, 64*(2, Supplement), 200–205.

Gelso, C. L., & Samstag, L. W. (2008). The therapeutic relationship. In *Handbook of Counseling Psychology* (4th ed., pp. 267–287). NY: John Wiley.

George, R., & Cristiani, T. (1995). *Counseling: Theory and practice* (4th ed.). Boston: Allyn and Bacon.

Giallo, R., & Gavidia-Payne, S. (2006). Child, parent and family factors as predictors of adjustment for siblings of children with a disability. *Journal of Intellectual Disability Research, 50*(12), 937–948.

Gill, M. M. (1982). *The analysis of transference.* New York: International University Press.

Girolametto, L., & Weitzman, E. (2006). It takes two to talk—The Hanen Program for parents: Early language intervention through caregiver training. In R. McCauley & M. Fey (Eds.), *Treatment of language disorders in children* (pp. 77–103). Baltimore, MD: Paul H. Brooks.

Girolametto, L., Weitzman, E., & Greenberg, J. (2006). Facilitating language skills: In-service education for early childhood educators and preschool teachers. *Infants and Young Children, 19*, 36–48.

Gladding, S. (2009). *Counseling: A comprehensive profession* (6th ed.) Princeton, NC: Merrill.

Goetz, A. L., Gavin, W., & Lane, S. (2000). Measuring parent/professional interaction in early intervention: Validity and reliability. *Occupational Therapy Journal of Research, 20*, 221–241.

Goldenberg, I., & Goldenberg, H. (2007). *Family therapy: An overview* (7th ed.). Pacific Grove, CA: Brooks/Cole Publishing Co.

Goldfried, M. R. (1982). On the history of therapeutic integration. *Behavior Therapy, 13*, 572–593.

Goldfried, M. R., & Davison, G. C. (1976). *Clinical behavior therapy.* New York: Holt, Rinehart & Winston.

Goldfried, M. R., Davison, G. C., & McNeil, D. W. (1996). Clinical behavior therapy: Expanded edition. *Contemporary Psychology, 41*(5), 476.

Goleman, D. (1995). *Emotional intelligence: Why it can matter more than IQ.* New York: Bantam Books.

Goodman, G. S., Quas, J. A., & Ogle, C. M. (2010). Child maltreatment and memory. *Annual Review of Psychology, 61*, 325–351.

Goodwin, R. D., & Devinand, D. P. (2008). Stroke, depression, and functional health outcomes among adults in the community. *Journal of Geriatric Psychiatry and Neurology, 21*(8), 803–810.

Gordon-Brannan, M. E., & Weiss, C. E. (2007). *Clinical management of articulatory and phonological disorders.* Philadelphia: Lippincott Williams & Wilkins.

Gordon, T. (2000). *Parent effectiveness training.* New York: P. H. Wyden.

Granlund, M., Bjork-Akesson, E., & Alant, E. (2005). Family-centered early childhood intervention: New perspectives. In E. Alant & L. Lloyd (Eds.), *Augmentative and alternative communication and severe disabilities: Beyond poverty* (pp. 221–242). London: Whurr.

Green, S. E. (2007). "We're tired, not sad": Benefits and burdens of mothering a child with a disability. *Social Science and Medicine, 57*, 1361–1374.

Greenberg, J. (1999). *Sharing bad news: A module for the Hanen Program for Early Childhood Educators on sharing sensitive information with parents.* Toronto, Canada: The Hanen Center.

Greene, M. C., & Mathieson, L. (2001). *The voice and its disorders* (6th ed.). New York: Thieme.

Greenson, R. R. (1967). *The technique and practice of psychoanalysis.* Madison, CT: International Universities Press.

Gregory, H. H. (2003). *Stuttering therapy: Rationale and procedures.* Boston: Allyn and Bacon.

Groopman, J. (2004). *The anatomy of hope: How people prevail in the face of illness.* New York: Random House.

Gualtieri, L., Koriath, U., Van Bourgondien, M., & Saleeby, N. (1983). Language disorders in children referred for psychiatric service. *Journal of the American Academy of Child Psychiatry, 22*, 165–171.

Guitar, B. (2006). *Stuttering: An integrated approach to its nature and treatment* (3rd ed.). Baltimore: Williams & Wilkins.

Guitar, B. (2008). Starting to help yourself. In *Do you stutter: A guide for teens.* Memphis, TN: Stuttering Foundation of America.

Guitar, B., & Reville, J. (2006). Counseling school-age children in group therapy. In *Effective counseling in stuttering therapy.* Memphis, TN: Stuttering Foundation of America.

Gurman, A. E., & Messer, S. B. (Eds.). (2003). *Essential psychotherapies: Theory and practice.* New York: Guilford Press.

Gussy, M., & Kilpatrick, N. (2006). The self-concept of adolescents with cleft lip and palate: A pilot study using a multidimensional/hierarchical measurement instrument. *International Journal of Pediatric Dentistry, 16*(5), 335–341.

Hackney, H., & Cormier, L. (1999). *Counseling strategies and interventions* (5th ed.). Boston: Allyn and Bacon.

Hagen, C. (1998). *Rancho levels of cognitive functioning* (Rev. ed.). Downey, CA: Communication Disorders Department, Rancho Los Amigos Medical Center.

Haggen, P. (2002). Family resilience through sports: The family as a team. *Journal of individual psychology, 58*(3), 279–289.

Hahn, E. (1989). Directed home language stimulation program with infants with cleft lip and palate. In K. R. Bzoch (Ed.) *Communication disorders related to cleft lip and palate* (3rd ed.) (pp. 313–329). Boston: Little Brown & Co.

Haley, J., & Hoffman, L. (1968). *Techniques of family therapy.* New York: Basic Books.

Haley, W. E. (1997). The family caregiver's role in Alzheimer's disease. *Neurology, 48*, S25–S29.

Hall, E. T. (1996). *The hidden dimension.* Garden City, NY: Doubleday.

Hallenbeck, J. (2003). *Palliative care perspectives.* New York: Oxford University Press.

Hanna, K. & Rodger, S. (2002). Towards family-centered practice in pediatric occupational therapy: A review of the literature on parent-therapist collaboration. *Australian Occupational Therapy Journal, 49*, 14–24.

Hansson, R. O., & Stroebe, M. S. (2007). *Bereavement in late life: Coping, adaptation, and developmental influences.* Washington, DC: American Psychological Association.

Harris, S. F., Prater, M. A., Dyches, T. T., & Heath, M. A. (2009). Job stress of school-based speech-language pathologists. *Communication Disorder Quarterly, 30*(2), 103–111.

Harrison, R. L., & Westwood, M. J. (2009). Preventing vicarious traumatization of mental health therapists: Identifying protective practices. *Psychotherapy: Theory, Research, Practice, Training, 46*(2), 203–219.

Hasselkus, B. R. (1988). Meaning in family caregiving: Perspectives on caregiver/professional relationships. *The Gerontologist, 28*(5), 686–691.

Health Insurance Portability and Accountability Act (HIPAA). (1996). Office of the Federal Register, National Archives and Records Administration, United States Government Printing Office.

Hefferon, K., Grealy, M., & Mutrie, N. (2010). Transforming from cocoon to butterfly: The potential role of the body in the process of posttraumatic growth. *Journal of Humanistic Psychology, 50*(2), 224–247.

Helfer, T., Jordan, N., & Lee, R. (2005). Post deployment hearing loss in US Army soldiers seen at audiology clinics from April 1, 2003 through March 31, 2004. *American Journal of Audiology, 14*, 161–168.

Henry, W. P. (1997). Interpersonal case formulation: Describing and explaining interpersonal patterns using the structured analysis of social behaviors. In T. Eells (Ed.), *Handbook of psychotherapy case formulation*. New York: Guilford Press.

Henry, W. P., Schacht, T. E., & Strupp, H. H. (1986). Structural analysis of social behavior: Application to a study of interpersonal process in differential psychotherapeutic outcome. *Journal of Consulting and Clinical Psychology, 54*, 27–31.

Henry, W. P., Schacht, T. E., & Strupp, H. H. (1990). Patient and therapist introject, interpersonal process, and differential psychotherapy outcome. *Journal of Consulting and Clinical Psychology, 58*, 768–774.

Hess, S. A., Knox, S., & Hill, C. E. (2006). Teaching graduate students how to manage client anger: A comparison of three types of training. *Psychotherapy Research, 16*(3), 282–292.

Hibbs, E. D., & Jensen, P. S. (Eds.). (2005). *Psychosocial treatments for child and adolescent disorders: Empirically based strategies for clinical practice*. Washington, DC: American Psychological Association.

Hill, D. G. (2006). Counseling parents of children who stutter. In *Effective counseling in stuttering therapy*. Memphis, TN: Stuttering Foundation of America.

Hoffman, L. (1981). *Foundations of family therapy*. New York: Basic Books.

Hoffman, L. (2002). *Family therapy: An intimate journey*. New York: Norton.

Hoge, C. W., Castro, C. A., Messer, S. C., McGurk, D., Cotting, D. I., & Koffman, R. L. (2004). Combat duty in Iraq and Afghanistan, mental health problems, and barriers to care. *New England Journal of Medicine, 35*(1), 13–22.

Holland, A. L. (2007). *Counseling in communication disorders: A wellness perspective*. San Diego, CA: Plural.

Hollon, S. D., & Beck, A. T. (2004). Cognitive and cognitive behavioral therapies. In M. J. Lambert (Ed.), *Bergin and Garfield's handbook of psychotherapy and behavior change*. New York: John Wiley and Sons.

Holmes, R. M., & Holmes, S. T. (2005). *Suicide: Theory, practice, and investigation*. Thousand Oaks, CA: Sage.

Holmes, T., & Rahe, R. (1967). The social readjustment rating scale. *Journal of Psychosomatic Research, 11*, 213–218.

Holstein, J. A., & Gubrium, J. F. (2003). Inside interviewing: New lenses, new concerns. Thousand Oaks, CA: Sage.

Hooyman, N. R., & Kiyak, H. A. (2008). *Social gerontology: A multidisciplinary perspective* (5th ed.). Boston: Allyn and Bacon.

Horowitz, M., Marmar, C., Krupnick, J., Wilner, N., Kaltreider, N., & Wallerstein, R. (2001). *Personality styles and brief psychotherapy*. New York: Basic Books.

Hunt, O., Burden, D., Hepper, P., & Johnston, C. (2005). The psychological effects of cleft lip and palate: A systematic review. *European Journal of Orthodontics, 27*(3), 274–285.

Ievers, C., & Drotar, D. (1996). Family and parental functioning in cystic fibrosis. *Journal of Developmental and Behavioral Pediatrics. 17*, 48–55.

Iverach, L., Jones, M., O'Brian, S., Block, S., Lincoln, M., Harrison, E., et al. (2009). Screening for personality disorders among adults seeking speech treatment for stuttering. *Journal of Fluency Disorders, 34*(3), 173–186.

Ivey, A., Ivey, M. B., & Zalaquett, C. P. (2009). *Intentional interviewing and counseling: Facilitating client development in a multicultural society* (7th ed.). Clifton Park, NY: Cengage Learning.

Jeffreys, J. S. (2004). *Helping grieving people: When tears are not enough*. New York: Routledge.

Jerome, A., Fujiki, M., Brinton, B., & James, S. (2002). Self-esteem in children with specific language impairment. *Journal of Speech, Language, and Hearing Research, 45*, 700–714.

Jia, H., Damush, T. M., Quin, H., Reid, L. D., Wang, X., Young, L., & Williams, L. S. (2006). The impact of poststroke depression on healthcare use by veterans with acute stroke. *Stroke, 37*(11), 796–801.

Johnson, A., & Jacobson, B. (2006). *Medical speech-language pathology: A practitioner's guide* (2nd ed.). New York: Thieme.

Johnson, C., Beitchman, J., Young, A., Escobar, M., Atkinson, L., & Wilson, B. (1999). Fourteen-year follow-up of children with and without speech/language impairments: Speech-language stability and outcomes. *Journal of Speech and Hearing Research, 42*(3), 744–760.

Johnson, M., & Wintgens, A. (2001). *The selective mutism resource manual*. Milton Keynes, UK: Speechmark.

Johnson, S. M. (1994). *Character styles*. New York: Norton.

Johnson, W. (1939). The treatment of stuttering. *Journal of Speech Disorders, 3*, 170–176.

Joiner, T. E., Van Orden, K. A., Witte, T. K., & Rudd, M. D. (2009). *The interpersonal theory of suicide*. Washington, DC: American Psychological Association.

Kabat-Zinn, J. (2003). *Coming to our senses: Healing ourselves and the world through mindfulness*. New York: Hyperion Press.

Kahn, M. (1999). *Between therapist and client: The new relationship*. New York: W. H. Freeman and Company.

Kapp-Simon, K. A., & McGuire, D. E. (1997). Observed social interaction patterns in adolescents with and without craniofacial conditions. *Cleft Palate-Craniofacial Journal, 34*, 380–384.

Kappes, N. (1995). Matrix. In D. Meyer (Ed.), *Reflections on raising a child with a disability* (pp. 13–28). Bethesda, MD: Woodbine House.

Kashinath, S., Woods, J., & Goldstein, H. (2006). Enhancing generalized teaching strategy use in daily routines by parents of children with autism. *Journal of Speech, Language, and Hearing Research, 49*, 466–485.

Katz, S. (2002). When the child's illness is life threatening: Impact on the parents. *Pediatric Nursing, 28*(5), 453–463.

Katz, N., & Pattarini, N. (2008). Interest-based negotiation: An essential business and communication tool for the public relations counselor. *Journal of Communication Management, 12*(1), 88–97.

Katz, R. C., Flasher, L., Cacciapaglia, H., & Nelson, S. (2001). The psychosocial impact of cancer and lupus: A cross-validation study that extends the generality of "benefit finding" in patients with chronic disease. *Journal of Behavioral Medicine, 24*(6), 561–571.

Kaye, K., & Charney, R. (1981). Conversational asymmetry between mothers and children. *Journal of Child Language, 8*, 35–49.

Kazak, A. E. (2001). Comprehensive care for children with cancer and their families: A social ecological framework guiding research, practice, and policy. *Children's Services: Social Policy, Research, and Practice, 4*(4), 217–233.

Kazak, A. E., Segal-Andrews, A. M., & Johnson, K. (1995). Pediatric psychology research and practice: A family/systems approach. In M. Roberts (Ed.), *Handbook of pediatric psychology* (pp. 84–104). New York: Guilford.

Kelly, D. (2001). *Central auditory processing disorder: Identification and intervention*. Gaylord, MI: Northern Speech-National Rehab.

Kelly, K. (1991). Theoretical integration is the future for mental health counseling. *Journal of Mental Health Counseling, 13*(1), 106–111.

Keltner, N., Schwecke, L., & Bostrom, C. (2007). *Psychiatric nursing* (5th ed.). St. Louis, MO: Mosby.

Kenyon, B. (2001). Current research in children's conception of death: A critical review. *Omega: Journal of Death and Dying, 43*, 63–91.

Kernberg, O. (1965). Notes on countertransference. *Journal of the American Psychoanalytic Association, 13*, 38–56.

Kiesler, D. J. (1982). Confronting the client-therapist in psychotherapy. In J. Anchin & D. Kiesler (Eds.), *Handbook of interpersonal psychotherapy*. New York: Pergamon Press.

Kiesler, D. J. (1988). *Therapeutic metacommunication: Therapist impact disclosure as feedback in psychotherapy*. Palo Alto, CA: Consulting Psychologist Press.

Kiesler, D. J. (1996). *Contemporary interpersonal theory and research: Personality, psychopathology, and psychotherapy*. New York: Wiley & Sons.

Kincer, K., Zipper, J., Crenshaw, J., & Solley. Giving bad news. Retrieved February 6, 2010, from http://www.uky.edu (Stanford website).

Kindermann, S. S., & Brown, G. C. (1997). Depression and memory in the elderly: A meta-analysis. *Journal of clinical and experimental neuropsychology, 19*(5), 625–642.

King, G., Cathers, T., King, S., & Rosenbaum, P. (2001). Major elements of parents' satisfaction and dissatisfaction with pediatric rehabilitation services. *Children's Health Care, 30*, 111–134.

King, G., Rosenbaum, P., & King, S. (1997). Evaluating family-centered service using a measure of parents' perceptions. *Child: Care, Health, and Development, 23*(1), 47–62.

Klerman, G. L., & Weissman, M. M. (Eds.). (1993). *New application of interpersonal therapy*. Washington, DC: American Psychiatric Press.

Knijnik, D. Z., Salum, G. A., Blanco, C., Moraes, C., Hauck, S., Mombach, C. K., et al. (2009). Defense style changes with the addition of psychodynamic group therapy to clonazepam in social anxiety disorder. *Journal of Nervous and Mental Disease, 197*(7), 547–551.

Koepp-Baker, H., & Harkins, C. (1936). *The [cleft palate] child we have forgotten*. Philipsburg, PA: The Women's Club of Philipsburg, Pennsylvania.

Kottler, J. (2010). *On being a therapist* (4th ed.). San Francisco: Jossey-Bass.

Kottler, J., & Blau, D. (1989). *The imperfect therapist: Learning from failure in therapeutic practice*. San Francisco: Jossey-Bass.

Kranowitz, C. S. (2005). *The out-of-sync child: Recognizing and coping with sensory processing disorder*. New York: Skylight Press.

Kriege, M. (1993, October). *Managing the behavioral challenges of patients with traumatic brain injury and/or CVA: A workshop for rehabilitation specialists*. Paper presented at a workshop on Managing the Unmanageable, Long Beach, CA.

Krueckeberg, S., Kapp-Simon, K., & Ribordy, S. (1993). Social skills of preschool children with and without craniofacial anomalies. *Cleft Palate-Craniofacial Journal, 30,* 475–481.

Kubler-Ross, E. (1969). *On death and dying*. New York: Macmillan Publishing Co.

Kummer, A. W. (2008). *Cleft palate and craniofacial anomalies: Effects on speech and resonance* (2nd ed.) Clifton Park, NY: Thomson Delmar Learning.

La Greca, A., Silverman, W., Vernberg, E., & Roberts, M. (2002). *Helping children cope with disaster and terrorism*. Washington, DC: American Psychological Association.

Lafond, D., DeGiovani, R., Joanette, Y., Ponzio, J., & Sarno, T. (1993). *Living with aphasia: Psychological issues*. San Diego, CA: Singular.

Lambert, K. (2008). *Lifting depression: A neuroscientist's hands-on approach to activating your brain's healing power*. New York: Basic Books.

Lambert, M. J. (2004). *Bergin and Garfield's handbook of psychotherapy and behavior change* (5th ed.). New York: Wiley.

Lang, P., & McTeague, L. (2009). The anxiety disorder spectrum: Fear imagery, physiological reactivity and differential diagnosis. *Anxiety, Stress, and Coping, 22*(1), 5–25.

Langdon, H. (2002). Communicating effectively with clients during a speech-language pathologists/interpreter conference: Results of a survey. *Contemporary Issues in Communication Science and Disorders, 29,* 17–34.

Langlois, J. H., & Stephen, C. (1977). The effects of physical attractiveness and ethnicity on children's behavioral attributions and peer preferences. *Child Development, 48,* 1694–1698.

Langmore, S. E. (2000). An important tool for measuring quality of life. *Dysphagia, 15*(3), 134–135.

Lansdown, R. (2000). Meeting the psychosocial impact of facial disfigurement: Developing a clinical service for children and families. *Clinical Child Psychology and Psychiatry, 5*(4), 497–512.

LaPointe, L. L. (2005). *Aphasia and related neurogenic language disorders* (3rd ed.). New York: Thieme.

Larson, E. (1998). Reframing the meaning of disability to families: The embrace of paradox. *Social Science and Medicine, 47*(7), 865–875.

Law, J., Garrett, Z., & Nye, C. (2003). Speech and language therapy interventions for children with primary speech and language delay or disorder. *Cochrane Database of Systematic Reviews, 3,* Art. No.: CD004110. DOI: 10.1002/14651858.CD004110.

Law, M., Hanna, S., Hurley, P., King, S., Kertoy, M., & Rosenbaum, P. (2003). Factors affecting family-centered service delivery for children with disabilities. *Child: Care, Health, and Development, 29,* 357–366.

Lawrence-Lightfoot, S. (2003). Delivering difficult news to parents: Guidelines for school counselors. *Child: Care, Health and Development, 20,* 101–113.

Lazarus, A. (1996). The utility and futility of combining treatments in psychotherapy. *Clinical Psychology: Science and Practice, 3*(1), 59–68.

Lazarus, A. & Beutler, L. (1993). On technical eclecticism. *Journal of Counseling and Development, 71,* 381–385.

Leiter, V. (2004). Dilemmas in sharing care: Maternal provision of professionally driven therapy for children with disabilities. *Social Science and Medicine, 58,* 837–849.

Leonard, B. J., Brust, J. D., Abrahams, G., & Sielaff, B. (1991). Self-concept of children and adolescents with cleft lip and/or palate. *The Cleft Palate-Craniofacial Journal, 28,* 347–353.

Levenson, H. (1995). *Time-limited dynamic psychotherapy: A guide to clinical practice*. New York: Basic Books.

Levenson, H. (2010). *Brief dynamic therapy*. Washington, DC: American Psychological Association.

Levenson, H., Butler, S. F., Powers, T. A., & Beitman, B. D. (2002). *Concise guide to brief dynamic and interpersonal therapy*. Washington, DC: American Psychiatric Publishing, Inc.

Levine, M. (2002). *A mind at a time*. New York: Simon & Schuster.

Lew, H. L., Poole, J. H., Alvarez, S., & Moore, W. (2005). Soldiers with occult traumatic brain injury. *American Journal of Physical Medicine and Rehabilitation, 84*(6), 393–398.

Lew, H. L., Poole, J. H., Vanderploeg, R. D., Goodrich, G. L., Dekelboum, S., Guillory, S. B., et al. (2007). Program development and defining characteristics of returning military in a VA polytrauma network site. *Journal of Rehabilitation Research & Development, 44*, 1027–1034.

Lewis, K. E., & Goldberg, L. L. (1997). Measurement of temperament in the identification of children who stutter. *European Journal of Disorders of Communication, 32*, 441–448.

Leys, D., Bandu, L., Henon, H., Lucas, C., Mounier-Vehier, F., Rondepierre, P., & Godefrom, O. (2002). Clinical outcomes in 287 consecutive adults (15 to 45 years) with ischemic stroke. *Neurology, 59*, 26–33.

Lightsey, O. R., & Sweeney, J. (2008). Meaning in life, emotion-oriented coping, generalized self-efficacy, and family cohesion as predictors of family satisfaction among mothers of children with disabilities. *The Family Journal, 16*(3), 212–221.

Linehan, M. M. (1993). *Cognitive-behavioral treatment of borderline personality disorder.* New York: Guilford Press.

Lingiardi, V., Lonati, C., Delucchi, F., Fossati, A., Vanzulli, L. and Maffei, C. (1999). Defense mechanisms and personality disorders. *Journal of Nervous and Menal Disease, 187*(4), 224–228.

Lloyd, M., & Bor, R. (2004). *Communication skills for medicine.* Edinburgh, UK: Churchill Livingston.

Lubinski, R., Golper, L. A., & Frattali, C. (2007). *Professional issues in speech-language pathology and audiology* (3rd ed.). Clifton Park, NY: Thomson Delmar Learning.

Lubinski, R. & Orange, J. B. (2000). A framework for assessment and treatment of functional communication in dementia. In L. Worral & C. Frattali (Eds.), *Neurogenic communication disorders: A functional approach.* New York: Thieme.

Lukash, F. N. (2002). Children's art as a helpful index of anxiety and self-esteem with plastic surgery. *Plastic and Reconstructive Surgery, 109*(6), 1777–1786.

Luper, H. L. (2008). Some helpful attitudes underlying success in therapy. In *Advice to those who stutter* (2nd ed.). Memphis, TN: Stuttering Foundation of America.

Luria, A. R. (1973). *The man with a shattered world.* London: Jonathan Cape.

Luterman, D. (1987). *Deafness in the family.* Boston: Little, Brown.

Luterman, D. (1995). *In the shadows: Living and coping with a loved one's chronic illness.* Bedford, MA: Jade Press.

Luterman, D. (2008). *Counseling persons with communication disorders and their families* (5th ed.). Austin, TX: Pro-Ed.

Macharey, G., & von Suchodeletz, W. (2008). Perceived stigmatization of children with speech-language impairments and their parents. *Folia Phoniatrica and Logopedics, 30*, 256–263.

Mahoney, M. J. (1974). *Cognitive and behavior modification.* Cambridge, MA: Ballinger.

Mahoney, M. J. (2004). *Cognitive and constructive psychotherapies: Theory, research, and practice.* New York: Springer.

Malatesta-Magal, C., Jonas, R., Shepard, B., & Culver, L. C. (1992). Type A behavior pattern and emotion expression in younger and older adults. *Psychology and Aging, 7*, 551–561.

Malkin, J. (2002). *Medical and dental space planning: A comprehensive guide to design.* Hoboken, NJ: Wiley.

Manguno-Mire, G., Sautter, F. J., Lyons, J., Myers, L., Perry, D., Sherman, M., et al. (2007). Psychological distress and burden among female partners of combat veterans with PTSD. *Journal of Nervous and Mental Diseases, 195*, 144–151.

Manning, W. (2010). *Clinical decision making in fluency disorders* (3rd ed.). Clifton Park, NY: Cengage Delmar Learning.

Manning, W., Dailey, D., & Wallace, S. (1984). Attitude and personality characteristics of older stutterers. *Journal of Fluency Disorders, 9*, 207–215.

Marcusson, A. (2002). Facial appearance in adults who had cleft lip and palate treated in childhood. *Scandinavian Journal of Plastic and Reconstructive Surgery and Hand Surgery, 35*(1), 16–23.

Marcusson, A., Akerlind, I., & Paulin, G. (2001). Quality of life in adults with repaired complete cleft lip and palate. *The Cleft Palate-Craniofacial Journal, 38*(4), 379–385.

Margo, R. (2006). *After a parent's suicide: Helping children heal.* Sebastopol, CA: Healing Hearts Press.

Martin, D. (2000). *Counseling and therapy skills* (2nd ed). Prospect Heights, IL: Therapy Press.

Martin, D. J., Garske, J. P., & Davis, M. K. (2000). Relation of the therapeutic alliance with outcome and other variables: A meta-analytic review. *Journal of Consulting and Clinical Psychology, 68,* 438–450.

Martin, R. C., & Dahlen, E. R. (2005). Cognitive emotion regulation in the prediction of depression, anxiety, stress, and anger. *Personality and Individual Differences, 39,* 1249–1260.

Martin, T. & Doka, K. (1996). Masculine grief. In K. Doka (Ed.), *Living with grief: After sudden loss.* Washington, DC: Hospice Foundation of America.

Maslach, C. (2003). Job burnout: New directions in research and intervention. *Current Directions in Psychological Science, 12,* 189–192.

Maslach, C., & Leiter, M. P. (1997). *The truth about burnout: How organizations cause personal stress and what to do about it.* San Francisco: Jossey-Bass.

Mast, V. R. (1952). Level of aspiration as a method of studying personality of adult stutterers. *Speech Monographs, 19,* 196.

Masterson, J. F., & Lieberman, A. R. (2004). *A therapist's guide to the personality disorders: The Masterson approach.* Phoenix, AZ: Zeig, Tucker, and Theisen.

Matsakis, A. (1998). *Managing client anger: What to do when a client is angry at you.* Oakland, CA: New Harbinger.

Mattas-Curry, L. (2000). Eight factors found critical in assessing suicide risk. *Monitor on Psychology, 31*(2), 17.

Maurer, J., & Martin, D. (2001). Counseling the older adult who is hearing impaired. In R. Hull (Ed.), *Aural rehabilitation: Serving children and adults* (3rd ed., pp. 337–345). San Diego, CA: Singular.

Maxmen, J., & Ward, N. (1995). *Essential psychopathology and its treatment* (2nd ed.). New York: W. W. Norton and Company.

May, R. (1953). *Man's search for himself.* New York: Norton.

May, R. (Ed.). (1961). *Existential psychology.* New York: Random House.

May, R. (1975). *The courage to create.* New York: Norton.

May, R. (1994). *The discovery of being.* New York: Norton.

May, R., Remen, N., Young, D., & Berland, W. (1985). The wounded healer. *Saybrook Review, 5,* 84–93.

McBeth, J., & Silman, A. (2001). The role of psychiatric disorders in fibromyalgia. *Current Rheumatology Reports, 3*(2), 157–164.

McCann, I. L., & Pearlman, L. A. (1990). Vicarious traumatization: A contextual model for understanding the effects of trauma on helpers. *Journal of Traumatic Stress, 3,* 131–149.

McDevitt, S. C., & Carey, W. B. (1978). The measurement of temperament in 3 7-year-old children. *Journal of Child Psychology and Psychiatry and Allied Disciplines, 19,* 245–253.

McGonigel, M., Kaufman, J., & Johnson, B. (Eds.). (1991). *Guidelines and recommended practices for the individualized family service plan* (2nd ed.). Bethesda, MD: Association for the Care of Children's Health.

McHorney, C. A., Martin-Harris, B., Robbins, J., & Rosenbek, J. (2006). Clinical validity of the SWAL-QOL and SWAL-CARE outcome tools with respect to bolus flow measures. *Dysphagia, 21*(3), 141–148.

McHorney, C. A., Robbins, J., Lomax, K., Rosenbek, J. C., Chignell, K. A., Kramer, A. E., & Bricker, D. E. (2002). The SWAL-QOL and SWAL-CARE outcomes took for oropharyngeal dysphagia in adults: III. Documentation of reliability and validity. *Dysphagia, 17*(2), 97–114.

McLaughlin, E., Lincoln, M., & Adamson, B. (2008). Speech-language pathologists' views on attrition from the profession. *International Journal of Speech-Language Pathology, 10*(3), 156–168.

McLean, M., & Crais, E. (2004). Procedural considerations in assessing infants and toddlers with disabilities. In M. McLean, M. Wolery, & D. Bailey (Eds.), *Assessing infants and preschoolers with special needs* (3rd ed., pp. 45–70). Upper Saddle River, NJ: Pearson Merrill Prentice-Hall.

McWilliam, R. A., Synder, P., Harbin, G., Porter, P., & Munn, D. (2000). Professionals' and families' perceptions of family-centered practices in infant-toddler services. *Early Education and Development, 11*(4), 519–538.

McWilliam, R. A., Tocci, L., & Harbin, G.L. (1998). Family-centered services: Service providers' discourse and behavior. *Topics in Early Childhood Special Education, 18,* 206–221.

McWilliams, B. J., & Paradise, J. L. (1973). Educational, occupational, and marital status of cleft palate adults. *Cleft Palate Journal, 10,* 223–229.

Meichenbaum, D. (1999). *Cognitive-behavior modification.* New York: Plenum.

Meir, S., & Davis, S. (2000). *The elements of counseling* (2nd ed.). Pacific Grove, CA: Brooks/Cole.

Menahem, S. (1987). Teaching students of medicine to listen: The misdiagnosis from a hidden agenda. *Journal of the Royal Society of Medicine, 80*(6), 343–346.

Meretoja, R., Isoaho, H., Leino-Kilpi, H., & O'Neil, E. (2004). Parents' experiences of having a child with cleft lip and palate. *Journal of Advanced Nursing, 47*(2), 120–123.

Messer, S. B. (2004). Evidence-based practice: Beyond empirically supported treatments. *Professional Psychology: Research and Practice, 35*, 580–588.

Michallet, B., Tetreault, S., & Dorze, G. (2003). The consequences of severe aphasia on the spouses of aphasic people: A description of the adaptation process. *Aphasiology, 17*(19), 835–859.

Middleton, G., Lass, N., Starr, P., & Pannbacker, M. (1986). Survey of public awareness and knowledge of cleft palate. *Cleft Palate Journal, 10*, 367.

Millard, T., & Richman, L. C. (2001). Different cleft conditions, facial appearance, and speech: Relationship to psychological variables. *The Cleft Palate-Craniofacial Journal, 38*, 68–75.

Miller, S. Q., & Madison, C. L. (1984). Public school voice clinics, Part II: Diagnosis and recommendations—a 10-year review. *Language-Speech-Hearing Services in Schools, 15*, 58–63.

Miller, T. (2010). *Handbook of stressful transitions across the life span*. New York: Springer.

Millon, T., & Davis, R. (2004). *Personality disorders in modern life*. Hoboken, NJ: Wiley.

Minke, K., & Scott, M. (1995). Parent-professional relationships in early intervention: A qualitative investigation. *Topics in Early Childhood Special Education, 15*(3), 335–352.

Minuchin, S. (1974). *Families and family therapy*. Cambridge, MA: Harvard University Press.

Minuchin, S. (1978). *Psychosomatic families*. Cambridge, MA: Harvard University Press.

Minuchin, S., Nichols, M. P., & Lee, W. Y. (2007). *Assessing families and couples*. Boston: Pearson Education.

Mitrani, V. B., & Czaja, S. J. (2000). Family-based therapy for dementia caregivers: Clinical observations. *Aging Mental Health, 4*(3), 200–209.

Mohammed, J., & Girvin, J. P. (2002). The communication of neurological bad news to parents. *Canadian Journal of Neurological Sciences, 29*, 78–82.

Monat, A., & Lazarus, R. S. (1991). *Stress and coping: An anthology*. New York: Columbia Universities Press.

Moore, M. (2001). Amid chaos, Air Force major finds her role. *The ASHA Leader, 6*(20), 6.

Moore, R. (1999). *The creation of reality in psychoanalysis: A view of the contributions of Donald Spence, Roy Schafer, Robert Stolorow, Irwin Z. Hoffman and beyond*. Hillsdale, NJ: Analytic Press.

Mora, A. G., Ritenour, A. E., Wade, C. E., Holcomb, J. B., Blackbourne, L. H., & Gaylord, K. M. (2009). Posttraumatic stress disorder in combat casualties with burns sustaining primary blast and concussive injuries. *Journal of Trauma, 66*(4), 178–185.

Morrison, J. (1997). *Psychological symptoms that mask medical disorders*. New York: Guilford Press.

Morrison, J. (2008). *The first interview, revised for DSM-IV*. New York: Guilford Press.

Morrison, J., & Anders, T. (2001). *Interviewing children and adolescents: Skills and strategies for effective DSM-IV diagnosis*. New York: The Guilford Press.

Mosak, H., & Maniacci, M. (1998). *Tactics in counseling and psychotherapy*. Itasca, IL: F.E. Peacock Publishers, Inc.

Moursund, J., & Erskine, R. (2003). *Integrative psychotherapy: The art and science of relationship*. Pacific Grove, CA: Brooks/Cole.

Mueser, K. T., Rosenberg, S. D., & Rosenberg, H. J. (2009). *Treatment of posttraumatic stress disorder in special populations: A cognitive restructuring program*. Washington, DC: American Psychological Association.

Muran, J. C, Safran, J. D., Gorman, B. S., Samstag, L. W., Eubanks-Carter, C., & Winston, A. (2009). The relationship of early alliance ruptures and their resolution to process and outcome in three time-limited psychotherapies for personality disorders. *Psychotherapy: Theory, Research, Practice, Training, 46*(2), 233–248.

Murray, F. P. (2008). Toward freer speech. In *Advice to those who stutter* (2nd ed.). Memphis, TN: Stuttering Foundation of America.

Musiek, F. & Chermak, G. (1997). *Central auditory processing disorders: New perspectives*. San Diego, CA: Singular.

Nagy, T. F. (2005). *Ethics in plain English: An illustrative casebook for psychologists* (2nd ed.). Washington, DC: American Psychological Association.

Nath, U., Ben-Shlomo, Y., Thomson, R., Lees, A., & Burn, D. (2003). Clinical features and natural history of progressive supranuclear palsy. *Neurology, 60,* 910–916.

Nelson, L. A. (2006). How does our home life influence his stuttering? In *Stuttering and your child: Questions and answers.* Memphis, TN: Stuttering Foundation of America.

Niebuhr, R. (1987). *The essential Reinhold Niebuhr: Selected essays and addresses.* New Haven, CT: Yale University Press.

Nippold, M. A. (2001). Adolescents with language disorders: An underserved population. *New Zealand Journal of Speech-Language Therapy, 55,* 27–32.

Nissenbaum, M. S., Tollefson, N., & Reece, R. M. (2002). The interpretive conference: Sharing a diagnosis of autism with families. *Focus on Autism and Other Developmental Disabilities, 17,* 40–43.

Noam, G. G., & Recklitis, C. J. (1990). The relationship between defenses and symptoms in adolescent psychopathology. *Journal of Personality Assessment, 54,* 311–327.

Norcross, J. C. (2002). *Psychotherapy relationships that work: Therapist contributions and responsiveness to patients.* New York: Oxford University Press.

Norcross, J. C., & Guy, J. D. (2007). *Leaving it at the office.* New York: Guilford Press.

Norcross, J., & Newman, C. (2005). Psychotherapy integration: Setting the context. In J. Norcross & M. Goldfried (Eds.), *Handbook of psychotherapy integration* (pp. 3–45). New York: Basic Books.

Norcross, J. & Prochaska, J. (1988). A study of eclectic (and integrative) views revisited. *Professional Psychology: Research and Practice, 19*(2), 170–174.

Novak, J. (2002). Counseling: An approach for speech-language pathologists. *Contemporary Issues in Communication Science and Disorders, 29,* 79–90.

Nystul, M. (2005). *Introduction to counseling: An art and science perspective* (2nd ed). Boston: Allyn and Bacon.

Olson, T. R., Presniak, M. D., & MacGregor, M. W. (2009). Differentiation of depression and anxiety groups using defense mechanisms. *Journal of Nervous and Mental Disease, 197*(11), 834–840.

Orlinsky, D. E., Botermans, J. F., & Ronnestad, M. H. (2001). Towards an empirically grounded model of psychotherapy training: Five thousand therapists rate influences on their development. *Australian Psychologist, 36,* 139–148.

Ortony, A. (1979). *Metaphor and thought* (2nd ed.). Cambridge, UK: Cambridge University Press.

Oyler, M. E., & Ramig, P. T. (1996). *Vulnerability in stuttering children.* Session presented at the annual convention of the American Speech-Language-Hearing Association, San Francisco.

Palazzoli, M. S., Boscolo, L., Cecchin, G., & Prata, G. (1980). Hypothesizing-circularity-neutrality: Three guidelines for the conduct of the session. *Family Process, 19,* 3–12.

Palmieri, A., Abrahams, S., Soraru, G., Mattiuzzi, L., D'Ascenzo, C., Pegoraro, E., & Angelini, C. (2009). Emotional lability in motor neuron disease/amyotrophic lateral sclerosis: Relationship to cognition and psychopathology and impact on caregivers. *Journal of the Neurological Sciences, 278*(1), 16–20.

Parkinson, K., & Rae, J. (1996). The understanding and use of counseling by speech-language therapists at different levels of experience. *European Journal of Disorders of Communication 32*(2), 140–152.

Parks, S. M., & Novielli, K. D. (2000). A practical guide to caring for caregivers. *American Family Physician, 62,* 2613–2621.

Patel, Z., & Ross, E. (2003). Reflections of the cleft experience by South African adults: Use of qualitative methodology. *The Cleft Palate-Craniofacial Journal, 40*(5), 471–480.

Patterson, C. (1986). *Theories of counseling and psychology.* New York: Harper & Row.

Patterson, J. M. (2002). Understanding family resilience. *Journal of Clinical Psychology, 58*(3), 233–246.

Patterson, J., Budd, J., Goetz, D., & Warwick, W. (1993). Family correlates of a ten-year pulmonary health trend in cystic fibrosis. *Pediatrics, 91*(2), 383–389.

Patterson, J., Garwick, A., Bennett, C. F., & Blum, R. W. (1997). Social support in families of children with chronic conditions: Supportive and nonsupportive behaviors. *Journal of Developmental and Behavioral Pediatrics, 18*(6), 383–391.

Paul, D. R., Frattali, C. M., Holland, A. L., Thompson, C. K., Caperton, C. J., & Slater, S. C. (2004). *Quality of communication life scale.* Bethesda, MD: American Speech-Language-Hearing Association.

Paul, R. (2006). *Language disorders from infancy through adolescence: Assessment and intervention* (3rd ed.). St. Louis, MO: Mosby.

Pedersen, P. B., Crethar, H. C., & Carlson, J. (2008). *Inclusive cultural empathy: Making relationships central in counseling and psychotherapy.* Washington, DC: American Psychological Association.

Pedersen, P., Draguns, J., Lonner, W., & Trimble, J. (Eds.). (2002). *Counseling across cultures* (5th ed.). Thousand Oaks, CA: Sage.

Pelchat, D., Lefebrie, H., & Perreault, M. (2003). Differences and similarities between mothers' and fathers' experiences of parenting a child with a disability. *Journal of Child Health Care, 7,* 231–247.

Penn, P. (1992). Feed-forward: Future questions, future maps. *Child Welfare Journal, 71*(1), 19–35.

Peppard, R. C. (2000). Functional falsetto. In J. C. Stemple (Ed.), *Voice therapy: Clinical studies.* Clifton Park, NY: Thomson Delmar Learning.

Perlmann, R., & Berko-Gleason, J. (1994). The neglected role of fathers in children's communicative development. *Seminars in Speech and Language, 14,* 314–324.

Persons, J. B., Davidson, J., & Tompkins, M. A. (2001). *Essential components of cognitive-behavior therapy for depression.* Washington, DC: American Psychological Association.

Persson, M., Aniansson, G., Becker, M., & Svensson, H. (2002). Self-concept and introversion with cleft lip and palate. *Scandinavian Journal of Plastic and Reconstructive Surgery and Hand Surgery, 36*(1), 24–27.

Peter, J. P., & Chinsky, R. (1974). Sociological aspects of cleft palate adults: Marriage. *Cleft Palate Journal, 11,* 295–309.

Petersen, R. (2002). *Mayo Clinic on Alzheimer's disease.* Rochester, MN: Mayo Clinic.

Peterson-Falzone, S. J., Hardin-Jones, M. J., & Karnell, M. P. (2010). *Cleft palate speech* (4th edn.). St. Louis, MO: Mosby.

Pillemer, F. G., & Cook, K. V. (1989). The psychosocial adjustment of pediatric craniofacial patients after surgery. *Cleft Palate Journal, 26*(3), 201–207.

Pipes, R. & Davenport, D. (1998). *Introduction to psychotherapy: Common clinical wisdom* (2nd ed.). Englewood Cliffs, NJ: Prentice Hall.

Plante, T. G. (2009). *Spiritual practices in psychotherapy: Thirteen tools for enhancing psychological health.* Washington, DC: American Psychological Association.

Pope, A. W., & Snyder, H. T. (2004). Psychosocial adjustment in children and adolescents with a craniofacial anomaly: Age and sex patterns. *The Cleft Palate-Craniofacial Journal, 42,* 4–12.

Pope, A. W., & Ward, J. (1997a). Factors associated with peer social competence in preadolescents with craniofacial anomalies. *Journal of Pediatric Psychology, 22,* 455–470.

Pope, A. W., & Ward, J. (1997b). Self-perceived facial appearance and psychosocial adjustment in preadolescents with craniofacial anomalies. *The Cleft Palate-Craniofacial Journal, 34,* 396–401.

Potter, M. L. (2006). Loss, suffering, grief, and bereavement. In M. Matzo & D. Sherman (Eds.), *Providing competent nursing care at the end-of-life.* New York: Springer.

Pound, P., Parr, S., Lindsay, J., & Woolf, C. (2000). *Beyond aphasia: Therapies for living with communication disability.* Bicester, UK: Winslow.

Prizant, B., Audet, L., Burke, G., Hummel, L., Maher, S., & Theadore, G. (1990). Communication disorders and emotional and behavioral disorders in children and adolescents. *Journal of Speech and Hearing Disorders, 55,* 179–192.

Prizant, B., & Meyer, E. C. (1993). Socio-emotional aspects of communication disorders in young children and their families. *American Journal of Speech-Language Pathology, 2,* 56–71.

Prochaska, J., & Norcross, J. (2009). *Systems of psychotherapy: A transtheoretical analysis* (8th ed.). Pacific Grove, CA: Thomson-Brooks/Cole.

Prokhorov, A. V., Perry, C., Kelder, S., & Klepp, K. (1993). Lifestyle values of adolescents: Results from the Minnesota Heart Health Youth Program. *Adolescence, 28,* 119–127.

Pyszczynski, T., Solomon, S., & Greenberg, J. (2003). *In the wake of 9/11: The psychology of terror.* Washington, DC: American Psychological Association.

Ramig, P. R. (2008). Don't ever give up! In *Advice to those who stutter* (2nd ed.). Memphis, TN: Stuttering Foundation of America.

Ramig, P. R., & Dodge, D. M. (2010). *The child and adolescent stuttering treatment and activity resource guide* (2nd ed.). Clifton Park, NY: Cengage Delmar Learning.

Rammage, L., Morrison, M., & Nichol, H. (2001). *Management of the voice and its disorders* (2nd ed.). Clifton Park, NY: Thomson Delmar Learning.

Ramstad, T., Ottem, E., & Shaw, W. (1995). Psychosocial adjustment in Norwegian adults who had undergone standardized treatment of complete cleft lip and palate. *Scandinavian Journal of Plastic and Reconstructive Surgery, 29,* 251–257.

Reddy, L. A., Files-Hall, T. M., & Schaefer, C. E. (2005). *Empirically-based play interventions for children.* Washington, DC: American Psychological Association.

Reed, V. A. (2010). *An introduction to children with language disorders* (4th ed.) Boston: Pearson/Allyn and Bacon.

Reiter, M. D. (2008). *Therapeutic interviewing: Essential skills and contexts of counseling.* Boston: Pearson/Allyn and Bacon.

Rescorla, L., & Achenbach, T. (2002). Use of the Language Development Survey in a national probability sample of children 18 to 35 months old. *Journal of Speech, Language, and Hearing Research, 45,* 733–743.

Rice, M. L., Hadley, P. A., & Alexander, A. L. (1993). Social biases toward children with speech and language impairments: A correlative-causal model of language limitations. *Applied Psycholinguistics, 14,* 455–471.

Richman, L., & Millard, T. (1997). Cleft lip and palate: Longitudinal behavior and relationships of cleft conditions to behavior and achievement. *Journal of Pediatric Psychology, 22*(4), 487–494.

Ridley, C. R., & Lingle, D. W. (1996). Cultural empathy in multicultural counseling. In P. B. Pedersen, J. G. Draguns, W. J. Lonner, & J.E. Trimble (Eds.), *Counseling across cultures* (4th ed., pp. 21–46). Thousand Oaks, CA: Sage.

Riley, J. (2002). Counseling: An approach for speech-language pathologists. *Contemporary Issues in Communication Science and Disorders, 29,* 6–16.

Roberts, A. R. (2005). *Crisis intervention handbook: Assessment, treatment, and research.* New York: Oxford University Press.

Roberts, G. (1999). Introduction: A story of stories. In G. Roberts and J. Holmes (Eds.), *Healing stories: Narrative in psychiatry and psychotherapy.* New York: Oxford University Press.

Rock, E. E., Fessler, M. A., & Church, R. P. (1997). The concomitance of learning disabilities and emotional/behavioral disorders: A conceptual model. *Journal of Learning Disabilities, 30*(3), 245–263.

Roeser, R. J. & Downs, M. P. (2004). *Auditory disorders in school children: The law, identification, remediation* (4th ed.). New York: Thieme Medical.

Rogers, C. (1951). *Client-centered therapy.* Boston: Houghton Mifflin.

Rogers, C. (1957). The necessary and sufficient conditions of therapeutic personality change. *Journal of Consulting Psychology, 21,* 95–103.

Rogers, C. (1961). *On becoming a person.* Boston: Houghton Mifflin.

Rogers, C. (1980). *A way of being.* Boston: Houghton Mifflin.

Rogers, E. R. (1987). Professional burnout: A review of a concept. *The Clinical Supervisor, 5*(3), 91–106.

Rogers, J. M., & Read, C. A. (2007). Psychiatric comorbidity following traumatic brain injury. *Brain Injury, 21,* 1321–1333.

Rolland, J. (1994). *Families, illness, & disability: An integrative treatment model.* New York: Harper-Collins.

Rolland, J. (1998). Beliefs and collaboration in illness: Evolution over time. *Families, Systems, and Health, 16*(1–2), 7–25.

Rollin, W. (2000). *Counseling individuals with communication disorders: Psychodynamic and family aspects* (2nd ed.). Boston: Butterworth-Heinemann.

Roseberry-McKibbin, C. (2008). *Multicultural students with special language needs, practical strategies for assessment and intervention* (3rd ed.). Oceanside, CA: Academic Communication Associates.

Rosen, D. C., & Sataloff, R. T. (1997). *Psychology of voice disorders.* San Diego, CA: Singular.

Ross, A., Winslow, I., & Marchant, P. (2006). Evaluation of communication, life participation and psychological well-being in chronic aphasia: The influence of group intervention. *Aphasiology, 20*(5), 427–448.

Roy, N., Bless, D. M., & Heisey, D. (2000a). Personality and voice disorders: A superficial trait analysis.

Journal of Speech, Language and Hearing Research, 43, 749–768.

Roy, N., Bless, D. M., & Heisey, D. (2000b). Personality and voice disorders: A multivariate-multidisorder analysis. *Journal of Voice, 14*(4), 521–548.

Roy, N., McGrory, J. J., Tasko, S. M., Bless, D. M., Heisey, D., & Ford, C. N. (1997). Psychological correlates of functional dysphonia: An investigation using the Minnesota Multiphasic Personality Inventory. *Journal of Voice, 106*(12), 1012–1019.

Rubin, J. S., Sataloff, R. T., & Korovin, G. (Eds.). (2006). *Diagnosis and treatment of voice disorders* (3rd ed.). San Diegeo, CA: Plural.

Ryan, E. (1995). Normal aging and language. In R. Lubinski (Ed.), *Dementia and communication*. San Diego, CA: Singular.

Ryan, E., Bourhis, R., & Knops, U. (1991). Evaluating perceptions of patronizing speech addressed to elders. *Psychology and Aging, 6,* 442–450.

Ryan, E., Hummert, M., & Boisch, L. (1995). Communication predicaments of aging: Patronizing behavior toward older adults. *Journal of Language and Social Psychology, 14,* 144–166.

Ryder, A. G., McBride, C., & Bagby, R. M. (2008). The association of affiliation and achievement personality styles with DSM-IV personality disorders. *Journal of Personality Disorders, 22*(2), 208–216.

Saba, G., Karrer, B., & Hardy, K. (1995). *Minorities and family therapy.* New York: Haworth Press.

Sadock, B. J., Kaplan, H. I., & Sadock, V. A. (2007). *Kaplan and Sadock's synopsis of psychiatry: Behavioral sciences/clinical psychiatry, North American edition* (10th ed.). Philidelphia: Lippincott Williams & Wilkins.

Safran, J. D., & Muran, J. C. (2000). *Negotiating the therapeutic alliance: A relational treatment guide.* New York: Guilford Press.

Safran, J. D., & Segal, Z. V. (1990). *Interpersonal process in cognitive therapy.* New York: Basic Books.

Salas-Provance, M., Erickson, J., & Reed, J. (2002). Disability as viewed by four generations of one Hispanic family. *American Journal of Speech-Language Pathology, 11,* 151–162.

Samson, K. (2004). Iraq injuries challenge VA brain injury rehabilitation teams. *Neurology Today, 4*(11), 56–59.

Sanders, A. (2007). A cognitive-behavioral intervention for family members of persons with TBI. In N. Zasler, D. Katz, & R. Zafonte (Eds.), *Brain injury medicine: Principles and practices* (pp. 362–394). New York: Demos Medical Publications.

Sanders, C. (1998). Gender differences in bereavement expression across the life span. In R. Doka & J. Davidson (Eds.), *Living with grief: Who we are, how we grieve.* Washington, DC: Hospice Foundation of America.

Sanger, D. D., Hux, K., & Belau, D. (1997). Oral language skills of female juvenile delinquents. *American Journal of Speech-Language Pathology, 6,* 70–76.

Satir, V. (1976). *Making contact.* Berkeley, CA: Celestial Arts.

Satir, V. (1983). *Conjoint family therapy* (3rd ed.). Palo Alto, CA: Science and Behavior Books.

Sayer, N. A., Cifu, D., McNamee, S., Chiros, C. E., Sigford, B. J., Scott, S. G., & Lew, H. L. (2009). Rehabilitation needs of combat-injured service members admitted to the VA polytrauma rehabilitation center: The role of PM&R in the care of wounded warriors. *Physical Medicine & Rehabilitation 1*(1), 23–28.

Schaefer, E. (1965). Children's report of parental behavior: An inventory. *Child Development, 36,* 413–424.

Schafer, R. (1983). *The analytic attitude.* New York: Basic Books.

Schafer, R. (1992). *Retelling a life: Narration and dialogue in psychoanalysis.* New York: Basic Books.

Scheuerle, J. (1992). *Counseling in speech-language pathology and audiology.* New York: Macmillan Publishing.

Schon, D. (1983). *The reflective practitioner: How professionals think in action.* New York: Basic Books.

Schon, D. (1987). *Educating the reflective practitioner.* San Francisco: Jossey-Bass.

Schow, R., & Nerbonne, M. (2006). *Introduction to audiologic rehabilitation* (5th ed.). Boston: Allyn and Bacon.

Schultz, D., & Carnevale, F. (1996). Engagement and suffering in responsible caregiving: On overcoming maleficience in health care. *Theoretical Medicine, 17,* 189–207.

Schultz, D. S., & Flasher, L. V. (in press). Charles Taylor, phronesis, and medicine: Ethics and interpretation in illness narrative. *Journal of Medicine and Philosophy.*

Schwartz, J. P. (2002). Family resilience and pragmatic parent education. *Journal of Individual Psychology, 58*(3), 250–262.

Scott, C. D., & Hawk, J. (1986). *Heal thyself: The health of health care professionals.* New York: Brunner/Mazel.

Segebert-DeThorne, L., & Watkins, R. V. (2001). Listeners' perceptions of language use in children. *Language, Speech, and Hearing Services in Schools, 32*, 142–148.

Semans, C., & Cox, M. (1982). The stutterer and stuttering: Personality correlates. *Journal of Fluency Disorders, 7*, 141–158.

Shadden, B. B., & Agan, J. P. (2004). Renegotiation of identity: The social context of aphasia support groups. *Topics in Language Disorders, 24*(3), 174–186.

Shadden, B. B., & Toner, M. (Eds.) (1997). *Aging and communication.* Austin, TX: Pro-Ed.

Shames, G. (2006). *Counseling the communicatively disabled and their families: A manual for clinicians* (2nd ed.). Mahwah, NJ: Lawrence Erlbaum Associates.

Shapiro, S. L., & Carlson, L. E. (2009). *The art and science of mindfulness: Integrating mindfulness into psychology and the helping professions.* Washington, DC: American Psychological Association.

Shapiro, S. L., & Walsh, R. (2007). Meditation: Exploring the farther reaches. In T. G. Plante & C. E. Thoresen (Eds.) *Spirit, science, and health: How the spiritual mind fuels physical wellness* (pp. 57–71). Westport, CT: Praeger/Greenwood.

Sharpe, D., & Rossiter, L. (2002). Siblings of children with a chronic illness: A meta-analysis. *Journal of Pediatric Psychology, 27*(8), 699–710.

Sheehan, J. G. (1953). Theory and treatment of stuttering as an approach-avoidance conflict. *The Journal of Psychology, 36*, 27–49.

Sheehan, J. G. (1970). *Stuttering: Research and therapy.* New York: Harper & Row.

Sheehan, J. G. (1979). Level of aspiration in female stutterers: Changing times? *Journal of Speech and Hearing Disorders, 44*, 479–486.

Sheehan, J. G. (2008). Message to a stutterer. In *Advice to those who stutter* (2nd ed.). Memphis, TN: Stuttering Foundation of America.

Shiner, M., Scourfield, J., Fincham, B., & Langer, S. (2009). When things fall apart: Gender and suicide across the life-course. *Social Science and Medicine, 69*, 738–746.

Shipley, K. G., & McAfee, J. (2008). *Assessment in speech-language pathology: A resource manual* (4th ed.). Clifton Park, NY: Delmar Cengage Learning.

Shipley, K. G., & Roseberry-McKibbin, C. (2006). *Interviewing and counseling in communicative disorders: Principles and procedures.* Austin, TX: Pro-Ed.

Siegel, D. J. (2007). *The mindful brain.* New York: W.W. Norton & Company.

Silverman, F. H. (1996). *Stuttering and other fluency disorders.* Boston: Allyn and Bacon.

Simis, K. J., Verhulst, F. C., & Koot, H. M. (2001). Body image, psychosocial functioning, and personality: How different are adolescents and young adults applying for plastic surgery? *Journal of Child Psychology and Psychiatry and Allied Disciplines, 42*, 669–678.

Simons Michelson, L. A. (1985). The effects of chronic childhood illness on healthy siblings. *Electronic Doctoral Dissertations for UMass Amherst*, Paper AAI8509578.

Skinner, B. (1953). *Science and human behavior.* New York: Free Press.

Skinner, B. (1974). *About behaviorism.* New York: Vintage Books.

Skovholt, T. (2001). *The resilient practitioner: Burnout prevention and self-care strategies for counselors, therapists, teachers, and health professionals.* Boston: Allyn & Bacon.

Slade, P., Emerson, D. J., & Freedlander, E. (1999). A longitudinal comparison of the psychological impact on mothers of neonatal and 3-month repair of cleft lip. *British Journal of Plastic Surgery, 52*, 1–5.

Slaughter, V., & Griffiths, M. (2007). Death understanding and fear of death in young children. *Clinical Child Psychology and Psychiatry, 12*(4), 525–535.

Slifer, K., Amari, B., Diver, T., Hilley, L., Beck, M., Kane, A., & McDonnel, S. (2004). Social interaction patterns of children and adolescents with and without oral clefts during a videotaped analogue encounter. *The Cleft Palate-Craniofacial Journal, 41*, 175–184.

Slifer, K., Pulbrook, M., Amari, B., Vona-Messersmith, M., Cohen, J., Ambadar, Z., et al. (2006). Social acceptance and facial behavior in children with oral clefts. *The Cleft Palate-Craniofacial Journal, 43*(2), 226–236.

Smedegaard, L., Marxen, D., Moes, J., Glassou, E., & Scientsan, C. (2008). Hospitalization, breast-milk feeding, and growth in infants with cleft palate and cleft lip born in Denmark. *Cleft Palate Craniofacial Journal, 45*(6), 628–632.

Smith, P. (1981). Empirically based models for viewing the dynamics of violence. In Keltner, N., Schwecke, L., & Bostrom, C. (Eds.), *Psychiatric nursing* (3rd ed.). St. Louis: Mosby.

Snow, P. C., & Powell, M. B. (2004). Developmental language disorders and adolescent risk: A public-health advocacy role for speech pathologists? *Advances in Speech-Language Pathology, 6*(4), 221–229.

Snyder, H. T., Bilboul, M. J., & Pope, A. W. (2005). Psychosocial adjustment in adolescents with craniofacial anomalies: A comparison of parent and self-reports. *The Cleft Palate-Craniofacial Journal, 42*, 5–16.

Sommers-Flanagan, J., & Sommers-Flanagan, R. (1993). *Foundations of therapeutic interviewing*. Boston: Allyn and Bacon.

Sommers-Flanagan, R., & Sommers-Flannagan, J. (1999). *Clinical interviewing*. New York: Wiley.

Sourkes, B. M. (1982). *The deepening shade: Psychological aspects of life-threatening illness*. Pittsburgh, PA: University of Pittsburgh Press.

Sourkes, B. M. (1995). *Armfuls of time: The psychological experience of the child with a life-threatening illness*. Pittsburgh, PA: University of Pittsburgh Press.

Spears, R. A. (2006). *McGraw-Hill's dictionary of American idioms*. New York: McGraw-Hill.

Speltz, M., Armsden, G., & Clarren, S. (1990). Effects of craniofacial birth defects on maternal functioning post-infancy. *Journal of Pediatric Psychology, 15*(2), 177–196.

Speltz, M. L., Morton, K., Goodell, E., & Clarren, S. (1993). Psychological functioning of children with craniofacial anomalies and their mothers: Follow-up from late infancy to school entry. *Cleft Palate Craniofacial Journal, 30*, 482–489.

Sprenkle, D. (2005). Systemic assessment. In M. Cierpka, V. Thomas, & D. Sprenkle (Eds.), *Family assessment: An integrated approach* (pp. 211–230). Seattle, WA: Hogrefe.

St. Louis, K. O. (2008). Your life is too important to spend it worrying about stuttering. In *Advice to those who stutter* (2nd ed.). Memphis, TN: Stuttering Foundation of America.

Stahl, J. V., Hill, C. E., Jacobs, T., Kleinman, S., Isenberg, D., & Stern, A. (2009). When the shoe is on the other foot: A qualitative study of intern-level trainees' perceived learning from clients. *Psychotherapy Theory, Research, Practice, Training, 46*(3), 376–389.

Steele, C. M., Greenwood, C., Ens, I., Robertson, C., & Seidman-Carlson, R. (1997). Mealtime difficulties in a home for the aged: Not just dysphagia. *Dysphagia, 12*, 43–50.

Stemple, J. C. (2000). *Voice therapy: Clinical studies* (2nd ed.). San Diego, CA: Singular.

Stephens, R. J., Hopwood, D. J., Girling, D., & Machin, D. (1997). Randomized trials with quality of life endpoints: Are doctors' ratings of patients' physical symptoms interchangeable with patients' self-ratings? *Quality of Life Research, 6*(3) 507–511.

Stewart, C. J., & Cash, W. B. (2003). *Interviewing: Principles and practices*. New York: McGraw-Hill.

Stewart, W. (2005). *An A–Z of counseling theory and practice*. London: Chapman & Hall.

Stirling, J., & Elliot, R. (2008). *Introducing neuropsychology*. New York: Psychology Press.

Stolorow, R. D., Brandcraft, B., & Atwood, G. E. (1987). *Psychoanalytic treatment: An intersubjective approach*. Hillsdale, NJ: Analytic Press.

Stone, J. & Olswang, L. (1989). The hidden challenge in counseling. *ASHA, 31*, 27–31.

Stone, J., Shapiro, J., & Pasino, J. (1990). *The boundaries of counseling: Strategies for habilitation/rehabilitation professionals*. Paper presented at Counseling for Rehabilitation Professionals Conference, Reno, NV.

Strauss, R. P. (1991). Culture, health care, and birth defects in the United States: An introduction. *Cleft Palate Journal, 27*(3), 275–278.

Strauss, R., Sharp, M., Lorch, S., & Kachalia, B. (1995). Physicians' communication of "bad news": Parent experiences of being informed of their child's cleft lip/palate. *Pediatrics, 96*(1), 82–89.

Stricker, G. (2010). *Psychotherapy integration*. Washington, DC: American Psychological Association.

Stricker, G., & Gold, J. (2006). *A casebook of psychotherapy integration*. Washington, DC: American Psychological Association.

Stroebe, M., Hansson, R., Schut, H., & Stroebe, W. (2008). *Handbook of bereavement research and practice*. Washington, DC: American Psychological Association.

Strupp, H. H. (1992) The future of psychodynamic psychotherapy. *Psychotherapy, 29*(1), 21–27.

Strupp, H. H. (1996). The tripartite model and the consumer reports study. *American Psychologist, 51*(10), 1017.

Strupp, H. H., & Binder, J. L. (1984). *Psychotherapy in a new key*. New York: Basic Books.

Strupp, H. H., & Hadley, S. W. (1979). Specific versus nonspecific factors in psychotherapy: A controlled study of outcome. *Archives of General Psychiatry, 36*, 1125–1136.

Stuart, G. W. (2008). *Principles and practice of psychiatric nursing*. St. Louis, MO: Elsevier Health Sciences.

Sullivan, H. (1953). *The interpersonal theory of psychiatry*. New York: Norton.

Sullivan, H. (1972). *Personal psychopathology*. New York: Norton.

Surtee, P., Wainwright, N., Luben, R., Wareham, N., Bingham, S., & Khaw, K. (2008). Depression and ischemic heart disease mortality: Evidence from the EPIC-Norfolk United Kingdom Prospective Cohort Study. *American Journal of Psychiatry, 165*, 515–523.

Sweeny, K., & Shepperd, J. A. (2007). Being the best bearer of bad tidings. *Review of General Psychology, 11*(3), 235–257.

Sweet, A. A. (1984). The therapeutic relationship in behavior therapy. *Clinical Psychology Review, 4*, 253–272.

Tannen, D. (2007). *You just don't understand: Women and men in conversation*. New York: Harper Collins.

Tanner, D. (2008). *The family guide to surviving stroke and communication disorders*. Sudbury, MA: Jones & Bartlett.

Tanner, D. C. (2003). *The psychology of neurogenic communication disorders: A primer for health care professionals*. Boston: Allyn and Bacon.

Teasell, R., McRae, M. R., & Finestone, H. (2000). Social issues in rehabilitation of younger stroke patients. *Archives of Physical Medicine and Rehabilitation, 82*(2), 205–209.

Tennen, H., & Affleck, G. (1999). Finding benefits in adversity. In C. R. Snyder (Ed.), *Coping: The psychology of what works*. New York: Oxford University Press.

Teyber, E. (2005). *Interpersonal process in psychotherapy* (5th ed.). Belmont, CA: Brooks/Cole, Thomson Learning.

Thomas, P., Turner, S., Rumsey, N., Dowell, T., & Sandy, J. (1997). Satisfaction with facial appearance among subjects affected by a cleft. *Cleft Palate-Craniofacial Journal, 34*(3), 226–231.

Thompson, K. (1998). Early intervention services in daily family life: Mothers' perceptions of "ideal" versus "actual" service provision. *Occupational Therapy International, 5*(3), 206–221.

Tian, Y., Kanade, T., & Cohn, J. (2005). *Handbook of facial recognition*. New York: Springer.

Tiegerman, E., & Siperstein, M. (1984). Individual patterns of interaction in the mother-child dyad: Implications for parent intervention. *Topics in Language Disorders, 4*, 50–61.

Tobiasen, J. M., & Hiebert, J. (1993). Combined effects of cleft impairment and facial attractiveness on social perception: An experimental study. *Cleft Palate Craniofacial Journal, 30*, 82–86.

Tomm, K. (1987). Interventive interviewing: Part II. Reflexive questioning as a means to enable self-healing. *Family Process, 26*, 167–183.

Tomm, K. (1988). Interventive interviewing: Part III. Intending to ask linear, circular, strategic, or reflexive questions? *Family Process, 27*, 1–15.

Toner, M., & Shadden, B. (2002). Counseling challenges: Working with older clients and caregivers. *Contemporary Issues in Communication Sciences and Disorders, 29*, 68–78.

Topolski, T. D., Edwards, T. C., & Patrick, D. L. (2005). Quality of life: How do adolescents with facial differences compare with other adolescents: The *Cleft Palate-Craniofacial Journal, 42*(1), 19–24.

Trapp, P. E., & Evans, J. (1960). Functional articulatory defect and performance on a nonverbal task. *Journal of Speech and Hearing Disorders, 25*, 176–180.

Travis, L. E. (1931). *Speech pathology*. New York: Appleton-Century-Crofts.

Trombly, T. (1965). Responses of stutterers and normal speakers to a level of aspiration inventory. *Central States Speech Journal, 16*, 179–181.

Truscott, D. (2010). *Becoming an effective psychotherapist: Adopting a theory of psychotherapy that's right for you and your client.* Washington, DC: American Psychological Association.

Trute, B., & Hiebert-Murphy, D. (2002). Family adjustment to childhood developmental disability: A measure of parent appraisal of family impacts. *Journal of Pediatric Psychology, 27*(3), 271–280.

Tschudin, V. (2003). *Ethics in nursing: The caring relationship* (3rd ed.). Edinburgh, UK: Butterworth-Heinemann.

Turnbaugh, K., Guitar, B., & Hoffman, P. (1981). The attribution of personality traits. *Journal of Speech and Hearing Research, 24*, 288–291.

Turner, S. R., Rumsey, N., & Sandy, J. R. (1998). Review of psychological aspects of cleft lip and palate. *European Journal of Orthodontics, 20*, 407–415.

Tye-Murray, N. (2009). *Foundations of aural rehabilitation, children, adults, and their family members* (3rd ed.). Clifton Park, NY: Thomson Delmar Learning.

Umweni, A., & Okeigbemen, S. A. (2009). Gender issues in parenting cleft lip and palate babies in the southern Nigeria: A study of the University of Benin Teaching Hospital. *Early Child Developmental Care, 179*(1), 81–86.

Vaillant, G. E. (1994). Ego mechanisms of defense and personality psychopathology. *Journal of Abnormal Psychology, 103*, 44–50.

Vaillant, G. E., Bond, M., & Vaillant, C. O. (1986). An empirically validated hierarchy of defense mechanisms. *Archives of General Psychiatry, 73*, 786–794.

Van Riper, C. (1957). Symptomatic therapy for stuttering. In L. E. Travis (Ed.), *Handbook of speech pathology.* New York: Appleton-Century-Crofts.

Van Riper, C. (1982). *The nature of stuttering* (2nd ed.). Englewood Cliffs, NJ: Prentice-Hall.

Van Riper, C. (2006). The severe young stutterer. In *Effective counseling in stuttering therapy.* Memphis, TN: Stuttering Foundation of America.

Van Riper, C. (2008). Putting it all together. In *Advice to those who stutter* (2nd ed.). Memphis, TN: Stuttering Foundation of America.

Van Riper, C., & Erickson, R. (1996). *Speech correction: An introduction to speech pathology and audiology.* Englewood Cliffs, NJ: Prentice-Hall.

Van Riper, M. (1999). Maternal perceptions of family-provider relationships and well-being in families of children with Down Syndrome. *Research in Nursing and Health, 22*, 357–368.

van Staden, F., & Gerhardt, C. (1995). Mothers of children with facial cleft deformities: Reactions and effects. *South American Journal of Psychology, 25*(1), 39–46.

Vaughn, S., Elbaum, B, & Broardman, A. G. (2001). The social functioning of children with learning disabilities: Implications for inclusion. *Exceptionality, 9*(1–2), 47–65.

Veterans Health Administration. (June 2005). *Polytrauma rehabilitation centers* [VHA Directive 2005-024]. Washington, DC: Department of Veterans Affairs.

Veterans Health Administration. (2008, January). *Analysis of VA health care utilization among US global war on terrorism (GWOT) veterans: Operation Enduring Freedom, Operation Iraqi Freedom.* Washington DC: Veterans Health Administration, Office of Public Health and Environmental Hazards.

Visser-Meily, A., Post, M., Meijer, A., Maas, C., Ketelaar, M., & Lindeman, E. (2005). When a parent has a stroke: Clinical course and prediction of mood, behavior problems, and health status of their children. *Stroke, 36*, 2436–2440.

Visser-Meily, A., Post, M., Meijer, A., van de Port, I., Maas, C., Forstberg-Warleby, G., & Lindeman, E. (2009). Psychological functioning of spouses of patients with stroke from initial inpatient rehabilitation to 3 years poststroke: Course and relations with coping strategies. *Stroke, a Journal of Cerebral Circulation, 40*(4), 1399–1404.

Wachtel, E. F. (1994). *Treating troubled children and their families.* New York: Guilford Press.

Wachtel, P. L. (1977). *Psychoanalysis and behavior therapy.* New York: Basic Books.

Wachtel, P. L. (1993). *Therapeutic communication: Principles and effective practice.* New York: Guilford Press.

Wachtel, P. L. (2007). *Relational theory and the practice of psychotherapy.* New York: Guilford.

Wachtel, P. L., & Messer, S. B. (Eds.). (1997). *Theories of psychotherapy: Origins and evolution.* Washington, DC: American Psychological Association.

Wagner, P. J., Lentz, L., & Heslop, S. D. (2002). Teaching communication skills: A skills-based approach. *Academy of Medicine, 77*(11), 1164.

Wallace, D. (2006). Military TBI during the Iraq and Afghanistan wars. *Journal of Head Trauma Rehabilitation, 21*(5), 398–402.

Wallace, M. (2007) *Essentials of gerontological nursing.* New York: Springer.

Ward, D. (2006). *Stuttering and cluttering: Framework for understanding and treatment.* East Sussex, UK: Psychology Press.

Warden, D. (2006). Military TBI during the Iraq and Afghanistan wars. *Journal of Head Trauma Rehabilitation, 21,* 398–402.

Warschausky, S., Kay, J., Buchman, S., Halberg, A., & Berger, M. (2002). Health-related quality of life in children with craniofacial anomalies. *Plastic and Reconstructive Surgery, 110*(2), 409–414.

Wasserman, G. A., & Allen, R. (1985). Maternal withdrawal from handicapped infants. *Journal of Child Psychology and Psychiatry, 26,* 381–387.

Wasserman, G. A., Allen, R., & Solomon, C. (1985). At-risk toddlers and their mothers: The special case of physical handicap. *Child Development, 56,* 82–85.

Watt, F., & Whyte, M. N. (2003). The experience of dysphagia and its effect on the quality of life of patients with esophageal cancer. *European Journal of Cancer Care, 12*(2), 183–193.

Watts Pappas, N., & McLeod, S. (2009). *Working with families in speech-language pathology.* San Diego, CA: Plural.

Watts Pappas, N., McLeod, S., McAllister, L., & McKinnon, D. H. (2008). Parental involvement in speech intervention: A national survey. *Clinical Linguistics and Phonetics, 22*(4), 335–344.

Watzlawick, P. (1978). *The language of change.* New York: Basic Books.

Watzlawick, P., Weakland, J., & Fisch, R. (1974). *Change: The principles of problem formation and problem resolution.* New York: Norton.

Wayne, C., Cook, K., Sairam, S., Hollis, B., & Thilaganathan, B. (2002). Sensitivity and accuracy of routine antenatal ultrasound screening for isolated facial clefts. *British Journal of Radiology, 75,* 584–589.

Weakland, J. (1976). Communication theory and clinical change. In P. J. Guerin, Jr. (Ed.), *Family therapy: Theory and practice.* New York: Gardner Press.

Wehman, T. (1998). Family-centered early intervention services: Factors contributing to increased parent involvement and participation. *Focus on Autism and Other Developmental Disabilities, 13*(2), 80–86.

Weiss, L. (2004). *Therapist's guide to self-care.* New York: Routledge Mental Health.

Weissman, M. M., & Klerman, G. L. (1991). Interpersonal psychotherapy for depression. In B. D. Beitman & G. L. Klerman (Eds.), *Integrating pharmacotherapy and psychotherapy.* Washington, DC: American Psychological Association.

Weismann, M. M., Markowitz, J. C., & Klerman, G. L. (2007). *Clinician's quick guide to interpersonal psychotherapy.* New York: Oxford University Press.

Wepman, J. (1951). *Recovery from aphasia.* New York: Ronald Press.

West, R. (1938). The function of the speech pathologist in studying cases of dysphonia. *Journal of Speech Disorders, 3,* 81–84.

West, R. (1942). The pathology of stuttering. *The Nervous Child, 2*(2), 96–106.

Wetchler, J. L., & Gutenkunst, G. (2005). First contact and preconditions for the initial interview: Conducting the first interview. In M. Cierpka, V. Thomas, & D. Sprenkle (Eds.), *Family assessment: Integrating multiple clinical perspectives* (pp.35–52). Cambridge, MA: Hogrefe.

White, K. R., Taylor, M. J., & Moss, V. D. (1992). Does research support claims about the benefits of involving parents in early intervention programs? *Review of Educational Research, 62*(1), 91–125.

White, M. (2007). *Maps of narrative practice.* New York: Norton.

Wiig, E. H. (1995). Assessment of adolescent language. *Seminars in Speech and Language, 16(1),* 14–30.

Wiig, E. H., & Semel, E. (1984). *Language assessment and intervention for the learning disabled.* Columbus, OH: Charles E. Merrill.

Williams, D. E. (2005). *The genius of Dean Williams.* Memphis, TN: Stuttering Foundation of America.

Williams, D. E. (2006). Talking with children who stutter. In *Stuttering and your child: Questions and answers.*

Williams, D. E. (2008a). Coping with parents. In *Do you stutter: A guide for teens.* Memphis, TN: Stuttering Foundation of America.

Williams, D. E. (2008b). Some suggestions for those who want to talk easily. In *Advice to those who stutter* (2nd ed.). Memphis, TN: Stuttering Foundation of America.

Williams, L. S., Weinberg, M., Harris, L. E., Clark, D. O., & Biller, J. (1999). Stroke-Specific Quality of Life Scale: Development of a stroke-specific quality of life scale. *Stroke, 30,* 1362–1369.

Wilson, D. K. (1987). *Voice problems of children* (3rd ed.). Baltimore: Williams & Wilkins.

Wilson, G. T., & Franks, C. M. (Eds.). (1982). *Cognitive behavior therapy: Conceptual and empirical foundations.* New York: Guilford Press.

Wolpe, J. (1958). *Psychotherapy by reciprocal inhibition.* Stanford, CA: Stanford University Press.

Wolpe, J. (1987). *Essential principles and practices of behavior therapy.* Phoenix, AZ: Milton H. Erickson Foundation.

Woods, R. T., Bruce, E., Edwards, R. T., Hounsome, B., Keady, J., Moniz-Cook, E. D., et al. (2009). Reminiscence groups for people with dementia and their family carers, *Trials, 10,* pp. 64–71.

Worden, J. W. (2008). *Grief counseling and grief therapy* (4th ed.). New York: Springer.

World Health Organization. (1998). *World Health Organization Quality of Life-BREF.* Geneva, Switzerland: World Health Organization, Programme on Mental Health.

Worrall, L., & Frattali, C. (2000). *Neurogenic communication disorders: A functional approach.* New York: Thieme.

Yairi, E. (1970). *Perceptions of parental attitudes by stuttering and by nonstuttering children.* Unpublished doctoral dissertation, University of Iowa, Iowa City.

Yairi, E., & Williams, D. (1971). Reports of parental attitudes by stuttering and by nonstuttering children. *Journal of Speech and Hearing Research, 14,* 596–603.

Yalom, I. (2004). *Existential psychotherapy.* New York: Basic Books.

Ylvisaker, M., & Feeney, T. (1998). *Collaborative brain injury intervention: Positive everyday routines.* San Diego, CA: Singular.

Young, J. L., O'Riordan, M., Goldstein, J. A., & Robin, N. (2001). What information do parents of newborns with cleft lip, palate, or both want to know? *The Cleft Palate-Craniofacial Journal, 38,* 55–58.

Yu, Y., Chamorro-Premuzic, T., & Honjo, S. (2008). Personality and defense mechanisms in late adulthood. *Journal of Aging Health, 20*(5), 525–544.

Zanarini, M. C., Weingeroff, J. L., & Frankenburg, F. R. (2009). Defense mechanisms associated with borderline personality disorder. *Journal of Personality Disorders, 23*(2), 113–121.

Zaner, R. (1993). *Troubled voices.* Cleveland, OH: The Pilgrim Press.

Zaner, R. (2004). *Conversations on the edge: Narratives of ethics and illness.* Washington, DC: Georgetown University Press.

Zaro, J., Barach, R., Nedelman, D., & Dreiblatt, I. (2000). *A guide for beginning psychotherapists.* Cambridge, UK: Cambridge University Press.

Zebrowski, P. M. (2002). Counseling: An approach for speech-language pathologists. *Contemporary Issues in Communication Science and Disorders, 29,* 91–100.

Zebrowski, P. M. (2006). Understanding and coping with the emotions: Counseling teenagers who stutter. In *Stuttering and your child: questions and answers.* Memphis, TN: Stuttering Foundation of America.

Zebrowski, P. M., & Kelly, E. M. (2002). *Manual of stuttering intervention.* Clifton Park, NY: Thomson Delmar Learning.

Zingeser, L. (1999, September/October). Communication disorders and violence. *Hearing Health, 15*(5), 26–30.

Zuckerbrot, R. A., Cheung, A. H., Jenson, P. S., & Stein, R. E. K. (2007). Identification, assessment, and initial management guidelines for adolescent depression in primary care. *Pediatrics, 120,* 1299–1312.

Zur, O. (1993). Avoiding the hazards of your profession. *The California Psychologist, 26*(3), 16.

INDEX